Fitness: Theory & Practice

The Comprehensive Resource for Group Fitness Instruction

Fifth Edition

Editor

Laura A. Gladwin, MS

Published by
Aerobics and Fitness Association of America
15250 Ventura Blvd., Suite #200
Sherman Oaks, California 91403-3297
(818) 905-0040 FAX (818) 990-5468
www.afaa.com
contactafaa@afaa.com

AFAA's Mission: AFAA provides comprehensive cognitive and practical education for fitness professionals grounded in research, reflecting a commitment to quality distance education that upholds safe and effective fitness practice.

The Aerobics and Fitness Association of America (AFAA) is accredited by the Accrediting Commission of the Distance Education and Training Council (DETC), which is listed by the U.S. Department of Education as a nationally recognized accrediting agency and a recognized member of the Council for Higher Education Accreditation (CHEA).

AFAA and logo, Aerobics and Fitness Association of America, AFP Fitness Practitioner, Fitness Triage, Fitness Gets Personal, Mat Science, American Fitness, FitMarkers, Multitraining Live, Multitraining, and Fitness Management for Life are registered trademarks of the Aerobics and Fitness Association of America. The Sunrise Yoga Format, and AFAA 5 Questions are trademarks of the Aerobics and Fitness Association of America. Other marks referenced in this book may be trademarks or registered trademarks of other companies, and are used only for informational purposes and to the owner's benefit, without intent to infringe.

 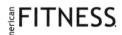 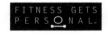 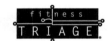

Fifth Edition, revised 2011
Copyright © 2010 by Aerobics and Fitness Association of America
All rights reserved.

First Edition, 1993   Third Edition, 1997
Second Edition, 1995   Fourth Edition, 2002, revised 2005

ISBN 0-9638168-9-6

Printed in the United States of America
10 9

Acknowledgements

The editor wishes to acknowledge the guidance and talents of the following people in the creation of this book.

From the AFAA Organization

President and CEO: Linda D. Pfeffer, RN

Educational Director: Kathy Stevens, MA

Director of Operations/Fulfillment: Tom Hamlin

Publisher, *American Fitness* magazine: Tom Ivicevic

The AFAA Education Advisory Board

Board Chair: Laura A. Gladwin, MS; William Beam, PhD; Nancy Clark, RD; James Gavin, PhD; Nancy Gillette, MA; Dave Herbert, JD; William Herbert, PhD; C. Jessie Jones, PhD; Michael Phelan, MD; Mark Pierce, DC; J.P. Saleeby, MD; Kathy Stevens, MA

The AFAA Certification Board

Marcia Ditmyer, PhD; Meg Jordan, PhD, RN; Dorette Nysewander, EdD; Gwen Uman, PhD; Gregory Welch, MS

Editorial Production

Editor-in-Chief/Managing Editor: Laura A. Gladwin

Assistant Managing and Text Editor: Lindsay Stieber

Layout, Design, and Graphics Editor: Laura Carrington

Cover Design: Tom Ivicevic

Illustrators: Michael Aniel, Andrew Bonsall, Laura Carrington, Gina Urwin

Photographers: Nancy Gillette, Tom Ivicevic

Aqua Fitness Photos: Tracy Frankel, Courtesy of WaterFit.com and the YMCA of the USA

Healthy Back–Fit for a Lifetime Photos: Shannon Burbridge

Sample Workout for Active Seniors Photos: Nancy Gillette

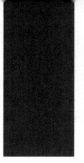

AFAA's Notice

PLEASE READ BEFORE USING AFAA PROGRAMS AND MATERIALS

The courses and materials offered by the Aerobics and Fitness Association of America (AFAA) are intended to provide general educational information to you in your efforts to educate yourself, obtain relevant professional certification, secure continuing education credits if available to you and to work with your clients to reach definable goals. "You," as used here, includes, but is not limited to, fitness trainers and other fitness professionals of all kinds, fitness trainer students and other professional fitness students of all kinds, providers of continuing education services, AFAA educational contractors, and all other readers and users of the courses and materials offered by AFAA. The courses and materials of AFAA are intended to provide what is believed to be accurate information. However, please note the following important cautions before making use of AFAA courses and materials.

- To the best of the knowledge of the authors, publishers, and presenters of AFAA courses and materials, the contents of such courses and materials were accurate as of the date of publication and/or presentation. However, you are strongly encouraged to keep yourself informed of new developments in the field to make sure that the contents are still accurate when you consult the courses and materials.

- AFAA courses and materials are made available with the understanding that the authors, publishers, and presenters are not engaged in rendering legal, medical, or other professional services by reason of their authorship, publication, or presentation of such courses and materials. You are strongly encouraged to consult an appropriate legal, medical, or other expert if you are seeking such advice or assistance. This is an especially important precaution in the field of fitness and exercise, personal fitness training, and fitness practice.

- AFAA courses and materials are made available without warranties or guarantees of any kind, express or implied, all of which are disclaimed. By way of example only, and without limiting the general disclaimer given above, the authors, publishers, and presenters of AFAA courses and materials cannot and do not promise or guarantee that the contents of such courses and materials are appropriate for every reader or user, or that use of such courses and materials will result in certification or in obtaining employment, or that, if you are certified, you will be able to obtain third-party insurance payments for any services that you may render to your clients.

- You acknowledge that all of the above-referenced authors, publishers, and presenters are independent contractors whom AFAA has engaged for their respective purposes, and that consistent with their independent contractor status, AFAA neither has nor had any right of control over the manner or methods by which they provide their services, and is not legally responsible for their acts or omissions while performing services in their respective capacities.

- The laws that define the practice of medicine or other health care fields specify that the provision of delineated services are reserved for provision by those who are licensed to provide such services. These laws vary from state to state, and the delivery of service is dependent upon specific circumstances which require independent judgment and decision making. In some states, and under some circumstances, the rendering of services by those who are not so licensed may be actually or potentially in violation of law. For that reason, you are cautioned to obtain specific professional advice about the laws and regulations that may apply to you and your delivery of service in a particular locality.

- The documents, forms, and other content found in AFAA courses and materials are offered as illustrative examples only. No such documents, forms, graphs, or other content should be used or adapted for use in violation of copyright or other applicable law. Since the use of these documents, forms, and other content may have legal implications, you are strongly cautioned to consult a qualified attorney before using or adapting them.

- AFAA courses and materials are not intended to establish or define any specific professional standards that apply to all fitness trainers or other fitness professionals and their clients in all circumstances or to limit the exercise of your independent professional judgment as to what is in the best interest of any particular client. The standard of care that you must observe may change from time to time or vary from place to place, and you are strongly cautioned to familiarize yourself with the standard of care that applies to you.

- All of these cautions apply to you regardless of your location. However, since AFAA courses and materials were prepared for use in the United States, special care should be taken if you are outside the U.S. to make sure you are familiar with the laws and regulations that apply in your country and locality or where services are provided by you.

- Participation in AFAA courses, use of AFAA materials, and/or any certification of a fitness trainer or other fitness professional that may result do not qualify you to approve, endorse, or recommend dietary supplements or other ingestibles, ergogenic aids, or any other products or services that claim to enhance physical performance or appearance, nor does AFAA itself issue any such approvals, endorsements, or recommendations. AFAA disclaims any responsibility or liability for any claim resulting from any such approvals, endorsements, or recommendations that you may offer.

- By participating in and/or using courses and materials offered by AFAA, and as condition for providing and presenting such materials and courses to you, you are acknowledging and agreeing that (a) you are solely responsible for all aspects of the conduct of your business and your practice as a fitness trainer or other fitness professional; (b) you are not sponsored or endorsed by or otherwise affiliated with AFAA by reason of any certification that AFAA may issue to you; (c) AFAA is not responsible or liable in any manner whatsoever for claims or liabilities arising from the conduct of your business; and (d) AFAA disclaims any liability, loss, or damages that may result from the conduct of your business or practice, and/or your use of such courses and materials, and/or the information, advice, and techniques embodied in such courses and materials.

- You acknowledge that you retain sole control over and responsibility for the development and implementation of any course that you develop or engage others to develop for you ("Your Course"), including the responsibility for ensuring that such courses do not infringe or violate the intellectual property rights or contract rights of any third party, and that AFAA's approval of such courses is based strictly on its approval criteria, which cannot and does not consider any such third-party rights. You agree to indemnify and hold harmless AFAA, its owners, shareholders, directors, officers, employees, agents, successors, and assigns from and against any third party claims, demands, liabilities, costs, or expenses, including without limitation reasonable attorney's fees and expenses, resulting from or attributable to any third-party claims that involve or relate to you or your provision of service or your participation in any course.

Part of the foregoing was adapted from a Declaration of Principles of the American Bar Association and a Committee of Publishers and Associations.

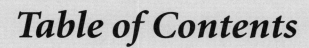

Table of Contents

Part 5 How to Teach—Basics

Part 6 How to Teach—Multitraining®

Part 7 Mind/Body Considerations

Part 8 Special Populations

Aerobics and Fitness Association of America

Reviewers & Contributors

Reviewers

William C. Beam, PhD, FACSM

    Exercise physiologist; professor, Department of Kinesiology, California State University, Fullerton (CSUF); co-founder and director, the Employee Wellness Program, CSUF; co-author with Gene Adams, *Exercise Physiology Laboratory Manual* (McGraw-Hill, 2008); fellow, American College of Sports Medicine (ACSM); former president, Southwest Regional Chapter of ACSM; research interest in bioenergetics and acute and chronic changes associated with exercise and sport.

Val Gokenbach, DM, RN, MBA

    Doctoral degree, management and organizational leadership; master's degree, business administration; bachelor of science, nursing; fellow, RWJ Executive Nurse; has held administrative healthcare positions for over 30 years; managed nursing and support departments such as radiology, respiratory therapy, radiation oncology, nuclear medicine, oncology services, neurodiagnostic services, employee health, schools of allied health, patient service departments, and emergency services; under her leadership her nursing team was recipient of the prestigious Magnet accreditation (2003) for nursing and organizational excellence; professional dancer, consultant, and fitness instructor for over 40 years; AFAA workshop presenter/specialist; guest host, QVC sales network and Shopping Channel, Ontario; developed exercise video series called "You Can Do This;" co-creator of Safety City USA, dedicated to the reduction in pediatric trauma; author, *Tap Dancing Through Life: Seven steps to finding your rhythms and the life of your dreams;* featured in *Chicken Soup for the Nurse's Soul: A second dose;* and *Nurse Executive: The four principles of Management from Springer Publishing;* lecturer and presenter.

David L. Herbert, JD

    Senior member, David L. Herbert & Associates, LLC, Attorneys & Counselors at Law, Canton, Ohio; co-editor, *Exercise Standards and Malpractice Reporter* and *Sports Medicine Standards and Malpractice Reporter;* represents a variety of fitness, exercise, and sports medicine organizations; author of 15 books, over 20 book chapters, and over 600 articles on various issues concerning health club operations and the law, standards of practice, negligence, and malpractice; frequent speaker/resource for such groups as ACSM, NSCA, AHA, as well as other organizations; regular contributor to *Fitness Management Magazine, OnSite Fitness,* and *ACE Certified News;* a Trustee of the NBFE; helped draft standards and guidelines for ACSM, AFAA, NSCA, and is in the process of assisting NSF International to draft new standards for health and fitness facilities.

William Herbert, PhD, FACSM

    Professor Emeritus, Department of Human Nutrition, Foods and Exercise, Virginia Tech, Blacksburg, VA; clinical physiologist, Virginia Tech for 38 years; conducted studies on exercise testing and training with cardiovascular disease patients and adults with obstructive sleep apnea; developed first comprehensive cardiac rehabilitation program in Virginia; fellow, ACSM; founding fellow, the American Association of Cardiovascular and Pulmonary Rehabilitation; national and international lecturer; renowned author of numerous peer-reviewed scientific journal articles and book chapters.

Contributors

Ken Alan

Current lecturer, Department of Kinesiology, California State University, Fullerton; chapter co-author, *Physical Activity Instruction of Older Adults*, Human Kinetics; chapter author, *Fitness for Travelers*; co-presenter, Time-Life Medical exercise video series (4); program design/choreographer, Richard Simmons videos (7); holds certifications from ACE , AFAA, and ACSM; former exercise director, Cedars-Sinai Medical Center Employee Wellness, Development & Training; Outpatient Weight Control Program; authored articles for *Men's Fitness, Oprah, Shape, Men's Journal, Men's Health, Longevity*, and *Weight Watchers*; owner, Ken Alan & Associates; renowned IDEA award winner and international presenter.
Chapter 19

William C. Beam, PhD, FACSM

Exercise physiologist; professor, Department of Kinesiology, California State University, Fullerton (CSUF); co-founder and director, Employee Wellness Program, CSUF; co-author with Gene Adams, *Exercise Physiology Laboratory Manual* (McGraw-Hill, 2008); fellow, American College of Sports Medicine (ACSM); former president, Southwest Regional Chapter of ACSM; research interest in bioenergetics and acute and chronic changes associated with exercise and sport.
Chapters 3, 4, 5

Lawrence Biscontini, MA, NC, CPT

AFAA international certification specialist; AFAA contributing author, American Fitness magazine; author, industry articles and texts such as *Morning Cardio Workouts, Running the Show*, and *Cream Rises*; creator, land & water Yo-Chi®; star, internationally-selling fitness videos; presenter at most global fitness conventions; winner of Instructor of the Year Awards: ACE (2002), IDEA (2004), CanFitPro (2004), and ECA (2005); faculty member for AFAA, ACE, AEA, ACSM, and NASM.
Chapter 42, Appendix A

Jill Boyer-Holland

AFAA senior trainer, master certification specialist and consultant, certified personal trainer, continuing education provider; ski instructor and amateur ski racer; specialties include injury prevention, mid-life fitness, kickboxing, resistance training, instructor training and certification, sports conditioning, and rebounding.
Chapters 25, 30

Lynne G. Brick, BSN

Co-founder and owner, Brick Bodies Fitness Services, Inc., Baltimore, MD; awarded Ernst and Young Maryland Entrepreneur of the Year (2004) and IDEA (The Association for Fitness Professionals) Instructor of the Year (1990); first woman to be inducted into the Baltimore County Chamber of Commerce Business Hall of Fame; technical advisor, BodyVive™; featured in over a dozen exercise videos including *Buns of Steel* series; practiced nursing for 7 years, Maryland's Shock Trauma Center; sits on IHRSA's (International Health Racquet and Sportsclub Association) Board of Directors.
Chapter 21

Meryn G. Callander

Social worker; co-author with John Travis, *Wellness for Helping Professionals*; co-director, Wellness Associates, a non-profit educational corporation; co-founder, Alliance for Transforming the Lives of Children.
Chapter 2

Sharon Cheng, MBA, MSPT

Director, Baylor All Saints Medical Centers, Fort Worth, TX; physical therapist; health/fitness instructor with an emphasis on working with special populations; author; international presenter; trainer for group fitness, personal training, and physical medicine and rehabilitation.
Chapter 7

Janie Clark, MA

President, American Senior Fitness Association; winner of the National Council on Aging, Health Promotion Institute, Best Practice Award (2009); author, *Seniorcise, Full Life Fitness, Brain Fitness for Older Adults*, and *Quality-of-Life Fitness*; chapter author, *Physical Activity Instruction of Older Adults, Exercise for the Frail Elderly, Functional Fitness for Older Adults*, and *Exercise for Older Adults*; national scientific advisory board member on the LifeSpan functional fitness assessment study; co-author and contributor, national and international guidelines for preparing senior fitness professionals.

Chapter 38 (sub-chapter)

Nancy Clark, MS, RD, CSSD

Board Certified Specialist in Sports Dietetics (CSSD); private practice at Healthworks Fitness Center, Chestnut Hill, MA; member, AFAA Advisory Board; featured columnist, *American Fitness* magazine; fellow, American Dietetic Association; fellow, ACSM; author, *Nancy Clark's Sports Nutrition Guidebook* and *Nancy Clark's Food Guide for New Runners*.

Chapter 9

Susan O. Cooper, MA

Founder and owner, BodyBusiness Health Clubs & Spas, Austin, TX; BodyBusiness won seven Nova 7 Awards for excellence in service and programming and was voted Best Health Club, 2003, 2004, 2005, 2006; recognized as a top 25 women owned businesses; former Nike sponsored fitness athlete; first female president, THRSA (Texas Health, Racquet, & Sportsclub Association); member, IHRSA Board of Directors (International, Health, Racquet, and Sportsclub Association); global fitness professional trainer; video producer of "P.U.M.P.," "P.U.M.P. Bench," "The Upper Cut," and "Below the Belt;" holds certifications from ACE, ACSM, AFAA, and IAR.

Chapter 28

Julie Cornelius, BS

Nutritionist living and working in Tucson, AZ; bachelor's degree in nutritional sciences from the University of Arizona, Tucson; specializes with endurance athletes through her nutrition consulting business; an avid athlete who enjoys cycling, weight lifting, and yoga.

Chapter 8

Troy DeMond, MA

Owner, Fitness on the Move Lifestyle Center, Ft. Myers, FL; author of two fitness books for the fitness professional; contributing writer for several health and fitness magazines; starred in 5 exercise videos.

Chapter 26

Marcia M. Ditmyer, PhD, MS, MBA, CHES

Assistant professor, the University of Nevada, Las Vegas, School of Dental Medicine, with PhD in public health education from the University of Toledo, OH; consulted for many nationally-recognized health/fitness organizations developing, editing, and conducting certification and continuing education workshops; commissioner, Division Board for Certification for the National Commission for Health Education Credentialing (NCHES); member, AFAA Certification Board; AFAA master certification specialist.

Chapter 16

Tere Filer, MS, MPH

Owner, Action Plus Consulting Services, Los Angeles, CA, providing health education seminars, coordinating and implementing wellness programs, special events, and health fairs at the worksite, and conducting risk appraisals and follow-up counseling for employees; master's degrees in nutritional sciences and public health; currently a PhD candidate in behavioral psychology.

Chapter 26

Judy Gantz, MA, CMA

Director and founder, the Center of Movement Education and Research (CMER), a non-profit movement organization; international movement specialist, teacher, and lecturer; associate adjunct professor, University of California, Los Angeles (UCLA), Department of World Arts & Cultures from 1982–2005; specialized in anatomy for dancers, Laban movement analysis, somatic movement, dance kinesiology, and creative dance/movement education; worked on numerous professional certification programs, Laban/Bartenieff Institute of Movement Studies, New York, NY, Westwood Charter Elementary, and Palms Middle School, Los Angeles, CA; former fitness editor for Shape magazine; former co-editor, *Kinesiology for Dance*; latest writings on dance kinesiology, published by Oxford Press, *International Encyclopedia of Dance*.

Chapters 22, 23

James Gavin, PhD, ABPP, FACP

Full professor of applied human sciences and director of the professional coaching program, Concordia University, Montreal, Quebec, Canada; work focuses on the psychological aspects of sports and exercise; author of 8 books and over 150 professional articles including the landmark, *Lifestyle Fitness Coaching* (Human Kinetics, 2005); a competitive swimmer, triathlete, and modern dancer; former instructor, aerobics and yoga; holds a black belt in aikido.

Chapters 10, 11

Nancy Gillette, MA

Physical educator with two California State teaching credentials and a master's degree in adaptive physical education, University of Southern California (USC), Los Angeles, CA; workshop presenter, author, and lecturer; serves on several school and educational boards; owner, ATG International, a consulting company; member, AFAA Education Advisory Board; AFAA lead presenter and master certification specialist.

Chapters 17, 18, 34, 43

Laura A. Gladwin, MS, MAFP, FNBFE

Owner, LGA Consulting, Marana, AZ, specializing in wellness educational program development and implementation; bachelor's degree, physical education, Michigan State University, East Lansing, MI; master's degree with specialties in gerontology and exercise physiology, California State University, Fullerton (CSUF); chair, AFAA Education Advisory Board; fellow, National Board of Fitness Examiners; member, National Advisory Board, American Senior Fitness Association; coalition member, *National Standards for Preparing Senior Fitness Instructors*; coalition member, *International Curriculum Guidelines for Preparing Physical Activity Instructors of Older Adults*; editor-in-chief, AFAA's *Fitness: Theory & Practice*, 3rd, 4th, and 5th ed.; ACSM's former advisory board member, ACSM's *Health & Fitness Journal*; former associate professor, CSUF; former special advisor to the California Governor's Council on Physical Fitness and Sports; author, presenter, and mentor.

Chapters 17, 29, 38

Tracy Gordner-Cherry, RD, CDE, CDN

Former outpatient nutrition counselor, ViaHealth of Wayne, Newark, NY; AFAA certified fitness instructor; former co-owner, Fitcompany, which provided classes for corporations in and around Rochester, NY.

Chapter 8

Sandy Greger, MEd, ATC

Certified athletic trainer, physical and occupational therapist, Sports Medicine Lehigh Valley, Bethlehem, PA; ski racing coach and competitor; alpine ski instructor; certified level one ski racing coach with the U.S. Ski Coaches Association; member, Camelback Alpine Team.

Chapter 30

David L. Herbert, JD

Senior member, David L. Herbert & Associates, LLC, Attorneys & Counselors at Law, Canton, Ohio; co-editor, *Exercise Standards and Malpractice Reporter* and *Sports Medicine Standards and Malpractice Reporter*; represents a variety of fitness, exercise, and sports medicine organizations; author of 15 books, over 20 book chapters, and over 600 articles on various issues concerning health club operations and the law, standards of practice, negligence and malpractice; frequent speaker/resource for such groups as ACSM, NSCA, AHA, as well as other organizations; regular contributor to *Fitness Management Magazine*, *OnSite Fitness*, and *ACE Certified News*; a Trustee of the NBFE; helped draft standards and guidelines for ACSM, AFAA, NSCA, and is in the process of assisting NSF International to draft new standards for health and fitness facilities.
Chapter 44, Appendix B

Gail Johnston

Owner, Progress! Health Coaching & Consulting, Durango, CO; former vice president, SOF (Speaking of Fitness), Inc., a marketing, advertising, and health education publishing firm, Durango, CO.
Chapter 36

Meg Jordan, PhD, RN

Clinical medical anthropologist; international health journalist; registered nurse; editor-in-chief, AFAA's *American Fitness* magazine; department chair and professor, Integrative Health Studies, California Institute of Integral Studies, San Francisco, CA; known as the Global Medicine Hunter®, she searches the world for healing remedies; former director, integrative practice, Health Medicine Center, Northern California, where she specialized in behavioral health; host, weekly morning newscast "Healthy Living" for Global TV; host, daily radio program "The Dr. Meg Jordan Show" on Health Radio Network; former health reporter, FOX-KTVU, San Francisco, CA; former health commentator, CNN and "Today Show;" her columns have appeared in over 800 newspapers; authored several books in health and fitness, including *The Fitness Instinct*; serves on numerous advisory boards, including the National Wellness Institute and AFAA; recipient of awards such as the Healthy American Fitness Leader and the National Wellness Institute Service and Leadership Circle.
Foreword, Chapters 1, 32

Deanna Lowe, MA

Master's degree in physical education; instructor at California State University, Chico and Butte Community College, Oroville, CA; currently certified and has served as both a workshop coordinator and instructor for ACSM's health fitness specialist and personal trainer certifications.
Chapters 35, 40

Joelle Mancuso

Owner, Mancuso Fitness Consultants, Simi Valley, CA; former director of education and master instructor for the Spinning program worldwide, Mad Dogg Athletics, Inc., Venice, CA; ACE certified personal trainer; ACE and AFAA continuing education provider; national and international lecturer and workshop presenter; owner, Joe's Gym, Brentwood, CA.
Chapter 27

Patti Mantia, EdD

Owner/director of education, The Fitness Firm, Mansfield, MA, providing education and training for fitness professionals and personal trainers; AFAA master certification specialist; original developer, AFAA's step and strength training programs; professor and faculty chair, Department of Physical Education, Holyoke Community College, Holyoke, MA.
Chapters 6, 12, 31

Linda Mason, PT

Physical therapist specializing in pulmonary rehabilitation, orthopedics, and sports medicine; lecturer and presenter.
Chapter 12

Diana McNab, MEd

Adjunct professor, Daniels College of Business, Denver, CO; co-director, Wellness and Sports Psychology for the Professional Sports Wives Association; presents Destination Location Stress Management courses, former professor and sports psychologist, Seton Hall University, South Orange, NJ; former member, Canadian National Ski Team.

Chapter 19

Kathy F. Normansell, MS

Co-developer, adaptive fitness guidelines for AFAA in conjunction with the former National Handicapped Sports (NHS) in Washington, DC; former director, adaptive fitness instructor workshop, NHS.

Chapter 34

Dorette Nysewander, EdD, AFP, NBFE

Owner, dgroup Consulting Services, Inc., Jacksonville, FL, providing clients with wellness education and curriculum design focusing on accreditation services; doctorate in educational leadership with an emphasis in health care education, Nova Southeastern University, Fort Lauderdale, FL; master's degree, health services administration, Central Michigan University, Mount Pleasant, MI; over 25 years in the wellness field; member, AFAA Certification Board; fellow, National Board of Fitness Examiners; member, U.S. Department of Education, Human Services Committee; facilitated wellness trainings worldwide and met with industry leaders of many countries; holds numerous certifications in the field of wellness; author, facilitator, wellness coach, and career mentor.

Chapters 16, 17, 37, 39

Richard Michael Odom

Owner/director, Integrated Fitness Strategies, Sun Valley, ID; instructs at local YMCA; international yoga practitioner, instructor, trainer, consultant, presenter, and lecturer; former director of the Sun Valley Physical Fitness and Rehabilitation Center, Sun Valley, ID; former principal of Idaho's Yoga College of India.

Chapter 33

Michael T. Phelan, MD, FACOG, FACS

Board Certified Obstetrician-Gynecologist; fellow, American College of Obstetricians and Gynecologists (ACOG); fellow, American College of Surgeons; 30 years in private practice, Jacksonville, FL; a courtesy associate clinical professor, University of Florida, Shands Jacksonville; ACOG regional representative, Florida Ob-Gyn Society.

Chapter 39

Scott O. Roberts, Ph.D., FAACVPR, FACSM

Professor and coordinator, Exercise Science Program, California State University, Chico; over 15 years of clinical experience in a variety of hospital-based and free-standing exercise facilities; fellow, American Association of Cardiovascular and Pulmonary Rehabilitation; fellow, ACSM; author and co-author of numerous exercise and fitness books; currently an author and senior editor of ACSM's *Exercise Management for Persons with Chronic Diseases and Disabilities* (3rd ed.).

Chapters 35, 40

Linda Romaine, MS, MBA

AFAA personal fitness trainer, certification specialist, step specialist, emergency response specialist, certified personal fitness trainer, and continuing education provider; professor, Health Sciences Department, Raritan Valley Community College, North Branch, NJ; director of group fitness, Health Quest of Hunterdon County, Flemington, NJ.

Chapter 25

Jo-Ann Ross, MA, CCC

Licensed speech pathologist with private practice; co-founder of "Vocal Impact," a voice care program for aerobic instructors.

Chapter 14

Mary E. Sanders, Ph.D., FACSM

Associate professor, School of Medicine, University of Nevada, Reno; director, WaterFit®/Golden Waves®; associate editor, ACSM's *Health & Fitness Journal*; fellow, ACSM; advisory board member, International Council on Active Aging; columnist, *The Journal of Active Aging*; education director, Mizuno, Japan; conducts research in water fitness for health; certified, health & fitness instructor by ACE and ACSM; continuing education provider for a number of certification organizations.
Chapter 24

Linda Shelton, MS

Internationally recognized fitness and wellness consultant, certified trainer, speaker and health writer for 40 years; founding member, AFAA, co-authored the original 1983 Basic Exercise Standards and Guidelines and Primary Certification; authored and developed AFAA's Mat Science I and II programs; master's of science degree in exercise physiology; authored 8 books; produced, directed, and/or choreographed over 350 DVDs and co-produced three award winning television fitness shows; former fitness director, Weider/AMI fitness publications including *SHAPE* for 23 years; current fitness director, VIVmag, a digital women's lifestyle and fitness magazine; executive advisory board member, Elite Trainer; communications director, Beamfit; full partner, Worksite Wellness, a Pacific Northwest-based Corporate Wellness Company; president, LIFESTYLEscapes™ LLC, a multi-media online fitness and resource wellness company; inducted into the National Fitness Hall of Fame (2007).
Chapter 29

Arthur Siegel, MD

Chief, Department of Internal Medicine, McLean Hospital, Belmont, MA; assistant professor of medicine, Harvard Medical School, Boston, MA; original contributor to AFAA's first textbook, *Aerobics: Theory & Practice*; founding member of AFAA's Advisory Board.
Chapter 13

Kathy Stevens, MA, MAFP

AFAA's educational director; member, AFAA Education Advisory Board; master's degree in kinesiology; over 30 years experience in the development, implementation, and publishing of fitness programs, services, videos, and textbooks; college professor, fitness athlete, consultant, and global educator; former Reebok master trainer; dedicated presenter, author, mentor, and visionary.
Chapters 17, 28, 41, 44

Carol Swett, MA, CCC

Licensed speech pathologist; professor of English, director of International Programs, Benedictine University, Lisle, IL; specializes in presentation skills, oral communication and pronunciation dialect reduction, and second language acquisition; AFAA certification specialist; co-founder of "Vocal Impact," a voice care program for aerobic instructors.
Chapter 14

John Travis, MD, MPH

Pioneer in the field of wellness; founder of the first wellness center in the United States, Mill Valley, CA (1975); co-author, *Wellness Workbook, Simply Well,* and *Wellness for Helping Professionals*; co-director, Wellness Associates, a non-profit education corporation; co-founder, Alliance for Transforming the Lives of Children.
Chapter 2

Gregory L. Welch, MS

Exercise physiologist and owner of SpeciFit: An Agency of Wellness, Seal Beach, CA; over 20 years in the fitness industry with a focus on special needs population; author and lecturer; creator, SpeciFit Foundation, designed to further wellness concepts for adolescent women.
Chapter 20

Mary Yoke, MA, MM

Master's degree in exercise physiology, two degrees in music, and holds 22 certifications; adjunct professor, Adelphi University, NY; served as a fitness video consultant and reviewer for SHAPE, *Consumer Reports*, and *Good Housekeeping*, and has served as an expert witness in lawsuits involving injuries related to fitness videos; has worked in the areas of cardiac rehab, physical therapy, and corporate fitness and health promotion; former advisory board member, ACSM's *Health & Fitness Journal*; served 6+ years, ACSM's Credentialing Committee; AFAA master certification specialist for group and personal training; author of four books: AFAA's *A Guide to Personal Fitness Training*, 1996, 2001, *Functional Exercise Progressions*, 2004, *Methods of Group Exercise Instruction*, 2nd ed. 2009, and AFAA's *Personal Fitness Training: Theory and Practice*, 2006; featured in six educational videos.

Chapters 13, 15, 35, 36

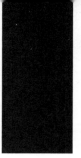

Foreword

Fitness instruction is an exciting profession that has continued to evolve since the Aerobics and Fitness Association of America (AFAA) published its first edition of *Fitness: Theory & Practice* in 1985 (originally entitled *Aerobics: Theory & Practice*). This extensively revised and updated fifth edition for students and practitioners promises to be another tried-and-true winner as the most widely used fitness instructor manual in the world. With now over three million copies sold, AFAA's *Fitness: Theory & Practice*, has been recognized globally as the groundbreaking resource for the fitness industry. May it serve as your much used, dog-eared, never-collecting-dust "bible"—just as it has for over 500,000 group exercise instructors and fitness professionals throughout the world.

Today, AFAA has grown into a widely respected international presence in over 72 nations, with licensed, fully operational organizations from China and Japan to Brazil and Turkey. The dream of founder and president, Linda D. Pfeffer, RN, and a handful of concerned instructors in 1983 has blossomed into the world's largest fitness educator today through the hard work, selfless contributions, and unbridled enthusiasm of thousands of AFAA Specialists and Presenters. To give you an idea of this massive scope, AFAA hosts over 2,500 workshops every year in health clubs, community centers, colleges, and military posts. But what is more amazing is that AFAA has retooled its online education offerings to keep pace with the explosive demand for digital media. Through e-learning platforms, AFAA offers over 150 opportunities to gain new knowledge, video-check practical skills, and submit your continuing education lessons.

Still, with all this expansive growth, online presence, and international reach, the typical fitness professional appreciates a good book in hand—and that's what this version promises: a way to curl up, hunker down, find some quiet time, and dive into the pages of this book. Take your time with these chapters—they're densely packed and designed to lead you, step by step, into a comprehensive education of the most effective ways to attain optimal fitness.

AFAA certified fitness professionals not only teach aerobics and group exercise classes, they counsel clients on everything from strength training for older adults to postpartum exercises for nursing mothers. Today, an accomplished fitness professional may teach advanced yoga for seasoned exercisers, and tomorrow, receive medical referrals for clients looking to decrease risk for chronic disease and improve quality of life. They are, in fact, fitness practitioners, new advocates in the making—professionals who play a key role in the future of health promotion.

The entire gamut of AFAA-trained fitness professionals—from the newly certified instructors to the top-of-the-ladder AFAA Fitness Practitioners (AFP)—fulfills a life span of fitness needs for diverse populations. The public has come to count on AFAA professionals for exercise safety, effectiveness, guidance, and accuracy. Because of that comprehensive coverage, they not only need a book that presents and deciphers the explosion of research and practical knowledge developed over the past decade—they need a book that clearly speaks their language, a book that takes the theory from the exercise laboratory and brings it where it is needed most—the fitness center, the home gym, the street.

This anthology presents recognized leaders and authors in fields that impact fitness instruction: (a) exercise physiology, (b) anatomy, (c) biomechanics, (d) sports medicine, (e) nutrition, (f) weight management, (g) sports psychology, (h) exercise adherence, (i) personal fitness training, (j) business management, and (k) instructional technique. Their professional knowledge and hard-earned practical wisdom is passed onto you with the intention that you will use them to develop your own rewarding fitness career or perhaps simply to pursue your personal fitness dreams.

As always, we include the latest version of AFAA's Basic Exercise Standards and Guidelines, which has guided exercise instructors since AFAA's inception in 1983. In that same year, about 200 spanking new instructors gathered at a gym in Northridge, California for the first AFAA Aerobic Exercise Certification workshop. Three examiners looked for proper biomechanics, knowledge of exercise modification for various limitations, well-timed cues, and AFAA's hallmark standard—both *theoretical* and *practical* knowledge of fitness concepts. Over the years, the level of sophistication has taken an exponential leap forward. However, the fundamental AFAA 5 Questions™ have stood the test of time. Some things just don't have to change—they grow better with age.

AFAA's *Fitness Theory & Practice* continues to open up a new world of quality instruction to fitness professionals. It is AFAA's sincere intention that this resource becomes just as dog-eared and relied upon as the original. May it help you put the latest fitness theory into a rewarding practice!

Meg Jordan, PhD, RN
Editor, AFAA's *American Fitness* magazine

Aerobics and Fitness Association of America

Part 1

Essentials of Exercise

The Fitness Evolution

Wellness: The Big Picture

Improving Health and Performance Through Aerobic Fitness

Energy Production During Exercise

Developing and Maintaining Aerobic Fitness

The Cardiorespiratory System: Structure, Function, and Exercise Application

The Musculoskeletal System: Structure, Function, and Exercise Application

1

The Fitness Evolution

Meg Jordan, PhD, RN

Ever-Changing Concept

In 1983, the Aerobics and Fitness Association of America (AFAA) set out to address the needs of an enthusiastic, emergent profession of fitness instructors. So new and unproven, yet they were several steps ahead of a growing body of research for group exercise. AFAA gathered the best and the brightest among exercise physiologists, cardiologists, physical educators, sports medicine experts, physical therapists, and fitness professionals to compile the first-ever exercise standards and guidelines for group exercise instructors so they could deliver safe and effective classes for their participants and themselves.

On the heels of developing AFAA's *Basic Exercise Standards and Guidelines*, AFAA published its first textbook in 1985, offering a definition of fitness that focused on cardiorespiratory endurance, muscular strength, and flexibility. That definition has significantly broadened since those first offerings, keeping pace with research in healthy aging, multicultural interests, and the exponential growth and popularity of the fitness movement worldwide. Today, some 25 years later, the definition of fitness includes the greater attributes of an active and fit body and a positive mind and spirit. In addition to the basic trio of endurance, strength, and flexibility, fitness training also encompasses agility, power, speed, balance, and mind/body wholeness.

Most importantly, fitness instruction has earned a seat at the preventive health table, recognized as one of the best "medicines" available. AFAA certified fitness professionals have forged alliances within the health care system, and function in rehabilitation settings and hospital-based wellness programs. When working in rehabilitation or hospital-based environments, fitness professionals are supervised by licensed medical personnel and generally work with clinically stable individuals helping them reduce risk factors.

Many clinical settings contract with certified fitness professionals to teach modified classes for people living with chronic conditions such as diabetes, multiple sclerosis, and stroke. In these cases, fitness professionals follow the lead of licensed physical therapists or advanced degreed exercise physiologists working with physicians and nurses.

Public and private elementary and secondary schools have also benefitted from contracted and volunteer hours donated by fitness professionals. In an age of severe budget cuts, some schools have lost their physical education specialists, and local fitness professionals have filled in the gaps with age-appropriate cardio or strength training programs. They serve critical roles supplementing physical education in schools, and providing stress reduction, conditioning, and ergonomic advice in corporate wellness programs. More than ever, fitness is viewed as an essential component for overall physical and psychoemotional wellness.

Explosive Growth of a Profession

To appreciate just how far fitness has come in the past decade or so, it helps to bring the historical view into focus. In the early 1980s, fitness professionals were called "aerobic instructors," and teaching classes was often viewed as a "part-time hobby" to earn a little extra money and stay in shape—not a *real* profession. Not anymore. Fitness professionals are now recognized as providing one of the most effective services to enhance health, reduce risk for chronic disease, maintain muscle mass and bone density, and prevent premature aging as well as a host of additional physical, emotional, and psychological benefits.

At its onset in 1983, AFAA was devoted to the safe and effective instruction of aerobic classes, and that generally meant whatever it took to keep a conventional dance exercise class injury-free and enjoyable. Today, AFAA offers eight certifications, eight specialty trainings, and approximately 4,000 workshops per year. The AFAA certified group exercise instructor is joined by an entire career ladder of professionals, including personal fitness trainers, exercise specialists, certified consultants, and AFAA Fitness Practitioners (AFP). AFAA certified professionals interface with physicians, health clinics, managed care providers, and corporate health networks to assure clients receive a seamless program of lifestyle management.

Ever-Evolving Aerobics

Group exercise as a fitness activity has now been in existence for over 25 years, evolving into a number of truly remarkable forms. Today, fitness workouts encompass everything from aqua to interval, step to pump, seated to slide, and yoga to Pilates. While the definition of fitness reaches out to broader horizons, instructors scramble for new research and emerging guidelines in order to maintain a vision of teaching the most effective and exciting class possible.

This book is the culmination of widespread efforts, spanning several years, to discover the leading developers and professionals in these expanding fields of fitness. As a fitness professional, you will encounter both the theoretical foundation from which they draw and the innovative practices that spring forth. You will even have a chance to put into action specific examples of those practices, which are provided throughout the text.

Capturing the Trends

In each edition, AFAA's *Fitness: Theory & Practice* has attempted to capture the leading research and effective practices in exercise instruction. By far, the number one concern is that over two-thirds of Americans are considered over-weight, and almost 70% of the population is not engaging in regular, moderate, or even light physical activity, according to the American Heart Association. This trend in unhealthy weight gain has been chronicled in both post-industrial and developing countries worldwide, as a result of the overconsumption of processed, calorie-dense foods and inadequate physical activity. The human and economic costs from physical inactivity and unhealthy diets are staggering.

As medical experts try to reverse the nation's climbing obesity rates, they have looked at potential causes, such as overeating, fat metabolism, dietary fats, and lifestyle change. Very little has made a difference for people who are unable to keep the weight off for the long term. Now, a new report in *Obesity Research* shows that exercise is the key factor in weight loss regimens because it can lead to an increased expenditure of energy. That in itself is nothing new. However, what is new is the fact that physical activity can also inhibit food intake in overweight people. Plus, it seems to be the critical factor in maintaining a desirable weight.

Physical activity, more so than weight loss, also reduces the risk of coronary heart disease. This same report examined the decline in the amount of non-exercise energy expended for chores, moving about, work, as well as transporting kids, friends, and individuals. These hidden numbers—insidious little reductions accumulated here and there—are a major culprit in the fattening of America over the last decade.

Finally, decreasing the fat stores in obese people has been exasperatingly difficult for them when they have tried to follow exercise routines that suggest a moderately paced walk of 30 minutes once a day. Now, a new report from the Institute of Medicine suggests that for the obese to truly lose and maintain weight loss, exercise duration should stretch to 2 hours or more. It's up to fitness instructors to know how to do that safely. Another new report in *Medicine & Science in Sports & Exercise* confirms what researcher Ralph Paffenbarger, Jr., PhD. discovered with his 20-year study on over 16,000 Harvard University alumnae. A growing body of evidence supports the theory that moderate physical activity (e.g., gardening, bowling, housework, yard chores) not only reduces the risk of disease and extends the lifespan, it can help the "never-exercised" cross over the line for the first time.

How can fitness professionals counter this troubling trend toward obesity? First, keeping up to date with latest research will help fitness professionals approach clients who struggle with extra pounds in a more compassionate and realistic manner. Fitness professionals need to know that weight loss is a multifaceted challenge, and that efforts to reduce and maintain fat loss through exercise alone have only been modestly successful. The latest guidelines from both the American Dietetic Association and the American Society for Nutrition indicate that the key for shedding fat and maintaining its loss is both a modest reduction in caloric intake and an increase in physical activity.

Another way fitness professionals can help stem the rising tide of obesity is to promote activity in innovative ways. Talk about the positive benefits of exercise that flow into other aspects of one's life: (a) more confidence in relationships, (b) renewed interest in play and leisure, and (c) greater productivity at work. Keep programs fresh and exciting. It's crucial to employ the latest in motivational techniques. But most of all, knowing that the exercises and modalities you're teaching are the most effective means for accomplishing your clients' goals will really pay off. You need to know how to move larger bodies safely and strategically with the best warm-up techniques, and the most effective and well-targeted fat-burning choreography and strength-training styles. The chapters in this book are loaded with top-notch advice, insight, research, and rich experience.

In addition, fitness professionals can play an active role outside the studio. Fitness professionals can serve as advocates for community strategies to broaden safe walking and cycling paths; restore comprehensive physical education to primary and secondary education; and be a visible, proactive presence in healthy cities campaigns and health fairs. New research indicates that the built environment can either promote or hinder physical activity in communities. Are there walkways and well-lighted recreation areas, courts, playgrounds, and bike paths in your community? If not, you can be a community advocate working toward the establishment of policies that provide safe and enjoyable access to residents. Fitness is usually not achieved in a studio alone. It requires a 360° commitment to how we engage with our physical environment every day.

Another demographic trend that this textbook addresses is teaching to an aging population. Fitness professionals constantly look for applications to draw from exercise science for the older client as well as the frail elderly. New thinking is presented on how this population can benefit from bone and muscle strengthening classes, programs for improving balance and flexibility, modified yoga, and rhythmic dance for non- and low-impact aerobic conditioning. New research on exercise for seniors is among the most encouraging in our field. Senior-supportive exercise programs not only help prevent falls, ward off muscle loss and osteoporosis, build upper body strength for activities of daily living, and slow down the effects of aging, but they have been shown to also enhance memory, concentration, and cognitive abilities.

Attention to body shaping and contouring is another trend that is most visible in the high-volume markets of major cities. That is where floor work and specialized equipment classes, such as Pilates, are making waves. Quality of movement is being emphasized together with the elongation and strengthening of muscles. What was once a private session for ballerinas has now grown to accommodate millions who are seeking formerly esoteric concepts, such as core conditioning, stabilization, and micro-movements.

At the same time, the demand is up for high-powered workouts that take people to the top of their potential. Cardio kickboxing and indoor cycling classes are leading the charts in terms of group calorie burn, and AFAA is right there, often a step ahead of the game, supplying instruction, guidelines, and new certifications for each of the emerging trends.

It is obvious that the contemporary fitness professional needs to remain up-to-date in research, trends, and consumer interest. This latest edition of AFAA's *Fitness: Theory & Practice* promises to keep fitness professionals informed and prepared.

Expanding Needs of the Public

Today, most people live increasingly hectic and stressful lifestyles with overburdened schedules and a shrinking amount of recreational time. In such circumstances, fitness is more important than ever, and its definition has shifted to include time for pleasurable activities as well as physical training for endurance, strength, and flexibility. As a result, people have come to expect more from their workouts than a fast-paced drill for their hearts. They want their fitness professional to be knowledgeable in the latest best practices to reduce the deleterious effects of stress, and to follow guidelines supported by valid research and high quality standards.

Fitness professionals realize their clients need to both unravel knotted muscles and have a good workout in order to achieve optimal health benefits. This new attention to the total well-being of clients has blossomed into the creation of programs focusing on mind-body movement, yoga, and creative stretch, as well as basic starter programs for various segments of the population (e.g., seniors, youth, cardiac patients, the overweight and obese, and those who are pregnant, arthritic, or diabetic).

Risk Reduction for Chronic Disease

As stated earlier, fitness is now recognized as a fundamental component for overall health and longevity. Specifically, exercise is proving to be the number one "action" of choice by some medical researchers who have found that exercise may have beneficial effects on a variety of actual or potential disease processes, including heart disease, stroke, diabetes, and obesity. The research accumulated in the last 5 years is simply overwhelming. Some of the latest findings related to physical activity include changes in chronic inflammatory condition, which lay the groundwork for the development of chronic diseases. These include metabolic disorders such as hyperglycemic and hyperlipidemic conditions, metabolic syndrome, type 2 diabetes, certain cancers, cardiovascular disease, arthritis, stroke, migraines, irritable bowel syndrome, and osteoporosis. While the implementation of such measures to treat these conditions lies with licensed health care providers, the research findings represent exciting news for fitness professionals and their clients.

Responding to Social Forces

Finding ways to exercise "more, better, faster" is only part of the fitness picture. The real revolution within the fitness world over the past few years has been directed at ways in which fitness professionals sought the new recruit—the under-served, the dropouts, the non-converted. In the early days, aerobic dance definitely had its fans in a white, middle-class demographic, but four social factors have influenced how aerobics is practiced today.

First of all, a multicultural dynamic is alive and well in much of the world, especially in the United States. This new multiculturalism has energized the cardio (aerobic) class with fresh, downbeat sounds and rhythms of African dance, Salsa, hip-hop, funk, Caribbean movement, and Eastern oriented martial arts. With these exciting additions, classes are popular and well attended again in the major cities.

Secondly, more people are taking advantage of the skills of personal fitness trainers. No longer viewed as the exclusive territory of the elite or the wealthy, obtaining the services of a personal fitness trainer is a life-enhancing, good sense move for millions. Some innovative trainers have created the small group instruction model, making their services more affordable, or found clubs with which they could partner to provide a mutually beneficial service. Increasing their knowledge base for special health concerns is of paramount importance for trainers working one-on-one with people at midlife. This health-conscious part of the population often suffers from an old ski injury, runner's knees, a back disability, or a nagging sports injury.

Thirdly, the abundance of new research on the benefits of muscle strengthening for premenopausal women has alerted the professional group exercise instructor to provide a variety of excellent conditioning choices, such as step-plus-weights, tubing classes, and bands-plus-aerobics. Retaining lean muscle is not only great for body shaping, but it has taken a top standing in the struggle to ward off increasing weight gain. Strength training is being embraced by everyone from adolescents to the senior population, making a demand for personal fitness trainers and well-informed group exercise instructors alike.

Lastly, the benefits of cross-training have been well documented in the past few years. Not only does it provide a much-needed motivational diversion, cross-training allows the neurological and musculoskeletal systems to be challenged in new ways. The rich bounty of classes and guidelines presented in the following pages are designed to present a world of new ideas to interested readers.

From toddlers to seniors, from the overweight beginner to the wheelchair user—everyone deserves the right to wear a "fit" label, and be supported and taught with the latest, safest information. It requires a real shift in thinking to realize it is not that we have a host of unfit people out there—it is just that we have not thought of the right fitness program to spark their imaginations and get their pulses racing. Every time we expand our definition of fitness, we get to flex our creativity and commitment within a wonderful profession.

Fitness professionals should make it a priority to teach people to move like their lives depend on it—and AFAA's *Fitness: Theory & Practice* is their primary text on how to do just that.

References

1. American College of Sports Medicine. (2010). *ACSM's guidelines for exercise testing and prescription* (8th ed.). Baltimore, MD: Lippincott Williams & Wilkins.
2. American Dietetic Association & American Society for Nutrition. *Obesity, reproduction, and pregnancy outcomes.* Retrieved on July 28, 2009, from http://www.nutrition.org/media/news/fact-sheets-and-position-papers/ObesityReprodPreg.pdf
3. Daussin, F.N., Zoll, J., Dufour, S.P., Ponsot, E., Lonsdorfer-Wolf, E., Doutreleau, S., Mettauer, B., Piquard, F., Geny, B., & Richard, R. (2008). Effect of interval versus continuous training on cardiorespiratory and mitochondrial functions: Relationship to aerobic performance improvements in sedentary subjects. *American Journal of Physiology: Regulatory, Integrative, Comparative Physiology.* July, 295(1), R264-272.
4. Powers, S.K., & Howley, E.T. (2009). *Exercise physiology: Theory and application to fitness and performance* (7th ed.). Boston, MA: McGraw-Hill.
5. U.S. Department of Health and Human Services. *2008 Physical activity guidelines for Americans.* ODPHP Publication No. U0036, October 2008. Retrieved May 15, 2009 from http://www.health.gov/paguidelines
6. U.S. National Institutes of Health. *Physical activity and cancer*, March 2004. Retrieved May 15, 2009 from http://www.cancer.gov/newscenter/benchmarks-vol4-issue1/page2/

John Travis, MD, MPH
and Meryn G. Callander

2

Wellness: The Big Picture

Focus

While many people think of **wellness** only in physical terms (e.g., nutrition, fitness, stress reduction), its originators envisioned it as a multidimensional concept, also incorporating the mental, emotional, and spiritual aspects of a human being.

At its core, wellness emerges from a paradigm that stands in direct contrast to the prevailing **treatment paradigm**. The **wellness paradigm** promotes self-responsibility, compassion, and collaboration between client and practitioner. With the practitioner's help, the client recognizes "dis-ease" as a message, drawing attention to an aspect of life that needs healing, rather than something to be overcome, rejected, or fixed. In this way, the wellness paradigm empowers individuals to continue developing their unique potential as human beings.

This chapter assists the fitness professional in broadening his or her thinking on health and disease, offering a vantage point from the wellness paradigm.

Addressing the Underlying Attitudes and Behaviors

The word "wellness" caught on in the hospital and corporate worlds in the '70s and '80s, but at the cost of its proponents' watering down the original concept in order to fit wellness into the existing medical/treatment paradigm.

Similarly, many fitness programs are based on a modified treatment (authoritarian) paradigm, focusing on preventing problems/symptoms or attempting to overpower them. Great attention is placed on human *doing* (action/behavior change), but little attention is placed on human *being* (the underlying beliefs/feelings). The present emphasis on quick results and easy fixes falls short of addressing the fundamental issues that can lead to despair and self-destructive behaviors (that in turn have driven our illness-care system to bankruptcy).

Authentic well-being requires addressing the underlying self-destructive attitudes and behaviors rampant throughout society. Popular definitions of wellness need to be expanded beyond their narrow focus on individual fitness or nutrition. Without addressing the underlying causes of dis-ease, such programs are only Band-Aids, providing no more than symptomatic relief.

The wellness of an individual cannot be addressed in any meaningful way unless viewed within the context of the prevailing consciousness of our world. The impact of this consciousness is universal, manifesting in every realm of our society—the medical, economic, environmental, psychological, and the spiritual. It is inseparable from our well-being.

From Discountability to Accountability

The treatment paradigm mirrors the prevailing cultural norms. It is a **paradigm of discountability**. The roles open to us in this paradigm are the victimized, the dominator, and (of special interest to the helping professions) the rescuer (a driving need to "fix" people/problems). Even the language of the treatment paradigm (compliance, regimen, or more revealing—"regime," "battling," "overcoming") reveals its fundamentally adversarial mindset.

This approach is also perpetuated through many professionals' desires for only practical tools, with minimal questioning of the underlying assumptions inherent in the system in which they operate. To many people, this system appears to be bankrupt—financially and emotionally. Frustration and burnout among practitioners continues to climb. Clearly, another approach is needed to balance it, and attention to the dehumanization that has occurred in many treatment disciplines needs to be addressed.

The wellness paradigm offers a fundamentally different orientation to disease and health. Sustainable well-being, personal and planetary, calls for a shift into a **paradigm of accountability**—the wellness paradigm. The roles available in the wellness paradigm focus on life as a learning experience full of endless possibility. The results are self-responsibility with love/compassion, cooperation, and conscious co-creation (see *Wellness for Helping Professionals, Creating Compassionate Cultures* under References).

What is Wellness?
- A choice—a decision you make to move toward optimal health.
- A way of life—a lifestyle you design to achieve your highest potential for well-being.
- A process—a developing awareness that there is no endpoint, but that health and happiness are possible in each moment, here and now.
- A balanced channeling of energy—energy received from the environment, transformed within you, and returned to affect the world around you.
- The integration of body, mind, and spirit—the appreciation that everything you do, think, feel, and believe has an impact on your state of health.
- The loving acceptance of yourself.

Most people think in terms of illness and assume that the absence of illness indicates wellness. There are actually many degrees of wellness, just as there are many degrees of illness.

The Illness/Wellness Continuum
The **Illness-Wellness Continuum** (Figure 2-1) illustrates the relationship of the treatment paradigm to the wellness paradigm. Moving from the center to the left shows a progressively worsening state of health. Moving to the right of center indicates increasing levels of health and well-being. The treatment paradigm (which is designed to overcome unwanted conditions) can bring you up to the neutral point, where the symptoms of disease are minimized. The wellness paradigm, which can be entered at any point on the Continuum, helps you move toward higher levels of wellness. The wellness paradigm is not intended to replace the treatment paradigm, but to work in harmony with it. If you are sick treatment is important, but don't stop at the neutral point. Use the wellness paradigm to move to greater degrees of wellness.

While people often lack physical symptoms of illness, they may still be bored, depressed, tense, anxious, or generally unhappy with their lives. Such emotional states often set the stage for physical and mental disease. Today, it is well understood that cancer can be brought on through the lowering of the body's resistance from excessive stress. Negative emotional states can also lead to abuse of the body through smoking, overdrinking, overeating, and not exercising. But these symptoms and behaviors represent only the tip of an iceberg. They are usually substitutes for other more basic human needs, such as recognition from others, a more nurturing environment, caring and affection from friends, and greater self-acceptance.

The "well" being is not necessarily the strong, the successful, the young, or even the illness-free being. People can be living a life of wellness and yet be physically handicapped, aged, in pain, imperfect. Conversely, they can be physically healthy and still functioning from an illness mentality—constantly worrying and judging themselves. Regardless of where on the Illness-Wellness Continuum people perceive themselves to be, what matters most is the direction he or she is facing.

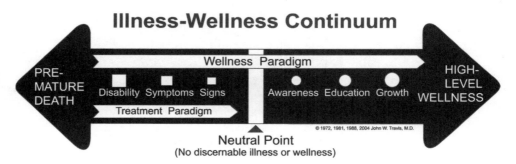

Fig. 2-1. The Illness/Wellness Continuum
(Reprinted with permission from the *Wellness Book* [3rd ed.] by John W. Travis, MD and Regina Sara Ryan; Celestrial Arts, Berkeley, CA.)

The Iceberg Model

Icebergs reveal only about one-tenth of their mass above the water. The remaining nine-tenths remain submerged. Your current state of health—be it one of disease or vitality—is just like the tip of an iceberg (Figure 2-2). This is the apparent part—what shows. If you don't like it, you can attempt to change it, do things to it, chisel away at an unwanted condition. But, whenever you chip some off, more of the same comes up to take its place.

To understand all that creates and supports your current state of health, you have to look under the surface. The first level is the **lifestyle/behavioral** level—what you eat, how you use and exercise your body, how you relax and let go of stress, and how you safeguard yourself from the hazards around you.

Many people follow lifestyles that they know are destructive, both to their own well-being and to that of the planet. Yet, they feel powerless to change them. To understand why, you must look still deeper, to the **psychological/motivational/cultural** level. Here lies what moves you to lead the lifestyle you've chosen. You can learn what payoffs you get from being overweight, smoking, driving recklessly, or from eating well, being considerate of others, and getting regular exercise (refer to Chapters 3, 8, 10, & 11).

Exploring below the psychological/motivational level, you encounter the **spiritual/being/meaning level**. This is really more of a realm than a level because it has no clear boundaries. It includes the mystical and mysterious, and everything else in the unconscious mind. Your level of wellness is closely tied to how you address (or ignore) such issues as your reason for being, the real meaning of your life, or your place in the universe. The answers you choose underlie and permeate all of the layers above. Ultimately, this realm determines whether the tip of the iceberg, representing your state of health, is one of disease or wellness.

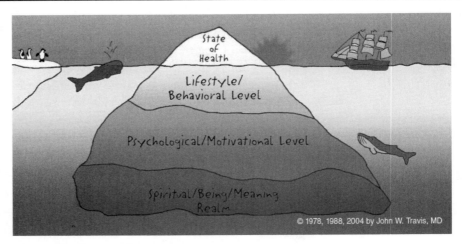

Fig. 2-2. The Illness/Wellness Continuum
(Reprinted with permission from the *Wellness Book* [3rd ed.] by John W. Travis, MD and Regina Sara Ryan; Celestrial Arts, Berkeley, CA.)

The Wellness Energy System

Energy Input. Imagine yourself receiving energy from three major sources: (a) breathing (oxygen), (b) sensing (stimuli in your environment), (c) and eating (food that is oxidized by cells and is used to build and repair body tissues). You convert some of the energy you take in to maintain the channel—your body— by generating heat and nerve impulses; replenishing and distributing blood, nutrients, and hormones; and repairing tissues.

Energy Output. Now think of your body as a pipeline or conduit of energy. You channel this energy through your body, mind, and being, converting it to forms of energy before returning it to the environment around you. Wellness results from the balanced flow of these energies through you.

The nine different outflows of energy to the environment are as follows.

- **Self-responsibility and Love**. This is a form of energy that manifests as the attitude you choose in living your life. Wellness is enhanced by living your life with self-responsibility and love.
- **Moving**. Not only do you move your body through your external environment (exercise and fitness), but you move internal muscles to provide blood circulation, digestion, reproduction, and so forth.
- **Feeling**. Energy is also used for expressing emotions.
- **Thinking**. The brain is a major user of energy for thought processing, intuition, and dreaming.
- **Playing/Working**. How you spend most of your waking hours.
- **Communicating**. A complex form of energy encompassing many of the preceding forms of energy.
- **Intimacy and Sex**. Covers the whole spectrum of life-energy, not just genital feelings.
- **Finding Meaning**. Seeking purpose and direction to the above forms of energy.
- **Transcending**. Beyond the rational and connects us with all-that-is.

Putting together the input and output, we have the complete wellness energy system of a human being. This system is an alternative to the usual piecemeal way of looking at health. It offers an integrated overview of all human life functions, seeing them as various forms of energy. The harmonious balancing of these life functions results in good health and well-being.

Summary

Every single aspect of life is interdependent (connected) with every other, and so even small changes have a ripple effect—throughout your being and throughout the web of life. You can't wear tight shoes for very long before you start to notice that everything about your world feels cramped. When you are worried about something, you're likely to have an upset stomach, too. What may appear to be separate events or individual symptoms are really interconnected aspects of a much larger and more complex system. Since there are many of us, and we are all interacting and exchanging energy with each other and everything else in our environment, the picture is very large. Taken together as a whole, our picture can be no smaller than the whole planet. But remember that small changes can have big results. Through small changes, we can heal ourselves and our world.

References

1. Travis, J.W., & Regina, R.S. (2001). *Simply well.* Berkeley, CA: Ten Speed Press.
2. Travis, J.W., & Regina, R.S. (2004). *Wellness workbook* (3rd ed.). Berkeley, CA: Celestial Arts.
3. Travis, J.W. & Callander, M.G. (1990). *Wellness for helping professional creating compassionate cultures.* Asheville, NC: Wellness Associates Publications.

William C. Beam, PhD

3

Improving Health and Performance Through Aerobic Fitness

Focus

A sufficient degree of aerobic fitness provides numerous benefits. Many of these are health-related and result in an improved state of overall wellness. To achieve wellness does not require an excruciating, drop-dead workout regimen. Wellness can be achieved, enhanced, and maintained with a consistent program of regular, moderate-intensity exercise. However, some benefits of exercise, those that improve an individual's aerobic exercise performance and optimal health, do require more vigorous workouts. Therefore, the benefits of aerobic exercise will be discussed first as they relate to improving wellness, and second as they relate to improving aerobic exercise performance.

Considerations Before Starting an Exercise Program

Before anyone starts an exercise program, several considerations should be made. The first is to assess whether the individual is a good candidate for an exercise program. The best candidates are individuals described by the American College of Sports Medicine (ACSM) as "low risk." This phrase denotes an adult who has no documented cardiovascular, pulmonary, and/or metabolic disease, no signs or symptoms of such diseases (e.g., chest pain, heart rhythm abnormalities, breathlessness, etc.), and no more than one primary risk factor for atherosclerotic cardiovascular disease (CVD). The ACSM recognizes the following eight primary risk factors for CVD, including (a) age, (b) high blood pressure ($\geq$ 140/90 mmHg), (c) high serum cholesterol ($\geq$ 200 mg/dL), (d) cigarette smoking, (e) prediabetes, (f) family history of CVD (especially premature death of family members due to heart attack or stroke), (g) obesity, and (h) physical inactivity. Low risk adults may engage in a moderate exercise program with very little risk of cardiovascular complications.

Those adults who are free of known cardiovascular, pulmonary, and/or metabolic disease and signs/symptoms, but who have two or more primary CVD risk factors, are classified as "moderate risk" individuals. It is especially important that these individuals are evaluated thoroughly before engaging in an exercise program. A third classification ("high risk") includes those subjects who are known to have signs/symptoms of, or diagnosed with, cardiovascular, pulmonary, and/or metabolic disease. They should only exercise on the advice of their physicians, preferably within some supervised exercise setting, such as a cardiac rehab program or a corporate, community, or commercial fitness program staffed by appropriately trained and certified personnel.

Other considerations include deciding on an appropriate exercise program, setting short- and long-term goals, creating a social support system of family and friends, and developing a method of monitoring the effectiveness of the program. The exercise program must fit into an existing schedule that may very well include work, school, family, friends, church, hobbies, social commitments, and more. The program must allow the participant to derive some personal, physical, psychological, and social benefits. Goals may be set, including physical goals, such as attaining a particular body weight, body composition, resting blood pressure, or improved blood lipid profile; stress reduction goals, such as feeling more relaxed; or social goals, such as exercising twice a week with a spouse or friend. The early goals should be easily monitored and reasonably attainable.

Once the potential exerciser has been assessed as a good candidate for an exercise program, the most important goal is to begin and continue the workouts. The expected benefits of exercise will occur only if a regular habit of physical activity is established.

Adaptations to Aerobic Exercise that Improve Health and Well-Being

Many adaptations that lead to improved health take place as a result of physical activity. Changes occur in resting blood pressure, serum cholesterol, body composition, and other health-related factors that enhance the overall wellness of the participant. Many of the health benefits associated with regular physical activity are included in Table 3-1.

What is Wellness?

A significant adaptation to continuing aerobic exercise is an increased volume of the left ventricle, the main pumping chamber of the heart. This volume allows the heart to pump more blood per beat, so that it does not have to beat as often, thereby improving its mechanical efficiency. This improved efficiency results in the low, resting heart rates characteristic of aerobically trained individuals. Changes in the lungs allow oxygen and carbon dioxide to exchange more efficiently. Increased blood flow through the lungs and increased lung diffusion lead to improved oxygen delivery to various body tissues. Several other changes leading to improved aerobic exercise performance are described in a later discussion.

Changes that Lower Risk of Cardiovascular Disease

The main complication of cardiovascular disease is an increased risk of premature heart attack or stroke. Exercise has been found effective at lowering the risk of cardiovascular disease by affecting two primary risk factors: (a) arterial blood pressure, and (b) total serum cholesterol. Exercise is most effective in lowering the blood pressure of those subjects who already have elevated blood pressure (systolic at or above 140 mmHg or diastolic at or above 90 mmHg).

Aerobic exercise may reduce blood pressure (systolic and diastolic by 5–6 mmHg), and may also reduce the need for antihypertensive medications. Favorable changes have also been observed in blood lipids or blood fats. Regular, continuous aerobic exercise has little to no effect on total serum cholesterol, but results in mild to moderate increases in high-density lipoprotein (Table 3-1).

High-density lipoprotein (HDL), a component of cholesterol metabolism and known as "good" cholesterol, actually serves to protect an individual from developing disease. The higher the HDL, the better protection provided. Aerobic exercise, especially in combination with a low-fat diet and weight loss, significantly increases the proportion of HDL in the blood, thereby lowering the risk of disease. It might be interesting to note that increases in HDL have also been observed in individuals who have stopped smoking and in people who partake of alcohol in moderation.

Body Composition and Metabolic Changes

Body composition can be improved dramatically through a program of proper exercise and dietary intake. Body composition is best improved by a combination of (a) daily, prolonged (30–60 minutes), low-to-moderate intensity aerobic exercise; (b) mild caloric restriction (300–500 fewer kcal per day); (c) resistance exercise (two to three times weekly); and (d) slow weight loss (1–2 lb per week). Crash dieting and semi-starvation, especially without exercise, are not suggested

Table 3-1. Health Benefits Associated With Regular Physical Activity for Adults and Older Adults

Strong evidence
- Lower risk of early death
- Lower risk of atherosclerotic cardiovascular heart disease
- Lower risk of coronary heart disease
- Lower risk of stroke
- Lower risk of high blood pressure
- Lower risk of adverse blood lipid profile
- Lower risk of type 2 diabetes
- Lower risk of metabolic syndrome
- Lower risk of colon cancer
- Lower risk of breast cancer
- Prevention of weight gain
- Weight loss, particularly when combined with reduced calorie intake
- Improved cardiorespiratory and muscular fitness
- Prevention of falls
- Reduced depression
- Better cognitive function (for older adults)

Moderate to strong evidence
- Better functional health (for older adults)
- Reduced abdominal obesity

Moderate evidence
- Lower risk of hip fracture
- Lower risk of lung cancer
- Lower risk of endometrial cancer
- Weight maintenance after weight loss
- Increased bone density
- Improved sleep quality

Source: U.S. Department of Health and Human Services, 2008.

due to the related loss of muscle and lean tissue. Weight loss can be estimated on the assumption that the loss of 1 pound of fat requires that a subject expends 3,500 kcal more than consumed over some given length of time, preferably about a week. The typical changes in body composition observed with appropriate exercise and diet include a loss of body weight, a loss of body fat, and no change or an increase in muscle and lean weight. Weight loss, as previously discussed, may help promote a reduction in blood pressure and serum cholesterol. In individuals with type 2 diabetes or those at high risk of diabetes, there is strong evidence that physical activity and weight loss improves glucose metabolism, reducing the dependency on medication, insulin, or the risk of developing the disease.

Metabolic syndrome is a relatively new diagnosis defined by the combination of numerous conditions, including abdominal adiposity (waist girth > 102 cm in men or > 88 cm in women), blood fat disorders (high LDL, high triglycerides, low HDL), high blood pressure ($\geq$ 140/90 mmHg), impaired fasting glucose (fasting blood glucose $\geq$ 100 mg/dL) or insulin resistance, and other potential blood and inflammatory conditions. There is strong evidence that regular physical activity can significantly lower the risk of metabolic syndrome. Other metabolic changes associated with physical activity are also likely related to the reduced risk of certain cancers in active individuals. There is strong evidence that regular physical activity can lower the risk of colon and breast cancer by as much as 30–40%. There is moderate evidence that physical activity can also lower the risk of lung and endometrial cancer (Table 3-1).

Neuromuscular and Bone Changes

There may be modest changes in skeletal muscle, connective tissue, and bone associated with regular and continuing aerobic exercise. The loss of muscle tissue and bone mineral content is a significant problem among the elderly. It leads to an increased likelihood of immobility and bone fracture, and a reduction in the degree of independence the older adult is able to maintain. Active, older adults are generally more capable of maintaining their physical independence, and therefore maintain a higher quality of life. However, aerobic exercise may not be enough. The ACSM recommends that regular resistance exercise (2–3 days per week) be included in the average adult's exercise regimen with the specific purpose of maintaining muscle mass and bone mineral content over the life span.

Interval Training to Improve Aerobic Performance

Aerobic training can be done either continuously or intermittently. When training for prolonged activities, more than 45–60 minutes in duration, such as the marathon or triathlon, continuous aerobic exercise can be used almost exclusively. Training for activities of shorter duration, however, should also include some higher intensity, interval training. Such activities might include running a 5K or 10K race, competing in a mini-triathlon, or competing in an aerobic competition. All of these types of activities require a high degree of aerobic power that is maximally developed only by the addition of interval training.

Interval training generally refers to any type of training that is intermittent or discontinuous in nature. It consists of a bout of exercise of varying duration and intensity interspersed with varying periods of recovery. Interval training is not necessary for the non-athletic population because most of the beneficial effects of exercise can be achieved with continuous aerobic exercise alone. Some subjects may still use interval training, however, to help minimize the boredom associated with long, continuous exercise. But then again, what some consider boring, others may find an enjoyable experience and a good way to relax and relieve stress.

If the interval training is being done simply as an alternative to continuous exercise and not to improve performance, there is no reason to highly structure the intervals. The subject runs, or swims, or cycles, or performs harder for 2–5 minutes until the exercise becomes stressful, then reduces the intensity for several minutes to allow a sufficient recovery. The recovery periods should be of a duration equivalent to the exercise interval. These intervals of alternating exercise intensity are continued for the same duration as discussed previously (20–60 minutes).

In preparation for competition, interval training is used to maximize aerobic power, and when done at higher intensity, to increase aerobic endurance and anaerobic power. Interval training to improve performance is done with relatively long exercise intervals, lasting anywhere from a minimum of about 2–3 minutes to a maximum of 4–5 minutes. It should be done two to three times per week during the time leading up to the competition as a supplement to aerobic or distance training, rather than as a substitute or alternative form of training. Appropriate training intervals for events, such as 5K and 10K runs, include repeated runs of 800–1,500 meters (about 1/2–1 mile), with a total distance per workout of around 5–7 kilometers (3–5 miles). Some general interval training guidelines for improving aerobic performance are provided in Table 3-2.

See Chapter 26 on "Interval Training" for specific exercise class models and intensities.

Table 3-2. Interval Training Guidelines for Improving Aerobic Performance					
Intensity (%HRR)	Number of intervals	Exercise duration	Recovery duration	% Contribution by Aerobic system	Anaerobic systems
80–85%	3–5	4–5 minutes	2–5 minutes	75–85%	15–25%
85–90%	6–8	2–3 minutes	1–5 minutes	50–60%	40–50%
90–95%	10–20	30 seconds–1 minute	1–3 minutes	20–25%	75–80%

NOTE: Interval training for the purpose of improving performance is advocated only for "low- risk" individuals with a good aerobic training base.)

Adaptations that Improve Exercise Performance

Numerous adaptations occur in the heart, lungs, and skeletal muscle that enhance the delivery of oxygen, speed the removal of carbon dioxide, and thereby contribute to improvement in aerobic exercise performance. A laboratory assessment of the elite aerobic athlete clearly demonstrates that many physiological variables are significantly improved as a result of regular, continued aerobic training.

Increased Maximal Blood Flow

As discussed earlier, performing aerobic exercise forces the left ventricle to pump large volumes of blood, which gradually causes an enlargement of the chamber. The heart, thus, pumps more blood each beat, or in other words increases stroke volume. The maximal stroke volume attained during exercise is increased as well, which increases maximal cardiac output, and therefore the maximal heart rate may actually decline somewhat with training. The increased stroke volume more than compensates, however, for the lower maximal heart rates.

Increased Oxygen Delivery and Carbon Dioxide Removal

While maximal heart rate frequently declines with training, the opposite is true of maximal breathing rate. Maximal breathing rates in trained aerobic athletes reach 45–55 breaths/minute compared to 40–45 breaths/minute in non-athletes. In combination with a larger tidal volume (i.e., the volume of air exhaled per breath), the increased maximal breathing rates allow trained athletes to possess high pulmonary ventilations during maximal aerobic exercise. The cardiorespiratory system saturates the blood coming through the lungs with oxygen very efficiently. In fact, the blood fully saturates with oxygen in less than 1 second. The high pulmonary ventilation appears to assist more with the removal of carbon dioxide during exercise. If carbon dioxide is not removed, the acidity of the muscle increases which reduces the muscle's ability to contract. Trained aerobic athletes, by possessing very high maximal pulmonary ventilations, are able to remove carbon dioxide at a higher rate, thereby better maintaining appropriate acid/base balance.

Increased Maximal Oxygen Uptake and Aerobic Power

The adaptations that occur in trained skeletal muscle consist of two types: (a) structural and functional changes that allow increased blood flow, and (b) biochemical changes that increase the capacity and power of the aerobic system. These changes, observed with aerobic training, usually occur more frequently in slow-twitch muscle fibers than in fast-twitch muscle fibers.

Maximal blood flow during exercise in trained skeletal muscle is determined by the extent to which the vascular system or blood vessels have developed in that particular muscle. Regular aerobic exercise causes an increase in the number of capillaries per muscle fiber. Highly trained endurance athletes may possess 30% more capillaries per muscle fiber than untrained subjects. The increased vascularization provides a richer supply of oxygen and nutrients, removes carbon dioxide and other wastes more rapidly, and therefore allows a higher maximal rate of aerobic energy production. The higher maximal cardiac outputs in trained athletes are also due in part to the 20–25% increases in total blood volume observed.

The capacity and power of the aerobic system are increased by many biochemical changes resulting from regular, continuous aerobic training. Significant increases, as much as 50–100% or higher, in both carbohydrate (glycogen) and fat (triglyceride) storage in skeletal muscle have been observed. The increased fuel storage increases the total capacity of the system. Aerobic power increases primarily through an increase in mitochondrial volume and activity. The mitochondrial adaptations translate into a significant increase in many key enzymes associated with aerobic metabolism. The concentration and activity of all of the enzymes associated with fat oxidation, the Krebs cycle, and electron transport are augmented by as much as 100% in comparison to untrained subjects. These adaptations are reflected in the superior maximal oxygen uptakes observed in elite aerobic athletes along with other related physiological variables (Table 3-3).

Table 3-3. Values for Untrained Subjects, Trained Subjects, and Elite Athletes Demonstrating the Adaptations to Aerobic Training

Variable (units)	Untrained M/W	Trained M/W	Elite M/W
Max cardiac output (L/min.)	24/20	27/21	38/30
Max pulmonary ventilation (L/min.)	120/96	135/108	193/154
Max oxygen uptake (L/min)	3.2/2.3	3.9/2.9	5.3/4.0
Max oxygen uptake (ml/kg/min)	45/40	55/50	75/70

NOTE: M: Men; W: Women.

Summary

Those individuals who maintain a regular program of aerobic exercise and physical activity derive significant physical, physiological, and psychological benefits. When accomplished with sufficient regularity, exercise of even a relatively low intensity can promote health benefits and enhance wellness. Exercise performed at a higher intensity not only provides health benefits, but can lead to structural adaptations in the body, which can, in turn, result in improved aerobic exercise performance.

To maximize the benefits and enjoyment of exercise, it is recommended that many different types of exercise be used, including aerobics, walking, running, cycling, swimming, and more.

References

1. American College of Sports Medicine. (2010). *ACSM's guidelines for exercise testing and prescription* (8th ed.). Baltimore, MD: Lippincott Williams & Wilkins.

2. American College of Sports Medicine. (2010). *ACSM's resource manual for guidelines for exercise testing and prescription* (6th ed.). Baltimore, MD: Lippincott Williams & Wilkins.

3. Heyward, V.H. (2006). *Advanced fitness assessment & exercise prescription* (5th ed.). Champaign, IL: Human Kinetics.

4. Nelson, M.E., Rejeski, W.J., Blair, S.N., Duncan, P.W., Judge, J.O., King, A.C., et al. (2007). Physical activity and public health in older adults: Recommendation from the American College of Sports Medicine and the American Heart Association. *Medicine & Science in Sports & Exercise*, 8, 1435–1445.

5. Powers, S.K., & Howley, E.T. (2009). *Exercise physiology: Theory and application to fitness and performance* (7th ed.). Boston, MA: McGraw-Hill.

6. U.S. Department of Health and Human Services. *2008 Physical activity guidelines for Americans.* ODPHP Publication No. U0036, October 2008. Retrieved May 15, 2009, from http://www.health.gov/paguidelines

7. U.S. National Institutes of Health. *Physical activity and cancer,* March 2004. Retrieved May 15, 2009, from http://www.cancer.gov/newscenter/benchmarks-vol4-issue1/page2/

4

Energy Production During Exercise

William C. Beam, PhD

Focus

Human skeletal muscle contains a variety of fuels and enzymes that allow it to provide energy in a number of ways. Exercise physiologists have categorized these fuels and enzymes into "energy systems" and have described their importance for different types of exercise. Changes within the muscle itself, dependent on the duration and intensity of the exercise, control which of the energy systems is most active at any one time. As a result, energy is produced automatically, in the most efficient manner possible, to meet the energetic needs of the exercising muscle. The study of how energy is released and transformed in the body is referred to as **energetics**.

Basic Principles of Energetics

The term **energy** is most simply defined as the ability to do work. Various forms of physical or biological work that require energy include contraction of skeletal muscle that allows us to move, walk, and exercise; the growth of new tissue in children or healing adults; and the conduction through our bodies of electrical impulses that control heart rate, release hormones, or constrict blood vessels. Ultimately, the source of energy for all of these bodily functions comes from the sun. It is hard to imagine, in the middle of a cardio kickboxing session, that the energy you are using to contract your muscles has actually originated in the sun, but it is true. You cannot simply exercise in the sunshine, however, and absorb the energy. The energy needs to be transformed from light energy into a form of chemical energy that your body can use.

Energy Flow to Humans

The transformation of light energy begins with its absorption by green plants through the process of **photosynthesis**. Plants begin with very simple forms of synthetic compounds, such as water and carbon dioxide, and in the presence of light, produce complex food molecules that contain a large supply of stored chemical energy. Plants can form and store various types of carbohydrates, fats, and proteins. Animals and humans can derive energy by ingesting these plants and using them as sources of fuel. Vegetarians derive all their energy from plant sources alone. Those humans and animals who consume meat, derive a portion of their energy by consuming the protein and fat stored in the meat of other animals.

During this energy flow from the sun, neither plants nor humans are creating the energy. It is being transformed by plants from light energy into a form of stored chemical energy. Humans, after ingesting the plants, then transform the energy again. At this point, it is used for biological work or it is stored, primarily in adipose tissue, skeletal muscle, and the liver, for later use. None of these transformations are particularly efficient. In fact, humans use or store less than half of the original energy that was available from the food. The unused or lost energy escapes in the form of heat. When large amounts of energy are released, as is the case during exercise, the energy lost as heat is enough to increase body temperature. Equation 4-1 expresses the relationship or balance between the energy flowing into the body, and that which is used, stored, and lost.

Eqn. 4-1	Energy consumed = Energy used + Energy stored + Energy lost

Significance of Adenosine Triphosphate

In most cases of biological work, the source of energy is specific. Energy must first be transferred into a compound called **adenosine triphosphate** (ATP) before it can be used. A molecule of ATP possesses a significant amount of stored energy. ATP possesses this energy largely because of its structure. The last phosphate group attaches to the remainder of the molecule by way of a "high-energy" bond. When the bond breaks, the phosphate group is released, and at the same time a substantial amount of energy is released. The end result is adenosine diphosphate (ADP) and phosphate (P), as seen in Figure 4-1.

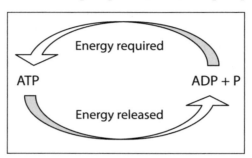

Fig. 4-1. ATP releases energy necessary for muscular contraction by releasing a phosphate (P). Energy is required to reform ATP from ADP and P.

This breakdown of ATP provides the only source of energy for muscular contraction. Any energy stored in the body in the form of carbohydrate or fat, must first be converted into ATP before it can be used for exercise. As may also be observed, this reaction is reversible. That is, ATP can be replenished if there is a source of ADP, P, and energy.

The actual amount of energy released from the breakdown of ATP can be estimated. When a specific amount of ATP, described as " 1 mole" of ATP, reacts in a test tube under standard conditions of temperature and acidity, it consistently releases about 7 kilocalories (kcal) of energy. In the body, however, the amount of energy released from 1 mole of ATP is about 10 kcal due to the increase in body temperature and acidity during exercise. To put this amount of energy in perspective, let us assume that walking 1 mile requires about 100 kcal of energy. One mole of ATP could supply enough energy to walk only about one-tenth of a mile.

Overview of Energy Production

The body possesses three separate systems for the production of energy. Each muscle cell in the body contains these energy systems. The systems differ considerably in their complexity, regulation, capacity, power, and the types of exercise for which they are the predominant supplier of energy. They are called upon to provide energy at a rate dependent upon the intensity and duration of the exercise performed. The three energy systems are (a) the **phosphagen system**, (b) the **lactic acid system**, and (c) the **aerobic system**. The goal of each system is to release energy from chemical or food sources, and transform that energy into ATP that can subsequently be used for muscular contraction and exercise (Figure 4-2).

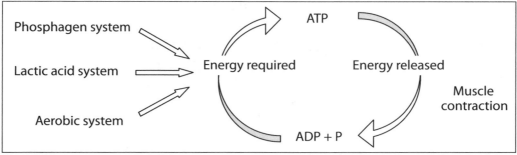

Fig. 4-2. The common goal of all three energy systems is to release the chemical energy from food that can be used to make ATP, which subsequently breaks down and supplies energy to the muscle.

The energy systems are discussed in this chapter beginning with the simplest and moving toward the most complex. The phosphagen system is a simple system of coupled reactions; the lactic acid system is more complex involving a sequence of reactions; and finally, the aerobic system is a complex and intricate combination of several pathways. In terms of their significance in everyday life, however, the order of discussion would be reversed. Most of our energetic needs throughout the day (and night) are met by the aerobic system alone. It is only activities that require a significant amount of muscular effort, such as moderate to intense exercise, heavy manual labor, climbing several flights of stairs, carrying a baby, or changing a tire, that require the recruitment of the lactic acid or phosphagen systems.

Anaerobic Energy Systems

There are two energy systems in the body—the phosphagen system and the lactic acid system—that can operate in the absence of oxygen. Because of this, they are frequently referred to as **anaerobic** energy systems. It is probably more important, however, to identify them as systems that are capable of producing ATP energy at a high rate or fast. They are utilized when the rate of energy production demanded of the exercise exceeds that of the aerobic system alone. The main limitation of these systems is the relatively small amount of ATP that can be made before fatigue ensues.

Phosphagen System (ATP-CP System)

The **phosphagen** system supplies energy very rapidly. It relies entirely on a chemical source of fuel, however, and because of this its total capacity for producing energy is severely limited. It is the primary source of energy for very high-intensity exercise.

Description

Biochemically, the phosphagen system is by far the simplest of the three systems. Energy for the production of ATP comes by way of a coupled reaction involving the breakdown of **creatine phosphate**. The compound creatine phosphate (CP), also referred to as phosphocreatine, is similar to ATP. Because of this similarity, CP and ATP are referred to collectively as "phosphagens." The structure of CP consists of a creatine base molecule with one phosphate group attached by way of a "high-energy" bond. The splitting of CP into creatine (C) and phosphate (P) results in the release of enough energy to attach a phosphate onto an ADP molecule thereby producing ATP (Figure 4-3). During high-intensity exercise, at almost the same instant ATP is produced, its terminal phosphate group is lost. The energy is then transferred into the contractile mechanism of the muscle. This mechanism transforms the chemical energy now available into the mechanical energy necessary for rapid or forceful muscular contractions.

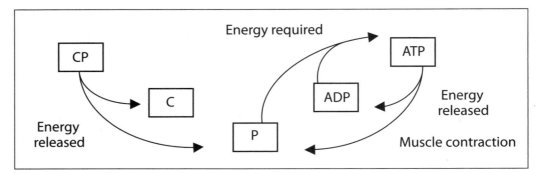

Fig. 4-3. The energy released from the breakdown of creatine phosphate is coupled to the production of ATP, which subsequently breaks down and supplies energy to the muscle for exercise.

The regulation of the phosphagen system—and the other energy systems—relies in large part on the activity of its specific regulatory enzyme(s). **Enzymes** are protein molecules that speed up a chemical reaction by lowering the amount of energy necessary for the reaction to initially occur. Every reaction in a biological system has an associated enzyme. An enzyme is considered regulatory if it possesses the ability to alter or regulate the rate at which an entire series of reactions occurs.

The enzyme most responsible for the rate at which the phosphagen system operates is **creatine kinase** (CK), also called creatine phosphokinase. Any condition that stimulates or speeds CK will increase the rate at which the phosphagen system produces energy. Conversely, any condition that inhibits or slows CK will reduce the maximal rate of energy production of the system. The most significant stimulatory factor is the rapid accumulation of ADP within the muscle cell. This is a signal to the muscle that ATP is being consumed rapidly. In an attempt to maintain the concentration of ATP, creatine kinase is activated, and creatine phosphate is rapidly broken down. The energy released from CP is used to replace the ATP being consumed.

Capacity and Power

The **capacity** of the phosphagen system can be estimated by measuring the amount of fuel available in the muscle. Heavy physical exercise can be sustained only while CP and ATP are available. Once the level of phosphagen is depleted, fatigue will rapidly ensue. To determine the capacity of the system requires the measurement of the total amount of phosphagen stored in skeletal muscle. For years, the only way of making such measurements was through the use of a needle muscle biopsy in which a small piece of muscle is removed from the body for analysis. More recently a method of quantifying CP, ATP, ADP, and P from outside the body has been developed. It is called nuclear magnetic resonance (NMR) spectroscopy.

Throughout this chapter, whenever estimates of the capacity or power of any of the energy systems are made, they are based on the following assumptions. The proposed subjects are a young man and woman who are healthy, active, and trained. The man is assumed to weigh 70 kg (154 lb) with 30 kg (66 lb) of muscle. The woman is assumed to weigh 57 kg (126 lb) with 20 kg (44 lb) of muscle. Any changes in body weight, muscle mass, or level of training will significantly affect the estimated capacities and powers.

It has been estimated, using NMR spectroscopy, that the average amount of phosphagen (combined CP and ATP) in a man with 30 kg of muscle is about 1 mole. Therefore, the capacity of the phosphagen system would be limited to 1 mole of ATP, or equivalent to about 10 kcal of energy. This is a very small amount of energy, barely enough to sprint 200 m in 20–30 seconds before it is exhausted. The capacity in a woman with 20 kg of muscle is less, about 0.7 mole of ATP or 7 kcal, due to the smaller muscle mass. The difference in capacity is actually less a gender issue and more a muscle mass issue. Those people with more muscle mass will have a higher capacity, and those with less muscle mass will have a lower capacity.

The **power** of the system expresses its ability to produce energy at a particular **rate**, usually in moles of ATP per minute, or in kcal of energy expended per minute. Thus, a system that is characterized as possessing a high power is able to produce ATP very rapidly. To estimate the power of the phosphagen system another assumption must be made. Assume that with maximal exercise, the total phosphagen in the body (1.0 mole) would last for no longer than about 15 seconds. The power of the system then is equal to the total phosphagen used divided by the amount of time required to utilize the fuel as seen in Equation 4-2. Therefore, the power of the phosphagen system is about 4.0 moles/min of ATP production, or 40 kcal/min of energy expenditure. With no frame of reference, this value has little significance. However, as will soon be seen, the power of the phosphagen system is twice that of its nearest competitor, the lactic acid system.

$$\textbf{Eqn. 4-2} \quad \frac{1 \text{ mole of ATP}}{15 \text{ seconds}} \times \frac{60 \text{ sec}}{} = 4.0 \text{ moles/min (40 kcal/min)}$$

Types of Exercise

Because of its ability to supply energy immediately, the phosphagen system is most important in exercise in which energy is required immediately. Such exercises would include sprinting, jumping, throwing, kicking, and lifting heavy weights. Sports that include these activities would rely at least in part on the phosphagen system. The common factor of analysis is the **time** involved. If the activity can be sustained for no more than 15–20 seconds, the phosphagen system is the primary source of energy (supplying over 50% of the energy).

Shorter exercise (1–5-second duration) that requires even higher energy production relies more heavily on the phosphagen system. Exercise sustained slightly longer (30–45-second duration) relies less on phosphagen metabolism. Good examples of specific events that rely on the phosphagen system for their primary source of energy include 100 and 200 meter running sprints, 50 meter swimming sprints, high jump and long jump, shot put and discus, and power lifting.

Many other activities and sports are more difficult to analyze due to their variable, intermittent nature. Even with these complicating factors, however, it can be concluded that the more intense sections of an aerobics routine; the sprinting and kicking in soccer; the jumping and spiking in volleyball; and the sprinting, jumping, and shooting in basketball, all rely heavily on the phosphagen system.

Lactic Acid System (Fast Glycolysis)

The **lactic acid system** also provides a rapid source of energy. Its fuel source is glucose, the usable form of carbohydrate in the body. Because the supply of glucose exceeds that of muscle phosphagen, the lactic acid system produces more ATP than the phosphagen system. But still, its capacity is limited because of the production of its end product, **lactic acid**, which is not tolerated well by the body. The lactic acid system is the primary source of energy for sustained high-intensity exercise lasting no longer than a few minutes.

Description

Glycolysis is a process that occurs in the sarcoplasm or fluid portion of the muscle cell. It involves a sequence of reactions that partially breaks down glucose into a simpler compound called pyruvate. Once pyruvate is formed, it can take one of two pathways, depending on the need for energy or the presence of oxygen in the muscle. If the level of oxygen in the muscle is sufficient and the demand for energy is low, glycolysis operates in such a way that pyruvate enters the mitochondria and is combusted aerobically. This is referred to as "aerobic" or "slow" glycolysis. But if the level of oxygen is insufficient, or the demand for energy is high, the pyruvate is transformed into lactate (lactic acid). Under these circumstances, the process is referred to as "anaerobic" or "fast" glycolysis, and is also described as the "lactic acid system."

The foods that we typically eat can be separated into three categories: (a) carbohydrates, (b) fats, and (c) proteins. Carbohydrates are the only form of food that can be used as fuel in the lactic acid system. Furthermore, the only form of carbohydrate that can be used is glucose, a simple six-carbon sugar. The glucose used for fuel can come either from the blood glucose or from stored **glycogen** within the muscle. In either case, the glucose enters glycolysis initiating a sequence of nine or more reactions resulting in the production of lactate. A simplified version of glycolysis is presented in Figure 4-4. It is believed that this sequence developed into the most efficient way of rapidly transforming food energy (from glucose) into ATP.

As mentioned previously, the source of fuel for glycolysis is provided by blood glucose through a phosphorylation (addition of phosphate) made possible by the breakdown of ATP. This is considered a "priming step." It is analogous to priming a pump. Energy must first be added before any work can be done resulting in the flow of water. In this case, before any ATP can be made, one phosphate group is removed from ATP and attaches to glucose-making glucose phosphate. This priming step is not necessary if glycogen is the source of fuel. (Keep in mind, however, that the glucose had to proceed through this step to be stored as glycogen in the first place.)

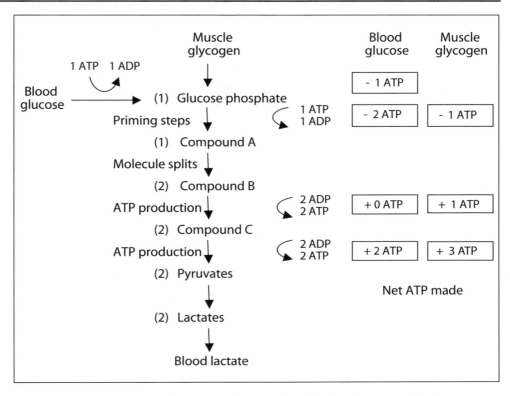

Fig. 4-4. A simplified version of the lactic acid system (fast glycolysis). Note that (a) glucose can come from blood glucose or muscle glycogen, (b) priming steps are required, (c) the glucose splits into two equal parts, (d) ATP is produced, and (e) lactate is made in the muscle and diffuses into the blood. The increase in blood lactate indicates that the system is active.

Next, a second priming step occurs, with another mole of ATP donating its phosphate group. The compound then **splits** into two equal parts. Therefore, from this point on, every reaction actually occurs twice for every one glucose that originally entered glycolysis. The next step is the first reaction in the sequence in which ATP is produced. There is sufficient energy released during this reaction (10 kcal) to combine an ADP and P to produce ATP. There are actually two ATP formed from the input of one glucose. Another reaction now occurs in which ATP is formed. Again, two ATP are made since this reaction occurs twice.

The final step in glycolysis is the conversion of pyruvate to lactate. Also indicated in Figure 4-4 is the net production of ATP from blood glucose and muscle glycogen, which is summarized in Equations 4-3 and 4-4.

Eqn. 4-3	1 Glucose + ADP + P + Energy $\longrightarrow$ 2 Lactate + 2 H_2O + 2 ATP (20 kcal)
	(from blood glucose)

Eqn. 4-4	1 Glucose + ADP + P + Energy $\longrightarrow$ 2 Lactate + 2 H_2O + 3 ATP (30 kcal)
	(from muscle glycogen)

Regulation

The regulation of the lactic acid system is considerably more complex than that of the phosphagen system. It still depends, however, on the activity of regulatory enzymes, of which there are several. The most important regulatory enzyme in glycolysis is **phosphofructokinase** (PFK). Its importance lies in the fact that it exists in the lowest concentration and possesses the lowest activity of any enzyme in the sequence. Because of these characteristics, the reaction that PFK catalyzes is considered the "rate-limiting step" of glycolysis. It is analogous to the strength of a chain being determined by its weakest link. PFK, and hence the lactic acid system, is stimulated by the rapid accumulation of ADP and by the rapid depletion of CP that occur during very high-intensity exercise.

The lactic acid system is inhibited under resting conditions due to an interaction effect with the aerobic system. Specific intermediates in aerobic metabolism that are in relatively high concentration in skeletal muscle at rest inhibit PFK and suppress the use of carbohydrate and anaerobic metabolism at rest.

Capacity and Power

The primary limiting factor in the **capacity** of the lactic acid system is not fuel depletion, but the accumulation of lactic acid. If used to its fullest extent, the lactic acid system would fatigue before using 1 mole of glucose. If it is assumed that the average person stores at least 2.0–2.5 moles of glucose, this means that as much as 50% of the fuel remains in the body at the time of fatigue. It does not seem likely, therefore, that the level of fuel limits the capacity of the system.

What is important to remember about this system is that while producing ATP, it simultaneously produces lactic acid. As the lactic acid is formed it rapidly loses a proton or hydrogen ion (H+) and becomes lactate. The problem is the neutralization or "buffering" of the excess hydrogen ions. The result is the muscle becomes too acidic to operate, many of the enzymes are inhibited and the actual mechanism of muscular contraction is affected.

The maximal capacity of a person's lactic acid system is determined by his or her ability to neutralize and tolerate lactic acid. Research suggests that the highest level of lactic acid that can be tolerated by a trained 70 kg person is about 90 grams (or about 1 mole of lactic acid). Based on Equation 4-4, this means that at the same time the person makes 1 mole of lactic acid they have concurrently made 1.5 moles of ATP. So the capacity of the system, or the total amount of ATP that can be made, is about 1.5 moles, corresponding to a total energy expenditure of 15 kcal. This amount of energy would allow for only about 45–90 seconds of high-intensity exercise.

The maximal **power** of the system again depends on the time required to produce a given amount of ATP. If it is assumed that the lactic acid system can be exhausted in as little as 45 seconds of intense exercise, the theoretical rate at which ATP energy is produced through the lactic acid system can be determined as seen in Equation 4-5. The estimated power of the system in our trained person turns out to be around 2.0 moles/min or 20 kcal/min.

$$\textbf{Eqn. 4-5} \quad \frac{1.5 \text{ mole of ATP}}{45 \text{ seconds}} \times \frac{60 \text{ sec}}{1 \text{ min}} = 2.0 \text{ moles/min (20 kcal/min)}$$

Types of Exercise

Because of the relative simplicity of glycolysis, and because oxygen is not needed, the lactic acid system produces ATP rapidly. It provides the primary supply of energy for physical activity that results in fatigue in 45–90 seconds. Shorter, more intense exercise would rely to some degree on the phosphagen system, while longer, less intense exercise would begin to require aerobic metabolism. The lactic acid system is very important in prolonged sprints (400–800 meters running, 100–200 meters swimming or 1,000–2,000 meters cycling). It also provides much of the energy for sustained, high-intensity rallies in soccer, field hockey, ice hockey, lacrosse, basketball, volleyball, tennis, badminton, and other sports. The floor routine in gymnastics relies in part on this system, with intermittent bursts of higher energy production from the phosphagen system. The common denominator in all of these activities is a sustained, high-intensity effort lasting from 1 to 2 minutes.

Aerobic Energy System (Oxidative Metabolism)

The **aerobic system** is a complex collection of several different components sometimes collectively called oxidative metabolism. Because of its ability to use carbohydrates, fats, and proteins as sources of fuel, and because it produces only carbon dioxide and water as end products, the aerobic system has a virtually unlimited capacity for making ATP. Its complexity and its need for a constant supply of oxygen, however, limit the rate at which ATP is produced. The aerobic system supplies all of the energy for low- to moderate-intensity exercise. It supplies energy for sleeping, resting, sitting, walking, and other forms of low-intensity, long duration physical activity. As the activity becomes more intense, to the point that it can only be sustained for a matter of a few minutes, the aerobic system can no longer provide energy at a sufficient rate. At this stage, ATP production is supplemented by the lactic acid and phosphagen systems.

Description

The term "aerobic system" refers to a complex series of reactions that, for the purpose of description, can be divided into three components (Figure 4-5). The first component can actually be one of three pathways depending upon whether the source of fuel is carbohydrate, fat, or protein. When carbohydrate is used, the first component is **glycolysis**, which under these conditions operates slowly or aerobically. As a result, lactate is not formed and the end product is pyruvate. When fat is used, the first component is a process called **fat oxidation**, in which large molecules of fat are made into much simpler molecules that fuel subsequent reactions in the system. If the source of fuel is protein, the first component pathway is **protein metabolism**. While a minimal amount of ATP is formed directly in each of these pathways, the main purpose of the first component is to produce acetyl groups (small two-carbon compounds) and a supply of electrons for subsequent reactions.

The second component is a cyclical process called the **Krebs cycle** and is common to all types of fuel. The main purpose of the Krebs cycle is to remove electrons and protons for subsequent reactions. The final component, also common to all types of food fuel, is the **electron transport system** (ETS). The electron transport system, because of a coupled process called oxidative phosphorylation, accounts for over 85% of the total ATP produced by the aerobic system. A good way to begin to understand the components of the aerobic system is to follow 1 mole of glucose from start to finish throughout the entire system.

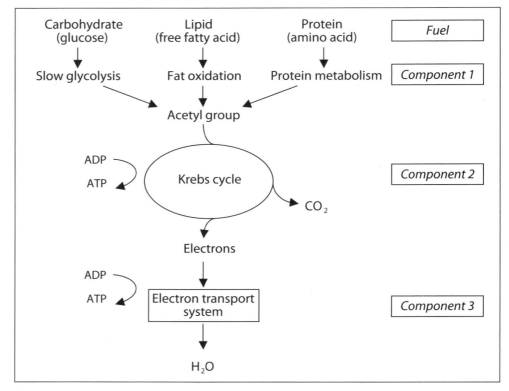

Fig. 4-5. An overview of the pathways involved in the aerobic system. Complex food molecules (e.g., glucose, free fatty acid, amino acid) are broken down into much simpler molecules of CO_2 and H_2O. In the process, energy is released that can be used to produce ATP.

ATP Production from Carbohydrates

The aerobic production of energy from carbohydrate begins with "slow" or "aerobic" glycolysis as seen in Figure 4-6. The enzymes and intermediate compounds of glycolysis are simply dissolved in the sarcoplasm (fluid portion) of the muscle cell. Although they are not physically arranged in any particular order, the compounds react in the specific sequence described previously. The muscle cell is also composed of subcellular (within the cell) structures called **mitochondria**. The mitochondria are oval-shaped structures, existing separately or possibly in "networks" that contain the enzymes associated with the Krebs cycle and electron transport system (ETS). It is within the mitochondria that most of the ATP is produced aerobically.

The difference between "fast" and "slow" glycolysis is the utilization of the electrons and pyruvates produced. If the activity of the mitochondria (which relies in part on the supply of oxygen and the rate at which energy is being produced) is sufficient, the electrons and pyruvates formed enter the mitochondria. The electrons flow directly to the ETS, while the pyruvates are oxidized (lose electrons) and decarboxylated (lose CO_2) forming acetyl groups that enter the Krebs cycle. Because of the entry of the pyruvates and electrons into the mitochondria, there is no lactate produced under these conditions.

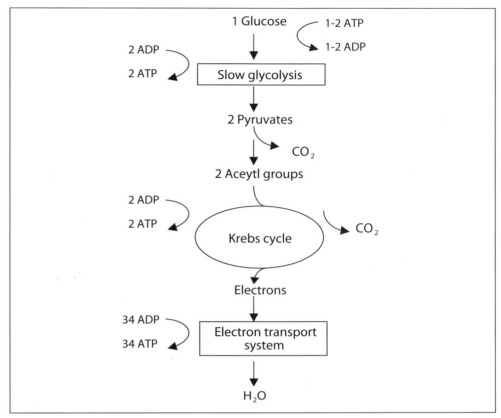

Fig. 4-6. Overview of the aerobic system using carbohydrates as a source of fuel. Glycolysis produces pyruvates that are converted into acetyl groups and enter the Krebs cycle. Electrons are sent from many sources to the electron transport system where most of the ATP is actually made.

Krebs Cycle

The **acetyl groups** formed from the pyruvates enter into the Krebs cycle. The combination of the acetyl with other compounds results in the production of citric acid, the first intermediate in the Krebs cycle. Once citric acid is formed it goes through a series of reactions, including several oxidations in which more **electrons** are removed. These electrons are very important, because they are the driving force for the electron transport system (ETS). The electrons are actually shuttled into the ETS by something called coenzymes. A significant portion of the structure of the coenzymes consists of two B vitamins called niacin and riboflavin. Severe vitamin deficiencies could lead to reduced aerobic function.

Electron Transport System

The final sequence of reactions in the aerobic production of ATP is the electron transport system. This system consists of a number of reusable electron-carrying compounds that can exist in either oxidized or reduced form. These compounds are arranged into specific "complexes" and are physically located within the mitochondrial membrane. They are arranged so that an electrical gradient (difference) exists between the beginning and the end of the system. The gradient created by this arrangement allows the electrons to pass from one intermediate to the next, or in other words to "flow" through the system. This flow, through a very complicated chemical process beyond the scope of this explanation, supplies the energy necessary to make a tremendous amount of ATP. The entire aerobic breakdown of glucose can be summarized as seen in Equation 4-6.

Eqn. 4-6   1 Glucose + O_2 + ADP + P + Energy $\longrightarrow$ CO_2 + H_2O + 38 ATP

ATP Production from Fat

Fats are stored in the body in adipose tissue and within skeletal muscle in the form of **triglycerides**. For fat stored in adipose tissue to be used for exercise, it must first be mobilized and transported to the muscle. The fats must then be converted into a form the muscle can use as fuel. This usable form of fat is called a **free fatty acid**. A fatty acid is a molecule much longer than glucose that can contain as many as 26 carbons in a long chain. Typical fatty acids used by humans for energy production include the saturated fats—stearic acid (18 carbons) and palmitic acid (16 carbons), and the unsaturated fats—oleic acid and linoleic acid (each possessing 18 carbons).

The utilization of fat as a fuel begins with a cyclical process called the **fat oxidation cycle**, which occurs within the mitochondria. The fatty acid is first "activated" through a priming step involving the input of 1 mole of ATP. This priming step is not required for every revolution of the cycle, only for the initial entry of the fatty acid into the cycle. Three significant reactions occur during fatty acid oxidation. Two oxidations occur feeding electrons into the electron transport system, and the third involves the cleaving of an acetyl group from the carbon chain of the fatty acid. The fatty acid (less two carbons) then revolves a second time through the cycle.

This process will continue until only two carbons remain in the skeleton of the fatty acid. At this point, the two-carbon remnant (an acetyl group) enters the Krebs cycle leaving nothing of the fatty acid. It has been completely oxidized to carbon dioxide and water through the aerobic system with a considerable amount of ATP-energy produced in the process as seen in Figure 4-7. When stearic acid (an 18-carbon fatty acid) is used as a source of fuel, the combination of eight full revolutions of the fat oxidation cycle and the remaining acetyl group remnant results in the production of nearly 150 moles of ATP (or nearly 1,500 kcal of energy). A fatty acid with a longer carbon chain (> 18 carbons) results in greater energy production, while a shorter carbon chain (< 18 carbons) produces less energy. The aerobic breakdown of stearic acid can be summarized as seen in Equation 4-7.

Eqn. 4-7   1 Stearic acid + O_2 + ADP + P + Energy $\longrightarrow$ CO_2 + H_2O + 147 ATP

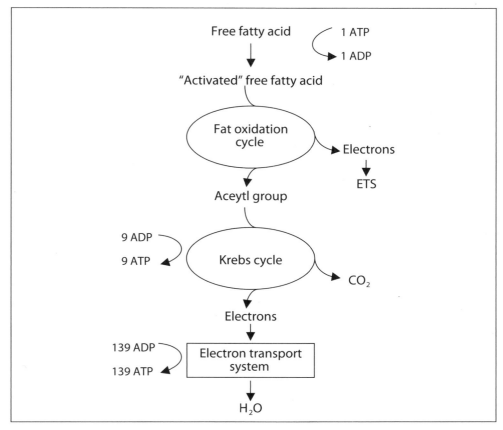

Fig. 4-7. Overview of the aerobic system using free fatty acids as a source of fuel. One revolution of the fat oxidation cycle produces an acetyl group that enters the Krebs cycle. Electrons are sent from many sources to the electron transport system where most of the ATP is actually made.

ATP Production from Protein

Finally, a brief word about the use of protein as fuel is in order. Protein usually does not provide more than 10–15% of the total energy requirement of an activity. As such, protein does not play as significant a role as carbohydrate or fat as a fuel for exercise. The main source of stored protein in the body is muscle. It is obviously not advantageous to use this source for fuel during exercise. Some dietary protein (from animal or vegetable origin) is used for fuel. It must first be broken down into amino acids—its simpler, more usable form. Typically, amino acids consumed through the diet include alanine, leucine, valine, and tryptophan. One mole of alanine, metabolized aerobically, produces one acetyl group and one pair of electrons, which result in the production of 15 ATP. In summary then, a mole of carbohydrate (glucose) produces 38 ATP, a mole of fat (stearic acid) produces 147 ATP, and a mole of protein (alanine) produces 15 ATP when combusted by the aerobic system.

Regulation

The regulation of the aerobic system is more complex than that of the lactic acid system. This complexity is understandable given the vast number and nature of the reactions involved in aerobic metabolism. The discussion of the regulatory factors focuses on the control of the Krebs cycle, fat and carbohydrate metabolism, and the electron transport system.

The rate at which the Krebs cycle operates depends primarily on the activity of its enzymes. All of these enzymes are stimulated by elevated concentrations of ADP, and inhibited by high concentrations of ATP. The enzyme that assumes the key regulatory role within the cycle is isocitrate dehydrogenase, which regulates the oxidation of isocitrate. Under resting conditions, the level of ATP in the mitochondria is high. To avoid the overproduction of ATP, which cannot be stored, the elevated mitochondrial ATP inhibits the regulatory enzyme and slows the Krebs cycle. During low- to moderate-intensity aerobic exercise, the amount of ADP entering the mitochondria rises. This has a stimulating effect on isocitrate dehydrogenase which speeds up the Krebs cycle.

Determining which gets burned—fat or carbohydrate—has been a subject of much concern to fitness instructors. The control of fat and carbohydrate entry into the aerobic system is intimately involved with its overall regulation. Under resting conditions, fatty acids are readily available and provide the primary source of fuel. The presence of high concentrations of fatty acid and citric acid inhibit glycolysis by inhibiting PFK.

Therefore, under these resting conditions, fat metabolism flourishes while carbohydrate metabolism is inhibited. During prolonged, moderate-intensity exercise ($< 75\%$ HR_{max}), subtle changes occur in the level of secretion of several hormones. The secretion of epinephrine (adrenaline) from the adrenal glands rises and the secretion of insulin from the pancreas decreases. These hormones influence the rate of fat and carbohydrate uptake by muscle in such a way that fat metabolism still predominates and is further enhanced naturally or endogenously during prolonged work.

With higher intensity exercise ($> 85\%$ HR_{max}), changes occur that begin to inhibit the use of fats. The most significant inhibitor is the lactic acid produced. It reduces the availability of fatty acids by slowing their release from triglycerides. As a result, fat metabolism is inhibited and carbohydrate becomes the preferred source of fuel, used by the aerobic system and the lactic acid system.

The status of the electron transport system also influences the overall regulation of aerobic metabolism. Oxygen must be in constant supply for the proper functioning of the system. The increase in blood flow to the muscle during aerobic exercise ensures a sufficient oxygen supply and allows the aerobic system to increase its rate of energy production. The increased influx of ADP into the mitochondria during exercise also stimulates the enzymes associated with ETS, further enhancing its performance. The system is inhibited, on the other hand, by reduced blood flow resulting in reduced oxygen availability. A strong, isometric muscular contraction, caused by exerting pressure on blood vessels, causes a brief restriction of blood flow. This results in the temporary inhibition of the aerobic system so that the muscle relies more on the lactic acid and phosphagen systems.

If all fuels are considered, including the total carbohydrate, fat, and protein stored in the body, the aerobic system has a virtually unlimited capacity for producing ATP energy. Its complexity and its need for oxygen, however, limit the maximal power at which the system can operate.

Capacity and Power

The only practical limit to the capacity of the system comes when analyzing prolonged, continuous aerobic exercise. The best example of this type of exercise is a marathon completed in competitive time (under 3 hours). A marathon run at this pace requires significant reliance on carbohydrate metabolism. If the competitor is not careful, the carbohydrate within the muscle can be depleted before the end of the race, resulting in premature fatigue or "hitting the wall." The total amount of ATP that can be produced aerobically from stored muscle glycogen can be estimated. If the same assumptions are used regarding the level of training, body weights, and muscle weights, a male subject may store about 450 grams (1 lb) of glycogen. This much glycogen would theoretically produce nearly 100 moles of ATP, equivalent to 1,000 kcal of energy, or sufficient energy to walk or run about 10 miles. A female subject, with a muscle mass of 20 kg and a similar glycogen concentration would have a capacity of approximately 65 moles of ATP upon glycogen depletion.

The capacity of the aerobic system grows tremendously if stored fat is included as a potential source of energy. For example, a 70 kg male of above average body composition (15% body fat) possesses just over 10,000 grams of stored body fat. Since 1 gram of fat yields 9 kcal of energy, the amount of energy available from the complete combustion of stored fat would result in over 90,000 kcal of energy, or 9,000 moles of ATP. Theoretically, this would be enough energy to walk from New York City to Chicago (900 miles) without eating. A 100 kg subject with 31% body fat would have enough stored energy to walk from New York City to Los Angeles (2,800 miles) without refueling.

The power of the aerobic system depends on the maximal rate at which the body can transport and consume oxygen. The maximal rate of oxygen uptake (VO_{2max}) is determined by a graded exercise test to exhaustion. If done on a treadmill, the protocol usually consists of increasing the speed and grade of the treadmill every 2–3 minutes during the exercise test. Oxygen uptake and other physiological variables are measured throughout the test. Testing continues until the subject can no longer maintain the speed of the treadmill belt and voluntarily stops due to exhaustion.

An average value for maximal oxygen uptake in an untrained 70 kg person is about 3 liters/min. If it is assumed that for every liter of oxygen consumed, about 5 kcal of energy are expended, the VO_{2max} can be converted into a maximal energy expenditure of about 15 kcal/min. Finally, if 1 mole of ATP is required for each 10 kcal of energy expenditure, an estimated maximal rate of ATP production would be about 1.5 moles/min. Thus, when producing energy at a maximal rate (15 kcal/min), the aerobic system produces energy 75% as fast as the lactic acid system (20 kcal/min) and less than 40% as fast as the phosphagen system (40 kcal/min).

Types of Exercise

The aerobic system, because of its limited power, provides energy primarily for low- to moderate-intensity exercise. Virtually all of the energy necessary for resting activities, including sitting, reading, studying, watching television, surfing the Internet, and sleeping, comes by way of the aerobic system. With slightly higher intensity activity, like walking, leisurely bicycling, shopping, and office work, the aerobic system still supplies most of the energy. It is not until the intensity reaches a moderately high level (above 75–85% of maximum heart rate) that the limit of the aerobic system is reached and other energy systems need to be recruited to provide supplemental energy. Such activities would include aerobics, running, swimming, cycling, rowing, skating, and others that are performed above 75–85% of maximum intensity. This intensity is such that the activity could be sustained continuously for at least 5 minutes without fatigue, yet requires a significantly elevated heart rate to accomplish.

The best examples of exercises relying primarily on the aerobic system for energy include 40–60 minutes of aerobics, distance running (> 5,000 meters), distance swimming (> 1,500 meters), distance cycling (> 10 kilometers), cross-country skiing (> 5,000 meters), and the triathlon. Any activity, providing it is sustained continuously for a minimum of 5 minutes, relies primarily on the aerobic system. This encompasses portions of several team or more complex individual sports, including soccer, field hockey, lacrosse, basketball, tennis, and squash, to name a few. All of these sports, however, also periodically require energy production from the lactic acid and phosphagen systems for more intense rallies and bursts of sprinting, jumping, and kicking.

Summary

"Aerobic system" is a term used by exercise physiologists to refer to a complex system of metabolic reactions. The system is capable of using any form of food, including carbohydrate, fat, or protein, as a source of fuel. The first component of the system, which is different depending on the source of fuel, begins with large food molecules and breaks them down so that pyruvates, acetyl groups, and/or electrons are produced. This provides the fuel for the Krebs cycle and for the subsequent reactions associated with electron transport and oxidative phosphorylation.

With a sufficient supply of oxygen, the aerobic system can completely catabolize these food fuels into carbon dioxide and water, while saving much of the energy released through the formation of ATP. (On the assumption that someone could utilize most of the carbohydrate and fat stored in the body, the aerobic system has a virtually unlimited capacity.) However, because of its complexity and the need for oxygen, the power of the system is somewhat limited. These characteristics make it an ideal source of energy for prolonged activity of a low to moderate intensity (< 65–75% HR_{max}).

Summary and Comparison of Energy Systems

A full appreciation of the energetics of exercise requires a fundamental understanding of the energy systems. Conclusions can be drawn as to the significance of each system with regard to many sports based on the system's characteristics.

Summary of Energy Systems

Energy is produced within the body in response to demands placed upon it. The body attempts to produce energy in the most efficient manner possible and at the necessary rate. When conditions permit, the body produces energy aerobically because of the efficiency with which this process is completed. However, when exercise is performed at an intensity that exceeds the capability of the aerobic system, the energy requirement is met through anaerobic metabolism.

Capacity and Power

The aerobic system produces a virtually limitless supply of energy through the catabolism of carbohydrate, fat, and protein stored within the body. The combustion of these fuels occurs in such a way that the only remaining end products (CO_2 and H_2O) are easily removed by exhalation from the lungs. The lactic acid system is more limited in its energy-producing capacity due to the disruption of the normal acid-base balance that it creates. Hydrogen ions produced by dissociation from lactic acid quickly saturate the body's buffer systems and fatigue ensues. The phosphagen system provides an immediate source of readily available energy. The amount of usable fuel is so limited, however, that the capacity is minimal and can be completely exhausted within a matter of seconds.

The significance of the anaerobic energy systems lies more in their ability to produce energy at high speed. The phosphagen system, because of its simplicity, is able to provide energy immediately for forceful muscular contractions. It produces energy at least twice as fast as either of the other systems. Anaerobic glycolysis, the sequence of reactions constituting the lactic acid system, is similarly simple and, as such, provides a rapid source of energy as well. The complexities of the aerobic system and its reliance on oxygen as an acceptor of electrons limit its rate of energy production to below that of the anaerobic systems.

Types of Exercise

Any sport, exercise, or physical activity that can be accomplished with a level of exertion not exceeding 65–75% of one's maximal capability (as indicated by heart rate for example) can be accomplished almost exclusively with aerobic metabolism. Frequently in sports, however, the athlete cannot exercise at a constant intensity, but instead must alternate between low ($< 65\%$ HR_{max}), moderate (65–75% HR_{max}), high (80–90% HR_{max}), and very high ($> 90\%$ HR_{max}) intensities. When this is the case, the body frequently shifts between energy systems, taking advantage of the differing characteristics of each.

Comparison of Energy Systems

The characteristics of the systems are compared in Table 4-1. Based on these characteristics, conclusions are made as to the types of exercise for which each system is best suited. The basic facts contained within this chapter provide a foundation for developing a training program for any sport. Through proper training, the capacities and powers of each of the systems can be improved with the accompanying expectation of improved sport performance.

Table 4-1. Summary of the Characteristics of the Three Energy Systems			
Characteristic	**Phosphagen system**	**Lactic acid system**	**Aerobic system**
Fuel used	Creatine phosphate	Carbohydrate only	CHO, fat, protein
Location	Sarcoplasm	Sarcoplasm	Mitochondria
Fatigue due to:	Phosphagen depletion	Lactate accumulation	Glycogen depletion
Capacity	Very limited	Limited	Unlimited
	7–10 kcal	10–15 kcal	> 100,000 kcal
Power	Very high	High/moderate	Moderate/low
	30–40 kcal/min	15–20 kcal/min	12–15 kcal/min
Intensity	Very high	High/moderate	Moderate/low
	> 90% max	75–90% max	< 75% max
Time to fatigue	Very short	Short/medium	Medium/very long
	1–15 s	45–90 s	> 3–5 min
Running distance	< 100 m	400–800 m	> 1,500 m
Swimming	< 25 m	100–200 m	> 400 m
Cycling	< 175 m	750–1,500 m	> 3,000 m
Rowing	< 50 m	250–500 m	> 1,000 m
NOTE: Assume person is healthy and trained with 30 kg of muscle mass. Distances are estimated based on various published performance times.			

References

1. McArdle, W.D., Katch, F.I., & Katch, V.L. (2007). *Exercise physiology: Energy, nutrition and human performance* (6th ed.). Philadelphia: Lippincott Williams & Wilkins.

2. Powers, S.K., & Howley, E.T. (2009). *Exercise physiology: Theory and application to fitness and performance* (7th ed.). Boston, MA: McGraw-Hill.

3. Spencer, M.R., & Gasti, P.B. (2001). Energy system contribution during 200- to 1500-m running in highly trained athletes. *Medicine & Science in Sports & Exercise*, 33, 157-162.

4. Wilmore, J.H., & Costill, D.L. (2004). *Physiology of sport and exercise* (3rd ed.). Champaign, IL: Human Kinetics.

Developing and Maintaining Aerobic Fitness

William C. Beam, PhD

5

Focus

There is little doubt that a conscientious program of physical activity, especially aerobic exercise, significantly improves the health and wellness of the exerciser. What is more, evidence is mounting that the benefits of regular and continuing exercise can be enjoyed over an entire life span. It has been proven fairly convincingly that individuals who maintain an active lifestyle may actually add years to their lives while significantly enhancing the quality of life in later years as well. Physical activity reduces the premature, deleterious effects of degenerative diseases, especially cardiovascular disease. Individuals of all ages, from children to the elderly, should be encouraged to exercise. It is never too late to begin a regular exercise program, but the best time to start is usually now. Clearance by a health care provider is always recommended prior to the commencement of an exercise program.

General Principles of Aerobic Exercise

Aerobic exercise is generally recognized as exercise that is rhythmic, uses the major muscle groups, and is maintained at a fairly continuous intensity for a prolonged period of time. Provided the intensity is such that the exercise is maintained without undue fatigue for at least 10–15 minutes, the aerobic system serves as the predominant source of energy. Because of the significant role the cardiovascular and respiratory systems play in aerobic exercise, adaptations occur in the heart, lungs, blood vessels, and skeletal muscles with regular and continued aerobic training. These adaptations can lead to significant health benefits and to an improvement in aerobic exercise performance.

Modes of Aerobic Exercise

Most authorities consider the best aerobic exercises to be those that consistently maintain intensity at a constant level. This is especially true for individuals who are just beginning an exercise program or for those individuals who may experience symptoms of cardiovascular disease, including chest pain, abnormal heart rhythms, or unusually high blood pressure. Many other exercise modes, in which the intensity is more variable, also provide significant aerobic benefits, but may not be recommended for all people.

Constant Intensity Exercise

Some of the best examples of aerobic exercise, in which the intensity can be maintained at a constant level, include walking, hiking, jogging, running, stepping, aerobics, step aerobics, stationary cycling, road cycling, mountain biking, rowing, roller skating, inline skating, and cross-country skiing. All of these exercises, provided they are performed at the appropriate frequency, duration, and intensity, improve the performance of the heart and lungs to an equal degree. However, some might be considered more beneficial than others because they train a larger portion of the body's muscle mass as well. The important factor is not which of these modes is used, but that any mode practiced consistently will result in beneficial health and performance changes.

Variable Intensity Exercise

Other modes of exercise, in which the intensity is less predictable and more variable, also have the potential for providing aerobic benefits. These include recreational pursuits, such as tennis, racquetball, squash, handball, soccer, basketball, roller hockey, and ice hockey. However, these sports must be played in a continuous manner. In the racquet sports, the time spent serving and receiving a serve must be intentionally reduced, and the players must have levels of skill that enable them to maintain longer rallies. In the team sports, penalties and play stoppages must be eliminated or severely restricted, so that the level of activity is more evenly maintained. For example, if basketball is played recreationally, if no free throws are taken, and the ball is quickly put back into play after each foul or basket, it can provide significant aerobic benefit. As it is played competitively at the collegiate or professional level, however, basketball is very intermittent and highly dependent on anaerobic metabolism.

Before and After Exercise

To maximize safety, certain precautions should be taken before and after exercise. Adequately warming up prior to the aerobic exercise session may prevent damage to skeletal muscle, connective tissue, and the heart. A sufficient cooldown is necessary after exercise to alleviate a potential rapid drop in blood pressure that could cause lightheadedness, dizziness, or fainting. Proper warm-up and cool-down are increasingly important before and after higher intensity exercise.

Warm-up

Prior to aerobic exercise, low-intensity, dynamic exercise is performed to gradually prepare the body for the exercise and to prevent damage to skeletal muscle, connective tissue, and the heart. The main benefits of the warm-up are to increase blood flow to the previously mentioned tissues and to increase body temperature. Skeletal muscle and connective tissue become more pliable, stretching more easily, and thus become more resistant to tearing. The gradual increase in exercise intensity allows adequate blood flow to the heart. Without proper warm-up, especially in older adults, exercise can result in an inadequate blood flow to the heart which can lead to chest pain, tissue damage, or an irregular heartbeat.

Inappropriate changes in blood pressure can be observed with inadequate warm-up. The large blood vessels in the arms and legs are constricted (narrow) at rest and provide a high resistance to blood flow. If exercise is started at a low intensity, it allows time for the blood vessels to slowly dilate and for the resistance to drop. If however, the exercise intensity is increased too fast, the blood vessels are still constricted and blood pressure rapidly rises to very high levels. Exercise blood pressures of 250/115 mmHg are considered too high, and increase the likelihood of stroke and the rupturing of other blood vessels throughout the body. Proper warm-up makes the working skeletal muscles warm and acidic, which makes it easier for the muscles to extract more oxygen from the circulating blood.

Typically, two different types of exercise are performed during the warm-up session. Mild, dynamic exercise is used to increase blood flow and body temperature. This exercise is usually of the same mode as the exercise used for the aerobic conditioning, but is performed at a very low intensity (30–40% of maximum). Prepartory stretching exercises are a second type of exercise that can be included in the warm-up to prepare muscles and help minimize the risk of soft tissue injury. For instance, cycling should be preceded by preparatory stretches emphasizing the muscles in the legs; swimming is preceded by stretches emphasizing the arms and upper body. While emphasizing particular muscle groups is a good idea, it should not be done at the exclusion of other muscles throughout the body. (For more information, see Chapter 17 in this text on "Basic Exercise Standards and Guidelines.")

Cool-down

The cool-down period following exercise is used primarily to prevent a rapid drop in arterial blood pressure. Many arteries are fully dilated following exercise due to changes that have occurred in the skeletal muscle around them. This significantly reduces the resistance to blood flow. If heart rate, stroke volume, and cardiac output are allowed to drop rapidly after exercise, the reduced blood flow, in combination with the reduced resistance, can result in very low blood pressure. As a result of inadequate blood pressure, an insufficient supply of blood reaches the brain, which can cause lightheadedness, dizziness, or fainting. To avoid rapid drops in blood pressure, it is important to continue some type of dynamic exercise during recovery. Due to the rhythmic muscular contractions, blood flow back to the heart is enhanced maintaining stroke volume and cardiac output. Standing or sitting still after exercise should be avoided because of the pooling of blood in the legs that will occur due to gravity. The blood pooling reduces stroke volume, which reduces cardiac output and thereby leads to a significant drop in arterial blood pressure.

During the cool-down period, heart rate, breathing rate, oxygen consumption, and caloric expenditure remain elevated above resting levels and gradually decline. This period of increased oxygen consumption and energy expenditure after exercise has traditionally been called oxygen debt. This name was given because the increased expenditure during recovery was thought to "pay back" the deficit incurred during the warm-up (the first 3–5 minutes) when the anaerobic pathways predominate. Today, oxygen debt is called excess post-exercise oxygen consumption, or EPOC. The length of the extra oxygen consumption and corresponding increased caloric expenditure depends on the intensity and the duration of the exercise. The harder and longer the exercise, the greater the EPOC, as the body works to restore resting levels and homeostasis.

Before and After Exercise

In this discussion, aerobic training is assumed to consist of continuous aerobic exercise. It is generally performed by healthy adults at 64–94% of **maximum heart rate** (HR_{max}) or 40–85% of **heart rate reserve** (HRR). The main purpose of aerobic exercise is to improve the ability of the cardiorespiratory system to deliver oxygen and to improve the aerobic endurance of the skeletal muscle used during the exercise. This type of training is highly recommended for the general public because of the associated health benefits provided by such activity. It is believed to facilitate a normalization of blood pressure, to lower body fat, to improve glucose utilization, to reduce psychological stress, and to reduce the risk of heart attack and stroke.

Three important characteristics of exercise must be considered. The **frequency**, **duration**, and **intensity** of the exercise are all interrelated and must be monitored and adjusted to provide maximal aerobic benefits. As discussed previously, to ensure the safety of the exercise, careful consideration must be given to the activity used in warming up prior to the exercise and in cooling down afterward. Provided all of these principles are followed correctly, they may be applied to improve the aerobic fitness of any apparently healthy adult or athlete.

Frequency

In order to see improvement in aerobic power, the exercise should be performed at least 3–5 days per week. Exercising only once or twice a week has been shown to maintain fitness for the most part, but does not provide enough stimulus to achieve significant gains in aerobic fitness. On the other hand, performing the same mode of exercise too frequently has a tendency to increase both the possibility of exhaustion and the risk of overuse injuries. It is recommended that 1–2 days per week be rest days with no hard training. Cross-training, using more than one primary mode of exercise (e.g., aerobics, running, cycling, swimming), is also a popular way of exercising more frequently with less risk of injury. It also relieves, for many people and athletes, much of the boredom associated with long months of training. In addition to aerobic training, it is strongly recommended that strength training (or resistance training) be done at least 2 days a week to gain the added benefits it provides, including increased strength, improved glucose utilization, and increased bone mineral content.

Duration

The duration of the exercise must be at least 20 minutes to achieve gains in aerobic endurance. More significant gains are observed when the duration is extended to 30–60 minutes per session. There is nothing wrong with exercising continuously for over an hour if it is tolerated well. Some individuals, however, become chronically fatigued and are prone to overuse injury due to exercising for too long with insufficient rest. Long training sessions, of over an hour in duration, should be divided into bouts of differing modes of exercise, or should be limited to two to three times per week. While exercise bouts of less than 20 minutes have not proven useful in improving aerobic endurance, there is recent evidence they may still result in health benefits and in psychological and emotional benefits. In other words, benefits can be gained by taking advantage of brief exercise breaks, such as walking the dog, walking during your lunch break, or riding your bike to work.

Intensity

The intensity of the exercise is more difficult to monitor than frequency or duration. With less experienced exercisers, intensity is best monitored by using heart rate as an indicator of stress. An added benefit of using heart rate is that it is sensitive to environmental changes the exerciser may encounter. To improve aerobic power (determined by your VO_{2max}), the intensity of the exercise should be maintained between 55% and 85% of heart rate reserve (HRR) in order to stimulate structural changes in your heart and peripheral changes in your skeletal muscles, which in turn lead to an increase in VO_{2max}. Keep in mind that the benefits of aerobic exercise (e.g., reduction in blood pressure, decrease in body fat) can occur at intensity thresholds as low as 40% HRR.

The **heart rate reserve** (HRR) method is based on the number of beats between resting heart rate (HR_{rest}) and a measured or estimated **maximal heart rate** (HR_{max}). HR_{rest} is simply the lowest palpable heart rate achieved while resting. It is usually suggested that HR_{rest} be taken in the morning, but it can be measured at any time during the day provided the subject is well rested and free from stress. Although HR_{max} is best obtained through the use of a graded exercise test, it can also be estimated based on the subject's age. Table 5-1 demonstrates the method for calculating training heart rates at 55%, 65%, 75%, and 85% of HRR using a HR_{max} estimated from age. A directly measured HR_{max} is preferred, but because it is infrequently measured, a HR_{max} estimated from age will suffice. (This calculation of intensity is one way to determine an appropriate training HRR. For more information, see Chapter 20 in this text on "Monitoring Exercise Intensity.")

Table 5-1. Equations for Calculating Training Heart Rates at Various Exercise Intensities by the Heart Rate Reserve (HRR) Method

(Example is for a 40-year-old subject with a HRmax of 180 bpm and HRrest of 80 bpm.)

Equations	Sample Calculations
HR_{max} = 220 – age	HR_{max} = 220 – 40 = 180 bpm
HR_{max} = 206.9 – (0.67 x age)	HR_{max} = 206.9 – (0.67 x 40) = 180 bpm
$HR_{reserve}$ (HRR) = HRmax – HRrest	$HR_{reserve}$ (HRR) = 180 – 72 = 108 bpm
$HR_{55\% HRR}$ = (HRR x .55) + HRrest	$HR_{55\% HRR}$ = (108 x .55) + 72 = 131 bpm
$HR_{65\% HRR}$ = (HRR x .65) + HRrest	$HR_{65\% HRR}$ = (108 x .65) + 72 = 142 bpm
$HR_{75\% HRR}$ = (HRR x .75) + HRrest	$HR_{75\% HRR}$ = (108 x .75) + 72 = 153 bpm
$HR_{85\% HRR}$ = (HRR x .85) + HRrest	$HR_{85\% HRR}$ = (108 x .85) + 72 = 164 bpm

NOTE: Example is for a 40-year-old exerciser with a HR_{rest} of 72 bpm. HR_{max} predicted from age is 180 bpm by both prediction equations. $HR_{reserve}$ (HRR) is a method of defining exercise intensity as a percentage of the difference between HR_{max} and HR_{rest}. It is analogous to using oxygen uptake reserve (VO_2R) to define exercise intensity. *Source*: Modified from ACSM, 2010.

The minimum intensity believed necessary to produce moderate fitness gains in a healthy adult is about 40–60% HRR. Increasing the intensity of the exercise to 65–85% HRR causes adaptations to occur more quickly, resulting in faster increases in aerobic fitness and aerobic exercise performance. By increasing the intensity still further, however, to over 85% HRR, the exercise now requires anaerobic energy production. Consequently, the exercise leads to fatigue too rapidly and, as such, is not suggested for inclusion in an aerobic program. More experienced exercisers usually do not need to monitor heart rate each time they exercise. Instead, they can eventually rely on their experience to perceive and maintain a level of exertion that produces the desirable heart rate within a minimal range of error.

The most appropriate exercise intensity is determined based on the participant characteristics, fitness level, and exercise program goals. Fitness level may be assumed based on the exercise history of the subject or can be measured using a graded exercise test. Intensity should be kept low (40–55% HRR) for apparently healthy individuals who are in poor to fair condition. In certain populations, such as previously sedentary, elderly, or symptomatic participants, even this level of intensity may be too high. In these populations it may be recommended that very low-intensity exercise (30–40% HRR) be performed until the subject reaches a sufficient level of fitness. The main advantage of very low- and low-intensity exercise is found in the health benefits achieved. It can result in weight loss, an improvement in body composition, a modest reduction in blood pressure, improved glucose utilization, and possible improvement in blood lipids. Because of the low intensity, however, it needs to be practiced more frequently and for a longer duration to obtain the desired benefit.

For those in fair to average condition, low- to moderate-intensity exercise (55–65% HRR) is recommended, but this intensity should not be attempted until some initial level of fitness is attained. Exercise of this type results in health benefits as well as some adaptations that may lead to moderate gains in aerobic fitness. For participants who are in average to good shape, with a previous history of regular aerobic exercise, moderate- to high-intensity exercise (65–75% HRR) or high-intensity exercise (75–85% HRR) is required to ensure sufficient stress for continued improvement in aerobic fitness and performance. Exercise of this intensity can lead to significant training effects in the heart, lungs, and skeletal muscles that can improve aerobic exercise performance.

A summary of determining training heart rates based on participant characteristics, fitness level, and exercise program goals is presented in Table 5-2.

Table 5-2. Choosing an Appropriate Exercise Intensity (%HRR) Based on Participant Description, Fitness Classification, and Exercise Program Goals

Intensity (%HRR)	Participant Description	Fitness Classification	Exercise Program Goals
30–40% (very low)	Sedentary, elderly, symptomatic	Poor	Health benefits only
40–55% (low)	Sedentary, elderly, symptomatic	Poor-Fair	Health benefits and modest gains in fitness
55–65% (low/moderate)	Sporadic physical activity	Fair-Average	Health benefits and moderate gains in fitness
65–75% (moderate/high	Regular physical activity	Average-Good	Health benefits and moderate gains in fitness/performance
75–85% (high)	High levels of physical activity	Good-Excellent	Health benefits and significant gains in fitness/performance

Source: Modified from ACSM, 2010.

Two other means of measuring intensity include the talk test and rating of perceived exertion. Both of these methods, along with a discussion on finding and calculating heart rates, are covered extensively in Chapter 20, "Monitoring Exercise Intensity."

Summary of Exercise Principles

To appreciate the relationship between frequency, duration, and intensity of exercise, a brief summary is necessary. When beginning an exercise program, it is best to maintain a conservative approach and start at the suggested minimums of three times per week, 20 minutes per session, at no more than 55–65% HRR. (This corresponds to an exercise heart rate of 131–142 bpm when considering the example in Table 3-1 for a 40-year-old exerciser.) Provided this level of activity is tolerated well, the next step consists of gradually increasing the duration to 30 minutes, while maintaining the same frequency and intensity. The intensity should not be increased until the subject can exercise for 30–45 minutes without becoming overly tired. At this point, the intensity can be increased to 65–75% HRR (e.g., 142–153 bpm).

The frequency may now also be increased to four to five times per week if so desired. Once the subject feels comfortable exercising 30–45 minutes, three to five times per week, at 65–75% intensity, the intensity may be raised toward the recommended maximum of 75–85% HRR (e.g., 153–164 bpm). If the purpose of the exercise is to maintain aerobic fitness in a healthy non-athlete, the previous recommendations of frequency (three to five times per week), duration (20–60 minutes), and intensity (55–85% HRR) apply.

It may be beneficial to consider a combination of exercise frequency, duration, and intensity almost as a "volume" of exercise per week. Table 5-3 includes key guidelines for physical activity that incorporate all three of these exercise principles. The minimal volume of exercise for substantial health benefits is 150 min of moderate intensity exercise (55–70% HRR) per week. This could be done as 30 min/day for 5 days, as 50 min/day for 3 days, or as any combination of duration and frequency. Or it could be 75 min of vigorous exercise (70–85% HRR). The goal eventually for more extensive benefits would be to increase the volume of aerobic exercise to 300 min of moderate intensity exercise (55–70% HRR) per week, or 150 min of vigorous exercise (70–85% HRR) spread throughout the week.

Table 5-3. Key Guidelines for Physical Activity in Adults and Older Adults

- All adults should avoid inactivity. Some physical activity is better than none, and adults who participate in any amount of physical activity gain some health benefits.

- For substantial health benefits, adults should do at least 150 minutes (2 hours and 30 minutes) a week of moderate-intensity aerobic physical activity (55–70% HRR), or 75 minutes (1 hour and 15 minutes) a week of vigorous-intensity aerobic physical activity (70–85% HRR), or an equivalent combination of moderate- and vigorous-intensity aerobic physical activity. Aerobic activity should be performed in episodes of at least 10 minutes, and preferably, it should be spread throughout the week.

- For additional and more extensive health benefits, adults should do 300 minutes (5 hours) a week of moderate-intensity aerobic physical activity (55–70% HRR), or 150 minutes a week of vigorous-intensity aerobic physical activity (70–85% HRR), or an equivalent combination of moderate- and vigorous-intensity aerobic physical activity. Additional health benefits are gained by engaging in physical activity beyond this amount.

- Adults should also do muscle-strengthening activities that are moderate or high intensity and involve all major muscle groups on 2 or more days a week, as these activities provide additional health benefits.

Source: U.S. Department of Health and Human Services, 2008.

If the purpose is to increase the aerobic power and endurance of a young athlete, more appropriate recommendations might include exercising a minimum of 45–60 minutes per session, 4–6 days per week, at 80–85% HRR. The same basic principles of frequency, duration, and intensity apply to virtually any subject; it is only the level at which they are performed that differs, depending upon the purpose and application of the exercise program.

References

1. American College of Sports Medicine. (2010). *ACSM's guidelines for exercise testing and prescription* (8th ed.). Baltimore, MD: Lippincott Williams & Wilkins.

2. American College of Sports Medicine. (1998). Position stand on the recommended quantity and quality of exercise for developing and maintaining cardiorespiratory and muscular fitness in healthy adults. *Medicine & Science in Sports & Exercise*, 30, 975–991.

3. Gellish, R.L., Gosline, B.R., Olson, R.E., McDonald, A., Russi, G.D., & Moudgil, V.K. (2007). Longitudinal modeling of the relationship between age and maximal heart rate. *Medicine & Science in Sports & Exercise*, 39, 822–829.

4. Heyward, V.H. (2006). *Advanced fitness assessment & exercise prescription* (5th ed.). Champaign, IL: Human Kinetics.

5. Nelson, M.E., Rejeski, W.J., Blair, S.N., Duncan, P.W., Judge, J.O., King, A.C., et al. (2007). Physical activity and public health in older adults: Recommendation from the American College of Sports Medicine and the American Heart Association. *Medicine & Science in Sports & Exercise*, 8, 1435–1445.

6. Pate, R.R., Pratt, M., Blair, S.N., Haskell, W.L., Macera, C.A., et al. (1995). Physical activity and public health: A recommendation from the Centers for Disease Control and Prevention and the American College of Sports Medicine. *Journal of the American Medical Association*, 273, 402–407.

7. U.S. Department of Health and Human Services. *2008 Physical activity guidelines for Americans*. ODPHP Publication No. U0036, October 2008. Retrieved on May 15, 2009, from www.health.gov/paguidelines

6

The Cardiorespiratory System: Structure, Function, and Exercise Application

Patti Mantia, EdD

Focus

This segment examines the cardiovascular system, the pulmonary system, and how they work together to maintain vital processes.

Heart Location and Structure

The heart is a muscular organ located in the chest, or thoracic cavity, diagonally behind the breastbone, or sternum. Shaped and sized similarly to that of a clenched fist, this relatively small organ performs a tremendous amount of work to maintain life processes.(1) Even at rest, the amount of blood pumped by the heart per minute (cardiac output) is an average of 5 liters.(5)

The structure of the heart (Figure 6-1) allows for an efficient mechanism to perform vital processes. The heart is divided, anatomically and functionally, into right and left sides by a partitioning wall, or septum. The right side of the heart receives deoxygenated blood as it is returned from the body through the venous system and pumps the blood to the lungs, or pulmonary system. The left side of the heart receives the oxygenated blood from the lungs and pumps it, via the arterial system, throughout the body. Because the heart performs two distinct functions, this singular organ is often referred to as a double-pump.

The heart is further broken down into upper and lower chambers called the atria (atrium, singular) and the ventricles, respectively. The superior **atria** (right and left) are the blood-receiving units of the heart. The blood is then forced through an efficient one-way system of valves, known as atrioventricular, or AV valves, to the inferior ventricles. The contraction of the **ventricles** forces blood through the semilunar valves and into the great arteries of either the pulmonary or systemic circulation. The familiar "lub-dub" sounds of the heart are produced by the closing of the atrioventricular and semilunar valves.

The heart is entirely contained within a loose yet protective sac, the pericardium, which prevents the beating heart from brushing against the chest wall. The heart itself is composed of three specialized layers of tissue: (a) the epicardium, (b) the myocardium, and (c) the endocardium (Figure 6-2). The **epicardium** is a thin membrane located on the outermost layer of the heart. The primary work of the heart is performed by the next layer of muscular tissue, the myocardium. The **myocardium** is thicker and stronger in the left ventricle as it is responsible for pumping blood into the systemic circulation, a much higher pressure system than the pulmonary circulation. The coronary arteries are the primary source of nourishment for the epicardium and myocardium, as only the endocardium is enriched by the blood-filled chambers of the heart. The term myocardial infarction, or heart attack, refers to a dysfunction of the tissues of the myocardium usually due to ischemia or a lack of blood flow to the myocardium. The **endocardium** is a smooth membrane that lines the cavities within the heart.

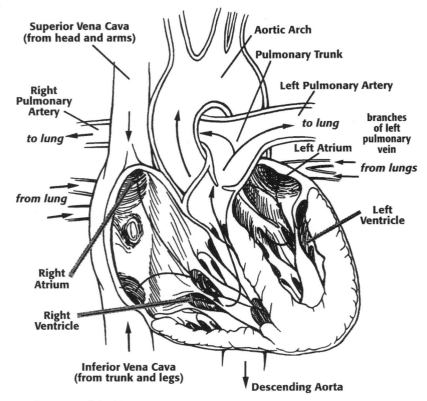

Fig. 6-1. Structure of the Heart

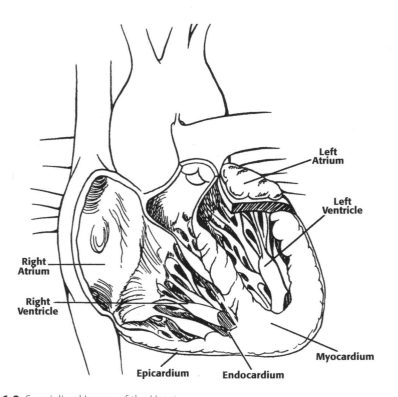

Fig. 6-2. Specialized Layers of the Heart

Conduction System

The conduction system of the heart (Figure 6-3) is "autorhythmic" in nature and controlled by a specialized nerve center in the brain. This center receives signals from the body and relays commands to the heart. Conduction begins with an electrical impulse of the **sinoatrial (SA) node** within the right atrium. The SA node, because of its rapid and spontaneous impulses, dictates regulation of contractions of the heart and is therefore referred to as the "pacemaker." On an average, the adult's heart, at rest, beats 60–80 times per minute.(6) The electrical impulse of the SA node causes both atria to contract synchronously and, consequently, blood is forced into the ventricles. Almost immediately after the SA node fires, the electrical charge travels through specialized conduction tissue to reach the **atrioventricular (AV) node**. The AV node consists of slow-conducting muscle cells and delays the impulse before it excites the ventricular conductors, through the bundle of His (pronounced: hiss). The conduction system continues through the branches of the bundle of His into the Purkinje fibers. This chain of electrical events results in a simultaneous and powerful contraction of the ventricles. The blood is then forced from the ventricles into the major arteries. It is the contraction of the ventricles that constitutes a heartbeat.

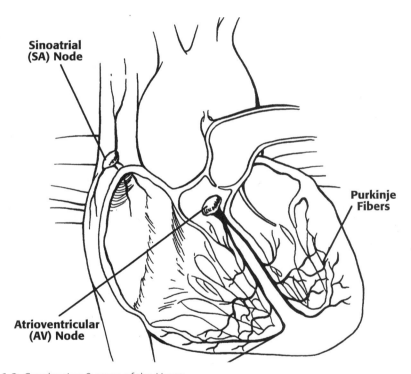

Fig. 6-3. Conduction System of the Heart

Cardiac Cycle

The contraction/relaxation pattern produced in the heart is known as the cardiac cycle. The contraction phase is called systole and the relaxation phase is diastole. Generally, these terms refer to the contraction/relaxation of the ventricles. It is important to understand that the atria have a separate contraction/relaxation phase. Fundamentally, atrial contraction (systole) occurs during ventricular relaxation (**diastole**) and ventricular **systole** occurs as the atria relax. The time interval of the cardiac cycle decreases as the cardiac rate increases, as would occur with vigorous exercise.

The contraction/relaxation phases of the cardiac cycle create pressure changes adequate to produce blood flow through the arteries. Arterial blood pressure increases from 80 to 120 mmHg within the systemic circulatory system as a result of ventricular systole.(6) The pressure in the pulmonary circulation is significantly lower. Simply stated, the contraction/relaxation of the ventricles causes a squeezing action that produces blood flow through the arteries.

Blood Pressure

Measurement of arterial blood pressure provides significant information concerning heart function. With the use of a device called a sphygmomanometer, the qualified technician can easily record blood pressure. First, an inflatable cuff is fastened around the arm, just above the elbow. Air is then pumped into the cuff to apply pressure sufficient enough to cut off blood circulation. As the air is slowly released from the cuff, the technician listens for the first pulsing sounds with a stethoscope. When the first sounds are heard, the pressure within the arteries can be determined by the reading shown on the dial attached to the cuff. This is the systolic blood pressure. The diastolic blood pressure is viewed on the dial when the technician can no longer hear the pulsing sound with the stethoscope. These figures reflect the pressures being exerted on the arterial walls during the contraction and relaxation of the heart.

Resting blood pressure of the healthy person averages around 120/80 mmHg. A resting blood pressure of 140/90 is considered by health care professionals to be high blood pressure, or hypertension, and often relates to serious health problems, such as cardiac arrest, stroke, aneurysm, and kidney failure.

The Circulatory System

The system that allows the blood to flow through the heart, lungs, and body is called the circulatory system. The circulatory system consists of the blood-carrying vessels: (a) the arteries, (b) capillaries, and (c) veins. As a unit, these vessels produce a circuit of blood flow throughout the body. That is, they work together as a closed system to provide a specific function in circulation. Arteries carry blood away from the heart to capillaries, which work as exchange vessels for nutrients and gasses, and veins transport blood from the capillaries back to the heart. Figure 6-4 illustrates the blood flow pattern of the circulatory vessels.

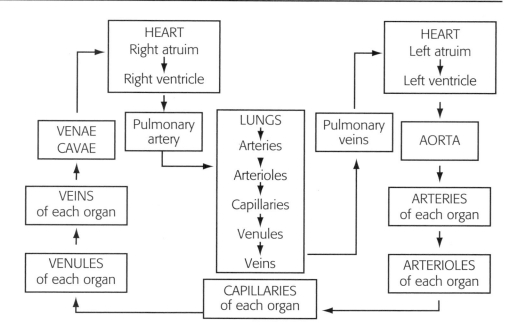

Fig. 6-4. Blood Flow Patterns of the Circulatory Vessels

Pulmonary Circulation

As previously stated, arteries constitute a major part of our blood transportation system and function to direct blood flow away from the heart. With each ventricular contraction, blood is pumped into the largest arteries (the aorta and pulmonary arteries). The pulmonary arteries receive **deoxygenated** blood from the right ventricle and direct it to the lungs where carbon dioxide is exchanged for fresh oxygen. This newly oxygenated blood leaves the pulmonary circulation, returns to the heart (left atrium and ventricle), and is then forced through the aorta, to the body, by a network of arteries. The primary arteries of this network are the carotid arteries in the neck and head, the abdominal arteries, and the axillary and iliac arteries of the arms and legs, respectively. A great number of smaller arteries branch off the large arteries, each yielding smaller and smaller units until the blood passes into the smallest arteries, called arterioles. The elastic, muscular structure of arterial walls is capable of expansion and contraction to regulate a smooth continued blood flow.

Exchange Vessels

Once again, the purpose of the pumping action of the heart and transportation mechanisms of the circulatory system is to exchange oxygen and other nutrients for waste products. This exchange takes place in microscopic vessels, called **capillaries**, which connect the arterioles to the smallest branches of the veins, the **venules**.

The structure of the capillaries is significant in that the single-celled composition of their walls allows for an easy transfer of materials to nearby tissue cells. It is here at the capillary level that the blood gives up its oxygen, food, and fluids to the tissues and the tissues give up carbon dioxide and fluid wastes to the blood. The blood leaving the capillaries, now laden with waste products and oxygen poor, returns to the heart through the venous system.

Venous System

The veins complement the arteries in function. Structurally, veins resemble the arteries, however, they are thinner walled and less muscular. The venous blood is returned to the heart under low pressure and is often forced to move against gravity. To keep a steady blood flow to the heart, veins contain a one-way system of valves that prevent backflow of blood. Additionally, the massaging action of the muscles in the legs and arms helps move blood back to the heart (**venous return**). This is why we must include a cool-down period after vigorous exercise. The muscular action will help prevent the blood from pooling in the extremities. Blood return begins in the venules, the smallest venous unit. The venules combine to form larger structures facilitating blood return to the right atrium through the largest veins, the superior and inferior vena cava. The blood is now returned to the heart and the circulatory process repeats itself.

The Pulmonary System

Of all systems required to maintain life, the pulmonary system is one of the most crucial. We can survive for weeks without food, days without water, but live only a few minutes without oxygen. The exchange of gasses, such as oxygen and carbon dioxide, is of the utmost importance. It is the pulmonary, or respiratory, system that provides these life-sustaining processes.

Assisted by numerous integrated body systems, the pulmonary system is responsible for providing two major functions: (a) **air distribution**, and (b) **gas exchange**. Additionally, the pulmonary system effectively filters, warms, and humidifies the inhaled air. Organs associated with the pulmonary system also produce sound, speech, and provide us with a sense of smell.

The pulmonary system (Figure 6-5) is divided into two major components: (a) the conducting airways, and (b) the functional unit. The elements of these systems will be examined as we trace an inhalation through the pulmonary system. The conducting airways consist of the mouth, nose, pharynx, larynx, and the primary branches of the bronchial tubes.

Air enters the body through the mouth or nostrils into the nasal cavity where it is warmed and humidified. The oral and nasal passages lead to the throat, or pharynx. The **pharynx** allows for passage of air into the lungs. After passing through the pharynx, the inspired air enters the larynx. The **larynx** is composed of pieces of cartilage, the largest of which is known as the Adam's apple. The larynx is often referred to as the voice box because the

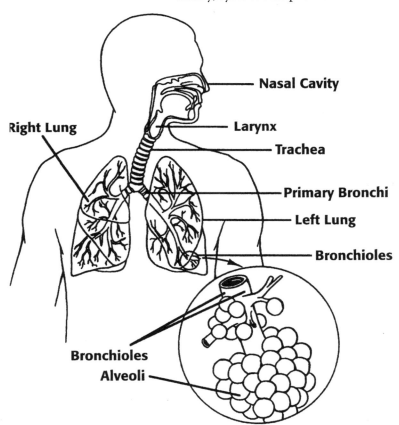

Fig. 6-5. Structures of the Pulmonary System

Nasal Cavity

Larynx

Trachea

Primary Bronchi

Left Lung

Bronchioles

Right Lung

Bronchioles

Alveoli

production of sound occurs as air passes the vocal cords which stretch across the interior of the larynx. Another cartilaginous structure found in the larynx is the **epiglottis**. The epiglottis partially covers the opening in the larynx and closes during swallowing to prevent food passage into the **trachea**. The epiglottis, or glottis, is the structure involved in the potentially dangerous Valsalva maneuver.

Valsalva Maneuver

The **Valsalva maneuver** occurs when a person deeply inhales and then holds his/her breath during strenuous activity, as in lifting weights or shoveling snow. The glottis is closed against pressure. This causes an increased thoracic pressure which interrupts venous return to the heart, blood flow to the coronary arteries, and oxygen supply to the brain. In healthy individuals, this may result in dizziness, slowing of the heart beat, or a temporary loss of consciousness. For the individual predisposed to cardiovascular disease, the Valsalva maneuver could trigger cardiac arrest and result in death. Therefore, proper breathing techniques are essential during heavy exercise.

Passage of Air

The air flows from the larynx into the trachea, or windpipe, which connects the larynx to the bronchi in the chest cavity. The trachea is structurally protected by cartilaginous rings. Sometimes, however, a blockage of the trachea occurs, such as in choking. The lifesaving Heimlich maneuver can be used to free the trachea of obstructions caused by food or other foreign bodies. The Heimlich maneuver is an easily acquired skill and, like CPR, should be learned by all professionals in the health/fitness field.

In the chest cavity, the trachea branches into two main bronchi, the right and the left bronchus, which travel into the respective lungs. In the lungs, the bronchus develops into smaller passageways for air known as the bronchioles. At this site, the functional unit of the pulmonary system begins.

The functional unit of the pulmonary system includes the bronchioles and alveoli, alveolar sacs within the lungs. The structure of this unit, as seen in Figure 6-5, resembles that of an upside down tree as it branches out into the terminal structures.

Pulmonary Airways

The bronchioles, found within the lungs, consist primarily of smooth muscle and elastic tissue in the walls. Excessive spasm in the **smooth muscles of bronchioles** creates breathing difficulties and associated diseases, such as asthma. Decreasing into respiratory units, the bronchioles lead to tiny tubes, or alveolar ducts. The ducts attach to a cluster of grape-like structures called alveolar sacs. The alveolar sacs are composed of millions of alveoli. The alveoli cover a large surface area and are extremely thin walled. The number, structure, and proximity of the alveoli to the structurally similar pulmonary capillaries allow for an efficient diffusion of gasses between air and blood. It is in the lungs that inhaled oxygen passes through the alveoli and enters the blood in the nearby capillaries. Some of the oxygen is absorbed in the blood, but most of it combines with the protein molecule called hemoglobin of the red blood cell. Oxygen is carried within the red blood cells to the tissues. Hemoglobin then releases oxygen to the tissues in exchange for carbon dioxide. Carbon dioxide is transported back to the alveoli for removal during exhalation.

The lungs are a pair of pine cone-shaped organs that lie within the chest cavity, one on either side of the heart. They are well protected by the surrounding structures: (a) the ribs, (b) intercostal muscles, (c) sternum, (d) spine, and (e) diaphragm. A thin layer of moist membranes, called pleura, covers the lungs and lines the chest cavity, which allows for smooth inflation/deflation of the lungs.

The protective structures surrounding the lungs also provide the mechanics of breathing. The breathing process begins with the respiratory center of the brain. Nerve impulses signal the muscles of respiration, the **diaphragm** and the **intercostal muscles**, to contract. The diaphragm is the pair of tent-like muscles that separates the lung cavity from the abdominal cavity like a bellows used to fan the flames of a fire. As the diaphragm contracts, it moves downward and increases the volume within the chest cavity. Contraction of the intercostal muscles pulls the ribs outward, causing further enlargement of the cavity. A vacuum is then created within the space and the negative pressure draws in the outside air. Exhalation occurs as the muscles relax and reverse the process, causing the lungs to contract and force air out.

The total amount of air exchanged between the body and the atmosphere per minute is referred to as minute ventilation. At an average of 12 ventilations per minute, approximately 6 liters of air are exchanged per minute.(6) During exercise, the demand for oxygen and amount of carbon dioxide to be removed increases. The respiratory center in the brain responds to the stimuli, and consequently increases the rate and depth of ventilations accordingly.

Summary

After a thorough analysis of the components of the cardiopulmonary system, we can better comprehend how the system functions collectively. In summary, air is inhaled from the atmosphere, through the conducting airways to the functional unit of the lungs. A gaseous exchange occurs between the alveoli and capillaries of the lungs. Carbon dioxide returns to the lungs and is exhaled. The newly inspired oxygen travels within the red blood cells from the lungs to the left side of the heart and is pumped throughout the body via the arterial circulation. Exchange of oxygen, carbon dioxide, and nutrients in the tissues occurs throughout the body at the capillary level. Oxygen-poor blood is then returned through the venous system to the right side of the heart. The heart contracts and forces blood back to the lungs whereby the process repeats itself.

How the Cardiopulmonary System Meets the Demands of Exercise

1. **Increased Heart Rate**

   Given an average resting heart rate (RHR) of 70 beats per minute (bpm), the heart can comfortably (assuming average fitness and without disease) perform at least twice its resting values. Aerobic exercise is generally performed between 40–85% of heart rate reserve (HRR). This is determined by subtracting your age from 220 minus RHR x % HRR plus RHR (see Chapter 20, "Monitoring Exercise Intensity"). The average adult at 20 years of age, for example, can comfortably train between 122–181 bpm.(1) This is a remarkable performance for such a small organ.

2. **Increased Stroke Volume**

   The amount of blood pumped by the heart per beat can increase as much as 50–60% above resting values to meet the physiological demands of exercise.(6) The tremendous increases in stroke volume are a result of fitness (adaptation) and are less significant in the untrained exerciser. That is, increased stroke volume is a training effect of aerobic exercise and allows the fit individual to pump more blood per beat, resulting in a lower heart rate for a given workload.

3. **Increased Cardiac Output**

    Cardiac output (Q), the amount of blood pumped by the heart per minute, is a product of heart rate (HR) times stroke volume (SV), that is, Q = HR x SV. The average adult heart at rest pumps approximately 5 liters of blood per minute. The cardiac output, in response to an exercise stimulus, can increase to almost eight times its resting values.(6) The increases are found within both the heart rate and stroke volume and depend tremendously on the efficiency of the system, that is to say, fitness. The sedentary individual will typically exhibit a cardiac output of 20–22 liters per minute during maximal exercise (four times resting values), whereas the elite athlete is capable of increases almost eight times the resting values, or 35–40 liters per minute.(3)

4. **Vasodilation and Vasoconstriction**

    An extraordinary physiological adaptation of the circulatory system is the ability to regulate direction of blood flow. The vessels have the capacity to constrict or dilate in order to redistribute blood flow to meet the physiological demands. During exercise, blood flow is diverted away from tissues that are less metabolically active, such as internal organs, and redirected to the active muscles. In fact, depending on the intensity of the exercise, as much as 88% of the blood flow is directed to the muscles during exercise.(6)

5. **Increased Extraction of Oxygen**

    Not only is the body capable of directing blood flow to the active tissues, but the ability to extract oxygen from the blood increases with exercise. Oxygen extraction at the capillary level increases from an average of 25% at rest to as much as 85% during exercise—another amazing adaptation.

6. **Vital Capacity**

    Vital capacity is defined as the greatest volume of air voluntarily moved in one breath, either during inhalation or exhalation, and the sum of the tidal volume and inspiratory/expiratory reserve volumes. Tidal volume is the amount of air inhaled or exhaled in an average breath. Reserve volume refers to the excess volumes that may be used in forceful inspiration or expiration. Research suggests that vital capacity is primarily based on body size and is not significantly influenced by training.(1,5) We do, however, increase the percentage of the vital capacity used during exercise. Figure 6-6 demonstrates the various lung capacities.

7. **Increase in Respiratory Rate**

    The rate of breathing plays a crucial role in delivery of oxygen during exercise. At rest, the adult averages 12 breaths per minute, compared to an exercise ventilatory rate of 35–40 breaths per minute, or an unbelievable rate of 60–70 breaths per minute of the elite athlete.(7) Considering both volume of air and ventilatory rate, we can observe increases in minute ventilation from 6 liters/min to 100 liters/min with exercise (or more).

For a more complete description of the physiological effects of exercise, see Chapter 5 on "Developing and Maintaining Aerobic Fitness."

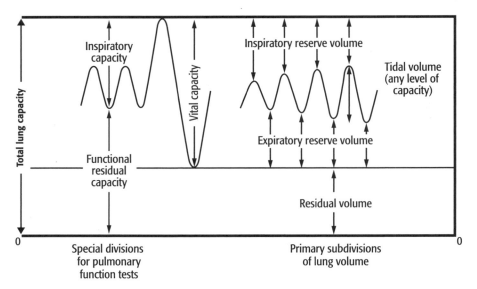

Fig. 6-6. Lung Volumes

Reference Notes

1. American College of Sports Medicine. (2010). *ACSM's resource manual for guidelines for exercise testing and prescription* (6th ed.). Baltimore, MD: Williams & Wilkins.
2. Anthony, C.P., & Thibodeau, G. (1984). *Structure and function of the body.* St. Louis, MO: Times Mirror/Mosby College Publishing.
3. Astrand, P., & Rodahl, K. (1986). *Textbook of work physiology.* New York, NY: McGraw-Hill.
4. Brooks, G., & Fahey, T. (1985). *Exercise physiology: Human bioenergetics and its applications.* New York, NY: Macmillan Publishers.
5. Frost, R. (1984). *Athletics and the heart.* Chicago, IL: Year Book Medical Publishers, Inc.
6. McArdle, W.D., Katch, F.I., & Katch, V.L. (2007). *Exercise physiology: Energy, nutrition and human performance* (6th ed.). Philadelphia: Lippincott Williams & Wilkins.
7. McClintic, J.R. (1985). *Physiology of the human body.* New York, NY: John Wiley & Sons.
8. Noble, B. (1986). *Physiology of exercise and sport.* St. Louis, MO: Times Mirror/Mosby College Publishing.

Sharon Cheng MBA,
MSPT

7

Part 1 Essentials of Exercise

The Musculoskeletal System: Structure, Function, and Exercise Application

Focus

This chapter will give a comprehensive overview of the anatomy and kinesiology of the musculoskeletal system as it relates to human exercise. Your applied knowledge of structure and motion is the cornerstone of safe fitness instruction.

Background

Scientists have always been interested in the structure and movement of the human body. The ancient Egyptians are believed to have been the first people to study anatomy. In the middle of the 4th century B.C., Hippocrates, the "Father of Medicine," continued these studies in Greece. Aristotle (384–322 B.C.), the "Father of Kinesiology," was the first scientist to describe and analyze the actions of muscles. Galen (131–201 A.D.) is credited with introducing the concept of muscle contractions and terms, such as agonist and antagonist muscles. Today, scientists continue to conduct research to learn more about how the human body works. Anatomy looks at the structure and function of the human body, while kinesiology addresses human motion by applying information from other sciences, such as anatomy, physiology, physics, and neurology.

When looking specifically at human motion, it is the musculoskeletal system that allows the body to move through space. Voluntary movements occur when muscles contract and pull on bony levers to cause movement at joints or fulcrums. The skeletal system, composed of bones and cartilage, provides the site of attachment for the muscles. The muscular system refers to the tissue that contracts and moves the bones. To study how voluntary movement occurs, it is necessary to understand both systems.

The Skeletal System

The skeletal system is composed of the bones and cartilage in the body. The basic functions of this system are (a) to provide a supportive framework for the body, (b) to protect its vital organs, (c) to act as levers in conjunction with muscles to cause movement, (d) to produce red blood cells, and (e) to store minerals such as calcium and phosphorus.

While bones are often thought of as lifeless, dry objects, they are actually living organs in the body that change as we age. They have an outer shell of compact bone encasing spongy bone which surrounds a medullary cavity. The spaces in the spongy bone and the medullary cavity are filled with bone marrow. Red bone marrow is where blood cells are made in a process known as hematopoiesis (Gr. hemato-blood; poiein, to make). As we mature, much of the red marrow is replaced with fatty yellow marrow except in parts of the ribs, skull, sternum, and vertebrae. The red marrow in these areas will continue to produce red blood cells throughout our lifetime. Like other organs of the body, bones also contain blood vessels, lymph vessels, and nerves.

To withstand the stresses of ordinary activities, bones must have a combination of elasticity and rigidity. Living bones are about 25–30% water, 60–70% mineral salts, and a small percentage of collagen. The collagen forms most of the organic matrix that provides elasticity and resilience. The inorganic minerals that give bone its hardness and rigidity are primarily composed of calcium and phosphate. If the inorganic materials were removed from a bone, it would keep its basic

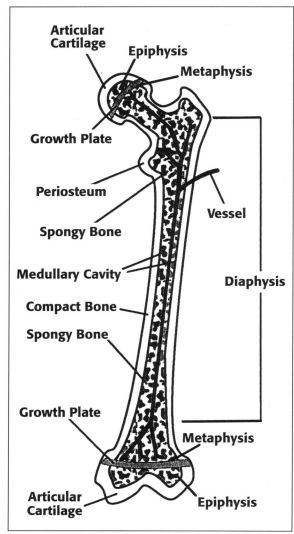

Fig. 7-1. Anatomy of a Femur

Labels on figure:
Articular Cartilage
Epiphysis
Metaphysis
Growth Plate
Periosteum
Vessel
Spongy Bone
Medullary Cavity
Diaphysis
Compact Bone
Spongy Bone
Growth Plate
Metaphysis
Articular Cartilage
Epiphysis

shape, but it would be so flexible, it could be tied into a knot. If all the organic materials were removed, the bone would be brittle and crumble easily. Therefore, the collagen fibers provide tensile strength while the bone salts give compressional strength. Bone strength can vary according to the changes in the amount of organic versus inorganic material as we age. The bones of a child have higher amounts of collagen and are slightly more flexible. As we mature, our bones become more rigid due to ossification (hardening) by an increase in salt crystals.

In addition to the changes in the amount of collagen and minerals, bones are constantly being broken down and repaired or remodeled throughout our lifetime. Wolff's Law states that bone increases or decreases its mass to adapt to functional stresses. The continual remodeling allows bones to become thicker and stronger in response to resistive activities. Conversely, the bones will also become weaker and thinner without any stress. If a leg is in a non-weight-bearing cast, the bones could become 30% decalcified in only a few weeks. That is why load-bearing or resistive activities are recommended to help increase bone density. However, studies have also shown that if the exercise is excessive, fatigue or stress fractures may develop. The amount of exercise that is considered excessive varies from individual to individual.

As we age, the rate of bone replacement gradually becomes slower than the rate of breakdown and our bones become less dense. In severe cases, **osteoporosis** (Gr. osteo-, bone; poros, passage; -osis, disease process) develops where there is a pathological decrease in both the collagen fibers and salt crystals. The osteoporotic bones become brittle, thin, and may fracture easily.

Bone Replacement

The basic structure of bone can be studied by looking at the anatomy of a long bone, such as the femur (thigh bone) shown in Figure 7-1. The main parts of the femur are the diaphysis (shaft or long portion), the epiphyses (ends of the bone; singular is epiphysis), the metaphysis (area between the diaphysis and epiphysis), the articular cartilage, and the periosteum. The articular (L. articulus, joint) cartilage covers the epiphyses (Gr. epi-, upon; phyein, to grow) and reduces the friction at a joint. The **periosteum** (L. peri-, around; L. osteum, bone) is a thin tissue-like covering around the surface of the bone that serves several purposes, including serving as the point of attachment for ligaments and tendons. Blood vessels and nerves supplying the bone are in the periosteum.

The **metaphysis** (Gr. meta-, between) is one of the areas that changes as we age. In a child, the metaphysis is cartilaginous, like columns of spongy tissue, joining the growth plate to the diaphysis. This is the area where the bone lengthens as the child increases in height. Once the bone reaches its adult length, the metaphysis ossifies and connects the diaphysis and epiphysis. If an injury to the growth plate causes premature fusion of the diaphysis and epiphysis, the bone will not grow to its normal length. This is one of the reasons why lifting with heavy weights is not recommended for children whose growth plates have not yet closed. While the diaphysis and epiphysis fuse at varying rates in different parts of the body, most of the bones are fused by about 20 years of age. X-rays, however, provide the most accurate method of determining whether or not the growth plates have closed.

The 206 bones in the human body are often grouped into two broad categories: (a) the axial skeleton (the skull, vertebral column, ribs, and sternum); and (b) the appendicular skeleton (the upper extremities, including the scapulae and clavicles, and the lower extremities, including the pelvic girdle). The **axial skeleton** provides the framework for the trunk and head while the **appendicular skeleton** consists of both arms and legs including the bones that connect these extremities to the axial skeleton. The appendicular skeleton contains trabecular bone, which has a faster turnover rate than the cortical bone found in the axial skeleton and ends of the long bones of the appendicular skeleton. Anterior and posterior views of the human skeleton are shown in Figures 7-2A and 7-2B, while the bones of the axial and appendicular skeleton are listed in Table 7-1.

Joints

Joints are the point at which two or more bones meet or articulate and where movement occurs. There are several different methods of classifying joints, but we will look at two general categories: (a) nonsynovial, and (b) synovial. Nonsynovial joints experience limited movement, while synovial joints are freely movable joints.

Nonsynovial joints are classified according to whether they are held together with fibrous connective tissue or cartilage. The fibrous or synarthrodial joints are immovable. Examples of fibrous joints include the joints between the bones of the skull and where the teeth fit into the mandible (jaw bone). The cartilaginous or amphiarthrodial joints are slightly movable. The amphiarthrodial joints, which are most important to the fitness professional, are the intervertebral joints (between the vertebrae). While there is little movement at one intervertebral joint, the vertebral column as a whole has a wide range of motion.

Synovial joints, also known as diarthrodial joints, are the most common type of joint. They have a small space between the articulating bones that allows a greater range of motion. Cartilage covers the weight-bearing surface of the bones, and the entire joint is enclosed by a capsule.

There are six types of synovial joints. Plane joints, such as those found between the carpal (wrist) bones, allow gliding or sliding movements. Ginglymus or hinge joints are found in the interphalangeal joints of the fingers and allow only flexion and extension movements. Pivot joints permit rotation to occur at places, such as the atlantoaxial joint, where the first cervical (neck) vertebra articulates with the second cervical vertebra. Condyloid joints allow flexion, extension, abduction, and adduction at joints, such as the metacarpophalangeal (knuckle) joints of the hand. Saddle joints, characterized by the carpometacarpal joint of the thumb, allow flexion, extension, abduction, and adduction. Spheroidal, or ball and socket joints, are highly mobile joints found in locations such as the shoulder and hip.

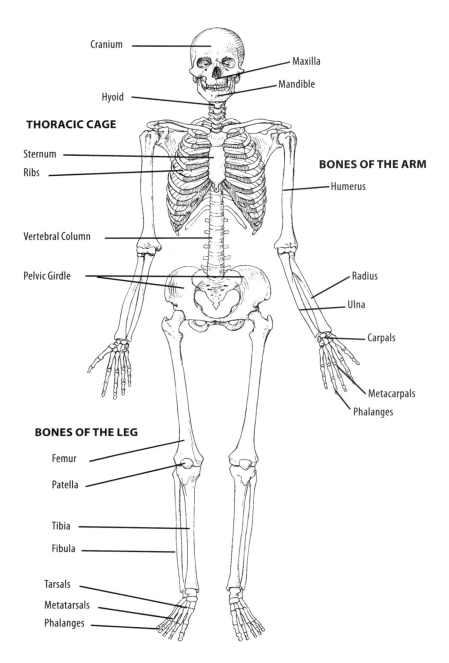

Cranium

Maxilla

Mandible

Hyoid

THORACIC CAGE

Sternum

Ribs

BONES OF THE ARM

Humerus

Vertebral Column

Pelvic Girdle

Radius

Ulna

Carpals

Metacarpals

Phalanges

BONES OF THE LEG

Femur

Patella

Tibia

Fibula

Tarsals

Metatarsals

Phalanges

Fig. 7-2A. Skeleton Anterior View

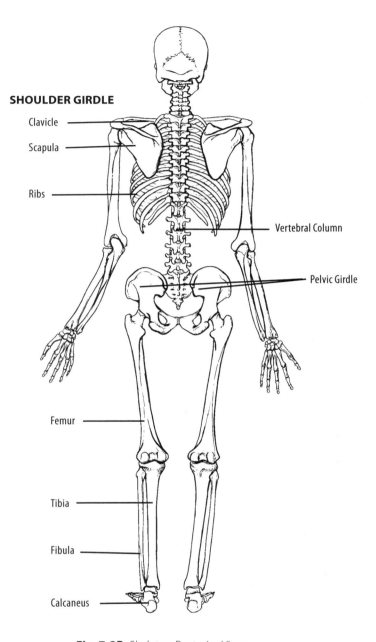

SHOULDER GIRDLE

Clavicle

Scapula

Ribs

Vertebral Column

Pelvic Girdle

Femur

Tibia

Fibula

Calcaneus

Fig. 7-2B. Skeleton Posterior View

Joint Capsule and Ligaments

The joint capsule has two layers: (a) the outer fibrous layer, and (b) the inner synovial membrane. The outer fibrous capsule is often reinforced with ligaments. The ligaments, which connect bone to bone, help prevent joint dislocation with the aid of the joint capsule. When injured or sprained due to excessive or continuous stress, ligaments can become permanently elongated. Once the ligaments across a joint are overstretched, the joint becomes less stable. The inner layer of the capsule, the synovial membrane, secretes synovial fluid. This fluid acts as a lubricant for the articulating surfaces and provides nutrients to the avascular (no direct blood supply) cartilage.

Table 7-1. Bones of the Human Skeleton

	Number of Bones		Number of Bones
AXIAL SKELETON	80	APPENDICULAR SKELETON	126
Skull	29	Upper Limb	64
Cranium (brain box)		Pectoral Girdle	
Parietal		Clavicle	
Temporal		Scapula	
Frontal		Arm	
Occipital		Humerus	
Sphenoid		Radius	
Ethmoid		Ulna	
Nasal		Carpal	
Lacrimal		Metacarpal	
Inferior nasal concha		Phalanges	
Vomer			
Face		Lower Limb	62
Zygomatic		Pelvic Girdle	
Palatine		Ischium	
Mandible		Ilium	
Others		Pubis	
Auditory ossicles		Leg	
Malleus		Femur	
Incus		Patella	
Stapes		Tibia	
		Fibula	
Vertebral Column	26	Tarsal	
Cervical vertebra (7)		Metatarsal	
Thoracic vertebra (12)		Phalanges	
Lumbar vertebra (5)			
Sacral vertebra (5 fused)		TOTAL BONES 206	
Coccygeral vertebra (2–4 fused)			
Rib Cage	25		
Rib (24)			
Sternum (3 fused)			

Range of Motion

The amount of motion that is available to a specific joint is referred to as the range of motion (ROM). In a healthy joint, the ROM is determined by factors such as the shape of the articular surfaces, musculotendinous connections, ligaments, and the joint capsule. The ROM can be pathological when the range is either greater or less than normal. A hypermobile joint is a joint where the available ROM exceeds normal limits. Conversely, a joint may have less than normal ROM or be hypomobile. This hypomobility may be due to many factors, including scar tissue, arthritis, lack of flexibility exercises, or aging. As we grow older, our ligaments and joint capsules, which are constantly being remodeled, are slowly replaced with less collagen. This leads to decreased flexibility. Either hypermobility or hypomobility of a joint can lead to injuries at the affected joint or at nearby joints. Because our joints are linked together in series, an altered movement in one joint can lead to altered movement at another joint.

Cartilage

There are two types of cartilage found in joints: (a) fibrocartilage, and (b) hyaline cartilage. Fibrocartilage is thick and heavy and forms structures, such as the menisci at the knees for a better fit of the femur (thigh bone) on the tibia (shin bone). Hyaline or articular cartilage is found on the articular surfaces of mobile joints. Its purpose is to reduce the friction between the bony surfaces and lessen the impact of the applied force that occurs on the articular surfaces during movement. Cartilage is avascular and aneural. Because it has no blood supply of its own, it depends on synovial fluid for nutrition. The synovial fluid can be distributed to the cartilage during full ROM movements. Immobilization or lack of full ROM at a joint decreases the flow of fluid to the cartilage and can lead to degenerative changes. While the hyaline cartilage has no nerve supply, the bone directly beneath it has many nerves. Therefore, with disease processes like chondromalacia (Gr. chondro-, cartilage; malakia, softness) of the articular cartilage of the patella, pain is felt along the posterior surface of the patella since the cartilage has worn away to expose the nerves of the periosteum covering the femur.

Bone and Joint Disorders

When working with bone and joint disorders, consult with a licensed healthcare professional, such as a physician, who has knowledge of your client's specific condition, abilities, and limitations.

Arthritis

There are two basic types of arthritis (Gr. arthro-, joint; -itis, inflammation of): (a) inflammatory arthritis, and (b) osteoarthritis (Gr. osteon, bone). Inflammatory arthritis, such as rheumatoid arthritis, often attacks synovial joints, such as the metacarpophalangeal joints (knuckles). The disease primarily affects the membrane in the joint capsule that releases synovial fluid. The inflammation of the synovial membrane leads to joint tenderness. During this stage, the swelling also limits the available range of motion. In severe cases, joint damage can lead to a permanent decrease in the range of motion at the joint. The disease is relatively rare and primarily affects women of childbearing age.

Osteoarthritis is the most commonly found joint disorder, and is often described as either a result of trauma or a normal result of aging and "wear and tear" on the joints. The articular cartilage slowly deteriorates while bony overgrowths may also occur within the joint. As the space in the joint cavity decreases, joint movements become more painful and restricted. Studies have shown that by 40 years of age, many people have some evidence of "wear and tear" osteoarthritis; by 75 years of age, almost everyone will have osteoarthritis in at least one joint. People who have injured a joint may develop osteoarthritis at an earlier age.

Herniated (slipped) Disc

A common cause of low-back pain is a herniated disc. The intervertebral disc, composed of the nucleus pulposus and annulus fibrosus (L. annulus, ring; fibrosus, composed of fibers), does not actually slip out of place. The gel-like center, the nucleus pulposus, may move posteriorly and either break through the annulus fibrosus or cause the fibrocartilage to press on structures, such as spinal nerve roots. The pressure can lead to various signs and symptoms, including low-back pain, decreased sensation, or muscle weakness in the lower extremities.

Osteoporosis

Osteoporosis refers to a condition where the bones have decreased calcium due to a decrease in osteoblastic activity to form new bone. The bones lose enough mineral salts to become more susceptible to fractures. It seems to be more common among middle-aged or elderly white females. Some of the factors that may contribute to osteoporosis include decreased levels of estrogen, calcium deficiency or malabsorption, and inactivity.

Sprain and Strain

Sprains refer to an overstretching of ligaments, while strains indicate that the damage occurred to a muscle.

Muscles

There are three types of muscle found in the human body: (a) skeletal, (b) smooth, and (c) cardiac muscle. Skeletal muscle is attached to bone via tendons and allows voluntary movement of the body. Because of its striped or band-like appearance under the microscope, skeletal muscle is also known as striated muscle tissue. Smooth muscle is nonstriated and is found in the walls of organs, such as the stomach and intestines. Because it does not require conscious control for a contraction, smooth muscle is also called involuntary muscle.

Cardiac muscle forms the walls of the heart. While cardiac muscle is striated in appearance, it does not require our conscious thoughts to contract and pump blood through the body.

Skeletal Muscle

Skeletal muscle makes up approximately 44–51% of total body weight in men and 35–42% total body weight in women. It is composed of contractile tissue, including muscle fibers, and connects to tendons surrounded by fascial sheaths. The muscle fibers are the portion that shorten or contract during muscular contraction. Tendons are noncontractile and connect the muscle to the periosteum of the bone or cartilage by Sharpey's fibers. Fascia is the thin, translucent covering that forms a sheath for an individual muscle or muscle group.

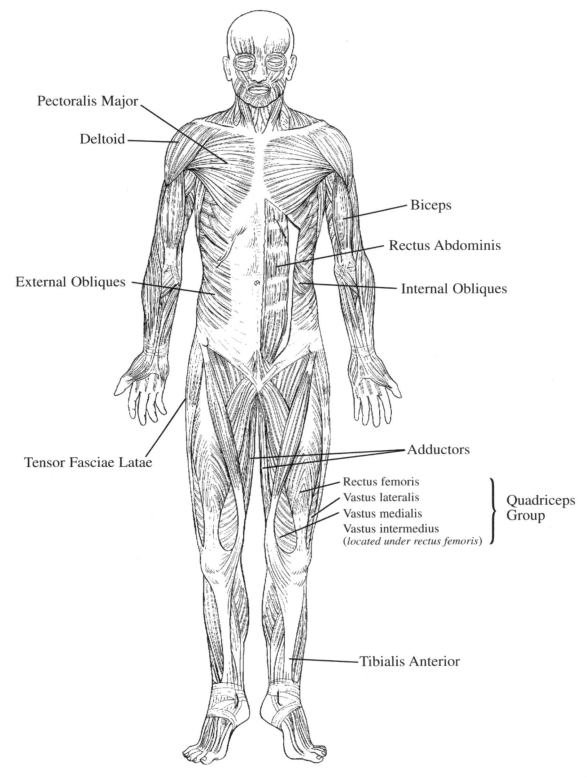

Pectoralis Major

Deltoid

Biceps

Rectus Abdominis

External Obliques

Internal Obliques

Adductors

Tensor Fasciae Latae

Rectus femoris
Vastus lateralis
Vastus medialis
Vastus intermedius
(*located under rectus femoris*)

Quadriceps
Group

Tibialis Anterior

Fig. 7-3A. Muscular System Anterior View

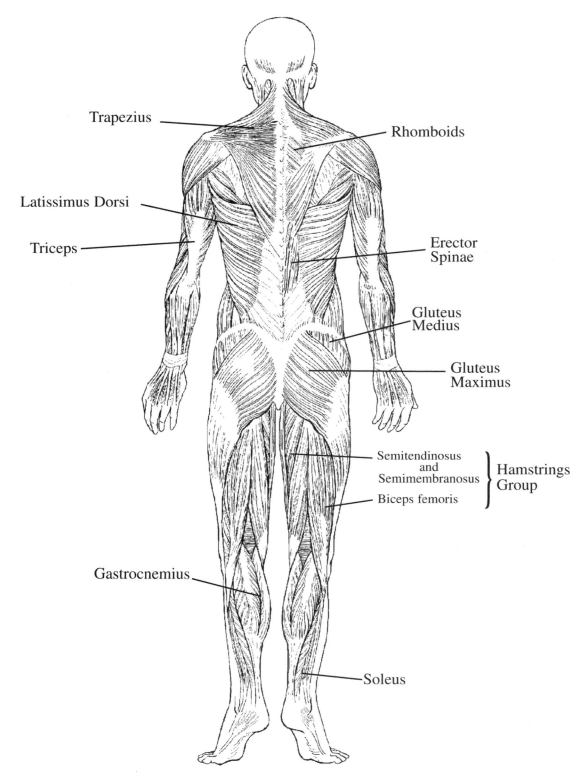

Fig. 7-3B. Muscular System Posterior View

Sliding Filament Theory

Each skeletal muscle is composed of thousands of muscle fibers or myofibers (Gr. myo-, muscle). The myofibers can be further broken down into functional units known as sarcomeres. Within the sarcomere are thick myofilaments (myosin) and thin myofilaments (actin). According to Huxley's sliding filament theory, these myofilaments are thought to be the structures that allow a muscle to contract or shorten (Figure 7-4). The myosin filaments have tiny crossbridges with a swivel head located at one end. These swivel heads have both an actin-binding site and an ATP-binding site. During a muscle contraction, the myosin head attaches itself to a myosin-binding site on the actin. With the energy from the ATP, the head swivels and draws the actin in toward the center of the sarcomere. As multiple myosin crossbridges simultaneously pull the actin inward, the entire sarcomere shortens. The shortening of the sarcomeres causes the muscle fibers to shorten and a muscle contraction occurs.

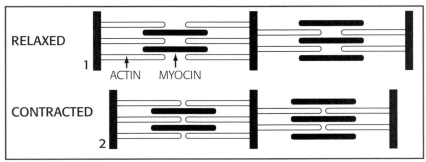

Fig. 7-4. Sliding Filament Theory

Types of Muscle Fiber

There are two basic types of muscle fibers found in skeletal muscle. Type I fibers are slow twitch or slow oxidative (SO) fibers, and Type II are fast twitch or fast glycolytic (FG) fibers. Slow twitch muscle fibers are designed for prolonged, submaximal aerobic activities and are slow to fatigue. These SO fibers are characterized by a large amount of myoglobin and a high number of mitochrondria that give a reddish color to the fibers. Aerobic energy metabolism occurs within the mitochrondria to generate ATP. The slow twitch muscle fibers are used for long-term, low- to moderate-intensity activities ranging from maintaining proper posture to long distance running. Fast twitch or FG muscle fibers are able to generate quick, high-intensity contractions, but are more easily fatigued. Because they rely predominantly on the anaerobic metabolic system for energy, they have less myoglobin and mitochrondria. Type II fibers are used in short-spurt activities, such as sprinting.

In humans, there appear to be several variations of the Type II fibers. Type IIa fibers have the capacity to use both aerobic and anaerobic energy systems and are known as fast-oxidative-glycolytic or FOG fibers. Type IIb fibers (also referred to as Type IIx) are the FG fibers previously described. Type IIc fibers are rare, undifferentiated fibers. Some research indicates that fibers may be able to change from one type to another as an adaptation to aerobic or anaerobic training. Therefore, with aerobic training, there may be an increase in Type I fibers; with anaerobic training there may be an increase in Type II fibers. Among elite competitors, endurance athletes have a high percentage of slow twitch muscle fibers while the groups trained for anaerobic-type sports exhibit more fast twitch fibers. What remains unclear, however, is how much was genetically predetermined, how much is due to increased efficiency of the original fibers from specific training, and how much is due to fiber transformation.

Muscle Innervation

The stimulus for a muscle contraction comes from a specialized nerve cell or motor neuron. Each motor neuron can transmit signals to a number of myofibers. One motor neuron and all the myofibers that it stimulates are called a motor unit. In areas needing fine motor control, such as the eye, a motoneuron may only connect with 5–10 muscle fibers. In larger muscles that require greater contractions, a single motor unit may have as many as 500 myofibers. Each motor unit follows the all-or-none principle. When the motoneuron is stimulated, all the muscle fibers in the unit will fire simultaneously. A contraction of only a portion of the fibers in an individual motor unit is not possible. However, to allow for smooth muscle contractions and to avoid fatigue, all the motor units in a muscle will not contract at the same time.

Recruitment refers to the number of motor units that are stimulated for a specific muscular response. The firing of the motoneurons will alternate to allow some motor units to contract while others relax. This system of recruitment allows the muscle to sustain a contraction for a longer period of time before fatigue sets in. It is also thought to contribute to muscle tone, where a muscle stays in partial contraction. In activities requiring power, where a high degree of force needs to be generated quickly, more motor units are fired simultaneously. However, since more of the units are being stimulated at any one time, fatigue will occur more quickly.

In a voluntary contraction, the brain sends a signal down through the spinal cord to the motoneurons to stimulate the appropriate motor units. According to the "size principle," the order of motor recruitment is usually from small to large. Therefore, the smallest motor units are normally recruited first. To recruit more motor units, it is necessary to increase the workload of the targeted muscles. When a muscle is overloaded or fatigued, assistor muscles will be recruited to help accomplish the task.

Proprioceptors

Proprioceptors in the muscle and tendon sense the degree of tension and the length of the muscle. The muscle spindle, the proprioceptive receptor that attaches to the sheaths of the surrounding muscle fibers, is parallel with the muscle. It sends afferent information to the brain about changes in muscle length and the speed at which the changes are occurring. When stimulated, the muscle spindles relay a message to the spinal cord to cause a contraction in the same muscle. The afferent or sensory neurons in the muscle spindle communicate with the motoneurons of the target muscle through interneurons in the spinal cord without requiring any conscious thought. This spinal reflex is known as the stretch reflex. When ballistic movements are used, the muscle spindles will sense the quick changes in muscle length and cause a muscular contraction. A physician checks the spinal reflex of the quadriceps by tapping on the patellar tendon to cause the knee to extend. Physical therapists use the stretch reflex to stimulate a muscle contraction when the patient is too weak to complete the movement.

The **Golgi tendon organ**, located in the tendon, is described as being in series with the muscle fibers. This proprioceptor protects the muscle from excessive contractions or stretches. It senses tension caused by muscular contraction or extreme stretching. When stimulated by excessive tension or stretching, the Golgi tendon organ inhibits contraction of the muscle from which it originates. This reflex inhibition is used in the proprioceptive neuromuscular facilitation (PNF) stretching technique known as hold-relax. With this PNF technique, the tight muscle is put on a light to moderate stretch. The client is asked to contract the target muscle isometrically for a few seconds. He or she is then asked to relax, and to further stretch the target muscle by contracting the opposing muscle group. This technique can be repeated several times until there are no further gains in range of motion or the client experiences any discomfort. To avoid muscle injury, the client should perform the movements without any additional resistance from external sources such as a fitness instructor. When done properly, the muscle will relax and increase its length due to the reflex inhibition from the Golgi tendon organ of the target muscle.

Types of Muscle Contractions

There are five types of muscle contractions (also referred to as muscle actions): (a) isometric (equal length), (b) concentric (shortening), (c) eccentric (lengthening), (d) isotonic (equal tension), and (e) isokinetic (equal or same motion). In an **isometric** (Gr. isos-, equal; metron, measure) contraction, no joint movement occurs. In physics, work is defined as force times distance. By this definition, no work is done because the bony lever has not been moved any distance. However, energy is expended and calories are burned to maintain the contraction. When using isometric contractions for strengthening, it is important to remember that the muscle will only be strengthened at the specific joint angle used in the exercise. To strengthen a muscle throughout its entire range, it will be necessary to do exercises throughout the full range of motion. Isometric contractions have also been found to increase blood pressure.

In a **concentric** contraction, the muscle fibers are shortening and positive work is done against gravity or an external resistance. On the other hand, an **eccentric** contraction, or negative work, occurs when the muscle fibers lengthen and the bony levers move into the direction of gravity. Strength gains throughout the range of motion can be achieved with either concentric or eccentric exercises. The difference is the amount of energy expended to perform the action. Eccentric contractions require the least amount of energy, isometric contractions use a moderate amount of energy, and concentric contractions require the most energy. Eccentric contractions also appear to be associated with delayed onset muscle soreness. Newcomers to step or high-impact aerobic classes sometimes experience delayed onset muscle soreness in their calves, which can be due to the repeated eccentric contractions of the gastrocnemius and soleus as the heel is lowered to the floor.

An **isotonic** contraction is one in which the tension remains constant as the muscle shortens or lengthens. It is rarely used during human performance, but is commonly referred to when describing dynamic free weight or resistance machine exercises.

Isokinetic contractions or movements are those in which the muscle shortens at a constant rate, and cannot be done without the use of specialized equipment. Due to the changing resistance of gravity and the ability of the muscle to contract, certain portions of a full-range-of-motion contraction are harder to perform than others. When working with free weights, the most difficult portion is often where a spotter is needed to assist with the exercise. Isokinetic equipment is designed to vary the resistance so that the speed of the movement is constant. Therefore, where a person would normally require a spotter with free weights, the isokinetic equipment makes the exercise easier to complete.

Levers

When looking at the forces required to perform a joint action, it is necessary to understand the three basic types of levers. Levers are rigid rods that move about a fulcrum or pivot point. Acting on the lever are two different types of forces: (a) resistance, and (b) effort. In the human body, the levers are the bones, the fulcrum is the joint, the effort force comes from the muscle, and the resistance force comes from gravity. The resistance force may also be increased with the use of training aids, such as weights or elastic bands.

The three types of levers are: (a) first-class, (b) second-class, and (c) third-class (Figure 7-5A). They are classified according to the placement of the fulcrum, the effort or applied force, and the resistance force on the lever. A **first-class lever** occurs when the fulcrum is in between the applied force (AF) and the resistance (R). The classic example of a first-class lever is the see-saw. A **second-class lever** is when the fulcrum or axis is at one end of the lever, resistance is in the middle, and the effort force is at the opposite end. The wheelbarrow is an example of a second-class lever. A **third-class lever** also has the axis at one end, but now the applied force is in the middle and the resistance is at the end. Using a hammer to drive a nail into a piece of wood is an example of a third-class lever.

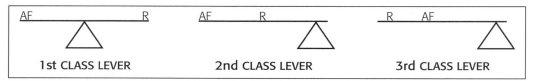

Fig. 7-5A. First-, Second-, and Third-Class Lever Systems

In addition to looking at the placement of the fulcrum, applied force, and resistance force, it is also important to understand the concept of mechanical advantage. The perpendicular distance from the pivot point to the line of action of the resistive force is known as the resistance arm. The effort or force arm would be the perpendicular distance from the fulcrum to the point of application of the applied force. Mechanical advantage refers to the relationship between the length of the effort arm and the length of the resistance arm. The equation for this relationship is Mechanical Advantage = Force Arm ÷ Resistance Arm.

As the length of the force arm increases, or as the resistance arm decreases, the mechanical advantage increases. In other words, the ease with which a task can be accomplished increases as the length of the force arm increases. Conversely, more muscular force is required if the force arm is shorter than the resistance arm. The patella, located in the quadriceps tendon, lengthens the force arm of the quadriceps muscle to increase the effectiveness of the muscle (Figure 7-6).

In a first-class lever, either the resistive force or the applied force may have the mechanical advantage depending on the exact placement of all three items. The force arm will always be longer in a second-class lever while the resistance arm will always be longer in a third-class lever. Gravity will always have a mechanical advantage in a third-class lever system. However, it is possible to achieve a greater range of motion at a faster speed at the distal end of a third-class lever system.

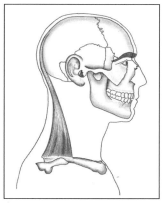

Fig. 7-5B. First-Class Lever at Skull and First Cervical Vertebra

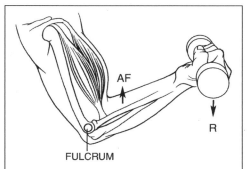

Fig. 7-5C. Typical Third-Class Lever System

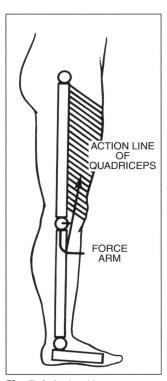

Fig. 7-6. Action Line

There are few examples of first- and second-class levers in the human body. Experts in biomechanics disagree about the exact number and examples of first- and second-class levers in the human body. The atlantooccipital joint, where the skull articulates with the first cervical vertebra, is an example of a first-class lever, shown in Figure 7-5B. The weight of the skull pulls the head forward while neck extensors, such as the trapezius, extend the head to keep it balanced on the vertebral column. In a full-body push-up, the entire body acts as a second-class lever. The toes are the axis, the rigid body is the lever, gravity is the resistive force and the arms supply the effort force. While there is general discussion about the clearest examples of first- and second-class levers in the human body, it is agreed that most of the musculoskeletal system is composed of third-class levers. While it requires more muscle force to move the body in a third-class lever system, it allows for greater speed and range of motion (Figure 7-5C).

When describing motions of the human body, it is common to assume that the movements are initiated with the body starting in anatomical position. According to K. Moore (2009), anatomical position is standing erect with the head, eyes, and toes directed forward, the heels and toes together, and the upper limbs hanging by the sides with the palms facing anteriorly. Motions are also named by the movement occurring at the joint rather than the segment that is moving. Therefore, "flexing the elbow" is more accurate than "bending the arm." Movements may be further described by the planes in which they occur. Figure 7-7 illustrates the three cardinal planes: (a) sagittal, (b) frontal, and (c) horizontal (or transverse). Table 7-2 indicates the joint, possible movements, and the planes in which the movements occur.

A muscle has at least two points of attachment on the skeleton. The most **proximal** (nearest to the center of the body) attachment is called the origin, and the more **distal** (L. distans, distant) attachment is referred to as the insertion. Conventionally, a muscle is said to bring the insertion closer to the origin during a concentric contraction. This is because the insertion is often on the most movable bone while the origin is located on the most stable bone. However, when muscle fibers contract, they simply shorten the distance between the ends of the sarcomeres. The least stable end of the joint will move toward the most stable end. In the arm, it is then easy to see how the insertion of the biceps on the radius (bone in the forearm) comes closer to its origin on the scapula during a biceps curl. However, in a pull-up, because the hands are fixed on an immovable bar, the rest of the body actually moves toward the insertion. Therefore, some fitness professionals will use the terms proximal and distal attachments rather than origin and insertion.

A straight line drawn between the centers of the proximal and distal attachments will indicate the direction of the muscle's line of pull or line of action (Figure 7-6). The power that a muscle can generate is partially dependent on its line of pull. Muscles with parallel fibers (fusiform muscles), such as the rectus femoris portion of the quadriceps, can lift a weight through a long distance at great speed (Figure 7-8A).

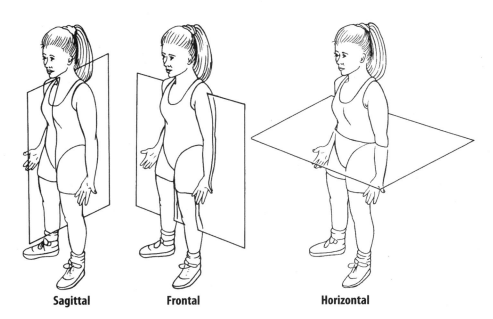

Sagittal   **Frontal**   **Horizontal**

Fig. 7-7. Sagittal, Frontal and Horizontal Planes

Some muscles have fibers that run obliquely to the long axis of the muscle. Because of their resemblance to a feather, they are called **pennate** (L. penna, feather) muscles. Pennate muscles may be unipennate, bipennate, or multipennate, such as the deltoid. The advantage of pennate muscles is that they can contract with greater force than fusiform muscles, but at the expense of speed (Figure 7-8B).

Muscles work together to accomplish a task. The muscle(s) performing the work are called **agonists** or primary movers. **Assistors** are muscles that help perform the same task. **Stabilizers** help prevent undesired or unnecessary motions. The muscle opposing the agonist is known as the **antagonist**. Because it has an action directly opposite to a primary mover, the antagonist must relax and elongate to allow the agonist to move the joint. This occurs due to a spinal reflex known as reciprocal innervation. In a biceps curl, during elbow flexion, the brachialis, biceps brachii, and brachioradialis are the agonists. The triceps must relax during elbow flexion since it is the antagonist. There is some disagreement among fitness professionals about the use of the word synergist. Some people use the word **synergist** to describe assistor muscles. Others describe synergists as muscles that complement the action of the primary mover by preventing unnecessary movements. For example, the anconeus prevents excessive supination by the biceps brachii as the elbow flexes. Fixator or stabilizer muscles steady the proximal joints to allow movement at distal joints. The deltoid is a fixator muscle that helps stabilize the humeral head during fine motor activities, such as writing.

The amount of tension that a muscle can develop is affected by its length. The optimal length for creating tension is close to the muscle's resting length. At this stage, the actin and myosin filaments are

Table 7-2. Joints, Possible Movements and Planes		
Joint	**Movement**	**Plane**
Vertebral Column	Flexion-Extension	Sagittal
	Lateral Flexion	Frontal
	Rotation	Horizontal
Shoulder	Flexion-Extension	Sagittal
	Abduction-Adduction	Frontal
	Inward-Outward Rotation	Horizontal
	Horizontal Abduction-Adduction	Horizontal
Elbow	Flexion-Extension	Sagittal
Radioulnar	Pronation-Supination	Horizontal
Wrist	Flexion-Extension	Sagittal
Hip	Flexion-Extension	Sagittal
	Abduction-Adduction	Frontal
	Inward-Outward Rotation	Horizontal
Knee	Flexion-Extension	Sagittal
	Inward-Outward Rotation (when knee is flexed at 90°)	Horizontal
Ankle	Dorsi-Plantar Flexion	Sagittal

capable of forming the greatest number of crossbridges to shorten the muscle. If the muscle is stretched beyond its normal limit, there is less overlap of the actin and myosin filaments to form crossbridges. When the muscle is in its shortened position, the crossbridges have already been formed so there are no more available actin and myosin filaments to generate any additional tension.

When a muscle is in a shortened position in which it cannot form any additional crossbridges, it is said to be in **active insufficiency**. The muscle cannot generate any additional tension because all of the crossbridges have been formed, and there are no additional actin and myosin filaments to slide across each other. Active insufficiency is easily demonstrated with biarticular or two-joint muscles. These muscles cross two or more joints and can cause motion at more than one joint. For example, because the hamstrings cross both the hip joint and the knee joint, they can extend the hip and flex the knee. However, when attempting to perform hamstring curls in the prone position with the hips extended, it is common to see people flex their hips near the end of the range of motion to bring their heels toward their buttocks. This is because their hamstrings are in active insufficiency since the hips are in extension and the knees are in flexion. In order to generate more tension, they flex their hips to allow more crossbridges to be formed to allow for knee flexion. Table 7-3 shows some biarticular muscles and the joints they cross.

Table 7-3. The Biarticulate Muscles and the Articulations They Cross	
Muscle	**Articulations**
Biceps Brachii	Shoulder/Elbow
Triceps	Shoulder/Elbow
Rectus Femoris	Hip/Knee
Semitendinosus	Hip/Knee
Semimembranosus	Hip/Knee
Biceps Femoris	Hip/Knee
Sartorius	Hip/Knee
Gastrocnemius	Knee/Ankle

Kinetic Chains

In engineering, kinetic (Gr. kinema, motion) chains are a series of rigid links interconnected by a series of pin-centered joints. Motion at one of the links will cause movement at the other joints due to their relationship to each other. In the body, it is possible to have open or closed kinetic chains. In an open kinetic chain, the terminal joint is free while it is fixed in a closed kinetic chain. Closed kinetic chains behave like the engineering kinetic chains—movement at one joint will cause motion in all the related joints. For example, if you keep both feet on the floor and bend your knees, you will also flex at the hips and dorsiflex at the ankles. Because the feet are fixed on the ground, the legs are operating as a closed kinetic chain. If you allow your foot to leave the floor as you bend one knee, no other joint movement has to occur. This is referred to as an open kinetic chain. The concept of closed chain exercises is important because muscles at other joints in the chain can substitute for the target muscle. In a push-up, the triceps muscle extends the elbow and the pectoralis major adducts the humerus to lift the body up against gravity. However, in this position, external rotation at the shoulders will also cause the elbows to extend and lift the body. The ability of the external rotators to assist in a push-up is easily demonstrated by first performing a push-up with both arms in the sagittal plane and the elbows close to the torso and pointed toward the feet throughout the entire exercise. Then, start with both arms in the horizontal plane and the elbows pointed away from the body and bring them in toward the torso as you lift. The second exercise will be less fatiguing to the triceps because the external rotators have assisted the movement.

We have now addressed the basic musculoskeletal anatomy and kinesiology of the human body. While a general understanding of how the body moves through space is useful, it is also important to look at specific joints that are used during exercise. A comprehensive look at the major joints of the body is beyond the scope of this book, but we will look at some specific details of the shoulder, the vertebral column, the hip and the knee.

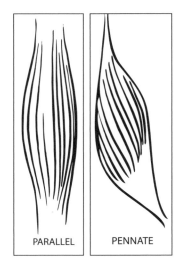

PARALLEL PENNATE

Fig. 7-8A & B.
Shapes of Muscles

The Shoulder Complex

The shoulder complex is composed of three bones: (a) the clavicle (collarbone), (b) the scapula (shoulder blade), and (c) the humerus (arm bone). These bones, together with the scapular and shoulder muscles and connective tissue, perform the complicated task of allowing dynamic stability. The shoulder complex has a larger range of motion than any other part of the body. At the same time, it has to provide a stable base for the rest of the upper extremity so the hand can perform fine motor skills.

The clavicles and the scapulae form the shoulder or pectoral girdle. The anterior portion of the pectoral girdle is formed by the clavicles while the posterior portion is comprised of the scapulae. The proximal end of a clavicle and the sternum (breast bone) form the sternoclavicular joint. This is the only bony attachment for the upper extremity to the axial skeleton. Muscles secure the shoulder girdle to the rest of the body.

The lateral portion of the scapula forms a small cup-like projection that is called the glenoid fossa (Gr. glene, a socket; L. fossa, trench or ditch). The head of the humerus (arm bone) articulates with the glenoid fossa and forms the glenohumeral joint. As a spheroidal or ball-and-socket joint, the glenohumeral joint provides a great deal of mobility to the upper extremity. However, the scapula can also move to further increase the available range of motion for the upper limb.

While the scapula moves along the thorax (rib cage), it is not a true anatomic joint because it has none of the characteristics of a joint. The movements of the scapula, however, are commonly described as motions of the scapulothoracic joint. The motions of the scapula include elevation/depression, abduction/adduction, and upward rotation/downward rotation (Figures 7-9A, B, C, D).

The dynamic stability of the shoulder complex can be demonstrated in the motions necessary to change a light bulb in the ceiling. In order to raise the hand over the head, the glenohumeral joint has to flex while the scapula rotates in an upward direction. Once the hand is in position, the muscles of the pectoral girdle have to stabilize the entire shoulder complex so the hand can unscrew the light bulb.

Because most motions of the shoulder complex involve both the scapulothoracic joint and the glenohumeral joint, a complete exercise program should include exercises for muscles that move the scapula and muscles that move the humerus. Table 7-4 shows the major muscles of the pectoral girdle and the glenohumeral joint.

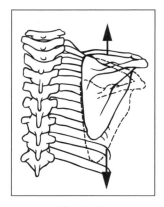

Fig. 7-9A.
Elevation/Depression

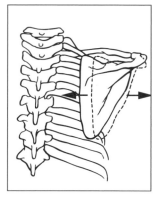

Fig. 7-9B.
Adduction/Abduction

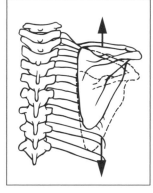

Fig. 7-9C.
Upward Rotation

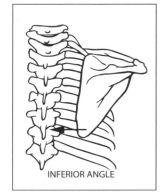

Fig. 7-9D.
Downward Rotation

The Vertebral Column

Figure 7-10 shows that the vertebral column is typically composed of 26 vertebrae: (a) 7 cervical (neck), (b) 12 thoracic (where the ribs attach), (c) 5 lumbar (lower back), (d) 5 sacral (fused to form the sacrum), and (e) 4 coccygeal (fused to form the coccyx or tailbone). The majority of the vertebrae have a body, a spinous process in the back, and transverse processes on either side. Behind the body is an opening or foramen through which the spinal cord passes. The spinal cord conducts **afferent**, or sensory, messages from the body up to the brain and **efferent**, or motor signals, down from the brain to various parts of the body. Certain afferent signals trigger specific motor responses in the spinal cord without going to the brain. These automatic responses that do not require our conscious thought are known as spinal reflexes.

Located between adjacent vertebral bodies to form the cartilagenous joints are the **intervertebral discs**. The discs have a soft, gel-like center called the nucleus pulposus surrounded by the annulus fibrosus (L. annulus, ring; fibrosus, composed of fibers). While the nucleus pulposus is usually found in the center of a disc, it is located more posteriorly in the cervical and lumbar regions. While each joint has limited movement, the intervertebral joints together contribute to the motions of the entire spinal column.

Table 7-4. Shoulder Joint and Pectoral Girdle Actions	
Shoulder Joint Actions	**Primary Mover**
Flexion	Deltoid
Extension	Latissimus Dorsi
Abduction	Deltoid, Supraspinatus
Adduction	Latissimus Dorsi
Internal Rotation	Subscapularis
External Rotation	Infraspinatus, Teres Minor
Horizontal Adduction	Pectoralis Major
Horizontal Abduction	Deltoid
Pectoral Girdle Actions	**Primary Mover**
Elevation	Trapezius, Levator Scapulae
Depression	Trapezius
Abduction	Serratus Anterior
Adduction	Trapezius, Rhomboids
Upward Rotation	Trapezius
Downward Rotation	Rhomboids

As a major portion of the axial skeleton, it is important that the vertebral column be properly aligned to protect the spinal cord, to bear the weight of the body and to provide, with the ribs, a framework for the attachment of our internal organs. There are four distinct curves in the normal vertebral column. Two of them, the cervical curve and the lumbar curve, are concave posteriorly (open to the back of the body). The thoracic and sacral curves are concave anteriorly. The purpose of these curves is to provide flexibility and shock-absorbing capacity to the spinal column. The spinal curves allow the vertebral column to handle axial compressive loads up to ten times greater than what could be expected from a straight spine. That is why proper alignment through the trunk is important during all of our regular activities including exercising.

Several structures work together to help maintain proper alignment of the spine. The shape of the vertebral bodies and the interver-

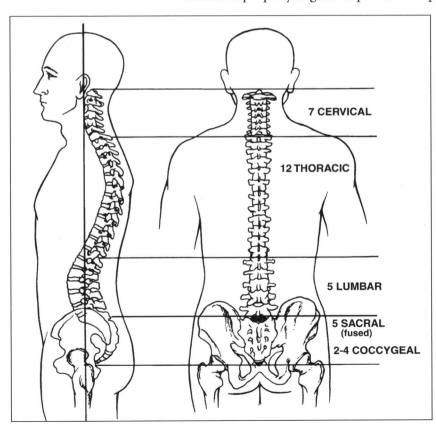

7 CERVICAL

12 THORACIC

5 LUMBAR

5 SACRAL (fused)

2-4 COCCYGEAL

Fig. 7-10. The Spinal Column

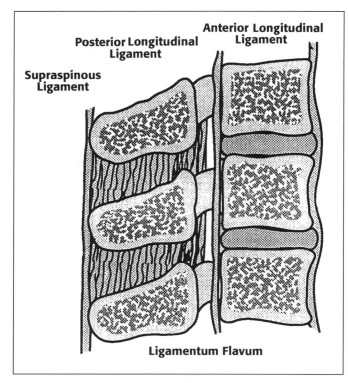

Fig. 7-11. Ligaments of the Vertebral Column

tebral discs is primarily responsible for the four spinal curves. The muscles that can affect the curves of the spine should be balanced in strength and flexibility. Many ligaments also provide stability throughout the length of the vertebral column (Figure 7-11).

Along the front of the vertebral bodies is the **anterior longitudinal ligament**, which is considered by some researchers to be the strongest ligament in the body. Along with the spinal muscles, the anterior longitudinal ligament limits spinal hyperextension and provides strength to the anterior portion of the intervertebral disc during lifting activities. The posterior longitudinal ligament reinforces the posterior annulus fibrosus and runs along the back side of the vertebral bodies. However, it is much narrower than the anterior longitudinal ligament and only attaches to the margins of the vertebral bodies to allow the blood vessels and lymph vessels to enter and exit the vertebrae. In the lumbar region, it is often narrowed to a cord-shaped filament and gives reduced support to the intervertebral discs. In the lumbar region, another posterior stabilizing ligament, the interspinous ligament, has been found to be weak or ruptured in 90% of the subjects studied who were over 40 years of age. The posterior longitudinal ligament, along with other ligaments and spinal muscles, such as the erector spinae, limit the degree of forward flexion.

In the United States, some studies have found that 80% of the general population will suffer from **back pain**. Back pain is currently the most expensive ailment among people in the 30–60-year-old category. While many disease processes can produce low-back pain, the primary causes of low-back pain appear to be poor posture, faulty body mechanics, stress, decreased flexibility, and poor physical fitness. Examples of poor posture include sitting in a slumped posture, leaning forward while standing, and standing with an excessive lumbar curve. Faulty body mechanics include one of the most common mechanisms for back injuries: bending forward and lifting while twisting.

All of these factors do not allow the vertebral column to maintain its natural spinal curves. Therefore, the flexibility and strength of the spine is compromised in these situations. While muscle contractions or spasms are commonly associated with low-back pain, some professionals do not believe that muscle spasms are the primary cause of the pain. These people believe that the back muscles tighten to prevent further movements that may aggravate the pain. Poor posture and faulty body mechanics can lead to back pain by causing intervertebral disc protrusions or herniations. Because the nucleus pulposus is a gel-like substance, it can protrude through the annulus fibrosus and irritate the spinal nerves as they exit the vertebral column. The higher incidence of intervertebral disc problems in the lumbar area may be due to the posterior position of the nucleus pulposus and the decreased strength of some of the posterior ligaments in this area. Both of these factors increase the opportunity for an intervertebral disc to bulge or herniate posteriorly. When a disc protrudes posteriorly, it can cause many

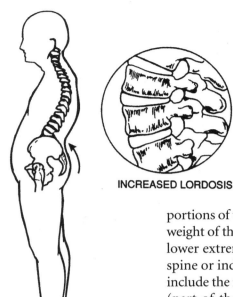

INCREASED LORDOSIS

Fig. 7-12A.
Anterior Pelvic Tilt

different signs and symptoms, including low-back pain, if it puts pressure on the spinal cord or spinal nerves in the area.

There is considerable controversy among health professionals about how much muscle weakness contributes to low-back pain. Some people feel that the erector spinae, as well as abdominal muscles and other spinal muscles, should be strengthened; others feel that muscle endurance is more important than strength; and still another group believes that there is not a clear cut relationship between muscle strength and endurance and low-back pain.

It is also important to look at the other muscles that can affect the lumbar curve. Near the bottom of the vertebral column is the sacrum, which is wedged between the two ileum (the posterior portions of the pelvic girdle). It is at this junction, the sacroiliac (SI) joint, that the weight of the head, upper body, and trunk is transferred to the pelvis and then the lower extremities. Muscles that can directly change the position of the lumbar spine or indirectly affect the spine by changing the position of the pelvic girdle include the rectus abdominus, the erector spinae, the iliopsoas, the rectus femoris (part of the quadriceps), and the hamstrings. These muscles need adequate strength and flexibility to maintain the pelvis in neutral alignment. Too much of an anterior tilt of the pelvis will lead to an increased lordotic curve (Figure 7-12A), while a posterior tilt (Figure 7-12B) can eliminate the normal curve of the lumbar spine (Figure 7-12C). Either extreme can be a contributing factor to low-back pain. Weak abdominals and hamstrings together with tight erector spinae and iliopsoas can cause an increased lordosis. Tight hamstrings with weak hip flexors and erector spinae can lead to a posterior tilt and lack of a normal lumbar curve. For muscle balancing, the tight muscles should be stretched and the weak muscles should be strengthened. AFAA's *Basic Exercise Standards and Guidelines* (found in Chapter 17 of this text) provides several recommendations for strengthening the erector spinae and stabilizing the torso safely and effectively.

The recommendations are designed for participants with normal, healthy backs. Instructors may wish to refer people with a predisposition for back problems to a licensed health care provider for more specific exercise prescriptions.

Abnormal curvatures of the spine, shown in Figure 7-13, include scoliosis, kyphosis, and lordosis. Scoliosis (Gr. skolios, twisted) is the most common of the three conditions and is a lateral bending of the spine. Kyphosis (Gr. kyphos, a hump) refers to an exaggerated curve in the thoracic area. Lordosis (Gr. lordos, bent backward) is an increased concave curve in the lumbar portion of the spine. This condition is often accompanied by an increased anterior tilt of the pelvis.

Core strengthening exercises are normally designed to increase the stability of the axial skeleton. Specialty programs like this require a deeper understanding of additional core muscles known as the pelvic floor muscles or the pelvic rotator cuff. These muscles work with the abdominal and spinal muscles to hold or move the trunk. Exercises that push the pelvic floor muscles downward or create a muscular imbalance among the core muscles can lead to pelvic or low-back pain, incontinence, and problems with balance. While considered a women's issue, both men and women can be affected by these conditions. If your participants have complaints of this type, refer them to a licensed professional with training in treating pelvic floor conditions.

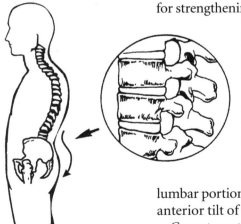

Fig. 7-12B.
Posterior Pelvic Tilt

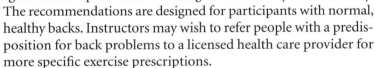

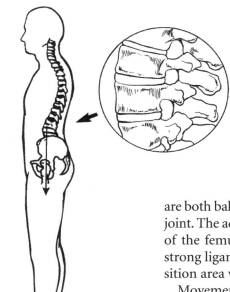

Fig. 7-12C.
Normal Curvature

The Hip

The hip is a spheroidal, or ball and socket, joint like the glenohumeral joint. The joint is formed where the pelvic girdle meets the femur (thigh bone) (Figure 7-14).

The pelvic girdle is composed of the two coxa or innominate (L. innominatus, nameless) bones. The innominate bones are united anteriorly at a fibrocartilagenous joint, the symphysis pubis. Posteriorly, the coxa bones meet the sacrum to form the sacroiliac joint. Each coxa bone is constructed from three fused bones: (a) the ilium, (b) the ischium, and (c) the pubis. The three bones meet and form a socket known as the acetabulum. This is where the femur articulates with the pelvis. While they are both ball and socket joints, the hip joint is more stable than the glenohumeral joint. The acetabulum forms a deeper socket than the glenoid cavity and the head of the femur forms a more complete sphere than the humeral head. Several strong ligaments add to further stability at the hip joint. The hips are the transition area where the weight of the body is transferred to the legs.

Movements of the hip include flexion/extension, abduction/adduction, and medial/lateral rotation. The primary muscle that flexes the hip joint is the iliopsoas assisted by the rectus femoris, a portion of the quadriceps that also crosses the hip. The hip extensors include the hamstrings and the gluteus maximus. The primary mover for **hip abduction** is the gluteus medius assisted by the tensor fasciae latae. The hip adductors include several different muscles, only one of which crosses the knee, the gracilis. The hip rotators include several smaller muscles that are beyond the scope of this chapter. As previously discussed, muscles that cross the hip joint may also lead to changes in the lumbar spine due to their attachments on the spine or their ability to affect changes through the pelvis.

The knee has two distinct purposes: (a) to provide stability in activities such as standing, and (b) to allow for mobility in movements such as sitting or squatting. The knee is actually two separate joints—the tibiofemoral joint (where the thigh bone meets the shin bone) and the patellofemoral joint (where the kneecap meets the thigh bone). The fibula, which is the bone at the lateral aspect of the lower leg, is not considered a part of the knee since it is not included in the joint capsule of the knee. Because the femur (thigh bone) and the tibia (shin bone) do not fit together particularly well, they are said to be somewhat incongruent. To increase the area of contact between the two

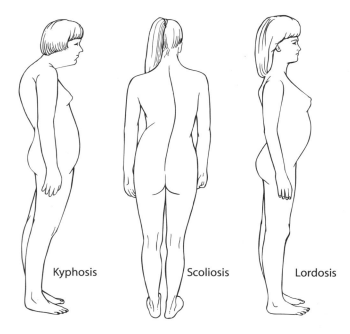

Kyphosis   Scoliosis   Lordosis

Fig. 7-13. Abnormal Curvatures of the Spine*

*Note: Among some medical professionals, kyphosis and lordosis refer to the normal curvatures found in the vertebral column. Curves that open toward the anterior portion of the body are kyphotic curves and are found in the thoracic and sacral areas of the spine. Lordotic curves are concave posteriorly and are located in the cervical and lumbar spine. Abnormal curvatures would be referred to as an exaggerated or increased lordotic or kyphotic curve in a particular area of the spine.

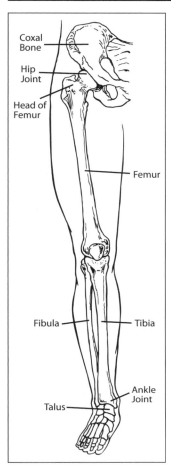

Fig. 7-14. Lower Extremity (Anterior View)

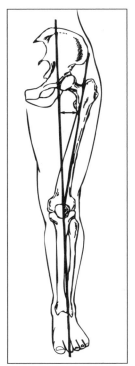

Fig. 7-15. Q-Angle

bones, there are the two fibrocartilagenous menisci on the superior surface of the tibia. Their purpose is to (a) serve as shock absorbers, (b) help lubricate and give nutrition to the knee, (c) decrease the friction, and (d) increase the area of contact between the femur and the tibia.

When looking at the leg anteriorly, you can see that the femur and the tibia do not form a straight line. The angle formed by these two bones is known as the Q-angle (Figure 7-15). To measure the angle, two lines should be drawn: (a) from the anterior superior iliac spine of the pelvis to the midpoint of the patella, and (b) from the tibial tuberosity to the midpoint of the patella. Figure 7-15 shows a normal Q-angle, which is approximately 15°.

Several ligaments and muscles that cross the knee joint also help provide stability. On either side of the knee are the medial collateral ligament and the lateral collateral ligament. Within the joint are the anterior cruciate ligament and the posterior cruciate ligament. The main muscles crossing the knee joint are the quadriceps (anteriorly) and the hamstrings (posteriorly).

The **quadriceps muscle** is composed of four parts: (a) the rectus femoris, (b) vastus lateralis, (c) vastus medialis, and (d) vastus intermedius. The rectus femoris (L. rectus, straight) runs down the front of the thigh and crosses both the hip and knee joints. As a biarticular muscle, the rectus femoris can flex the hip or extend the knee. The three vasti (L. vastus, large) muscles attach to the femur (thigh bone) and form the common quadriceps tendon that attaches at the tibial tuberosity (on the shin bone).

Embedded within the quadriceps tendon is the patella (L. patera, little plate), the body's largest sesamoid bone. Sesamoid bones are found in tendons, and they serve as a pulley and protect the tendon from excessive wear and tear. The main purpose of the patella is to increase the effective strength of the quadriceps by increasing its leverage or mechanical advantage.

The patella fits into the femur along the patellofemoral groove. The vastus lateralis, along with other structures, tends to cause the patella to track laterally during knee extension. A small, oblique portion of the vastus medialis appears to offset the lateral tracking to keep the patella centered in the patellofemoral groove. A weak vastus medialis oblique can lead to abnormal tracking of the patella in the **patellofemoral groove** and result in irritation of the lateral aspect of the patella.

The entire quadriceps muscle is worked in exercise programs that include standing, squatting, and stepping. It works concentrically to extend the knee from a squat position or to step up on a bench. The quadriceps muscle works eccentrically when lowering into a squat or stepping off of a bench. In both cases, all aspects of the quadriceps are working in a closed kinetic chain to support the weight of the body against gravity. It is important to balance the strength of the quadriceps with its opposing muscle group, the hamstrings. In an exercise program without additional equipment, it is difficult to strengthen the hamstrings as well as the quadriceps.

All three of the hamstring muscles cross the hip joint and help support the weight of the body against gravity in squats and stepping by concentrically extending the hips in a step up and eccentrically allowing the hips to flex in a squat. However, the short head of the biceps femoris does not cross the hip joint. Because it only crosses the knee joint, it is necessary to perform knee flexion against the pull of gravity to work this portion of the hamstring. Because this will be an open kinetic chain, you will only be lifting the weight of the lower leg against gravity rather than the trunk and upper extremities.

Research indicates that the trunk and upper extremities are about 60% of total body weight while the lower leg is only about 6%. Assuming that in a squat both legs work symmetrically, each quadricep supports about 45 pounds; in a hamstring curl, the weight lifted is only about 9 pounds in an individual weighing 150 pounds. Because of the difference in resistance provided by body weight alone, knee flexion with additional external resistance would help balance the strength of the quadriceps and hamstrings.

Exercise Application

Applying this knowledge of the musculoskeletal system is the cornerstone of safe fitness instruction. As you review Chapter 17, "AFAA's Basic Exercise Standards and Guidelines," you will find that many of the guidelines are based on human anatomy and kinesiology. With the diversity that we find in exercise programs today, it is essential that fitness professionals correctly apply these guidelines to ensure the safety and success of their participants.

Stability and Mobility

Moving the body is one of the most basic components of exercise. Movement requires that some joints remain stable while others are mobile. As a fitness professional, ensure that your participants understand the difference between stability and mobility. When they perform their exercises accurately, they decrease their risk of injury.

When using equipment, verify that the equipment fits the participant properly and is used correctly. For example, many weight training machines have specific instructions about how to align the participant's moving joint with the pivot point of the machine. By following the manufacturer's guidelines, you help ensure that non-moving joints are stabilized while mobile joints have the range of motion needed to perform effectively.

Various exercise programs prioritize joint stability and mobility differently. In performance sports, the actual performance is given more weight than the individual's musculoskeletal system. In core strengthening programs, the focus is on the stabilizing joints rather than on the moving joints. In aerobic programming, the priority is the individual's cardiac response. Giving different priorities to the body's musculoskeletal system is part of the diversity that the body needs to respond well to different situations.

Summary

By having a general understanding of anatomy and kinesiology, fitness professionals can plan effective exercise programs for their participants. It is easy to see why it is important that opposing muscle groups be balanced in strength and flexibility. Being able to understand how muscles work and the factors that affect their efficiency allows fitness professionals to design safe and effective muscle strengthening and endurance activities.

References

1. Adler, S.S., Beckers, D., & Buck, M. (2003). *PNF in practice: An illustrated guide* (2nd ed.). New York, NY: Springer.
2. Andreoli, T.E., et al. (2007). *Essentials of medicine* (7th ed.). Philadelphia, PA: W.B. Saunders Co.
3. Baechle, T.R., & Groves, B.R. (1998). *Weight training: Steps to success* (2nd ed.). Champaign, IL: Human Kinetics.

4. Bickley, L., & Bates, S. (2007). *Guide to physical examination and history taking* (9th ed.). Philadelphia, PA: J.B. Lippincott Co.

5. Brunnstrom, S. (1972). *Clinical kinesiology* (3rd ed.). Philadelphia, PA: F.A. Davis Company.

6. Fleck, J.F., & Kraemer, W.J. (1993). *Strength training for young athletes.* Champaign, IL: Human Kinetics.

7. Guyton, A.C. (2006). T*extbook of medical physiology* (11th ed.). Philadelphia, PA: W. B. Saunders Company.

8. Hamilton, N., Weimer, W., & Luttgens, K. (2008). *Kinesiology: Scientific basis of human motion* (11th ed.). Boston, MA: McGraw-Hill.

9. Hertling, D., & Kessler, R.M. (2005). *Management of common musculoskeletal disorders: Physical therapy principles and methods* (4th ed.). Philadelphia, PA: Lippincott, Williams & Wilkins.

10. Hulme, J.A. (2005). *Solving the mystery of the pelvic rotator cuff in human function and movement.* Missoula, MT: Phoenix.

11. Kapandji, I.A. (1974). *The Physiology of the joints: The trunk and the vertebral column* (2nd ed.). New York, NY: Longman, Inc.

12. Kisner, C., & Colby, L.A. (2007). *Therapeutic exercise: Foundations and techniques* (5th ed.). Philadelphia, PA: F. A. Davis Company.

13. Komi, P.V. (Ed.). (2002). "Strength and Power in Sport." The encyclopedia of sports medicine, international olympic committee (2nd ed.). Oxford, England: Wiley-Blackwell.

14. Kreighbaum, E., & Barthels, K.M. (1996). *Biomechanics, a qualitative approach for studying human movement* (4th ed.). Boston: Allyn and Bacon.

15. Knudson, D.V., & Morrison, C.S. (2002). *Qualitative analysis of human movement.* Champaign, IL: Human Kinetics.

16. McArdle, W.D., Katch, F.I., & Katch, V.L. (2007). *Exercise physiology: Energy, nutrition and human performance* (6th ed.). Baltimore, MD: Lippincott Williams & Wilkins.

17. McGinnis, P.M. (2005). *Biomechanics of sport and exercise* (2nd ed.). Champaign, IL: Human Kinetics.

18. McKenzie, R. (2006). *Treat your own back* (8th ed.) Waikanae, New Zealand: Spinal Publications, Ltd.

19. Moore, K.L. (2009). *Clinically oriented anatomy* (6th ed.). Baltimore, MD: Lippincott Williams & Wilkins.

20. Norkin, C., & Levangie, P. (2005). *Joint structure and function: A comprehensive analysis* (4th ed.). Philadelphia, PA: F.A. Davis Company.

21. Pollock, M.L., & Wilmore, J.H. (2002). *Exercise in health and disease: Evaluation and prescription for prevention and rehabilitation* (3rd ed.). Philadelphia, PA: W.B. Saunders Company.

22. Saunders, H.D. (2004). *Evaluation, treatment and prevention of musculoskeletal disorders* (4th ed.). Chaska, MN: Saunders Group.

23. Sullivan, P.E., Markos, P.D., & Minor, M.A. (1982). A*n integrated approach to therapeutic exercise: Theory & clinical application.* Reston, VA: Prentice-Hall.

24. Tortora, G.J. (2007). *Introduction to the human body* (7th ed.). Hoboken, NJ: John Wiley & Sons Inc.

Part 2

Essentials of Nutrition

General Nutritional Needs

Sports Nutrition

Tracy Gordner-Cherry,
RD, CDE, CDN and
Julie Cornelius, BS

8 *General Nutritional Needs*

Focus

This chapter introduces the instructor to nutritional needs that fuel exercise and sustain life. Class participants often ask their fitness instructors for nutritional advice. Sharing sound information encourages healthy eating habits, helps participants make the most of their workout sessions, and reduces risk of various diseases, such as heart diseases, some forms of cancer, type 2 diabetes, and osteoporosis. It is important to remember, however, that general nutritional information can be provided by fitness professionals and only licensed health care providers, such as a registered dietitian, can provide dietary recommendations and meal plans.

Nutrients

Nutrients are substances in food on which the body depends for proper functioning. There are six classes of nutrients: water, carbohydrates, protein, fat, vitamins, and minerals. Not getting enough of some nutrients can lead to health problems as can getting too much of other nutrients. The **Recommended Dietary Allowances** (RDA) and **Dietary Reference Intakes** (DRI), discussed later in this chapter, give recommended amounts of 23 vitamins and minerals. As scientific studies progress, additional nutrient recommendations will be announced. Other tools that help ensure a nutritious, balanced diet are also discussed.

Water

Water is the largest single component of the body. Muscle holds the highest concentration of water while fat tissue holds some of the lowest amounts. As a percent of body weight, water will vary from person to person depending on the proportion of muscle to fat tissue. An exercised individual will have a higher percentage of water compared to a less exercised person.

Water has a variety of functions that are essential to life. To name just a few, it acts as a transport medium for nutrients, aids in digestion and elimination, and directly maintains body temperature. Water has also been linked to the adequate functioning of the immune system and brain. Daily intake of water should be approximately equivalent to the amount lost (Table 8-1). When more water is lost than is taken in, dehydration develops. As little as a 5–10% loss can cause disorders, such as difficulty concentrating, dizziness, muscle spasms, and failing kidney function. An individual senses thirst when the body has already lost 5–10% of the needed water so it is important to proactively stay hydrated. Under normal circumstances, a reasonable daily water allowance for adults is 2.7–3.7 liters, with amounts based on the DRI for water. For additional information regarding water requirements during exercise, refer to Chapter 9, "Sports Nutrition."

Table 8-1. Daily Water Balance in Average Figures				
Intake		**Output**	**Normal Body Temperature**	**Prolonged Exercise**
Liquids consumed	64 oz.	Urine excretion	64 oz.	17 oz.
Water in solid food	25 oz.	Water in feces	4 oz.	4 oz.
Water from cellular		Perspiration	4 oz.	175 oz.
oxidation of food	8 oz.	Insensible losses*	25 oz.	35 oz.
TOTAL	97 oz.		97 oz.	231 oz.
*Respiratory tract and skin				

Carbohydrates

Carbohydrates provide much of the energy needed for physical activity and organ function. They vary from simple sugars, such as table sugar (sucrose), and the sugar in milk (lactose) and fruit (fructose), to **complex carbohydrates** found in grains, vegetables, and legumes. Fiber is a primarily indigestible type of carbohydrate found in fresh fruits, vegetables, and grains.

Glucose, the end result of carbohydrate digestion, is the sole energy for the brain under normal circumstances, and is essential in maintaining the functional integrity of nerve tissue. Carbohydrates are also necessary for the normal metabolism of fat. In the absence of carbohydrates, larger amounts of fat are used for energy than the body is able to handle. This could lead to a serious condition called acidosis, which can cause sodium imbalance and dehydration and in severe cases, serious metabolic imbalances.

There is no set recommendation for simple sugars. The Dietary Guidelines for Americans 2005, discussed later in this chapter, suggest keeping sugar intake moderate. The general recommendation for total carbohydrates is 45–65% of total calories. A 2,000-calorie diet calls for 225–325 grams of total carbohydrate per day. Some experts suggest maintaining added sugar intake to no more than 10–20% of total carbohydrates.

Simple sugars generally provide a quick source of energy that is not long lasting. They are categorized as monosaccharides and disaccharides. Glucose, fructose, and galactose are the **monosaccharides**, which are single units of sugar. Maltose, sucrose, and lactose are the disaccharides, which are made up of pairs of sugar units bound together.

Complex carbohydrates, also known as starches, are composed of long strands of glucose units called **polysaccharides**. Complex carbohydrates provide a longer lasting form of energy.

Fiber is categorized as soluble and insoluble, each playing important and distinctive roles in maintaining a healthy body. All fiber-rich foods contain a mixture of both types of fiber.

Fruits, vegetables, oat bran, barley, and legumes contain higher amounts of **soluble fiber**. This type of fiber has been shown to lower **blood cholesterol** levels, improve blood sugars in diabetics, and may help prevent overeating by providing an increased sense of fullness.

Insoluble fiber is found mostly in cereal grains, seeds, and the edible skins of fruits. This type of fiber has been shown to favorably affect diseases of the colon, namely diverticulosis and colorectal cancer. Insoluble fiber tends to normalize intestinal transit time, increasing it in persons with constipation, and delaying it in those with rapid transit, or diarrhea.

Whole grains offer more fiber, vitamins, and minerals than their processed counterparts. Whole wheat bread, oatmeal, brown and wild rice, and barley are all examples of whole grains.

Protein

Next to water, proteins are the most abundant substances in most cells. Proteins are needed for synthesis of enzymes, certain hormones, new tissue and some blood components, for maintenance and repair of tissue, and as energy when insufficient carbohydrates and fat are consumed. Proteins are an inefficient source of energy. The body prefers to utilize carbohydrates and fats for energy while sparing proteins for the variety of functions they are meant to perform.

Amino acids make up the structure of proteins, much like saccharides make up the structure of carbohydrates. There are 20 known amino acids of which nine are essential, meaning the body is unable to produce those on its own and they must, therefore be provided as part of the diet. Inadequate intake of any of the essential amino acids results in hair loss, impaired growth in infants and children, impaired physical recovery, and other clinical symptoms.

Protein is found most abundantly in animal sources—meat, poultry, fish, eggs, milk, and cheese. Animal products provide all the essential amino acids and, therefore are called complete proteins. Plant sources of protein, such as legumes, seeds, nuts, and grains, are incomplete proteins, meaning they are missing one or more essential amino acids or contain all of the essential amino acids in less than adequate quantities. However, when these foods are combined, with rice and beans for example, they provide the full complement of amino acids. What one plant food group is missing, another contains. It is recommended that 10–35% of calories come from protein for a 2000-calorie diet although protein requirements vary greatly depending on body size and activity level.

Fats

Fats are the major stored form of energy in the body. Despite their bad reputation, fats have many essential functions in maintaining health. Fat transports **fat-soluble vitamins**, forms the major materials of cell membranes, provides a protective covering for internal organs, provides an emergency energy source during times of lowered food intake, and insulates the body against cold temperatures. Additionally, dietary fats enhance the taste and smell of food and increase satiety of a meal.

Most natural fats are made up of about 95% **triglycerides**. Triglycerides earned their name because they are composed of three long chains. These chains are called fatty acids and are categorized as saturated, polyunsaturated, and monounsaturated. All fats are combinations of these fatty acids in differing concentrations.

Saturated fatty acids (SFA) are found in high concentrations in animal products and some vegetable oils—beef, pork, whole and 2% fat (reduced fat) dairy products, butter, poultry skin, palm oil, palm kernel oil, and coconut oil. The more saturated a fat is, the more solid it is at room temperature. Coconut oil, which remains liquid at warmer temperatures, is the exception due to its short-chain structure. Scientific studies have shown overconsumption of SFA to contribute to elevated blood cholesterol levels.

Polyunsaturated fatty acids (PUFA) make up most vegetable and fish oils, and are found in many types of nuts and seeds. Margarine, mayonnaise, soy products, and most salad dressings are also high in PUFAs. PUFAs can help lower blood cholesterol levels. However, they can also lower "good" cholesterol. Omega-3 fatty acids, a type of PUFA, help to lower blood triglyceride levels and reduce inflammation. Good sources of omega-3s are fatty fish (e.g., salmon, mackerel, lake trout, and sardines), walnuts, and flax seeds. Omega-3 fatty acids are considered essential fatty acids since they cannot be produced in the body. Omega-6, another PUFA, is an essential fatty acid found in nuts, seeds, and oils. Most Americans get enough Omega-6 fatty acids from processed foods, but not enough Omega-3 fatty acids. An imbalance in these two nutrients is believed to contribute to obesity, heart disease, asthma, depression, and even some forms of cancer.

Monounsaturated fatty acids (MUFA) are thought to be the healthiest types of fat for the heart. They decrease "bad" cholesterol without lowering "good" cholesterol as some PUFAs have shown. Foods high in MUFAs are olive oil, canola oil, peanut oil, peanuts, pecans, almonds, olives, and avocados. Both PUFA and MUFA are liquid at room temperature.

Trans **fatty acids** have received much attention in recent years. Trans fatty acids are formed during food processing when manufacturers change the chemical structure of unsaturated fats to make them semisolid at room temperature. This process is hydrogenation and it increases the stability of the product, which increases shelf life. The body processes trans fatty acids in such a way as to cause an increase in blood cholesterol levels. Major sources of trans fatty acids are stick margarine, shortening, commercial frying fats, high-fat baked goods, and salty snacks. As of January 2006, all food manufacturers are required to list trans fatty acids on nutrition labels.

Bear in mind that all types of fat mentioned above are pure or nearly pure sources of fat, and can lead to weight gain if over consumed since fats contain 9 calories per gram as compared to 4 calories per gram of proteins and carbohydrates. Leading authorities encourage Americans to consume 20–35% of calories from fat. That translates to about 46–71 grams depending on age and sex. A majority of that should come from MUFA food sources (e.g., nuts, seeds, olives, avocados).

Vitamins

Vitamins are non-caloric, organic compounds needed in small quantities to assist in such functions as growth, maintenance, and repair. These nutrients fall into one of two groups: **fat-soluble** and **water-soluble**. The fat-soluble vitamins (A, D, E, and K) can be stored in the liver. For that reason, mega dosing (10 times the RDA or DRI) may lead to toxic levels in the body. Water-soluble vitamins on the other hand are not able to be stored. The kidneys excrete excess intake, although toxicity has been reported with mega doses of vitamin C and vitamin B6.

Minerals

Minerals are inorganic compounds that assist processes, such as regulating activity of many enzymes and maintaining acid-base balance, and are structural constituents of body tissues. For example, iron is part of red blood cells, and calcium is found abundantly in bone and teeth.

The body best absorbs vitamins and minerals when provided through natural food sources rather than pill form. The potential for toxicity of fat-soluble vitamins is another reason to rely on food rather than supplements for nutrients.

Eating food triggers satiety, which prevents consuming toxic levels of nutrients, something pills cannot do.

Tools for Planning a Healthy Diet

There are many useful tools to assist in planning a diet that ensures adequate nutritional intake while attaining or maintaining a healthy weight. The following is a review of the U.S. Department of Health and Human Services (HHS) and the U.S. Department of Agriculture (USDA) Recommended Dietary Allowances, Dietary Reference Intakes, Dietary Guidelines for Americans, Food Guide Pyramid, and food label reading.

Recommended Dietary Allowance (RDA)

The Food and Nutrition Board of the National Academy of Sciences established RDAs over 50 years ago. These values were revised in 1997. RDAs are the average daily dietary intake levels for nutrients that would adequately meet the nutritional needs for nearly all healthy persons. Included are nutrients for which there is sufficient evidence that they are required for good health. RDAs are not appropriate for those with a diagnosed medical condition(s). In those cases, a doctor or dietitian provides specific recommendations.

Dietary Reference Intakes (DRI)

Scientific knowledge regarding the roles of nutrients has expanded dramatically since the inception of the RDAs. The Food and Nutrition Board has made fundamental changes in its approach to setting nutrient reference values. Dietary Reference Intakes is the new inclusive name given to this revised approach. DRIs include three sets of reference values: (a) Estimated Average Requirement (EAR), (b) RDA, and (c) Tolerable Upper Intake Levels (UL). EAR is part of the RDA calculation. UL is the maximum level of daily nutrient intake that is likely to pose no risk of adverse effects. Table 8-2 lists the RDAs which were revised between 1997 and 2002. Table 8-3 shows the most recent DRIs. Table 8-4 lists the currently established ULs. Along with the revised RDAs, the new DRIs include reference values for the macronutrients-fats, carbohydrates, and protein as well as for energy requirements and water intake.

Dietary Guidelines for Americans

These guidelines were developed by the U.S. Department of Health and Human Services and the U.S. Department of Agriculture. They are intended for healthy children, 2 years of age and older, and adults of any age. Figure 8-1 lists some of the key guidelines from the Dietary Guidelines for Americans, (6th edition). For more information, refer to http://www.dietaryguidelines.gov.

Fig. 8-1

Adequate Nutrients Within Calorie Needs

- Consume a variety of nutrient-dense foods and beverages within and among the basic food groups while choosing foods that limit the intake of saturated and trans fats, cholesterol, added sugars, salt, and alcohol.

Weight Management

- To maintain body weight in a healthy range, balance calories from foods and beverages with calories expended.
- To prevent gradual weight gain over time, make small decreases in food and beverage calories and increase physical activity.

Physical Activity

- Engage in regular physical activity and reduce sedentary activities to promote health, psychological well-being, and a healthy body weight.
- Achieve physical fitness by including cardiovascular conditioning, stretching exercises for flexibility, and resistance exercises or calisthenics for muscle strength and endurance.

Food Groups to Encourage

- Consume a sufficient amount of fruits and vegetables while staying within energy needs. Two cups of fruit and 2_ cups of vegetables per day are recommended for a reference 2,000-calorie intake, with higher or lower amounts depending on the calorie level.

- Choose a variety of fruits and vegetables each day. In particular, select from all five vegetable subgroups (e.g., dark green, orange, legumes, starchy vegetables, and other vegetables) several times a week.
- Consume 3 or more ounce-equivalents of whole-grain products per day, with the rest of the recommended grains coming from enriched or whole-grain products. In general, at least half the grains should come from whole grains.
- Consume 3 cups per day of fat-free, low-fat milk, or equivalent milk products such as low-fat yogurts and cheeses.

Fats

- Consume less than 10% of calories from saturated fatty acids and less than 300 mg per day of cholesterol, and keep trans fatty acid consumption as low as possible.
- Keep total fat intake between 20–35% of calories, with most fats coming from sources of polyunsaturated and monounsaturated fatty acids, such as fish, nuts, and vegetable oils.

Carbohydrates

- Choose fiber-rich fruits, vegetables, and whole grains often.

Sodium and Potassium

- Consume less than 2,300 mg (approximately 1 teaspoon of salt) of sodium per day.
- Choose and prepare foods with little salt. At the same time, consume potassium-rich foods,

such as fruits and vegetables (processed foods tend to have a higher sodium content).

Alcoholic Beverages

- Those who choose to drink alcoholic beverages should do so sensibly and in moderation—defined as the consumption of up to one drink per day for women and up to two drinks per day for men. One drink is defined as 12 ounces of beer, 5 ounces of wine, or 1.5 ounces of hard liquor.

Food Safety

- To avoid microbial foodborne illness:
  - clean hands, food contact surfaces, and fruits and vegetables. Meat and poultry should not be washed or rinsed.
  - separate raw, cooked, and ready-to-eat foods while shopping, preparing, or storing foods.
  - cook foods to a safe temperature to kill microorganisms.
  - chill (refrigerate) perishable food promptly and defrost foods properly.
  - avoid raw (unpasteurized) milk or any products made from unpasteurized milk, raw or partially cooked eggs or foods containing raw eggs, raw or undercooked meat and poultry, unpasteurized juices, and raw sprouts.

The full Dietary Guidelines for Americans 2005 is available at www.healthierus.gov/dietaryguidelines.

MyPyramid

In 2005, the USDA introduced MyPyramid (Figure 8-2), replacing the original Food Guide Pyramid. MyPyramid has the same goal of helping to translate grams and milligrams of nutrients into real food choices, but it is tailored to fit the Dietary Guidelines for Americans 2005. Each group provides some, but not all, of the nutrients a person needs. The newer MyPyramid is constructed with all of the food groups as vertical sections of the pyramid. This format is meant to show that all of the food groups are equally important to consume, but the width of the sections implies what portion of the diet should be consumed from each. MyPyramid also emphasizes the importance of physical activity in overall health with a set of stairs up one side of the pyramid and a figure climbing the stairs.

The far left section of MyPyramid is the largest portion for Grain with a recommendation to get half your grains from whole grains. The next section is the Vegetable section, and this section advises a consumer to "vary your veggies" by eating more dark green vegetables, more orange vegetables, and more dried beans and peas. After the Vegetable section is Fruits. MyPyramid advises to "focus on fruits," and to eat a variety of fruits including fresh; frozen; and dried fruit. The next section is Milk, and this section emphasizes getting calcium-rich foods such as milk, yogurt, and calcium fortified foods. The last section is Meat and Beans, and MyPyramid recommends to "go lean with protein" by eating lean meats and poultry, but also varying the diet with fish, beans, peas, nuts, and seeds. A small section of MyPyramid is designated for oils and sweets, and it is recommended that these be consumed in limited quantities.

NOTE:
MyPyramid recently changed to MyPlate. In 2011, the U.S. Department of Agriculture (USDA) introduced the new MyPlate image as an easy-to-understand visual cue to help consumers adopt healthy eating habits consistent with the 2010 Dietary Guidelines for Americans. The intent was to prompt all of us to think about building healthy eating patterns. In that regard, the USDA has set up a website with tools and resources to help Americans put the Dietary Guidelines into action. However, MyPyramid resources will remain available to health/fitness professionals and nutrition educators. For more information, go to www.ChooseMyPlate.gov (formerly MyPyramid.gov).

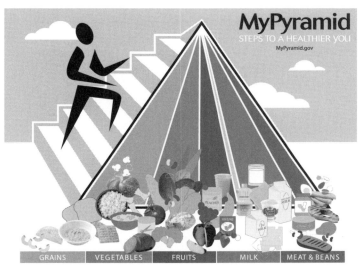

Fig. 8-2. MyPyramid

WHAT COUNTS AS A SERVING?	
Bread, Cereal, Rice, and Pasta Group • 1 slice bread • Approx. 1 cup ready-to-eat cereal • ½ cup cooked cereal, rice, or pasta	Milk, Yogurt, Cheese Group (Dairy) • 8 oz. cup milk or yogurt • 1½ oz. (1" cube) natural cheese • 2 oz. (2–3 slices) processed cheese • ½ cup cottage cheese

Vegetable Group
• 1 cup raw leafy vegetables
• ½ cup cooked or raw vegetables
• ¾ cup vegetable juice
	Meat, Poultry, Fish, Dry Beans, Eggs, & Nuts Group
	• 2–3 oz. cooked lean meat, poultry, or fish
	• The following are equivalent to
	    1 oz. meat:
	  ½ cup cooked beans, tofu
	  1 egg
	  2½ oz. soyburger
	  2 tablespoons peanut butter

Fruit Group • 1 medium piece of fruit • ½ cup chopped, cooked, or canned fruit • 1 cup melon or berries • ¾ cup juice	

Table 8-2. Recommended Dietary Allowances Revised 1997 (Abridged)

Designed for the maintenance of good nutrition of practically all healthy people living in the United States.

Category		Infants 0–6 (months)	6–12	Children 1–3 (years)	4–6	7–10	Males 11–14 (years)	15–18	19–24	25–50	51+	Females 11–14 (years)	15–18	19–24	25–50	51+	Pregnant	Lactating 1st 6 mo.	2nd 6 mo.
Weight*	(kg)	6	9	13	20	28	45	66	72	79	77	46	55	58	63	65			
	(lb)	13	20	29	44	62	99	145	160	174	170	101	120	128	138	143			
Height*	(cm)	60	71	90	112	132	157	176	177	176	173	157	163	164	163	160			
	(in)	24	28	35	44	52	62	69	70	70	68	62	64	65	64	63			
Protein	(g)	9.1	11.0	13	19	19	34	52	56	56	56	34	46	46	46	46	71	71	71
Vitamin A (µg RE)		400	500	300	400	600	600	900	900	900	900	600	700	700	700	700	770	1,300	1,200
Vitamin K (µg/d)		2.0	2.5	30	55	60	60	75	120	120	120	45	55	60	65	65	65	65	65
Iron	(mg)	0.27	11	7	10	10	8	11	8	8	8	8	15	18	18	8	27	9	9
Zinc	(mg)	2	3	3	5	5	8	11	11	11	11	8	9	8	8	8	11	12	12
Iodine	(µg)	40	50	70	90	120	150	150	150	150	150	150	150	150	150	150	175	200	200

*Weights and heights of reference adults are actual medians for the U.S. population of the designated age, as reported by NHANES II. The median weights and heights for those under 19 years of age were taken from Hamill, et al. (1979). The use of these figures does not imply that the height-to-weights ratios are ideal.

Table 8-3. Dietary Reference Intakes: Recommended Intakes for Individuals

Life Stage Group	Infants 0–6 (months)	6–12	Children 1–3 (years)	4–8	Males 9–13 (years)	14–18	19–30	31–50	51–70	70+	Females 9–13 (years)	14–18	19–30	31–50	51–70	70+	Pregnant < 18 (years)	19–30	31–50	Lactating < 18 (years)	19–30	31–50
Calcium (mg/d)	210	270	500	800	1,300	1,300	1,000	1,000	1,200	1,200	1,300	1,300	1,000	1,000	1,200	1,200	1,300	1,000	1,000	1,300	1,000	1,000
Phosphorous (mg/d)	100	275	460	500	1,250	1,250	700	700	700	700	1,250	1,250	700	700	700	700	1,250	700	700	1,250	700	700
Magnesium (mg/d)	30	75	80	130	240	410	400	420	420	420	240	360	310	320	320	320	400	350	360	360	310	320
Vitamin D (µg/d)	5	5	5	5	5	5	5	5	10	15	5	5	5	5	10	15	5	5	5	5	5	5
Fluoride (mg/d)	0.01	0.5	0.7	1	2	3	4	4	4	4	2	3	3	3	3	3	3	3	3	3	3	3
Thiamin (mg/d)	0.2	.03	0.5	0.6	0.9	1.2	1.2	1.2	1.2	1.2	0.9	1.0	1.1	1.1	1.1	1.1	1.4	1.4	1.4	1.4	1.4	1.4
Riboflavin (mg/d)	0.3	0.4	0.5	0.6	0.9	1.3	1.3	1.3	1.3	1.3	0.9	1.0	1.1	1.1	1.1	1.1	1.4	1.4	1.4	1.6	1.6	1.6
Niacin (mg/d)	2	4	6	8	12	16	16	16	16	16	12	14	14	14	14	14	18	18	18	17	17	17
Vitamin B_6 (mg/d)	0.1	0.3	0.5	0.6	1.0	1.3	1.3	1.3	1.7	1.7	1.0	1.2	1.3	1.3	1.5	1.5	1.9	1.9	1.9	2.0	2.0	2.0
Folate* (µg/d)	65	80	150	200	300	400	400	400	400	400	300	400	400	400	400	400	600	600	600	500	500	500
Vitamin B_{12} (µg/d)	0.4	0.5	0.9	1.2	1.8	2.4	2.4	2.4	2.4	2.4	1.8	2.4	2.4	2.4	2.4	2.4	2.6	2.6	2.6	2.8	2.8	2.8
Pantothenic (mg/d)	1.7	1.8	2	3	4	5	5	5	5	5	4	5	5	5	5	5	6	6	6	7	7	7
Biotin (µg/d)	5	6	8	12	20	25	30	30	30	30	20	25	30	30	30	30	30	30	30	35	35	35
Choline (mg/d)	125	150	200	250	375	550	550	550	550	550	375	400	425	425	425	425	450	450	450	550	550	550
Vitamin C (mg/d)	40	50	15	25	45	75	90	90	90	90	45	65	75	75	75	75	80	85	85	115	120	120
Vitamin E (mg/d)	4	6	6	7	11	15	15	15	15	15	11	15	15	15	15	15	15	15	15	19	19	19
Selenium (µg/d)	15	20	20	30	40	55	55	55	55	55	40	55	55	55	55	55	60	60	60	70	70	70

*In view of evidence linking folate to neural-tube defects in the fetus, it is recommended that all women capable of becoming pregnant consume 400 µg from supplements or fortified foods in addition to intake of food folate from a varied diet.

Table 8-4. Dietary Reference Intakes: Tolerable Upper Intake Levels (UL)

Life Stage Group	Infants 0–6 6–12 (months)		Children 1–3 4–8 (years)		Males 9–13 14–18 19–70 70+ (years)				Females 9–13 14–18 19–70 70+ (years)				Pregnant < 18 19–50 (years)		Lactating < 18 19–50 (years)	
Calcium (mg/d)	ND*	ND	2,500	2,500	2,500	2,500	2,500	2,500	2,500	2,500	2,500	2,500	2,500	2,500	2,500	2,500
Phosphorous (mg/d)	ND	ND	3	3	4	4	4	3	4	4	4	3	3.5	3.5	4	4
Magnesium (mg/d)	ND	ND	65	110	350	350	350	350	350	350	350	350	350	350	350	350
Vitamin D (µg/d)	25	25	50	50	50	50	50	50	50	50	50	50	50	50	50	50
Fluoride (mg/d)	0.7	0.9	1.3	2.2	10	10	10	10	10	10	10	10	10	10	10	10
Niacin (mg/d)	ND	ND	10	15	20	30	35	35	20	30	35	35	30	35	30	35
Vitamin B_6 (mg/d)	ND	ND	30	40	60	80	100	100	60	80	100	100	80	100	80	100
Folate (µg/d)	ND	ND	300	400	600	800	1,000	1,000	600	800	1,000	1,000	800	1,000	800	1,000
Choline (mg/d)	ND	ND	1.0	1.0	2.0	3.0	3.5	3.5	2.0	3.0	3.5	3.5	3.0	3.5	3.0	3.5
Vitamin C (mg/d)	ND	ND	400	650	1,200	1,800	2,000	2,000	1,200	1,800	2,000	2,000	1,800	2,000	1,800	2,000
Vitamin E (mg/d)	ND	ND	200	300	600	800	1,000	1,000	600	800	1,000	1,000	800	1,000	800	1,000
Selenium (µg/d)	45	60	90	150	280	400	400	400	280	400	400	400	400	400	400	400

*ND—No Data

Food Label Reading

The Nutrition Education and Labeling Act of 1990 improved label information by defining health claim terminology, requiring certain nutrients to be listed, and requiring uniform serving sizes for similar foods. Nutrient labels must appear on most foods with the exception of foods providing few nutrients (e.g., spices), restaurant foods, and ready to eat food prepared on site (e.g., deli items). Providing information for raw foods remains voluntary. Figure 8-3 shows and explains the Nutrition Facts panel of the food label.

More consistent serving sizes, in both household and metric measures, replaced those that used to be set by manufacturers.

Nutrients required on nutrition panel are those most important to the health of today's consumers, most of whom need to worry about getting too much of certain items (fat & sodium for example), rather than too few vitamins or minerals, as in the past.

Percent Daily Values (DV) are based on recommendations of a 2,000-calorie diet, shown below. %DV shows how a nutrient fits into the overall diet. An indication of 10% or more suggests an adequate or high source of that nutrient. While a 20% or more indicates an excellent or very high amount. This product is a good source of calcium and protein, but, it is also high in sodium.

Nutrition Facts

Serving size 1   Servings per container 1

Amount per Serving

Calories 310   Calories from Fat 80

% Daily Value*

Total Fat 8g	**12%**
Saturated Fat 3g	**15%**
Trans Fat 0g	
Polyunsaturated Fat 1.5g	
Monounsaturated Fat 3.5g	
Cholesterol 35mg	**10%**
Sodium 500mg	**23%**
Potassium 420mg	**23%**
Total Carbohydrate 35g	**12%**
Dietary Fiber 5g	**20%**
Sugars 3g	
Protein 22g	**44%**

Vitamin A	15%	Vitamin C	35%
Calcium	6%	Iron	10%
Vitamin E	8%	Thiamin	20%
Riboflavin	20%	Niacin	30%
Vitamin B6	6%	Folic Acid	15%
Vitamin B12	10%	Pantothenic Acid	8%
Phosphorus	30%	Magnesium	15%
Zinc	10%	Manganese	25%

*Percent Daily Values are based on a 2,000-calorie diet. Your daily values may be higher or lower depending on your calorie needs:

	Calories	2,000	2,500
Total Fat	Less than	65g	80g
Sat. Fat	Less than	20g	25g
Cholesterol	Less than	300mg	300mg
Sodium	Less than	2,400mg	2,400mg
Total Carbohydrate		300g	375g
Dietary Fiber		25g	30g
Protein		50g	65g

Calories Per Gram: Fat 9 • Carbohydrate 4 • Protein 4

Reference values help consumers gauge how much of these nutrients they should strive towards.

Conversion guide helps consumers learn caloric value of the energy producing nutrients.

Fig. 8-3. Nutrition Facts Panel

Summary

Simply stated, nutritious eating can be summarized as consuming enough vitamins and minerals without going overboard with fats and sodium. Foods are merely a combination of different nutrients and non-nutritive components. Balance, variety, and moderation are the keys. Choose a wide variety of foods to absorb all the nutrients needed by the body. Choose appropriate amounts, neither too restrictive nor excessive, and balance out foods higher in fat, sodium, and cholesterol with foods low in those nutrients. All foods can fit in a healthy diet. An occasional treat does not suddenly ruin an otherwise healthy diet, just as a one-time apple in a diet based on sweets and fast food does not render those eating habits nutritious. It is important for fitness instructors to know what constitutes healthful eating, and to pass this knowledge on to their class participants. Encourage nutritious, low-fat food choices. Be aware that many fat modified foods lack nutritional quality. The Nutrition Facts panel on food labels provides that information. Useful tools, such as the Food Guide Pyramid, are available to demonstrate how to plan meals and snacks for a healthy diet. Class participants, as well as instructors, will all benefit from combining their regular exercise with nutritious eating habits.

References

1. Food and Nutrition Board. (2000). Frequently asked questions about the DRIs. From http://www.4.nas.edu/IOM/IOMhome.nsf/pages/ FNB+FAQ+DRI *testing and prescription* (8th ed.). Baltimore, MD: Lippincott Williams & Wilkins.

2. Healthy People (2000). *National health promotion and disease prevention objectives.* Nutrition Priority Areas, U.S. Department of Health and Human Services, Public Health Service, U.S. Government Printing Office, Publications No. 017-001-00474.

3. International Food Information Council Foundation. (2002). Dietary reference intakes: An update. Retrieved May 4, 2009, from http://ific.org/publications/other/driupdateom.cfm?renderforprint=1

4. Mahan, L.K., & Escott-Stump, S. (1996). *Krause's food, nutrition, & diet therapy* (9th ed.). Philadelphia, PA: W.B. Saunders Co.

5. Monsen, E.R. (2000). Dietary reference intakes for the antioxidant nutrients: Vitamin C, vitamin E, selenium, and carotenoids. *Journal of the American Medical Dietetics Association, 100,* 637–640.

6. National Academy of Sciences. (2002). *Dietary reference intakes.* Retrieved May 4, 2009, from http://www.iom.edu/Object.File/Master/21/372/0.pdf

7. Stoker, H.S. (1998). *General organic and biological chemistry.* Boston, MA: Houghton Mifflin Co.

8. The American Dietetic Association. (1995). *Project lean resource kit.* Chicago, IL.

9. U.S. Department of Agriculture & U.S. Department of Health and Human Services. (2002). Nutrition and your health: Dietary guidelines for Americans (5th ed.). *Home and Garden Bulletin, 232.*

10. U.S. Department of Agriculture. (2008). Dietary guidelines for Americans, 2005: Key recommendations for the general population. Retrieved May 4, 2008, from http://www.health.gov/dietaryguidelines/dga2005/recommendations.htm

11. U.S. Food and Drug Administration. (2006). Questions and answers about trans fat nutrition labeling. Retrieved May 4, 2008, from http://www.cfsan.fda.gov/~dms/qatrans2.html#s3q1

12. Weil, A. (2007). Balancing omega-3 and omega-6. Retrieved May 4, 2008, from http://www.drweil.com/drw/u/QAA400149/balancing-omega-3-and-omega-6.html

9 *Sports Nutrition*

Nancy Clark, MS, RD, CSSD

Focus

This chapter offers practical sports nutrition information that addresses the nutrition questions commonly asked by fitness instructors, aerobic competitors, and other athletes. This information will help you guide your clients in the selection of a high-quality sports diet that (a) fuels the muscles for top performance, (b) nourishes the body, and (c) contributes to current health and future longevity. In general, athletic people do not need a diet substantially different from that recommended in the Dietary Guidelines for Americans and Eating Well for Canada's Food Guide (ACSM, 2009).

Carbohydrates— The Foundation of the Sports Diet

Athletes and fitness exercisers who do hard workouts should target 6–10 grams carbohydrate per kilogram body weight (2.7–4.5 g/lb) on a daily basis to ingest adequate carbohydrates for both training and competing (ACSM, 2009). This comes to about 270–450 grams carbohydrate per 100 pounds of body weight (~1,100–1,800 calories from carbohydrates), more easily visualized as carbohydrates (e.g., grains, fruits, vegetables) being the foundation of each meal and snack.

These carbohydrates are stored as (a) muscle glycogen, needed to perform exercise, and (b) liver glycogen, needed to maintain normal blood sugar level. Unfortunately, misconceptions about carbohydrates—what they are and what they aren't—keep many athletes from choosing the best carbohydrates.

Carbohydrates include both sugars and starches, and are found in fruits, vegetables, grains, and to a smaller extent, in milk. Both sugars and starches are stored equally as sources of fuel, but they have differing abilities to nourish the athlete with vitamins and minerals. The carbohydrates in sugary soda pop or sports drinks provide no vitamins or minerals, unlike the carbohydrates in wholesome fruits, vegetables, and grains that provide vitamins and minerals— the spark plugs that help the athlete's "engine" to perform at its best.

The average 150-pound active male has about 1,800 calories of carbohydrates stored in his liver, muscles, and blood in approximately the following distribution:

Muscle glycogen . . . . 1,400 calories
Liver glycogen . . . . . 320 calories
Blood glucose . . . . . . 80 calories

These carbohydrate stores determine how long an athlete can exercise. Depleted muscle glycogen is associated with "hitting the wall" and the inability to exercise energetically; depleted liver glycogen results in low blood sugar and causes the athlete to "bonk" or "crash," feeling lightheaded, uncoordinated, unable to concentrate, and overwhelmingly fatigued. Proper pre-exercise nutrition includes adequate carbohydrates and can reduce the likelihood of becoming glycogen depleted.

Carbohydrates are important for all athletes regardless of the sport. Both runners and bodybuilders alike need this fuel for performing their desired type of exercise. Weight-conscious athletes, such as runners and figure skaters, often try to "stay away" from carbohydrates, believing them to be fattening. Carbohydrates are not fattening. They supply only 4 calories per gram, as compared to fats that offer 9 calories per gram. Carbohydrates can become fattening if eaten with fatty foods, such as butter on bread, gravy on potato, and mayonnaise on a sandwich. Since carbohydrates are likely to be burned off rather than stored as fat, even weight-conscious athletes can and should include appropriate, but not excessive, amounts of them as the foundation of their sports diet.

The following menus are sample carbohydrate-based sports meals that offer at least 60% of the calories from carbohydrates. Some of the food items (e.g., soft drinks, milk shakes) are not generally recommended as part of an optimal daily diet, but they can be incorporated into a fast food meal on the road from time to time. The purpose of these sample meals is simply to offer the concept of what a carbohydrate-based sports diet "looks like," so that athletes can use it to guide their food choices. The menus are appropriate for active women and men who need 2,000–2,600+ calories per day. Food portions may be adjusted to suit individual needs.

Table 9-1. Sample High-Carbohydrate, Fast Food Meals	Total Cal.	Carb. Cal.
Breakfast		
McDonald's Fast Food		
Orange juice, 12 oz small	140	130
Egg McMuffin	300	120
English muffin w/jam	195	140
Total	635	(61% Carb.)
Bagel House, Bakery		
Bagel, whole wheat	320	250
Cream Cheese, light 2 T	60	--
Hot Cocoa, large	180	100
Total	560	(63% Carb.)
Family Restaurant		
Apple juice, large	145	145
Raisin Bran, 2 sm. boxes	220	200
Low-fat milk, 8 oz	110	80
Sliced banana, medium	125	120
Total	600	(91% Carb.)
Lunch		
Subway		
Turkey, 12" no mayo	580	370
Fruizle, Berry Lishus	110	110
Total	690	(70% Carb.)
Wendy's Fast Food		
Plain baked potato, 10 oz	270	245
Chili, large	280	115
Chocolate milk	170	115
Total	720	(66% Carb.)
Salad Bar		
Lettuce, 1 cup	15	10
Green pepper, 1/2	10	8
Broccoli, 1/2 cup	20	15
Carrots, 1/2 cup	20	17
Tomato, large	50	45
Chick peas, 1/2 cup	170	120
Feta Cheese, 1 oz	75	0
Italian dressing, 2 T	100	0
Bread, 1" slice	200	180
Total	660	(60% Carb.)

Table 9-1. Sample High-Carbohydrate, Fast Food Meals *(cont.)*		
	Total Cal.	**Carb. Cal.**
Dinner		
Pizzeria		
Cheese pizza, 4 sl. 13"	920	520
Large cola, 12 oz	150	150
Total	1070	(63% Carb.)
Italian Restaurant		
Minestrone soup, 1 cup	85	60
Spaghetti, 2 cups	400	320
Tomato sauce, 2/3 cup	120	60
Parmesan cheese, 1 T	30	0
Rolls, 2 large	280	240
Total	915	(74% Carb.)
Family Restaurant		
Turkey, 5 oz white meat	250	0
Stuffing, 1 cup	200	160
Mashed potato, 1 cup	95	65
Peas, 2/3 cup	70	60
Cranberry sauce, 1/4 cup	100	100
Orange juice, 8 oz	110	105
Sherbet, 1 scoop	120	110
Total	945	(63% Carb.)

Abbreviations: Carb. = carbohydrates, cal. = calories, oz = ounces, sm. = small, mayo = mayonnaise, T = tablespoon, sl. = slice.

To consume a daily carbohydrate-based sports diet, the athlete should opt for more grains and starches and fewer fatty, greasy foods. By working with a sports dietitian, the athlete can learn the appropriate food choices, such as bagels instead of croissants, oatmeal instead of cheese omelets, and pasta instead of fried chicken. Food labels, which list the grams of carbohydrates per serving, can assist with appropriate food selection. Some dedicated athletes "count carbohydrates" to reach their daily quota based on their body weight and level of activity, as explained above.

Fat

For both cardiovascular health and optimal sports performance, athletes should reduce their intake of fatty, greasy foods, such as donuts, pastries, butter, mayonnaise, French fries, and ice cream. These foods tend to fill the stomach, but leave the muscles unfueled. In addition, they also may contribute to heart disease if the foods are laden with saturated fat from greasy meats (e.g., bacon, spare ribs, greasy burgers) and creamy dairy products (e.g., butter, full-fat cheese). By trading in excessive fat calories for more carbohydrates (e.g., eating pasta with tomato sauce instead of Alfredo sauce), an athlete can enjoy better-fueled muscles, hence better athletic performance.

Although eating too much fat is a common problem among athletes, overly compulsive personalities may try to cut all fats out of their diet. They often become extremely restrictive with their food choices, eating only fat-free foods, such as rice cakes, broccoli, and non-fat yogurt. This restrictiveness, at times, may border on an eating disorder. Since 20–35% of the calories in a sports diet can appropriately come from fat, this entitles the athlete to a small amount of fat at each meal, which is easily consumed in the hidden fats in bran muffins, lean meats, granola, and other popular foods. The preferable sources of fats are the

Table 9-2. Protein in Commonly Eaten Foods

Although animal products generally provide the highest quality protein, eating a variety of plant proteins can provide the amino acids (building blocks of protein) the body needs to build and repair muscles. Note that you need to eat a generous portion (more calories) of beans and other plant protein to equal the protein in animal foods.

	Grams of protein/ standard serving		Grams of protein/ 100 calories (amount)	
Animal sources				
Egg white	3.5	from 1 large egg	20	6 egg whites
Egg	6	1 large	8	1.3 eggs
Cheddar cheese	7	1 oz	6	0.9 oz
Milk, 1%	8	8 oz	8	8 oz
Yogurt	11	1 cup	8	6 oz
Cottage cheese	15	1/2 cup	15	1/2 cup
Haddock	27	4 oz cooked	21	3 oz
Hamburger	30	4 oz broiled	10	1.5 oz
Pork loin	30	4 oz roasted	10	1.5 oz
Chicken breast	35	4 oz roasted	18	2 oz
Tuna	40	6 oz	20	3 oz
Plant sources				
Almonds, dried	3	12 nuts	3.5	14 nuts
Peanut butter	4.5	1 T	4.5	1 T
Kidney beans	6	1/2 cup	6	1/2 cup
Hummus	6	1/2 cup	3	1/4 cup
Refried beans	7	1/2 cup	7	1/2 cup
Lentil soup, Progresso	11	10.5 oz	6.5	6 oz
Tofu, extra firm	11	3.5 oz	12	4 oz
Baked beans	14	1 cup	7	1/2 cup

more healthful fats, such as in salmon, nuts, peanut butter, and olive oil.

Athletes with high-caloric demands who severely restrict their fat intake may have trouble consuming adequate calories and maintaining their weight if they rigidly limit their fat intake. The sheer volume of low-fat food that needs to get consumed poses a problem because one may tire of chewing before being adequately fed. Plus, a diet with less than 20% of calories from fat can hurt performance (ACSM, 2009). The body needs fat for not only fuel, but also to absorb vitamins A, D, E, and K, and to supply the essential fatty acids that optimize health. By working with a sports dietitian, the athlete can learn how to include appropriate amounts of peanut butter, olive oil, and other heart-healthy fats into their carbohydrate-based sports diet.

Protein

Traditionally, athletes have eaten high-protein sports diets, believing that if they eat extra meat, they'll build extra muscle. Excess protein does not build muscle; exercise does. To bulk-up, the athlete needs to perform resistance exercise, such as weight lifting and push-ups, in addition to eating a wholesome diet. To have adequate energy to perform the muscle-building exercise, the diet should be based on carbohydrates, with protein as the accompaniment to each meal and snack.

Protein recommendations for both endurance and strength-trained athletes range from 1.2–1.7 grams of protein per kilogram body weight per day (0.5–0.8 g/lb) (ACSM, 2009). Strange as it may sound, both bodybuilders and marathon runners should eat the same carbohydrate-based sports diet because both types of athletes need carbs to fuel their workouts.

It's hard to specify the exact protein requirement for athletes, because their needs vary according to total calorie intake (dieters need more protein/kg than athletes eating their full complement of food) and level of growth and training (athletes rapidly building muscles have higher protein needs).

When it comes to protein intake, athletes seem to fall into two categories: (a) protein pushers (e.g., the bodybuilders, weight lifters, football players who think they can't get enough protein), and (b) protein avoiders (e.g., the runners, triathletes, dancers who often limit their meat intake in their efforts to eat a low-fat, low calorie, and/or vegetarian diet). Both groups can perform poorly due to dietary imbalances.

Protein pushers, such as high school athletes who frequently eat protein shakes and protein bars for snacks plus meat-based meals, fail to consume enough carbs to fully fuel their muscles. If they choose fatty burgers, chicken wings, and other fast-food proteins, they consume a high-fat, high-cholesterol diet that not only leaves their muscles unfueled, but also contributes to heart disease.

Protein avoiders, such as athletes who believe that meat is bad for their health, tend to be deficient in not only protein, but also iron and zinc—two minerals important for top performance. The trick is to teach athletes how to obtain adequate, but not excess, portions of lean protein. If you suspect a protein imbalance, you might want to refer the client to a sports dietitian who will evaluate the current protein intake and teach the athlete how to make appropriate adjustments.

Vegetarian athletes who eat no meat or animal source of protein need to be sure to make the effort to incorporate adequate plant sources of protein into their diet. Rather than simply avoiding meat, they must conscientiously include beans, lentils, tofu, nuts, and other plant proteins to fulfill their protein needs. Yet, their diets may still be deficient in iron and zinc, two minerals found primarily in animal proteins, and particularly in red meats. Iron is important for preventing anemia; zinc is important for healing.

Iron

Athletes who become anemic due to an iron-deficient diet are likely to experience needless fatigue upon exertion. Those at highest risk of suffering from iron-deficiency anemia include female athletes who lose iron through menstruating, athletes who eat no red meats, marathon runners who may damage red blood cells via "footstrike hemolysis," endurance athletes who may lose a significant amount of iron through heavy sweat losses, and teenage athletes who are growing quickly and may consume inadequate iron to meet their expanded requirements. To boost and/or maintain a high-iron intake, an athlete can eat the following.

1. Lean cuts of beef, pork, and lamb (4-ounce portions), and the dark meat of chicken and turkey three to four times per week. (The heme-iron in these animal proteins is more bioavailable than the iron found in vegetable foods, such as spinach and raisins.)
2. Enriched and fortified breads and cereals (by reading the food label, the athlete can determine if the product has added iron) as well as whole grains, beans, and legumes. (The non-heme iron found in these plant foods has poor bioavailability.)
3. A food rich in vitamin C with each meal, such as a glass of orange juice or a vegetable, since vitamin C enhances iron absorption from both heme and non-heme iron sources.
4. Foods cooked in cast iron skillets, particularly acidic foods such as spaghetti sauce, since the acid attracts the iron and significantly increases iron content of a food.

Athletes who do not eat meat or iron-rich foods may wish to take an iron supplement as a "health insurance" to possibly reduce their risk of becoming anemic. They should be educated that the iron from a supplement may be poorly absorbed compared to that found in animal proteins, and that they are likely to still have a diet that's deficient in zinc, since the two minerals tend to be found in similar foods. Hence, a supplement that contains both iron and zinc is the better choice.

Vitamin/Mineral Supplements

Vitamins are big business among athletes and Americans in general. The reasons for taking supplements vary. Some take supplements to compensate for poor eating; others as "health insurance." Many athletes swallow the advertising claims that promise enhanced athletic prowess. Unfortunately, they don't realize that if a claim sounds too good to be true, it probably is! An athlete who takes vitamin supplements "for energy" is unlikely to notice increased performance, strength, or stamina, unless he or she was nutritionally deficient to start with, or perhaps experiences a placebo effect.

Supplement takers often fail to understand that they still need to eat a well-balanced diet, regardless of the amount of vitamins they take. A pill may contain only 8–12 of the more than 50 nutrients needed for top performance and none of the phytochemicals or fibers that protect health. Many athletes spend significant amounts of money on assorted pills and potions, when they could more wisely spend the money on wholesome foods. If clients are taking supplements because they question the adequacy of their diet, they should have a nutrition check-up with a registered dietitian who can teach them to get the nutrients they need from the foods they eat. (See www.SCANdpg.org to find a local sports dietitian.) In general, no supplements are needed if the athlete is consuming adequate calories from a variety of wholesome foods (ACSM, 2009). Yet, the recommendations unrelated to exercise should be heeded (e.g., folic acid for women who could become pregnant; mutivitamin/mineral pill for dieters restricting their food intake or eliminating a food group such as dairy.)

Although it seems logical that an active person would need more vitamins than a sedentary person, the research to date shows no evidence of dramatically increased vitamin needs that cannot be met through a wholesome diet. Most athletes can easily consume more than enough vitamins within 1,500–2,000 calories of a variety of wholesome foods. Hence, the hard-training athlete who consumes 3,000 to 4,000 calories can easily get more vitamins than needed. For example, the cyclist who drinks an 8 oz glass of orange juice gets 100% of the Daily Value (DV) for vitamin C. If the exerciser is extremely thirsty, such as after a workout, he or she is likely to drink 24 oz of juice—and get 300% of the DV for C from this snack alone, to say nothing of what is consumed in other fruits and vegetables throughout the day.

Amino Acid and Protein Supplements

Athletes who strive to develop muscles and increase strength often look to amino acid pills and protein supplements for beneficial effects. To date, there is no evidence that the consumption of these preparations results in greater muscular bulk. Exercise—not extra protein—is the key to building bigger muscles. Athletes who want to bulk up should spend time lifting weights and performing other forms of resistance exercise, rather than spending their money on expensive amino acid supplements.

The amount of protein or amino acids found in the special powders or pills can be far less than that obtained from foods. For example, an athlete would have to eat 5 tablespoons of one popular brand of protein powder to get the same amount of protein in a small can of tuna at half the price. Here's a comparison of the amounts of two essential amino acids (isoleucine and leucine) in food versus a popular protein supplement:

Protein source	Isoleucine grams	Leucine grams
Met-Rx Whey Protein, 1 scoop	1.4	2.3
Chocolate milk, 16 oz	.2	1.9
Tuna, 6 oz can	2.0	3.5
Cottage cheese, 1 cup	.6	2.9

Fluids

Drinking adequate fluids is essential for top sports performance. Fluids transport nutrients to and from the working muscles, dissipate heat, and eliminate waste products. Unfortunately, many athletes neglect this aspect of their sports diet and consequently hurt their performances. To maintain optimal hydration, athletes should do the following.

Prevent dehydration during training by drinking adequate fluids on a daily basis—preferably water, juices, and low-fat milk. Athletes can determine whether or not they're drinking enough fluid by monitoring their patterns of urination: the urine should be clear colored and copious, and they should be urinating frequently. Dark colored, scanty urine is a sign of dehydration and a signal for the athlete to consume more fluids throughout the day, as well as before and during the workout, to help prevent dehydration.

To increase awareness of sweat losses during exercise, athletes who sweat heavily should weigh themselves before and after a hard workout. A loss of 2 pounds equates to 32 ounces (1 quart) of sweat that needs to get replaced.

Before an event, athletes should drink extra water and other watery foods (e.g., fruit, soup, yogurt, low-fat milk), to be sure the body is well hydrated. They should drink two to three large glasses of fluid up to 2 hours before the start of the event. Since the kidneys require about 90 minutes to process fluids, this allows sufficient time to empty the bladder. Five or 10 minutes before start time, athletes should drink another 1–2 cups of water or sports drink.

Coffee is often used as a pre-exercise "perk me up." For some athletes, coffee seems to make the effort easier. It makes others needlessly nervous and jittery, plaguing them with a "coffee stomach" and excessive trips to the bathroom. Many studies suggest that caffeine enhances endurance performance, but each athlete responds differently to caffeine. Hence, the best bet is to be well fed, rested, and nutritionally prepared for competition.

If athletes ask about caffeine, they should be reminded that every person has a unique reaction to caffeine. Some "perk up" with a cup or two; others don't want to touch the stuff. Hence, each athlete has to experiment with pre-exercise caffeine to determine if he or she experiences any ergogenic benefits. Once thought to be a diuretic, we now know that caffeine does not have a dehydrating effect in people who regularly drink coffee (Armstrong, et al., 2005).

During hard exercise, athletes should prevent dehydration by drinking enough water or sports drink to quench their thirst, but not overhydrate. Athletes who sweat heavily should start drinking early in the event, consuming enough to match their predetermined sweat losses.

After exercise, athletes should drink enough fluids to quench their thirst, plus more, until the urine is light colored and copious. Monitoring urination is a good way to monitor hydration status (ACSM, 2007). If several hours pass before an athlete has urinated, he or she is still dehydrated.

For the recreational athlete, water is always an appropriate fluid replacer before, during, and after exercise. For endurance athletes who exercise for more than 90 minutes, as well as highly competitive athletes who exercise intensely for

Each pound of weight lost represents 2 cups (16 ounces) of sweat. Athletes should replace this accordingly during exercise, and strive to lose no more than 2% of their weight during a workout (e.g., 3 lb, 6 cups of sweat, for a 150-lb athlete). If they become 2% dehydrated, they have reduced their work capacity by 10–15%.

an hour or so (such as hockey, soccer, and basketball players), a sports drink or water plus carbs (e.g., gummy candy, gels, dried fruit, watermelon) is best during exercise because it will help to maintain normal blood sugar levels. A helpful recovery fluid after hard exercise is chocolate milk—a good source of not only carbs to refuel the muscles, but also high-quality protein to minimize muscle soreness, and repair and build muscles (Flakoll, et al., 2004).

Precompetition Nutrition

> *Since one single precompetition meal inadequately compensates for a poor training diet, athletes should eat a carbohydrate-rich sports diet every day to enhance daily muscle glycogen storage. The precompetition meal should be simply an extension of the tried-and-true daily training diet.*

The goals of the precompetition meal are to accomplish the following.

1. Help prevent hypoglycemia with its symptoms of lightheadedness, blurred vision, needless fatigue, and indecisiveness—all of which can interfere with top performance.
2. Abate hunger feelings, help settle the stomach, and absorb some of the gastric juices.
3. Provide energy for the muscles.
4. Provide adequate fluids to fully hydrate the body.

In preparation for competition, an athlete should eat a carbohydrate-rich diet (ideally, this is similar to their daily training diet) and drink additional fluids both the day(s) prior to the event and the day of the event, in combination with tapering off from exercise in order to allow the muscles the opportunity to store the carbohydrates as glycogen.

Athletes participating in endurance sports that last for longer than 90 minutes, such as marathon running or long-distance bike racing, should reduce exercise and emphasize carbohydrate-rich meals for 2–3 days prior to the event.

Athletes participating in events that last less than 90 minutes can store adequate glycogen with 1 or 2 rest days and a carbohydrate-rich diet.

Meal timing. When planning the time of the precompetition meal, the athlete should allow adequate time for the food to empty from the stomach, so that he or she can exercise comfortably without feeling weighted down. Since high calorie meals take longer to leave the stomach than lighter snacks, the general rule of thumb is for an athlete to allow:

- 3–4 hours for a large meal to digest.
- 2–3 hours for a smaller meal to digest.
- 1–2 hours for a blended or liquid meal to digest.
- less than an hour for a light snack to digest, as tolerated.

Since fatty foods delay gastric emptying, the meal should focus on carbohydrates, with small portions of lean protein also being appropriate as an accompaniment, such as oatmeal with milk, spaghetti with a little extra lean hamburger in the tomato sauce, or a turkey sandwich with thickly sliced bread and only a few ounces of turkey.

The night before **morning event**s, athletes should eat a hearty, high-carbohydrate dinner and bedtime snack. That morning, they should eat a light snack/breakfast to abate hunger feelings, replenish liver glycogen stores, and absorb some of the gastric juices. For example, a runner who is going to participate in a 10:00 a.m. road race may want only a light breakfast (such as a small bowl of cereal with low-fat milk @ 300–500 calories), since the primary fueling was done the night before by the hearty carbohydrate-rich dinner. Before **afternoon events**, athletes should plan a hearty carbohydrate-rich dinner and breakfast, to be followed by a light lunch. A runner racing at noon can enjoy a heartier breakfast (such as four or five pancakes @ 600–1,000 calories), as compared to when he races earlier in the day. Before **evening events**, athletes should plan a hearty carbohydrate-rich breakfast and lunch, followed by a light snack/meal 1–2 hours prior to the event. In addition to basing the meals on carbohydrates, athletes should also consume an additional glass of fluid with each meal, as well as between meals, to insure complete hydration. Water, low-fat milk, and juices are the recommended choices, although the less nourishing soft drinks and sports drinks are also popular, acceptable choices.

The importance of pre-exercise fueling should not be underestimated. According to one study (Gleeson, et al., 1986), subjects who ate about 280 calories of carbohydrate 45 minutes prior to hard exercise (73% VO_{2max}) improved their time to exhaustion by 12%. That's a lot!

Liquid meals. Since liquid foods leave the stomach faster than solid foods, the athlete may want to experiment with blended/liquefied meals or canned meal replacements (e.g., Carnation Instant Breakfast, Boost) to determine if they offer any advantages. Before converting to liquid meals, the athlete should experiment with any new food/fuel during training to determine if it settles well.

Pre-exercise sugar. Historically, athletes have been advised to stay away from sugary foods prior to exercise, with the belief that the "sugar high" will trigger a rebound hypoglycemic effect that will hinder performance. More recent studies suggest that pre-competition sugar may actually enhance stamina and endurance. The preferable strategy is to prevent the urge for a "sugar fix" by eating adequate, satiating meals on a regular basis that prevent hunger and the subsequent cravings for sugar and sweets.

The best advice regarding pre-exercise sugar is to avoid the need for a quick energy fix by consuming appropriately timed meals prior to the event.

For some athletes, pre-exercise sugar does result in a negative hypoglycemic feeling with lightheadedness, confusion, and fatigue. Hence, athletes who perceive themselves as being sugar sensitive should abstain from concentrated sweets and rely more upon hearty meals than sugary snacks for energy.

Psychological value of food. Precompetition food may have beneficial effects both physiologically and psychologically. If an athlete firmly believes that a specific food/meal (such as steak) enhances performance, then it probably does. The mind has a powerful effect upon the body's ability to perform at its best. Athletes who believe in a "magic food" that assures competitive excellence should take special care to be sure this food/meal is available pre-event. This is particularly important for athletes who travel. They should bring along tried-and-true precompetition foods, such as a favorite cereal, bagel, or sandwich. By doing this, the athlete will be worry-free about what he or she is going to eat and will be better able to focus on performance.

Eating During Exercise

Athletes who exercise for more than 90 minutes will have greater stamina and enhanced performance if they consume carbohydrates during the event. These carbohydrates help to maintain a normal blood sugar level as well as provide a source of energy for the exercising muscles. The athlete who weighs 150 pounds should target about 1 gram of carbohydrate per minute (240 calories of carbohydrates per hour) of endurance exercise (ACSM, 2009). This breaks down into 60 calories per 15 minutes (about 8 ounces of sports drink)—much more than most athletes are likely to consume.

The harder an athlete exercises, the less likely he or she will want to consume food. During intense exercise (> 70% VO_{2max}), the stomach may get only 20% of its normal blood flow (Brouns, et al., 1987). This slows the digestive process; any food in the stomach may feel uncomfortable or be distastefully regurgitated. Sports drinks or sugar solutions (5–7% carbohydrate) tend to be most readily accepted. Other popular choices include diluted juices, tea with honey, and defizzed coke taken along with water.

During moderate intensity exercise, the blood flow is 60–70% of normal; the athlete can still digest food (Brouns, et al., 1987). Hence, the solid food snacks, such as bananas, fig bars, and bagels, that recreational skiers, cyclists, and ultra-runners eat during exercise do get digested and contribute to lasting energy during long-term, moderate intensity events.

Postcompetition Eating: Recovery Foods

Many of the same athletes who carefully carboload prior to competition, neglect their recovery diet. Since muscles are most receptive to replacing muscle glycogen within the first 30 minutes after a hard workout, a low-carbohydrate post-event diet (e.g., cheese omelet, steak, fried chicken) can hinder optimal recovery. This, in turn, limits the athlete's readiness to compete again, an important factor in the case of repeated events in the same day, which occurs with swimming or track meets. A poor recovery diet can also delay the athlete's ability to return to intense training.

A carbohydrate-deficient recovery diet is selected by athletes who eat the following.

- Too much protein, which may happen at a post-event dinner that centers on meat as a change from the precompetition pasta meal.
- Too many greasy foods, such as cheeseburgers and French fries that are popularly eaten by athletes who frequent fast food restaurants.
- Too many sweets, when the "sweets" are actually fat-laden cookies, ice cream, and brownies that get at least half their calories from butter or margarine.
- Too few calories, such as may happen with diet-conscious athletes who skimp on carbohydrates (thinking that carbohydrates are fattening) and instead sustain themselves on protein-rich cottage cheese, tuna, and chicken.

To optimize the recovery process after a hard workout, an athlete should eat 200–400 calories of carbohydrates as soon as tolerable after the exercise bout, then repeat this dose another 2 hours later, and then again in another 2 hours (Ivy, 1988). A little protein combined with the carbs—as in yogurt, chocolate milk, cereal with milk, pasta with meat sauce—enhances the recovery process and can result in less muscle soreness.

This "dose" comes to about 0.5 grams carbohydrates per pound of body weight. For a 150-pound person this would be the equivalent of 300 calories of carbohydrates (75 grams) in a post-exercise snack (such as a fruit & yogurt smoothie); followed by a carbohydrate-rich meal after stretching, showering, and recovering from the workout (e.g., cereal/milk, bagel/peanut butter); followed by a snack of pretzels + yogurt or apple + crackers + low-fat cheese. A proper recovery plan is particularly important for the person who performs double-works or competes within 6 hours of the first exercise bout.

> *Examples of carb+protein snack/meals include the following.*
> - *Chocolate milk*
> - *Cereal with milk and fruit*
> - *Bagel with peanut butter/jam and a glass of milk*
> - *A dinner with generous servings of starch and vegetables*

Weight Gain

When thin, young athletes seek advice regarding weight gain, remind them that light athletes can be swift, skilled, and effective, and caution them that with age, they'll undoubtedly bulk up. Efforts to gain weight by eating large portions of steak, French fries, and ice cream may have negative future effects in terms of not only heart disease, but also food preferences. Many once thin high school athletes grow into obese coaches and businessmen with heart disease who love to eat fatty foods. Recommending healthful, high-energy diets in addition to appropriate exercise and a weight lifting program is by far preferable to encouraging the consumption of fatty, fattening diets.

Many athletes who desire to gain weight simply need to consistently eat three meals per day plus additional snacks. Thin athletes commonly are "too busy" to eat adequately to support their calorie needs for growth and training. With regular meals and snacks that include generous portions of wholesome foods, they can consume adequate calories to resolve this problem.

Some athletes do indeed have trouble gaining weight, despite their abundant food intake. In theory, athletes who eat an additional 500 calories per day will enjoy 1 pound of weight gain per week. In reality, some people are "hard gainers" and need to eat far more calories than that (Sims, 1976). For them, food becomes a medicine, and they must eat even if they don't feel hungry.

A sports nutritionist can suggest quick and easy snacks and meals that will help the busy athlete accommodate the higher calorie intake. Increasing consumption of juices and low-fat milk is often the easiest way to boost calories.

Weight Loss

Many athletes—and not just those in weight-related sports, such as running, dancing, and gymnastics—strive to lose weight. They believe that a lighter body will enhance performance and self-image (Rosen, et al., 1986). However, they commonly hurt their performances with crash diets and inappropriate weight reduction techniques.

"Diets" typically don't work. The best approach for successful weight loss that allows the athlete to lose fat and maintain energy for training is to incorporate appropriate portions of healthful, low-fat foods eaten evenly throughout the active part of the day, and then chip off a few hundred calories at the end of the day. Theoretically, eating 100 fewer calories at the end of the day will contribute to 10 pounds of fat loss a year. Strict diets based on sheer willpower result in feelings of denial (to say nothing of poorly fueled muscles).

A first step to successful weight reduction is for the athlete to keep greater food records and become aware of what, when, and how much they eat. Tracking food intake on Web sites such as www.fitday.com or www.MyPyramid.gov can be an eye-opener! Weight-conscious athletes typically "diet" during the day; then "blow it" at night. They are likely to have greater success if they eat the majority of their calories during the day so that they have energy to train, and then eat a lighter dinner. The higher daytime caloric intake prevents feelings of fatigue, to say nothing of the ravenous hunger that often results in overeating in the evening. Generally speaking, once dieters become too hungry, they don't care about what they eat—nor how much—and can too easily overeat.

A second step is to know how many calories/day are appropriate to eat. To roughly estimate caloric needs for weight maintenance, multiply the desired weight by 12–15 calories per pound for light to moderate activity; 15–20 calories per pound for higher levels of activity. This number offers a very rough estimate of daily calorie needs; the actual requirements will vary greatly, depending upon individual metabolic differences.

From this estimate of calories needed to maintain weight, the third step is to determine the number of calories appropriate for weight reduction by subtracting 10–20% of the maintenance calories per day. Divide this number into three, and you'll have a calorie target for each section of the day. For example, a 110-pound female runner who's moderately active with daily activities plus runs 5 miles per day may need 110 (lb) x 17 (cal/lb) = about 1,900 calories per day to maintain weight. To create a calorie deficit for weight loss, subtract about 10–20% of the maintenance calories, or about 200 to 400 calories, bringing the total to 1,600 to 1,800 calories per day or about 500 calories per meal and 100 to 300 calories for snacks. Weight loss should be no more than 1/2 to 2 pounds a week.

For best results with weight reduction, consult with a sports dietitian who can develop a personalized food plan for your lifestyle. (Use the referral network at www.SCANdpg.org to find a local sports dietitian.)

Special Nutritional Needs of Women

Female athletes should be particularly aware of their intake of iron (to replace menstrual losses) as well as calcium (to optimize bone mineralization). Unfortunately, many females are overly weight-conscious, think of food as the "fattening enemy" rather than as nourishing fuel, eat a very restrictive diet, and cheat themselves of important vitamins, minerals, and protein. Females who severely restrict their diets to the point of becoming amenorrheic place themselves at a much higher risk of suffering stress fractures and premature osteoporosis (ACSM, 2007).

Although there's no proof that the thinnest athlete will be the best athlete, most American women—athletes included—think of themselves as being too fat. This social problem has particularly detrimental effects upon female athletes, as evidenced by the surveys that suggest about 43% of collegiate female athletes report being "terrified of becoming overweight" (Beals, et al., 2002). To help reduce the incidence of eating disorders, sports nutrition counseling (which includes discussion of body image and differences in body types) should be an integral part of women's athletics, to help women determine their healthy weight (as opposed to a self-imposed ideal weight) and to fuel themselves optimally.

Summary

Since each athlete is metabolically unique and has personal food preferences and special "magic foods," it's hard to make specific rules and regulations regarding sports nutrition. During training, the athlete should experiment to determine the foods and fluids that settle best and contribute to top performance.

To ensure optimal sports nutrition among your athletes, work with a registered dietitian/sports nutritionist who has the time and expertise to educate the athletes about their nutritional needs and answer their nutrition questions with practical "how to" food suggestions. This sports nutritionist should be available for individual counseling with weight-conscious and eating-disordered athletes, and for group discussions with teams. The job of the sports nutritionist is to teach the athletes how to eat to win. Your job, as a fitness professional, is to reinforce that information and remind the athletes that everyone wins with good nutrition.

To find a local sports nutritionist, look at the referral network of the Sports and Cardiovascular Nutrition (SCAN) dietary practice group of the American Dietetic Association at www.SCANdpg.org. You can also ask for a referral from your state's dietetic association, your local sports medicine clinic, or your hospital's nutrition department.

References

1. American College of Sports Medicine, American Dietetic Association, & the Dietitians of Canada. (2009). Joint position statement on nutrition and athletic performance. *Medicine & Science in Sports & Exercise*, 41(3), 709–731.

2. American College of Sports Medicine. (2007). ACSM position stand on exercise and fluid replacement. *Medicine & Science in Sports & Exercise*, 39(2), 377–390.

3. American College of Sports Medicine. (2007). ACSM position stand on the female athlete triad. *Medicine & Science in Sports & Exercise*, 39(10), 1867–1882.

4. Armstrong, L., Pumerantz, A., Roti, M., et al. (2005). Fluid, electrolyte, and renal indices of hydration during 11 days of controlled caffeine consumption. *International Journal of Sport, Nutrition, & Exercise Metabolism*, 15, 252–265.

5. Beals K., & Manore, M. (2002). Disorders of the female athlete triad among collegeiate athletes. *International Journal of Sport, Nutrition, & Exercise Metabolism*, 12, 281–293.

6. Brouns, F., Saris, W., & Rehrer, N. (1987). Abdominal complaints and gastrointestinal function during long-lasting exercise. *International Journal of Sports Medicine*, 8, 175–189.

7. Flakoll, P., Judy, T., Flinn, K., Carr, C., & Flinn, S. (2004). Post exercise protein supplementation improves health and muscle soreness during basic military training in marine recruits. *Journal of Applied Physiology*, 96(3), 951–956.

8. Gleeson, M., Maughan, R., & Greenhaff, P. (1986). Comparison of the effects of pre-exercise feedings of glucose, glycerol and placebo on endurance and fuel homeostasis in man. *European Journal of Applied Physiology*, 55, 645–653.

9. Ivy, J. (1988). Muscle glycogen synthesis after exercise and effect of time of carbohydrate ingestion. *Journal of Applied Physiology*, 64, 1480–1485.

10. Rosen, L.W., McKeag, D.B., Hough, D.O., & Curley, V. (1986). Pathogenic weight-control behavior in female athletes. *The Physician Sportsmedicine*, 14, 79–86.

11. Sims, E. (1976). Experimental obesity, dietary induced thermogenesis and their clinical implications. *Endocrine Metabolic Clinics of North America*, 5, 377–395.

Additional Sports Nutrition Resources

TEXTBOOKS and PROFESSIONAL MANUALS

Beals, K. (2004). *Disordered eating among athletes: A comprehensive guide for health professionals.* Champaign, IL:Human Kinetics.

Burke, L. (2007). *Practical sports nutrition.* Champaign, IL: Human Kinetics.

Dunford, M. (2005). Sports nutrition: A practice manual for professionals (4th ed.). American Dietetic Association.

Manore, M., & Thompson, J. (2008). *Sport nutrition for health and performance.* Champaign, IL: Human Kinetics.

Wilmore, J., & Costill, D. (2008). *Physiology of sport & exercise* (3rd ed.). Champaign, IL: Human Kinetics.

BOOKS

For general nutrition: NCES (800) 445-5653
www.ncescatalog.com

For eating disorders: Gurze Eating Disorders Bookshelf (800) 756-7533
www.bulimia.com

For exercise books: Human Kinetics (800) 747-4456
www.hkusa.com

Clark, N. (2008). *Nancy Clark's Sports Nutrition Guidebook,*(4th ed.). Champaign, IL: Human Kinetics.

Clark, N. (2007). Nancy Clark's Food Guide for Marathoners: Tips for Everyday Champions (2nd Ed.). Germany: Meyer & Meyer Sport.

Clark, N. (2005). *The Cyclist's Food Guide: Fueling for the Distance.* Found at www.nancyclarrdrd.com

WEB SITES

www.gssiweb.com Gatorade Sports Science Institute; includes extensive sports nutrition information

www.sportsci.org Sportscience; an interdisciplinary site for research on human physical performance

www.supplementwatch.com Up-to-date scientific information about dietary supplements

wwwfindingbalance.com This website offers extensive resources for eating disorders as well as video interviews

Part 3

Psychological Aspects of Exercise

Understanding the Challenge of Behavior Change

How Sports and Exercise Influence Psychological Well-Being

Aerobics and Fitness Association of America

10

Understanding the Challenge of Behavior Change

James Gavin, PhD, ABPP, FACP

Focus

Change is the only reliable fact of life. Each moment differs from all others. We never step into the same river twice. People who join fitness centers or hire personal trainers are deliberately embarking on a path of change. The changes they seek may look like 5 pounds more or less, new muscles, or learning tennis. They may also take the form of significant lifestyle change—becoming active after decades of inactivity or locking onto a new fitness program with total commitment. Their change may be big or small, of minor or major life-altering consequence. Change may come about by accident, circumstance, or through a planned and conscious process. In all its variations, change represents a profound moment in a person's life (Gavin, 2005).

This chapter explores processes of behavior change related to the world of health and fitness. For the most part, the types of change we will consider involve intentional decisions whereby a person decides to alter his or her behavior, rather than having behavior change imposed by others or by circumstance. Two theoretical models will guide the presentation. The first is known as the Transtheoretical Model (TTM) originated by Dr. James Prochaska and his colleagues. The second is the Learning Process Model (LPM) developed by Dr. Marilyn Taylor. The first model helps us understand a client's readiness to change, while the second takes us to a deeper level of awareness about clients' inner processes and ways in which you can help them.

A Perspective about Change

As much as change can improve our lives, we normally gravitate toward homeostasis. We are driven by the desire to have things remain the same. We organize our lives to reflect a comforting quality of predictability. In this way, we feel safe, on track, and in alignment with our life's design.

Yet, change beckons and from time to time we enter a period of rebirth and renewal. As the renowned psychologist, Dr. Carl Rogers, said so many times and in so many different ways, "human beings are fundamentally motivated toward growth and wholeness, toward developing their full potential." Change is, at heart, a growth process—forward movement on the path of self-actualization.

The rumbling we feel inside, the itching in our soul that tells us something isn't quite right or that something else needs to happen, stems from a healthy, growth-oriented drive. These transformative urges move us from one plateau of our lives to the next stage in our evolution. They are the necessary stresses of our existence, the growth pains from stretching into the next dimension of ourselves (Bridges, 2004). In other words, life is a journey with no real end to desire which requires constant re-evaluation of goals and the need for more change. Even though most people do not like change, the human being is really quite good at it. Humans are constantly adapting to change and doing it very well. Examples of growth processes, school accomplishments, new jobs, moving, and marriage are all examples of change that is generally handled very well.

The Transtheoretical Model

How ready are your clients for change? The fact that someone has joined a health club, hired a personal fitness trainer, or begun exercising on his or her own provides concrete data that your client has moved beyond the starting gate of change. Even so, you may encounter someone who is committed to exercising, but smokes a pack of cigarettes each day or overeats at every meal. A person may be ready to change one behavior, yet completely unwilling to change another.

The Transtheoretical Model developed by James Prochaska, John Norcross, and Carlo DiClementi (1994) offers practical guidelines for understanding a person's readiness for change and what you can do to assist someone wherever he or she is in the process. The model describes six stages of change into which your clients can be classified. Imagine a behavior, such as exercising on a regular basis or quitting smoking. If you were to interview people about these behaviors, their readiness for change would enable you to classify them into one of six stages.

Stage 1. Precontemplation. Precontemplators have no current intention to change. They may have tried to change a particular behavior in the past and given up, or they may altogether deny they have a problem. Perhaps they are demoralized, having given up on the possibility of ever changing.

Stage 2. Contemplation. Contemplators acknowledge they have an issue and are willing to think about their need to change. While they are open to information and feedback, they can remain in this stage for years, realizing they have to alter their behavior, but are unable to generate sufficient energy to change.

Stage 3. Preparation. People in this stage are on the verge of action. They are developing plans, and may even have made small changes. They are focused on the possibilities for action more so than on the causes of their behavior.

Stage 4. Action. People in this stage are following an action plan they have developed. The better developed this plan is, and the more attention they have given to the work of the contemplation and preparation stages, the more successful they will be.

Stage 5. Maintenance. Maintainers have been continuously engaged in their change process for at least 6 months. While "just doing it" feels more natural in this stage, overconfidence and life stresses can lead to relapse.

Stage 6. Termination. In this stage, the new behavior has become an integral part of daily life, so much so that the likelihood of relapse is essentially nonexistent. Some professionals question whether people ever reach this stage, although Prochaska and colleagues say it is possible for a small percentage of individuals.

Begin with Empathy

When you encounter people who continue to engage in behaviors that put their lives at risk without the slightest inclination toward change, you may wonder what's wrong with them. How can anyone smoke cigarettes every day, never exercise, or drink excessively, and not want to change or at a minimum acknowledge that this behavior may be killing them? People who continue to engage in behaviors that are contrary to their best interests may be manifesting a deeper, more complicated dynamic involving their beliefs about themselves and ultimately their self-worth.

The more you work with people who say they want to change unhealthy behaviors, the more you come to appreciate what a heroic challenge they are confronting. Many of us manifest our psychic struggles in how we treat (or mistreat) our bodies. As fitness professionals, it is crucial to realize that whenever clients embark on a health-behavior change, such as commencing exercise or quitting smoking, they are likely to fail unless they also direct attention to their inner world and how profoundly rooted these behaviors are in their lifestyles. The best way for you to begin helping is by having empathy and by intervening in stage-appropriate ways.

Each of us has at least one behavior that we would like to change, yet we are either unable or unwilling to commit ourselves to the change process. Your clients may struggle with their motivation to change a behavior, such as exercise, that you have long ago confronted. Understanding your own resistance to changing an unhealthy pattern of your own will deepen your empathy for your clients' dilemmas. From this place of empathic understanding, you can intervene with clients in ways that are appropriate to your role and to the stage of change that your clients are in.

Intervention Strategies for the Six Stages of Change

How do you know which interventions are best suited to your clients? For each stage of change, there are recommended interventions. The following is a description of nine interventions that might be applied at different stages of change.

1. **Consciousness Raising.** Intentionally or unintentionally increasing knowledge about yourself and the nature of your problem by any means, including lectures, discussion groups, readings, advertisements, films, and unexpected life events (e.g., a disturbing medical diagnosis).
2. **Social/Environmental Control.** External social or environmental forces that control your behavior with or without your consent, including no-smoking areas, alcohol-free parties, and peer group pressure.
3. **Emotional Arousal.** Emotional arousal works on a deeper, feeling level than consciousness-raising. It can be generated through films, dramatic media presentations, and fear-arousing experiences, including graphic depictions of diseased lungs or lives ruined through substance abuse. It is important to note that this strategy may be more effective in the adult population that has had some life experiences that may have left a psychological effect as well. Adolescents and teens do not connect the fear approach to their own mortality.
4. **Personal Revisioning.** Looking toward the future by imagining your life after you have changed your problematic behavior. It enables you to appreciate how your behavior may conflict with core personal values, and thereby generates motivation for change.
5. **Commitment.** Choosing to change, accepting responsibility for your change, and then publicly announcing your commitment to change. This typically includes a clear delineation of the change through contracting or other means of making the commitment explicit.
6. **Rewarding.** Using praise and other forms of reward to reinforce the positive change in behavior. This involves helping clients structure incentives for small steps and achievements. It also speaks to your role as a source of positive reinforcement.
7. **Countering.** Substituting healthy behaviors for unhealthy ones (e.g., meditating instead of having a late night snack). It is based in the identification and control of internal reactions, such as being aware when an urge arises and then choosing a substitute behavior.
8. **Environmental Management.** Like countering, environmental management involves controlling your world, but here the focus is more on the external environment. It involves deliberately manipulating your

environment to support your change (e.g., removing alcohol, cigarettes, or certain foods from your home).

9. **Interpersonal Support.** Involving friends, families, colleagues, and professionals to assist you through the stages of change. Helping relationships offer understanding, acceptance, and guidance through the challenges of change.

Applying Intervention Strategies

Intervention strategies need to be aligned with the appropriate stages of change for maximum effectiveness. For example, consciousness raising is especially helpful for people in the stages of precontemplation and contemplation. It might take the form of giving a smoker a pamphlet on the health risks of smoking or suggesting that the client have an in-depth discussion about smoking with his or her doctor. Though beyond our control, unexpected events in a client's life, like a friend who is diagnosed with lung cancer, can serve as a major "wake up call."

Other interventions helpful in the early stages of change (precontemplation and contemplation) may involve social/environmental control. For instance, a client's behavior might be influenced by certain non-negotiable conditions of life. The prevalence of non-smoking laws throughout Western society provides a good example of how this strategy works. Of course, this type of control is often out of our hands. However, peer group pressure, a different form of social environmental control, may be a positive byproduct of clients' involvement in fitness activities. By changing their social networks to include people who are deeply concerned about high level wellness, clients may experience social pressure to engage in healthy habits.

Two other interventions become available in the contemplation stage: (a) emotional arousal, and (b) self-revisioning.

Causing clients to become emotionally aroused about their health status may result from your expression of concern. Fitness professionals are firsthand observers of the difficulties clients experience due to poor diet, smoking, and other unhealthy behaviors. Your empathic feedback in these moments can help heighten clients' emotional concern for their personal well-being. Imagine, for example, that your client becomes winded easily or coughs frequently during the aerobic part of training. You might say the following: "I'm concerned about your coughing. I sense it's pretty uncomfortable, especially when you begin picking up the pace." With consistent empathy, your client may eventually internalize your caring for his or her well-being.

Emotional arousal may also be created by reading stories or viewing films about lung cancer. As a fitness professional working with a client who is searching for motivation to change a life-threatening behavior, you might respond to that "cry for help" by recommending books, films, or discussion groups that can arouse emotions to bolster his or her energy toward commitment.

The second strategy, personal revisioning, builds on the effects of emotional arousal. Here, you might engage your client in imagining a positive future after a change has been affected. You could ask your client to consider life as a nonsmoker. This might sound as follows: "I'd like you to imagine yourself 6 months from now as a nonsmoker doing the same workout you did today. What do you think that would be like?"

Some interventions should be avoided in the early stages of the change process because they are likely to backfire. For example, encouraging someone to commit to action during the precontemplation or contemplation stage would most likely fail. The person hasn't connected to their internal resources for addressing the problem or developed an adequate strategy to deal with all the side effects of self-change.

Interpersonal support is a strategy that applies to all stages of change, and it can be exquisitely manifested in simple actions. Listening to clients with compassion and warmth enables them to open themselves to their inner wisdom and self-caring. Responding to clients without judgment or advice, but rather with concern and empathy, permits them to be their own judges and to find the strength to change.

The fact that many of your clients may be involved in exercising with some regularity means they have reached the stage of action or even maintenance in relation to fitness behaviors. In these latter stages of change, the most helpful strategies include rewarding clients for their accomplishments, helping them consciously manage their environments so they can show up for their workouts and train alone on days you don't work together, and enhancing their commitment through contracting.

People need feedback in order to grow—and positive feedback (reward) has the most beneficial effect on behavior. Even though your clients may be so routine about exercising that you may take their commitment for granted, it is crucial to regularly praise and reward their efforts. As part of your practice, you might set aside a 10-minute period every month to compliment and praise your clients for measurable and specific aspects of their training.

Another way to help your clients in the more advanced stages of action and maintenance is to periodically review and update their contracts, especially parts that deal with their training schedules and goals. In reviewing goals, you reinforce awareness of their commitments to exercise—and themselves. Since making public commitments increases adherence, encourage them to tell others about their training plans and goals.

A third strategy for the advanced stages is countering, which involves substituting positive behaviors for negative ones. Especially when clients are working on changing other health-related behaviors (e.g., eating habits), you might encourage them to use exercise as their "substitute" behavior. For example, instead of giving in to that urge for a late night snack, clients might perform a short, relaxing sequence of yoga stretches.

Although clients may be entirely reliable concerning their fitness commitments when they are on their normal schedules, holidays, vacations, and travel can create trouble spots for adherence. Working with your clients to factor fitness into travel plans will keep them on the right path. This might look like encouraging them to plan in advance for situations that previously led to inactivity. For example, you might advise them to book reservations in hotels with fitness centers when they are traveling, or help them design a space in their homes where they can exercise when time is limited or unexpected events keep them away from the gym.

Assessing clients' stages of change and applying appropriate intervention strategies implies that you work with them both as a trainer and as a coach (Gavin, 2005). In addition to the physical routines that you take your clients through, your role as a coach encompasses talking with clients about their plans, their commitments, how to shape their environments, and what they need to achieve their goals.

Learning Process Model

Committing to a lifelong exercise habit represents a major life change. So does altering one's diet or abstaining from alcohol and cigarettes. As observers, we may witness the outcome of a long internal struggle with change in a single moment when an individual takes her last puff or chews his last bite of red meat. By contrast, a commitment to exercise is manifested anew each time a person shows up to train. Whether repeatedly demonstrating a commitment to exercise each day a client shows up at the gym or definitively ending a pattern of substance abuse in that last cigarette, change is almost invariably a process that unfolds over time. It can, therefore, be depicted according to different phases or "seasons."

Marilyn Taylor (1980, 1999) described change as a process of learning. In her Learning Process Model (Figure 10.1), she identified four distinct phases or seasons. Progress or change can be seen as each season moves to the next season through what she calls a critical transition. Her model is based on the belief that mostly we live in a state of equilibrium where elements of our personal worlds are more or less in balance. The motivation for change may arise from an accumulation of experiences or from a single event. When our motivation reaches a critical mass, we venture out of our comfortable world to encounter a cycle of events that eventually returns us to a new equilibrium, which hopefully represents an improvement over our old way of being.

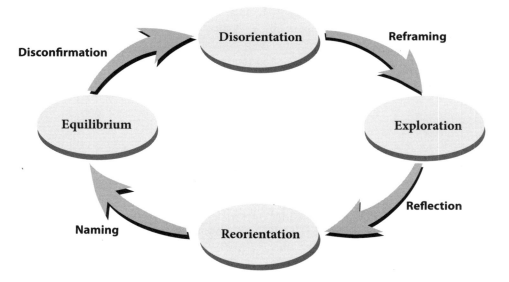

Fig. 10.1. Learning Process Model

Transition 1. Disconfirmation. Clients don't change without reason. Sometimes there is a big push like a medical report, although other times it may be a gradual accumulation of dissatisfactions that finally tips the scale and topples the person out of equilibrium. This first transition which takes clients from a phase of equilibrium to one of disorientation is called disconfirmation because some aspect of their old world no longer works or makes sense. For example, a client may deny the effects of smoking for years until an X-ray shows spots on the lungs. Less dramatically, a man may continue to believe he is in shape until his 10-year-old daughter easily beats him in a mad dash to catch a bus.

Phase 1. Disorientation. Once the excuses are exhausted, the rationalizations easily countered, or when the old reality no longer fits, clients may feel defenseless. They can't delude themselves any longer. They can't maintain their previous way of living. This first phase can be an emotional vortex where clients spin in confusion, anger, blame, sadness, frustration, or guilt. Taking a hard, cold look at themselves in the mirror, they may be saddened or repulsed to see what they have created over years of inactivity or personal neglect. They may look for someone to blame or they may be overcome by self-pity. When clients drop the mask behind which they have hidden certain dysfunctional habits, they may feel vulnerable. Even though they may try to make light of their new awareness, your best response is to show deep compassion for what they now realize. The first phase, disorientation, may last for days, weeks, or even months, depending on the nature and extent of the disconfirmation they have experienced. (The disorientation phase corresponds to the TTM's stage of contemplation.)

Transition 2. Reframing. Imagine someone who finally confronts the fact that she is out of shape and 50 pounds overweight. Perhaps she went to her 20th high school reunion and felt shamed by her athletic and slim former classmates. Such disconfirmation would pull her out of equilibrium and thrust her into the phase of disorientation. This phase normally lasts until the person is able to reframe what is upsetting her without self-blame and without blaming others. As long as she spins in self-rejection or fails to get to the root of what bothers her, she will continue to ride the emotional roller-coaster of disorientation. With empathic listening and compassionate feedback, you can help your client reframe what her developmental challenge is in a manner that implies neither self-blame nor blame of others.

Phase 2. Exploration. Imagine you have recently broken up with your lover. With the help of good friends, you move beyond blame and out of an emotional spin. Is this the time to get into a new relationship? Probably not—Dr. Taylor's model supports this. It's a time to explore what you need, what didn't work in your old way of being in a relationship, and what changes you need to incorporate in future relationships. Back to the world of health and fitness, after clients have identified an issue like sedentary living without blame and enter the phase of exploration, they can now consider options concerning how and when to exercise or, if it is another health change, what kinds of programs would be most beneficial. This is a phase where the right kind of social support is invaluable. Communicating with those who are at a similar phase of change, or perhaps a step ahead, validates the process of exploration. This is also a time when information from books or other sources is typically welcomed. Your clients will let you know they have entered this phase by their requests for information, by their need to talk to you about what they are doing, and by their efforts to connect with others who are walking a similar path. By having information readily at hand and by making time to talk with them, you will enable your clients to efficiently move through this phase. (The exploration phase corresponds to the TTM's stage of preparation.)

Transition 3. Reflection. The phase of exploration is typically an intensely social time when people who are trying to figure out new health habits and ways of functioning in a changed personal reality need other people with whom to examine ideas, plans, and proposals. The transition to the next phase in the cycle is marked by reflection. The client begins to withdraw into herself to consolidate thoughts and feelings, and to piece together a coherent strategy for action. From the outside, what you will notice is that the client has become more introspective. She may reduce her requests for feedback, and no longer ask for books and articles or other sources of information. It's important for you to be sensitive to this shift by allowing the person to withdraw, rather than continuing to flood your client with more ideas and suggestions.

Phase 3. Reorientation. Clients enter this phase with a plan. It may be a rudimentary one, but they will be committed to testing it out and determining how well it works. Maybe it is a particular schedule of exercising, coupled with a variable routine of exercises. Perhaps it is a healthy eating program that the client has derived from her exploration of how to sensibly lose weight and promote well-being. In the reorientation phase, you re-enter the picture by giving clients expert feedback and advice so they can fine-tune their programs. Your interventions represent a higher level of skill and conversation during this phase. You are no longer helping clients decide whether to take up running or to do weight training as you might have during the exploration phase. You are now engaged in providing more precise data about the program (e.g., weight training) that your client has committed to. There is a kind of shake down in this phase in which the client is making final adjustments to the plan before fully committing to an ongoing routine. (The reorientation phase parallels the occurrence of the TTM's stage of action.)

Transition 4. Naming. Have you ever come across someone who, in the recent past, succeeded in a smoking cessation program or who has become regular about exercise? Usually, these people enjoy broadcasting their success wherever they can. They want to help others who have struggled with what they have overcome. Clients who have made it through to this point are excited about their accomplishments, and they want others to feel as good as they do. You can help by validating their success, by acknowledging their achievements, and by making space for them to talk openly about their journeys. Creating opportunities for them to publicly name what they have learned and accomplished makes it more real for them, as well as providing them reason to celebrate. This transition is extremely important to implanting new behavior patterns.

Phase 4. Equilibrium. The Learning Process Model represents a cycle that begins and ends in equilibrium, although the new equilibrium hopefully represents a healthier and happier way of being. It represents the application of hard-earned learning that has been field-tested and refined. It demonstrates our capacity to grow and develop when we are confronted with challenges indicating that our old ways of being are no longer viable. At this point in the change process, your role as coach, confidant, cheerleader, and expert may be at an end—at least until the next challenge knocks at your client's door. (The equilibrium phase corresponds to the TTM's stage of maintenance.)

Summary: Your Role as Change Agent

Change is not an event, but a process. You can change your address, your hair color, your style of dress, but how do you change behavior? On the surface, change may look like doing something differently, exercising every day, or cooking healthy meals. Yet, habitual behaviors have deep roots, and changing these patterns requires effort and ongoing vigilance. How many smokers do you know who gave up smoking a dozen or more times only to resume after a stressful event or perhaps when they tested their willpower with a single cigarette?

As change agents or "coaches," it is important to realize that as your clients change, so do the ways in which they need to interact with you. If a client is in the emotional spin of Taylor's disorientation phase, he or she doesn't need a lot of well-intentioned advice. Perhaps the best thing you can do is to show compassion. Yet, as the client moves on to the exploration phase, you will want to have your portable library and expert advice on the ready.

Your clients often present themselves in the midst of a number of change processes. Defining yourself as a fitness professional means you will need to be as competent in encouraging your clients to think and plan as you are in motivating them into action. Choose your interventions based on your best estimates of where your clients are in the stages, or phases, of change. Know that action is not always the answer—sometimes people need to do "inside" work before they can act. Be aware that what may seem like little changes can have profound implications in a person's life—so avoid using your own standards in estimating the difficulty of another person's change. Recognize that listening only appears to be a simple task—most of us need to continually work at it in order to do it well. Finally, remember that ultimately you are only responsible for yourself; you can't take on the responsibility for "fixing" your clients. Remain in your heart— do your best. Care for them deeply; it's their job to change.

References

1. Bridges, W. (2004). *Transitions: Making sense of life's changes.* Cambridge, MA: Da Capo Press.
2. Gavin, J. (2005). *Lifestyle Fitness Coaching.* Champaign, IL: Human Kinetics.
3. Prochaska, J.O., & Norcross, J.C. (2002). "Stages of change." In J.C. Norcross (Ed.), *Psychotherapy relationships that work: Therapist contributions and responsiveness to patients.* New York, NY, US: Oxford University Press, pp. 303–313.
4. Prochaska, J.O., Norcross, J.C., & DiClemente, C. (1994). *Changing for Good.* New York, NY: William Morrow.
5. Taylor, M.M. (1980). Adult learning in an emergent learning group. Toward a theory of learning from the learner's perspective. *Dissertation Abstracts International,* 40, 8-a, p. 4358.
6. Taylor, M.M. (1999). *The Learning Process Model.* Montreal, Quebec: Centre for Human Relations and Community Studies.

James Gavin, PhD,
ABPP, FACP

Focus

11 *How Sports and Exercise Influence Psychological Well-Being*

Research has provided in-depth knowledge about the physical benefits of exercise, but a practical understanding of the psychology of exercise is only beginning to unfold. Sports science allows us to determine the calories we burn, the oxygen we consume, and the muscles we build as a result of an hour on the treadmill. But how much do we understand about the psychological payoffs of different exercise routines; what do we really know about how sports build character? This chapter offers an overview of the psychological benefits of exercise, and the way in which sports and fitness programs develop psychological skills.

Part I. Psychological Benefits

Sports science tells us that certain kinds of exercise will lift your mood, relieve your stress, and make you feel better about yourself, but exactly how does this happen, and what do you have to do to reap these benefits?(1,2) Research from literally thousands of studies will help us answer these questions. As a fitness professional, you have personal experiences of how exercise affects psychological well-being. Reflect on these experiences while reading this chapter as a way of personally validating the conclusions from research.

Psychological Well-Being

People with high levels of psychological well-being (PWB) report significant satisfaction with their life accomplishments and circumstances, they have a perceived relative absence of anxiety and depression, they are capable of dealing with daily stresses, and they show high levels of enjoyment and self-esteem. The overwhelming conclusion from research on the psychological outcomes of exercise tells us that people who exercise regularly tend to have higher levels of PWB than those who are sedentary.(3,4,5) Even with such strong evidence, researchers caution against making causal inferences. That is, while people who exercise tend to have higher levels of PWB than those who don't, scientists are reluctant to conclude that exercise causes high levels of PWB. It may be that people who choose to exercise have higher levels of PWB to begin with perhaps due to the fact that they feel in that they are maintaining a state of homeostasis through the achievement of personal control.

Since the concept of psychological well-being is made up of a number of distinct psychological outcomes, it may be more helpful to review how exercise relates to such components of PWB as psychological depression, anxiety, self-esteem, reactivity to stress, cognitive functioning, and positive moods.

Psychological Depression

Depression refers to an emotional state characterized by sadness and lethargy. It varies in degree from "feeling blue" to an extreme state of despair and suicidal thoughts. Can exercise help? The unequivocal answer is yes.(1,3,4,7,8) In fact, the more severe the depression, the more beneficial regular exercise can be. As you probably realize from your personal experience, common feelings of being down or "blue" dissipate during and after a good workout. While regular exercise can reduce depressive feelings, the consensus is that an ongoing and persistent depression is best responded to with a combination of exercise and psychotherapy. Fitness professionals may work in tandem with mental health specialists in promoting clients' return to health.

Are some forms of exercise better than others? In general, the answer is no. The critical factor is time. Within reason, the more regularly people exercise, the more benefits they experience. Remember, however, that extreme levels of exercise can induce feelings of depression, rather than alleviate them. The duration and intensity of exercise programs most beneficial to reducing depression correspond to guidelines from the American College of Sports Medicine (see Chapter 20, "Monitoring Exercise Intensity").

Anxiety

A person may experience momentary anxiety or be predisposed to anxious feelings in a wide variety of situations. Momentary feelings are referred to as state anxiety, while a general tendency to be anxious in a number of situations over a long period of time is defined as trait anxiety. Anxiety is generally represented by feelings of apprehension and tension. Research consistently shows that exercise helps reduce these anxious feelings and that benefits may persist for hours after the exercise session.(4,9) People with a predisposition to anxiety (trait anxiety) will also profit from a regular exercise program. Reaping these benefits requires regularity, generally in accordance with ACSM guidelines for intensity and duration. While there is some controversy about the type of exercise that may be helpful, it is generally thought that aerobic activities offer the best option to promote well-being. Severe or clinical anxiety needs to be evaluated and treated by mental health professionals, though exercise will often constitute as one of the treatment modalities. Also keep in mind that while exercise reduces anxiety, not all anxious feelings will be eliminated.

Self-Esteem

Self-esteem roughly translates as feelings of self-worth and competency. Of the hundreds of studies that have investigated the effects of exercise on self-esteem, none have reported negative effects.(4,10,11,12,13) In fact, the general conclusion is that people who exercise regularly tend to have higher levels of self-esteem than those who are sedentary. If someone is experiencing low self-esteem, what should you recommend? The most beneficial programs for low self-esteem individuals are likely to be those that allow the person to experience success, goal attainment, and feelings of physical competence. This means that the level of difficulty of the activity needs to be one that the individual can predictably master. It may also mean that competitive situations could be ill-advised for people whose self-worth is low.

Reactivity to Stress

Life is stressful, so it is normal to encounter stress in our daily lives. Stress results whenever we are expected to cope or adjust to situational demands. Stress itself isn't problematic; it is the frequency and intensity of stress reactions that cause difficulty. A regular program of exercise can help reduce the magnitude of stress reactivity that we might otherwise experience when life requires us to adjust, respond, or cope. Not only does exercise help lower our physiological reactions to stress, but it may also help reduce anxiety-related thoughts. People with highly stressful lives will fare better if they participate in regular exercise than if they are inactive.(4,14) Since exercise itself represents a stressful demand on our bodies, it makes sense that exercise programs designed to lower stress reactivity should not themselves be overly demanding, competitive, or frustrating.

Cognitive Functioning

There have been numerous claims that exercise can improve memory, increase intelligence, and sharpen mental acuity. While there may be more than a grain of truth in these assertions, research findings are generally more conservative in nature. Some studies have reported that people have quicker reactions to timed tasks, better mathematical performance, and better mental acuity after exercising than after a period of inactivity, yet the consensus of research is that these effects may be modest and are not always reliable.[1,4,15,16] Common sense tells us that moderate exercise may help us feel more alert, while high intensity and prolonged exercise sessions may temporarily reduce mental performance.

Positive Moods and Energy

It may seem almost paradoxical that when we expend energy in exercise, we feel more energetic as a result. Even short (10-minute) walks have been shown to increase an individual's perceived level of energy and vitality for up to 2 hours afterwards. It has also been demonstrated that people who exercise report an increase in positive affect, which may be experienced as tranquility, happiness, pleasure, or simply a sense of fun.[1,2,4,6,10,11] Some researchers think that this increase in positive affect could be due to the interactive nature of many exercise programs. This interpretation implies that we are more likely to experience positive feelings when exercise takes place in a social context.

Compulsivity and Addiction

To turn a phrase, can anything this good be bad for you? Over the past few decades, many reports have appeared on the "dark side" of exercise—addiction, compulsive behavior, and dependency. While these individual reports may have some basis, the case has been largely over represented. With population statistics highlighting the sedentary lifestyles of most North Americans, the problem is far more one of inactivity than of excessive activity. Only a minute fraction of the population manifest exercise habits that qualify as excessive and psychologically problematic.[1] Even in these cases, the "exercise addiction" tends to be part of a larger syndrome usually associated with such clinical disorders as anorexia nervosa and bulimia nervosa. The consensus of experts is that there is no clear evidence that people can become addicted to exercise the way they might to such substances as alcohol or drugs.[4] There is, however, a tendency for people who habitually exercise to experience some feelings of withdrawal when they are deprived of their opportunity to exercise. They may feel higher levels of anxiety and depression, or they may experience unpleasant physical symptoms during periods of inactivity.

Once again, common sense provides meaningful guidance for maintaining healthy exercise patterns. When a person's commitment to exercise begins to overshadow other critical life commitments or when severe anxiety and depression are encountered during short periods of exercise withdrawal, there would be reason to question whether the individual's exercise pattern is symptomatic of a more serious, underlying disturbance in need of referral to and evaluation by a mental health professional.

Explanations for Psychological Benefits

Sport scientists have not been satisfied knowing that exercise reliably offers such considerable psychological benefits to participants. Their inquiries have delved into the underlying mechanisms that might contribute to these effects. Results of hundreds of investigations have generated a number of factors, each with relative merit and explanatory potential.[17,18] One explanation is based on the increase in the body's temperature caused by exercising. This hyperthermic effect is thought to produce more relaxed peripheral musculature (a sense of physical calm) that can continue for hours after the exercise period.

Another theory proposes that increases in blood pressure and cardiovascular activity during exercise impacts the central nervous system in such a way as to reduce cortical stimulation and, over time, promote feelings of relaxation. Another physiologically-based model hypothesizes exercise may increase sensitivity of the right hemisphere of the brain which is associated with feelings of tranquility and nonlinear thinking.

One of the most popular explanations of psychological benefits is based on neuroendocrinal responses to exercise. Changes in chemical transmitter substances, such as norepinephrine and serotonin, alter communication between adjacent neurons in the brain and have profound effects on central brain processes. The end results of these transmitter changes, caused by physical activity, are often experienced in improved sleep, mood improvements, and anxiety reduction.

From a psychological perspective, a predominant theory regarding the benefits of exercise rests on the idea that when we exercise, we take "time out" from life issues and problems that demand our attention or require us to cope. In this respect, exercise periods constitute a mini-holiday from stress. The "time out" model applies not only to exercise, but to any recreational activity that provides a positive break from routine.

Summary: A full explanation of how exercise produces different psychological benefits is likely to require both physiological and psychological theories. Temperature, cardiovascular, and biochemical changes take place while we exercise, and as we take "time out" from the daily hassles and concerns of our lives. In combination, these changes bring about an enhanced sense of well-being including lower anxiety, decreases in depression, feelings of enjoyment, positive moods, and an increased ability to deal with stress.

Some Recommendations for Program Design

To maximize the psychological benefits of exercise, sports scientists have offered a number of helpful suggestions about program design. These are perhaps best captured in a model described by Dr. Bonnie Berger in which she recommends that psychological benefits are likely to be enhanced when exercise programs capture the following qualities or characteristics.[14]

1. **Enjoyment.** What one person finds enjoyable, another may find disagreeable. The definition of an enjoyable activity is highly subjective, yet the importance of doing something that one finds pleasing and enjoyable is critical to maximizing psychological payoffs.

2. **Rhythmic abdominal breathing or aerobic exercise.** There has been significant debate about whether exercise needs to be aerobic in order to produce reliable psychological benefits. Some studies have shown that activities like yoga, which involve rhythmical abdominal breathing, produce benefits similar to those from aerobic activities. Based on these findings, a regular fitness program will provide the best benefits, either

when it is aerobic in nature or when it involves rhythmical abdominal breathing.

3. **Absence of interpersonal competition.** Half the people involved in competitive activities lose. Along with the experience of losing, often go self-criticism and negative emotional states. If your self-esteem is at a high level, losing a game isn't as likely to throw you for a spin. Remember, however, that self-esteem waxes and wanes based on life experiences, and if you happen to be on a losing streak in life, involving yourself in a steady diet of competitively-oriented sports may accelerate your downward spiral. This highlights the need for a personal lifestyle fitness (or wellness) coach to create scenarios where the client can feel successful in a non-competitive setting.

4. **Closed or predictable activity.** When life circumstances are ambiguous, uncertain, and uncontrollable, having an exercise program that is predictable and contained may help. Swimming laps in a pool, doing a weight-training circuit, or going for a run on a well-worn path may allow your mind to release into free association. Such activities can also provide opportunities for solitude and reflection. While this may not work for all people or even at all times, this prescription can be important when the rest of one's life feels chaotic and stressful.

5. **Moderate intensity.** Throughout the literature on the psychological benefits of exercise are consistent recommendations for moderate, rather than light or intense, exercise. As a rule of thumb, engaging in a program that moderately taxes your body will more reliably produce beneficial psychological outcomes than participating in one that is either too hard or too easy.

6. **A minimum of 20–30 minutes.** More is not always better, and less is not always without benefit. Whenever possible, exercise sessions should be scheduled to last at least 20–30 minutes, remembering of course that even 10-minute exercise periods have been shown to have some psychological payoffs.

7. **Weekly scheduling.** The frequency of exercise sessions may vary according to preference, conditioning, and age. In general, the formula of being active on a daily basis—in one way or another—is a good one. When frequency drops below three times per week, psychological benefits usually decline as well.

Summary: When people participate in exercise and fitness programs as part of an ongoing effort to enhance physical and psychological well-being, their activities need to be chosen in a way that complements and respects other dimensions of their lives. A primary question to ask about fitness programs is whether or not they are enjoyable. If the answer is yes, exercise adherence is likely to remain high throughout the decades of life, and the considerable psychological benefits of exercise will continue to accrue.

The Big Picture— Keeping Benefits in Perspective

Exercise has been described as a kind of wonder drug that generates a sense of euphoria—experiences of creativity, sexual energy, mental powers, and stress resilience. With thousands of studies behind us, we are capable of putting exercise in perspective. What's the bottom line? It's a good thing, a very good thing. Yet, to over promote its benefits is to create disappointment. Exercise is part of a program for healthy living—it's not the whole package. One cannot exercise regularly, while eating poorly or neglecting other critical dimensions of living, and expect to feel good. Exercising wisely may be one of our most significant daily investments, yet it cannot compensate for inattention to other sound practices of health promotion. You don't need to sell clients on the psychological benefits of exercise. They will know them well enough through their personal experience. Your primary role is to help them shape programs that follow sensible guidelines for participation and sound principles of activity selection

Part II. How Sports Builds Character!

The expression "Sports builds character!" is so commonplace that it's true meaning may be overlooked. Consider how you and your clients unconsciously respond to physical activities based on their implicit "personalities." Just as you react positively or negatively to different people you meet, you may be drawn to or repelled by qualities embodied in particular sports and fitness programs. "Running is freeing!" "Martial arts are empowering!" "Tennis is fun!" "Yoga is relaxing!" Your clients carry certain projections of what it's like to play particular games or undertake specific physical activities. While there may be wisdom in their beliefs, the psychology of sports and fitness allows us to go beyond common perceptions to capture the specific psychosocial skills that different activities promote.(20,21,22)

A 20-year-old-woman who begins exercising for an hour each day will have logged more than 21,900 hours by the time she turns 80 years of age. If this woman understood how different sports and fitness programs emphasize the development of different psychosocial skills, she could use this information to choose activities that might assist her in mastering the psychosocial challenges that confront her at different phases of life.

How might this happen? Each sport you play or exercise you practice makes specific psychosocial demands of you. You may be asked to compete or to go it alone. You may be required to run full force to the finish line or dance balletically to choreographed steps. For each required movement or interaction, there is a corresponding psychological space that you enter within yourself so that you can stay in the "game." Over long periods of training, these spaces become home base—they give shape and structure to who you are. The longer and more intensely you participate, the deeper the personal change.

Each sport or activity represents a menu of emotional and behavioral experience that you elect to have as part of your life.(20) Over time, you may come to incorporate these elements into your definition of yourself and your behavioral strategy in the world. Knowing which psychosocial skills to emphasize comes through reflection on what your life needs in the moment in order for you to accomplish your goals and satisfy your needs. For example, if you are uncomfortable with competition, yet want to develop a greater sense of ease and personal competency when confronted with competitive situations, you can increase your personal effectiveness and life satisfaction by consciously choosing an activity that allows you to nurture your competitive potential. By choosing to condition your emotional response patterns in a self-managed process of change through sports and exercise, you create opportunities to enhance your potential in living, and thereby broaden your behavioral repertoire.(22)

You can characterize yourself based on how much you enjoy social interactions, competitive contests, or risky ventures. So too, you can describe any sport or fitness program based on the degree it requires you to interact socially, be competitive, or take risks. Choosing a fitness program might be based on which psychosocial traits you want to reinforce or bolster through participation.(22) Consider each of the dimensions as they are described below, and then refer to the Seven Dimensions Chart (Figure 11.1) to study how different activities rank on the dimensions in question.

1. **Sociability:** You may be a very social person or someone who prefers to do most things alone. In some cases, the choice to do things alone comes from a feeling of insecurity or discomfort with social interactions. Since exercise reduces anxiety, people who experience social anxiety will be less uncomfortable if they interact with others while exercising. In this regard, people can choose more social activities as a way of conditioning themselves to engage more freely in social encounters. The reverse is also true. If people want to develop a greater sense of independence, they can choose activities that require them to train on their own.

2. **Spontaneity:** You may be inclined to make spur-of-the-moment decisions or you may plan your life in great detail. Learning how to be more spontaneous or to exercise more control in your life can be assisted by choosing activities with the qualities you desire. Imagine taking an improvisational dance class to encourage your ability to be flexible in the moment. Or, by contrast, imagine designing a systematic weight training program to reinforce your feeling of self-management and self-control.

3. **Intrinsic/Extrinsic Motivation:** Some people need lots of support and encouragement to stick to a routine or to keep commitments (extrinsically motivated). Others manifest high levels of self-discipline in everything they do (intrinsically motivated). If you fall into the former category, choosing a fitness activity that has a number of built-in reinforcements for high-level participation will be critical while you are developing an exercise habit. However, once you have gotten into the habit of exercising, selecting activities that require you to rely on your internal motivation rather than external incentives for exercising can carry over in helping you gain a greater sense of self-sufficiency and personal reliability. On the other side of this equation, you may be missing out on a lot of fun activities if your intrinsic motivation always directs you to activities that are difficult and challenging.

4. **Aggressiveness:** This quality can be learned, as can a more relaxed and receptive stance toward life. Different fitness programs require you to act more or less aggressively. For example, it's generally not a good idea to be aggressive while practicing yoga, yet a racquet sport demands it. Depending on whether you need to learn to "go with the flow" or develop a more forceful character, your choice of activity can help you reinforce these qualities. Remember that aggression doesn't equate to violence. Substitute the term "assertiveness" which has to do with standing your ground, taking your place, and being strong in the face of conflict. Lots of sports foster assertive behavior.

5. **Competitiveness:** Some people thrive on competition, while others are traumatized by competitive interactions. Depending on who you are and what you need to function effectively in your present circumstances, you may want to choose an activity that encourages collaborative action or one that engages your competitive spirit. You may also want to choose an activity that takes you completely away from interactions with others, collaborative or competitive, so you can create opportunities for reflection.

Sports build character. What personal traits are you developing through your fitness program?
See how seven (7) psychosocial traits are developed by different sport and exercise programs in this chart.

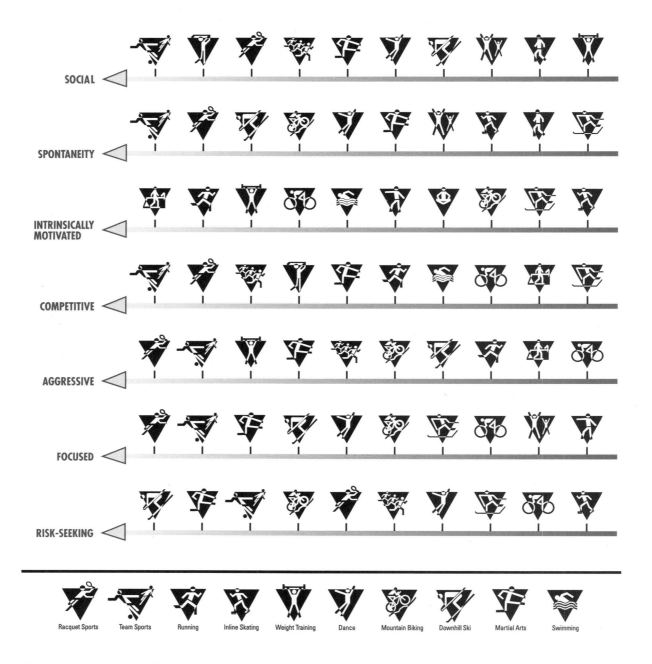

Fig. 11.1. Seven Dimensions Chart

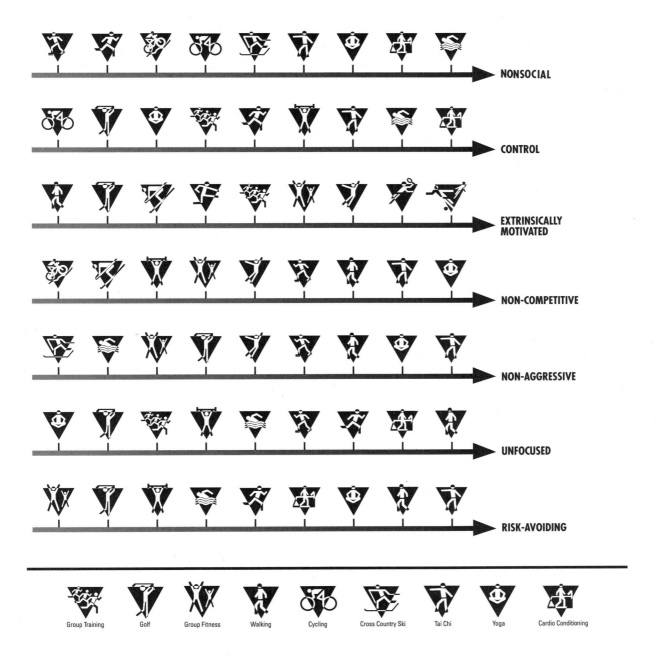

NONSOCIAL

CONTROL

EXTRINSICALLY MOTIVATED

NON-COMPETITIVE

NON-AGGRESSIVE

UNFOCUSED

RISK-AVOIDING

Group Training   Golf   Group Fitness   Walking   Cycling   Cross Country Ski   Tai Chi   Yoga   Cardio Conditioning

6. **Mental Focus:** Some sports or exercise programs resemble meditation in how they demand complete focus on what you are doing in the moment; others encourage free association by allowing your mind to wander wherever it wants. If you need an activity that will focus your mind, you can choose one (e.g., basketball) that rivets your attention in the moment. If you need time for your mind to wander at will, activities like distance running or swimming will create all the space you need for that to occur. A third possibility is intentionally bringing a meditative focus to activities that don't necessarily require it. You can run on a treadmill and watch TV, or you can drop into your breath and focus.

7. **Adventurousness:** You may be a risk-taker or you may be very cautious in all aspects of your life. Upon reflection, you may decide that you need to learn how to take more risks or perhaps that you need to create more personal safety. The sports you choose can be designed to reinforce either a more adventurous style or one that reduces your risks. Be aware that activities can be risky in either psychological or physical ways. Simply challenging yourself to do something new can be risky, and it allows you to stretch into new dimensions of your life. On the other hand, doing what is safe and known can increase your sense of personal boundaries and safety.

Guidelines for Application

The Seven Dimensions Chart provides guidance concerning the degree to which different activities emphasize each of the dimensions. There are essentially two principles for choosing activities based on the seven dimensions: (a) strategic matching, and (b) strategic mismatching.

Principle 1. Strategic Matching—When people don't have a well-ingrained exercise habit, activities should roughly match their psychosocial profiles. For example, if a man is very social and competitive, matching him with activities that are social and allow for competitive possibilities will improve adherence. Also when individuals have behavioral patterns that are working well for them, it's advisable—from a psychological perspective —to find programs that are essentially similar to their psychosocial style preferences.

Principle 2. Strategic Mismatching—When individuals exercise regularly, it may be opportune for them to use exercise programs as a mechanism for building their psychosocial skills. Let's assume a man has difficulty being assertive and thriving in a competitive work environment. If this person chooses to work on these psychosocial competencies, he can consciously design his fitness program so it incorporates more of these elements. This doesn't mean jumping into the most competitive game possible, but rather gradually introducing activities that incorporate these elements on a once or twice weekly basis. Having a coach or a trainer as he takes on this psychosocial challenge can be most beneficial both in mastering the activity and in keeping adherence at a high level.(22)

Summary: Recognizing the thousands of hours an active person will spend in physical activity over the course of his or her lifetime argues in favor of consciously designing fitness programs so they reinforce traits we want to either develop or maintain. Engaging in physical activity over all these years without conscious awareness of how they work on different facets of our personalities may represent a missed opportunity. Sports and exercise have traditionally been recognized for their physical development attributes, and only in the broadest way for their character building potential.(22,23) The seven psychosocial dimensions provide helpful guidance for understanding the specific traits that might be reinforced in different fitness programs.(22) You can be sure that the future of fitness will embrace a more comprehensive analysis of sports and exercise. Prescriptions for participants will include not only physiological parameters, but also the kind of character an individual wants to develop through practice.

Summary

The psychology of exercise is not just about the sense of psychological well-being that is promoted through regular participation; it is also about the potential exercise holds as a mechanism for personal growth and change. This chapter has overviewed the principal psychological outcomes that have been verified through thousands of research investigations. The overall conclusion is extremely positive. Sport scientists are in strong agreement that regular physical activity promotes psychological well-being, which is defined as including lower levels of anxiety and depression, higher self-esteem, greater resilience to stress, and a more positive outlook on life. Research also supports the idea that exercise can be used as part of a conscious plan to enhance psychosocial functioning according to needs that may arise at the various phases and stages of one's life. A well-rounded individual has the competency to be social and to work alone, to be competitive or collaborative as required, to be assertive or receptive, to take risks or to emphasize psychological and physical safety. Consciously varying one's sport or physical activity to enhance one's psychosocial competencies in life multiplies the reasons we have for exercising and the benefits we derive.

Reference Notes

1. Morgan, W.P. (1997). *Physical activity and mental health: Series in health psychology and behavioral medicine.* Washington, DC: Taylor & Francis..

2. Lutz, R.B. (2007). Physical activity, exercise, and mental health. In J.H. Lake & D. Spiegel (Eds.), *Complementary and alternative treatments in mental health care* (pp. 301–320). Arlington, VA: American Psychiatric Publishing.

3. Biddle, S.J.H. (1995). Exercise and psychosocial health. *Research Quarterly for Exercise and Sport,* 66(4), 292–297.

4. Gauvin, L., & Spence, J.C. (1996). Physical activity and psychological well being: Knowledge base, current issues, and caveats. *Nutrition Reviews,* 54(4), S53–S65.

5. Lox, C.L., Ginis, K.A., & Petruzzello, S.J. (2006). *The psychology of exercise: Integrating theory and practice* (2nd ed.). Scottsdale, AZ: Holcomb Hathaway.

6. Byrne, A., & Byrne, D.G. (1993). The effect of exercise on depression, anxiety and other mood states: A review. *Journal of Psychosomatic Research,* 37(6), 565–574.

7. Steptoe, A. (2007). Depression and physical activity. In A. Steptoe (Ed.), *Depression and physical illness* (pp. 348–368). New York, NY: Cambridge University Press.

8. Lambert, K. (2008). *Lifting depression: A neuroscientist's hands-on approach to activating your brain's healing power.* New York, NY: Basic Books.

9. Smits, J.A., et al. (2008). The promise of exercise interventions for the anxiety disorders. In M. J. Zvolensky & J. A. Smits (Eds.), *Anxiety in health behaviors and physical illness* (pp. 81–104). New York, NY: Springer.

10. Biddle, S.J.H. (1995). *European perspectives on exercise and sport psychology.* Champaign, IL: Human Kinetics.

11. Brown, D.R., et al. (1995). Chronic psychological effects of exercise and exercise plus cognitive strategies. *Medicine & Science in Sports & Exercise,* 27(5), 765–775.

12. Sonstroem, R.J., & Morgan, W.P. (1989). Exercise and self-esteem: Rationale and model. *Medicine & Science in Sport & Exercise*, 21(3), 329–337.

13. Duncan, M.J. (2008). Physical activity and self-esteem. In A. M. Lane (Ed.), *Sport and exercise psychology: Topics in applied psychology* (pp. 173–188). London, UK: Hodder Education Group.

14. Tsatsoulis, A., et al. (2006). The protective role of exercise on stress system dysregulation and comorbidities. In G. P. Chrousos & C. Tsigos (Eds.), *Stress, obesity, and metabolic syndrome* (pp. 196–213). New York, NY: New York Academy of Sciences.

15. Etnier, J.L., et al. (2006). A meta-regression to examine the relationship between aerobic fitness and cognitive performance. *Brain Research Reviews*, 52, 119–130.

16. Tomporowski, P.D. (2006). Physical activity, cognition, and aging: A review of reviews. In L.W. Poon, W. Chodzko-Zajko, & P.D. Tomporowski (Eds.), *Active living, cognitive functioning, and aging* (pp. 15–32). Champaign, IL: Human Kinetics.

17. Hatfield, B.D. (1991). *Exercise and mental health: The mechanisms of exercise-induced psychological states.* In L. Diamant (Ed.), Psychology of sports, exercise and fitness (pp. 17–43). New York, NY: Hemisphere Publishing.

18. Acevedo, E.O., & Ekkekakis, P. (Eds.). (2006). *Psychobiology of physical activity.* Champaign, IL: Human Kinetics.

19. Berger, B.G. (1996). Psychological benefits of an active lifestyle: What we know and what we need to know. *Quest*, 48, 330–353.

20. Gavin, J. (1988). *Body moves: The psychology of exercise.* Harrisburg, PA: Stackpole Books.

21. Gavin, J. (1992). *The exercise habit.* Champaign, IL: Human Kinetics.

22. Gavin, J. (2005). *Lifestyle fitness coaching.* Champaign, IL: Human Kinetics.

23. Vealey, R.S. (1989). Sport personology: A paradigmatic and methodological analysis. *Journal of Sport and Exercise Psychology*, 11(2), 216–235.

Part 4

Safety Guidelines

Common Injuries in Group Exercise

Risk Appraisal and Medical Considerations of Exercise

Voice Care for Instructors

Safe Foundations: Shoes and Floors

Emergency Response Guidelines for the Fitness Professional

Aerobics and Fitness Association of America

Patti Mantia, EdD and
Linda Mason, PT

12 Common Injuries in Group Exercise

Focus

> *Instructors sustain the majority of injuries due to overuse.*

The focus of this chapter is to create an awareness of injuries, the occurrence of which is somewhat common to the group exercise class setting. Recognition of injury potential, common injuries, and first-aid responses may be instrumental in protecting students, instructors, and even the activity itself. The decision to teach exercise programs comes with inherent responsibilities. These responsibilities include, yet are not limited to, the ability to instruct participants through a safe and effective exercise session, provide first-aid when appropriate, and refer participants to health care providers. Therefore, it is important for fitness professionals to be knowledgeable in exercise science, the various injuries that can occur during participation in physical activity, and trained in first-aid. However, it is just as important that fitness professionals do not go beyond their professional boundaries. Only health care providers can diagnose and treat injuries. Therefore, referral to a health care provider will always be necessary for service beyond first-aid.

Background

Probable causes of common injuries in group exercise classes:

- exercising on non-resilient floor surfaces
- use of improper footwear
- improper progressions
- improper or insufficient warm-up
- inferior choreography
- poor body mechanics
- postural misalignments/deviations
- inadequate muscular strength/muscle symmetry
- poor flexibility
- improper instruction, leadership, supervision
- overuse from teaching too many classes stressing the physical structure

In order to conduct a quality exercise program, the instructor must have a basic understanding of the exercise sciences (anatomy, physiology, and kinesiology), the principles of fitness conditioning and, in addition, must be able to recognize the potential for injury. Additionally, the instructor must have the skills necessary to transfer this knowledge into a practical setting.

Since its origin nearly two decades ago, group exercise programs have attracted millions of enthusiastic participants. The numerous benefits obtained from group exercise programs are well documented and demonstrate the validity of this sport. However, like any form of exercise, group exercise classes carry a certain potential for injury. Fortunately, the potential for injury can be minimized by the prudent instructor.

A review of the scientific studies performed regarding injuries in group exercise classes demonstrates similar findings. The majority of injuries sustained in group exercise classes are reported by the instructor. In fact, four times as many instructors than participants have suffered from the repetitive stresses of aerobics.[3] These findings concur with similar research in that overuse is most commonly associated with injuries in group exercise classes.[9,3,4] The injuries tend to occur in the lower extremities, with the majority reported in the lower leg and foot.[9,3]

Safety Considerations in Class

Floor Surface

The nature of group exercise classes provides movement patterns that multiply the gravitational forces on the body. Therefore, a resilient floor surface that will give and absorb impact is recommended. Exercise on concrete or other hard surfaces is never recommended. Texture of the floor also needs to be considered. Carpeted surfaces present a greater risk of hip, knee, and ankle torque if proper technique is not demonstrated and taught.

Footwear

See Chapter 15 on "Safe Foundations: Shoes and Floors."

Proper footwear is the most valuable piece of equipment for the group exercise participant. A shoe that provides adequate cushioning will help protect the lower extremities from impact shock. A shoe designed specifically for the biomechanical actions of cardiorespiratory fitness (aerobics) or other group exercise movement is preferred. That is, the shoe should provide support and cushioning in the metatarsal region where the initial impact lands. The longitudinal arch should be properly supported, and the heel counter should be firm and stable. Footwear must be carefully selected to accommodate the individual's foot structure and type of activity. A width sizing is recommended for a broad foot (refer to Chapter 15, "Safe Foundations: Shoes and Floors").

Progressions

Improper progressions are often exhibited by novice exercisers. Frequently, overzealous participants will begin with and/or rapidly advance to a regimen that is beyond their physical capacity (or at too high of an intensity). The result is, as one might suspect, muscle soreness, fatigue and possibly injury. This is the primary reason that new participants drop out. A recommendation of muscle conditioning and low-impact programs may be appropriate for the unconditioned participant. Certainly, the novice exerciser should begin with the minimum recommendations, such as 3 days per week, 20 minutes of aerobic activity performed at approximately 40 to < 60% of heart rate reserve (HRR).(11) Progressions that follow should be limited to one variable at a time, never increasing by more than one variable per week. The prudent instructor will not hesitate to advise students in this regard and help them modify when necessary.

Improper or Insufficient Warm-up

The warm-up period is designed to prepare the body for the exercise that will follow. The combination of rhythmic limbering exercises and short preparatory stretching is believed to reduce potential for injury. This, however, continues to be a debatable topic. In general, exercise selection for the warm-up period should mimic the work to follow and be appropriate for the group setting (modifications for some individuals may be required). Students should be advised of the importance of the warm-up period and encouraged to arrive to class on time to engage in such activity.

Inferior Choreography

Exercise selection should be carefully reviewed so that a training effect can be achieved with minimal stress to the body. This is, to some extent, specific to the population involved.

The experienced and prudent instructor will consider many factors to minimize injury potential in class.

- Choreography should be such that repeated stresses over one body part are avoided.
- Higher stress movements should be interspersed with lower stress activities, and should begin only after an appropriate warm-up.
- Movement patterns should be carefully choreographed to avoid sudden, rapid changes in direction.
- Modifications should be frequently included to accommodate all levels of fitness.

It is important to remember that the instructor's responsibility does not end with class design. Careful supervision and instruction is vital to ensure safety of exercise. Even the most carefully planned and well-executed exercise programs carry a certain potential for injury. It is important for instructors to be familiar with the common injuries associated with fitness programs. Instructors must also recognize the limits of their training, and refer all injuries to medical professionals for evaluation and treatment.

Student Physicality

See Chapter 7 on "The Musculoskeletal System: Structure, Function, and Exercise Application."

REFER TO PHYSICIANS
- all pain
- injuries
- misalignments and physical complaints leading to difficulty in exercising

Body Mechanics

Maintenance of proper posture and body mechanics are essential components of injury prevention. The body should be erect and a natural alignment should be maintained. Particular attention must be given to the knees and spine. Exercise selection should allow participants to maintain proper alignment and not place unnecessary stresses on vulnerable joints. For example, when weight bearing, the hip, knee, and foot should be facing one direction to avoid torque at the knee. Instructors should carefully monitor participants throughout the class for proper body alignment.

Postural Misalignments

Postural misalignments, such as genu valgum (knock-knees) or genu varum (bowlegs), may predispose participants to injuries. Students with known postural misalignments, who have had pain in the past, or who experienced an injury that has not completely healed as a result of exercise should be referred to a health care provider.

Postural deviations of the spine may lead to difficulties in exercise performance and/or injury to the participant. A certain degree of deviation is common as no two individuals are exactly alike. However, excessive spinal deviations, such as scoliosis, lordosis, or kyphosis, may result in increased injury potential (see Fig. 12-1). The injury may be a direct cause of the deviation itself, or a result of postural compensation.

Scoliosis, a lateral curvature of the spine, usually occurs in the thoracic region. This deviation often prevents the participant from maintaining proper spinal alignment and may result in pain or injury. However, not all individuals with scoliosis are symptomatic, as symptoms vary according to the degree or severity of the deviation. Although diagnosis should be made only by a health care provider, scoliosis may be recognized by observation of different shoulder heights of the individual when the individual bends forward and is observed from behind. The causes of scoliosis may be structural or functional.

Functional scoliosis is a result of a muscular imbalance between the right and left sides of the body. Exercise programs that address muscular imbalances are often used by the therapist to correct or alleviate functional scoliosis. Congenital, or structural, scoliosis is difficult to manage with exercise. Students with suspected scoliosis or who experience symptoms should be referred to a health care provider for evaluation prior to activity.

The low back, or lumbar spine, is designed to have a degree of curvature, known as posterior concavity. Excessive curve of this region, termed lordosis, is associated with an anterior tilt of the pelvis. Although lordosis may be congenital in nature, it is often a result of tight hip flexor and back extensor muscles and weak abdominals. Strengthening of the abdominal muscles and stretching of the hip flexors and back extensors may alleviate this condition. Individuals with

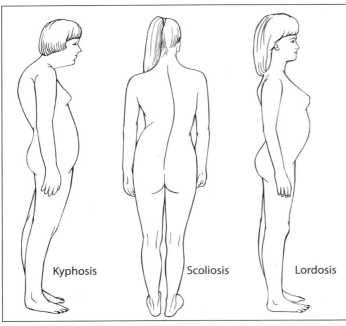

Fig. 12-1. Structural Deviations of the Spine

lordosis who experience musculoskeletal or neurological pain or discomfort should be referred for medical evaluation prior to activity.

Normal curve of the thoracic spine is known as posterior convexity. Excessive curvature of this region is properly termed kyphosis. Kyphosis is often seen in older women and could be a result of osteoporosis or osteoarthritis.(8) Other common causes of kyphosis include muscular imbalances, inflammation of the spine, and poor posture. Kyphosis may be identified with a rounded appearance of the shoulders, tight pectoral muscles, and overstretched middle trapezius and rhomboid muscles. Kyphosis is often accompanied by a forward head (cervical lordosis) as the individual must compensate the cervical spine to look in a forward direction. Treatment administered by a physician or other health care provider will vary according to cause and severity.

A review of Figure 12-1 will help familiarize the instructor with common postural deviations. If the instructor suspects that any postural deviation or misalignment is compromising the safety of exercise for the individual, a medical referral should be given.

Inadequate Muscle Strength/Muscle Symmetry

Group exercise classes, high-impact choreoghraphy in particular, present impact loads or stress to the body. Adequately developed musculature will help absorb and disperse the shock of impact throughout the body and will, therefore, reduce injury potential. It may be advisable for the novice exerciser to begin with a muscle conditioning program and/or low-impact activities to decrease injury potential.

Instructors should include exercises to help develop muscular endurance/strength and be aware of the agonist/antagonist relationship. Imbalances between opposing muscle groups may predispose participants to injury.

Poor Flexibility

Flexibility refers to range of motion and joint mobility, and is specific to joint design. Although flexibility does not directly relate to health, it is a key component of fitness. The importance of flexibility exercises is sometimes ignored. Just as hypermobility may compromise stability within a joint, inflexibility of the musculotendinous structures may predispose participants to injury. Acute muscle injuries are more likely to occur when the muscle fibers or surrounding tissues are taut and incapable of withstanding sudden forceful stretches.

Instructors should include a carefully planned series of static stretches at the end of each class and encourage participants to partake, and stay within their physical boundaries, in this very important segment.

If you strengthen the agonist, you must strengthen the antagonist.

Acute Versus Chronic Injury

Overuse Syndrome

The most common type of injury in group exercise is chronic or long term in nature. When excessive, repeated stress is placed on one area of the body over an extended period of time, the tissue may begin to fail. This failure results in a chronic injury, often called "overuse syndrome." There is no specific trauma or incident that causes the injury, and symptoms may persist for months with little change and/or frequent acute exacerbations.

An acute injury has a sudden onset due to a specific trauma, such as twisting your ankle. If the symptoms of an acute injury are ignored and the tissues continue to be stressed, the injury may become chronic. For example, a groin pull or hip adductor tendinitis can originate acutely from an excessive or fast lunging lateral movement. Rest, Ice, Compression, and Elevation (RICE) as first-aid responses should be implemented initially for such conditions. If these first-aid measures do not prove effective, the injury could become chronic. In such circumstances, participants should be referred to their health care provider.

Treatment

Providing a safe environment for participants is one of the primary responsibilities of a group exercise instructor. A safe environment includes the means to deal effectively with emergencies when they arise. The most basic of these means is a comprehensive first-aid kit for the response to minor injuries.

Response to an acute injury, as stated previously, consists of RICE: Rest, Ice, Compression, and Elevation. (NOTE: Instructors should recommend participants seek medical advice and/or care following any form of injury.)

Rest is necessary for proper healing to occur. Recommendations for rest depend upon the severity of the injury, and vary from modifications of the exercise program to complete non-use.

Ice is used to decrease swelling and diminish pain. Ice can be applied directly in the form of ice cups or ice packs, or indirectly through a plastic bag or towel. "Real ice," or a package of frozen vegetables (e.g., peas), are preferred over "chemical ice" which does not melt or freeze safely and may over-cool the tissues. Icing should be stopped (usually no longer than 10–20 minutes) when the skin begins to turn pink and can be applied repeatedly every 2–3 hours with breaks in between of 30–40 minutes in duration. Recommendations regarding the duration of ice application vary from 2–3 days, or until no further swelling is present. If ice application is not effective within that time period, the service of a health care provider should be obtained.

Compression also helps to decrease swelling. Ace bandages and elastic wraps are examples of compression devices, and they may be used in conjunction with ice. The area above and below the injury should also be included in the wrapping to ensure even compression. If the injury is in the foot or the ankle, do not remove the shoe as this provides compression. Removal of the shoe could also dislodge a fracture and cause further injury.

Elevation of the injured area helps to decrease swelling, so long as the afflicted area is raised above the level of the heart. For example, to sufficiently elevate the lower extremity, one must lie supine with the lower extremity elevated and supported versus sitting with the lower extremity at the same level as the hip.

For injuries that persist and/or increase in discomfort or swelling, a physician should be consulted as soon as possible. Also a health care provider should be consulted for any injury that involves joint pain or in which the affected area appears out of alignment.

Common Injuries

The following are the most commonly reported injuries in group exercise. Appropriate response is suggested for each injury, but it is strongly recommended that all pain be evaluated and treated under a physician's care. While fitness professionals cannot diagnose in a medical sense, the following may be helpful in rendering appropriate first-aid response to certain injuries.

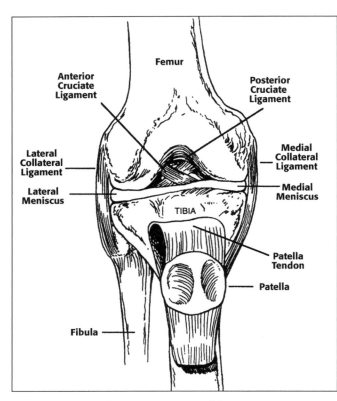

Fig. 12-2. Anatomy of the Leg

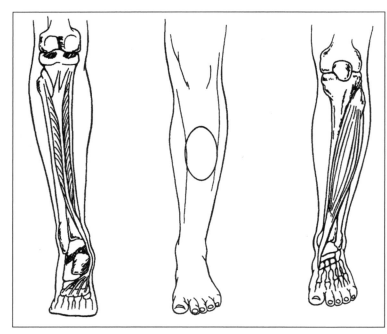

Fig. 12-3. Tibia/Fibia Pain

Patello Femoral Arthralgia (Chondromalacia patella) is an overuse injury affecting the articular cartilage of the posterior surface of the patella, or kneecap. Common symptoms are:

*   generalized pain that tends to increase with weight-bearing knee flexion activities (such as squats), walking up or down stairs, or sitting for a long period of time with bent knees
*   swelling
*   grinding or grating noises
*   pain in the knee with flexion or extention

The exact cause is unknown and may be multivariable. Abnormal lateral tracking of the patella in the groove of the femur is a contributing factor. Excessive weight bearing during knee flexion, an abnormally positioned or shaped patella, and ankle or hip deviations worsen the patellar tracking and cause inflammation. An effective response may include ice for acute exacerbations, and a change of activity may be required. Strengthening the quadriceps muscle group and correcting abnormal foot motion may also help. A health care provider's evaluation and treatment is required as necessary.

Shin splints is a catch-all term for pain occurring in the anterior or lateral lower leg, and is the most frequently reported injury in group exercise. The majority of the pain is located in the anterior tibialis muscle, resulting from tibial periostitis and/or stress fractures of the tibia. Treatment varies from RICE to immobilization with no weight-bearing activity allowed. If any numbness or weakness occurs in the foot distal to the site of anterior tibial pain, a condition called anterior compartment syndrome could be the cause which may need to be treated surgically. Participants with changes in sensation and strength of any body part should be referred immediately to a physician or other health care provider, as should any others who require more than simple first-aid attention.

Anterior compartment syndrome is a very common injury in running. It is a condition involving the three muscles in the anterior compartment of the leg: (a)

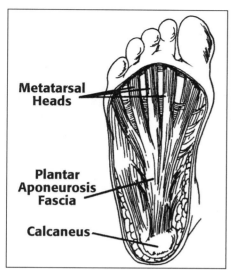

Fig. 12-4. Anatomy of the Plantar Aspect of the Foot

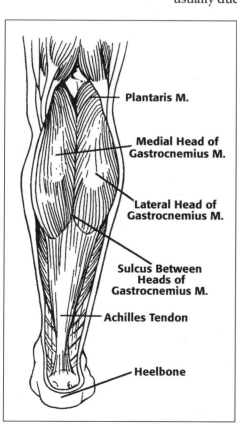

Fig. 12-5. Anatomy of the Posterior Leg

the tibialis anterior, (b) extensor hallucus longus, and (c) extensor digitorum longus. These muscles all perform ankle dorsiflexion. If these muscles are overworked, the condition may lead to swelling of the muscles and pressure to the fascia encompassing the muscles. This pressure may restrict blood flow to the muscle and lead to pain, numbness, and paralysis. This condition can be a medical emergency. If first-aid responses are not sufficient, health care intervention by a licensed provider is necessary.

Metatarsalgia is a term used for generalized pain and/or tenderness in the metatarsals, the heads of the long bones of the foot. Possible etiology is degenerative changes in the arches of the feet and/or excessive or repeated force on the ball of the foot, as in jumping. If first-aid does not relieve the pain, a health care provider's evaluation is needed.

Plantar fasciitis refers to inflammation of the fascia or connective tissue of the plantar or bottom surface of the arch of the foot. Pain commonly originates near the calcaneal insertion (heel) of the fascia and will progressively radiate towards the ball of the foot with increasing severity of inflammation. RICE, heel cushions, and arch supports are possible therapeutic measures. Again, if first-aid responses do not work (after a few days), medical evaluation is necessary.

Stress fractures are microscopic fractures that occur usually to a weight-bearing bone, such as tibia (leg bone) or metatarsals (foot bones). Pain is usually localized to one area and reaches a crescendo during activity. The fractures are usually due to repeated stress or overuse of the area. These fractures occur gradually and are not usually seen in X-rays during the early stages. Health care-provided treatment may vary from a recommendation of modifications in impact to complete non-weight bearing, by use of crutches. A stress fracture in the femur is a more serious form of stress fracture which may be present with diffuse hip pain. Potential or actual stress fractures always need medical evaluation.

Tendinitis is inflammation of the connective tissue that joins a muscle to a bone. The Achilles tendon is prone to this injury in group exercise. This is the common tendon of the gastrocnemius and the soleus muscles of the calf muscles. It inserts into the back of the heel bone. First-aid response (RICE) and a cushioned heel lift may assist. The underlying condition needs to be evaluated and treated by a licensed health care provider. Stretching before and after exercise may be key in prevention.

A **sprain** is a tearing or overstretching of a ligament. A ligament is connective tissue that connects bone to bone. Sprains are classified as first, second, or third degree depending upon the severity. Recovery length can vary from days to months. Ligaments may be permanently deformed, thereby increasing a participant's potential for injury in future activities. Fitness professionals should recommend first-aid and assessment by a physician to determine severity and need for bracing.

A **strain** is an overstretching or tearing of a muscle or tendon. Severity can range from a minimum of torn fibers up to complete tearing from the bone called an avulsion. First-aid should be recommended, followed by early assessment by a physician.

Summary

The injuries discussed in this chapter are the most prevalent in the group exercise class setting. The prudent instructor will regard this information as the basis for a medical referral and not diagnose injuries or recommend treatment.

Reference Notes

1. American College of Emergency Physicians. (2004). *First aid manual* (2nd ed.). DK Publishing. New York, NY.

2. Arnheim, D.D. (1997). *Modern Principles of Athletic Training* (9th ed.). St. Louis, MO: Times Mirror/Mosby College Publishing Company.

3. Francis, L.L., Francis, P.R., & Welshons-Smith, K. (1985). Aerobic dance injuries: A survey of instructors. *The Physician and Sportsmedicine*, 13(2), 105–111.

4. Garrick, J.G., Gillien, D.M., & Whiteside, P. (1986). The epidemiology of aerobic dance injuries. *American Journal of Sports Medicine*, 14, 67–72.

5. Gould, J.A., & Davies, G.J. (1990). *Orthopedic and sports physical therapy*. St. Louis, MO: C.V. Mosby Co.

6. Hillman, S.K. (2000). *Introduction to athletic training*. Champaign, IL: Human Kinetics.

7. Luttgens, K., & Hamilton, N. (1997). *Kinesiology: Scientific basis of human motion* (9th ed.). Boston, MA: McGraw-Hill.

8. Mutoh, M.D., et al. (1988). Aerobic dance injuries among instructors and students. *The Physician and Sportsmedicine*, 16(12), 81–86.

9. Van Gelder, N. (1990). Aerobic Dance-Exercise Instructor Manual. San Diego, CA: IDEA Foundation.

10. Vetter, W.L., et al. (1985). Aerobic dance injuries. *The Physician and Sports Medicine*, 13(2), 114–120.

11. Amercian College of Sports Medicine. (2010). *ACSM's guidelines for exercise testing and prescription* (8th ed.). Baltimore, MD: Lippincott Williams & Wilkins.

For information on vocal injury, see Chapter 14 on "Voice Care for Instructors."

Arthur J. Siegel, MD
and
Mary Yoke, MA, MM

13

Risk Appraisal and Medical Considerations of Exercise

Focus

The question is no longer "To exercise or not to exercise?" but how much, how often, and with what intensity to exercise in order to maximize fitness and well-being. For most people, the benefits of regular exercise far outweigh the risks. Benefits include a decreased risk for hypertension, diabetes, cardiovascular disease, colon cancer, breast cancer, and osteoporosis as well as improvements in mental health, functional capacity, and quality of life.[1] A majority of medical patients are encouraged to partake in regular physical activity, according to recommendations of the U.S. Preventive Services Task Force, although guidelines continue to be debated.[2] The purpose of this chapter is to review the cardiovascular and other potential complications of exercise to enable fitness professionals to make sound recommendations to their clients.

Broadened Guidelines

The 1996 *Surgeon General's Report on Physical Activity and Health* firmly established that regular physical activity prevents the major causes of mortality and morbidity among American adults.[1] But "activity" does not have to mean running or competing in a major sport. In fact, the American College of Sports Medicine (ACSM) differentiates physical activity from exercise, and defines physical activity as "bodily movement that is produced by the contraction of skeletal muscle and that substantially increases energy expenditure."[3] In 2007, ACSM and the American Heart Association published updated guidelines for physical activity which state that "all healthy adults aged 18 to 65 years need moderate-intensity aerobic physical activity for a minimum of 30 minutes on 5 days each week or vigorous-intensity aerobic activity for a minimum of 20 minutes on 3 days each week."[4] Currently, ACSM and AFAA agree that healthy adults should aim to exercise at 64–94% of maximal heart rate intensity (or 40/50–85% heart rate reserve). For those who are previously sedentary, lower levels of intensity should be undertaken at the outset. This recommendation translates into a strong mandate to counsel clients to introduce exercise slowly and incrementally. There are proven benefits for the cardiovascular system from regular, low-intensity physical activity. Recent research supports the conclusion that regular dynamic exercise has beneficial effects on cholesterol and blood pressure with energy expenditures as low as 40–60% of maximal heart rate. Sedentary subjects over 40 years of age, individuals with coronary heart disease, and those with risk factors at any age should be advised to undergo a physical examination and possibly an exercise electrocardiogram as determined by their health care professional before starting an aerobic exercise program. Once medical clearance has been obtained, exercise should be increased slowly with regard to intensity to avoid musculoskeletal injury and cardiovascular strain.[3,5]

The acute circulatory effects of dynamic exercise in untrained persons are shown in Table 13-1. Providing low-intensity exercise from moderate-paced walking to a conservative aerobic workout will enhance cardiovascular fitness including the cardiac and skeletal muscle effects as shown. With dynamic exercise, systolic blood pressure is raised, but diastolic pressure usually declines, producing an increase in cardiac output, oxygen delivery, and improved circu-

WITH EXERCISE
Systolic BP Rises
Diastolic BP Falls

Table 13-1. Acute Hemodynamic Effects of Upright Dynamic Exercise in Untrained Persons.

Increased values	
Arteriovenous oxygen difference	2–3x
Cardiac output	2.5–4x
Coronary flow	3–5x
Ejection fraction	10%
End-diastolic volume index	5%–10%
Heart rate	2–3x
Oxygen consumption	10x
Stroke volume	20–50%
Systolic blood pressure	60–80 mmHg
Decreased values	
Diastolic blood pressure	10–20 mmHg
End-systolic volume index	5%–10%
Peripheral vascular resistance	60–80%
Systemic vascular resistance	60–80%

latory parameters. In addition to producing beneficial effects on cholesterol, body weight, and body composition, exercise training lowers coronary risk by lowering resting heart rate and blood pressure.(6) As fitness improves during a regular exercise program, exercise intensity can be slowly increased with reduced injury risk and increased cardiovascular safety. Healthful exercise then becomes a part of an individual's life, with a positive effect on mental fitness and psychological well-being. Both young and old can obtain these benefits with an exercise program built around consistency and moderation.(4,5) This approach minimizes the acknowledged increase in cardiovascular risk that may be associated especially with prolonged strenuous exercise in susceptible individuals.(20)

Following the Exercise Prescription

A proper exercise prescription from a client's physician becomes even more important with advancing years given the underlying risk of cardiac, pulmonary, neurologic, oncologic, or musculoskeletal diseases which may make exercise difficult to initiate and potentially harmful if overexertion prevails.(7) Fitness professionals should make sure the prescription for exercise from the client's physician includes recommendations for type, intensity, duration, and frequency of exercise.

In some people with coronary artery disease (CAD), a target heart rate of 40–50% in a cardiorespiratory workout (once medically cleared) can provide cardiac and musculoskeletal conditioning with acceptable, if not dramatic, improvements in functional capacity. A modified Borg Scale of Perceived Exertion may be useful in regulating exercise intensity in low-impact aerobics classes for the elderly with levels of 12–14 corresponding to a 50% of maximal heart rate level. Exercise should be initiated on the light or low end of the Rate of Perceived Exertion Scale so that light conversation can also be conducted during workouts. Consistency over time maintains cardiovascular conditioning and may, with adequate dietary calcium, have a positive effect on bone by preventing post-menopausal osteoporosis.(8) Moderation in intensity and consistency over time are the foundation for an exercise program leading to enhanced well-being at any age and with most underlying medical conditions.

See Borg Scale in Chapter 20 on "Monitoring Exercise Intensity."

Hazards of Exercise

The professional fitness instructor needs to be fully aware of the following complications or hazards of exercise.

Heat Injury

Cardiorespiratory exercise involves the generation of internal heat through performance of muscular work. As the core temperature rises, an increased amount of cardiac output is delivered to the skin so heat can be dissipated in the form of sweating. Heat is lost principally through evaporation of sweat from the body surface, which cools the individual at the price of losing vital circulating fluids. Prolonged strenuous exercise invariably leads to dehydration, which may then lead to headache, muscle cramps, lightheadedness, fatigue, confusion, lethargy, and persistent elevated body temperature. Advanced stages of heat exhaustion from exercise may lead to coma and even cardiac arrhythmias and sudden death. These rare and extreme hazards can be prevented by knowing ways to avoid dehydration and hyperthermia during exercise. For the over-heated client, moistening the body surface by sponging or spraying to assist in the cooling process is advisable. Fans may aid evaporation. If the client appears week or disoriented or the skin is hot and dry, emergency medical intervention is necessary.

ACTIONS

1. Monitor hydration levels. Clients should drink approximately 8–12 oz of fluid shortly before exercise. For more information, see ACSM's position stand on exercise and fluid replacement.(9) Over-hydration, or exercise-associated hyponatremia (EAH), may occur if total fluid intake exceeds losses as may occur especially in slower runners and walkers after 2 or more hours of sustained exercise.(21) Drinking only to thirst is the best preventive measure, which will, for example, keep a runner from going into positive fluid balance.(21) Runners, or others engaged in prolonged workouts, should weigh themselves before and after workouts, adjusting fluid intake to lose 2–3% of initial body weight. While water is optimal for fluid replacement up to 1 hour, salt supplements and sports drinks may assist in preventing dehydration beyond that time frame especially in the heat. As dilute salt solutions, sports drinks do not prevent the onset of EAH if consumed over time in quantities greater than total fluid losses. Drinking to thirst remains the best approach with intake adjusted by changes in body weight if scales are available.

2. Insist on warming up. The warm-up phase of exercise allows the muscles and tendons to adapt to the biomechanics of exercise while the blood flow increases to the exercising muscles. As body temperature rises, the sweating mechanism kicks into place with the perception of "second wind."

3. Wear clothing that allows evaporation and ventilation. Appropriate dress during exercise is another important consideration in the prevention of heat stress. This involves dressing in light and loose-fitting clothing during hot weather exercise, especially on humid days when the sweating mechanism is less efficient.

4. Double digit sunscreen should be universally applied to protect exposed skin from ultraviolet injury and risk for neoplasia, including melanoma. Seek shade on very hot days. Utilize head coverings to guard against the sun's radiant energy and protect against dehydration as well as sunburn.

5. Avoid using saunas and hot tubs after strenuous aerobic exercise, which may enhance fluid depletion. Fainting from orthostatic hypotension and heat-induced vasodilation may occur in saunas after strenuous exercise, especially in warmer weather conditions.

Cardiovascular Complications and Risk Appraisal

In general, except as required by athletic or other sports association type standards, young healthy individuals require no medical clearance prior to undertaking a cardiorespiratory fitness program, but would benefit from a general medical screening. However, all fitness professionals should be aware of the ACSM atherosclerotic cardiovascular disease risk factors and the basic recommendations for medical clearance prior to exercise. The eight risk factors are (a) age, (b) family history, (c) cigarette smoking, (d) hypertension (high blood pressure), (e) dylipidemia (cholesterol abnormalities), (f) prediabetes, (g) obesity, and (h) sedentary lifestyle.(5) A physician's clearance is recommended if there are two or more risk factors present; or if there are symptoms of cardiovascular, pulmonary, or metabolic disease; or if there is known cardiac, pulmonary, or metabolic disease; or if the individual is male and 45 years of age or over; or if the individual is female and 55 years of age or over.(3)(5)

In addition, certain conditions, such as mitral valve prolapse, may run in families and be associated with serious arrhythmias and even with sudden cardiac death. Individuals with any of these factors in their family history should have a systematic medical evaluation prior to undertaking a vigorous exercise program.

If cardiac patients receive clearance from physicians to attend exercise class, an open line of communication should be maintained with them. If a patient is on cardiac or blood pressure medication, such as beta blockers, he or she should adhere to the prescribed target heart rate. **Beta blockers** will blunt the increase in heart rate and blood pressure, protecting the client from a risk for exercise induced ischemia.

The following are some first-stage actions fitness professionals can take in regard to preventing cardiovascular complications.

ACTIONS

1. Complete one or several of the following: (a) health risk appraisal, and/or (b) fitness assessment.
2. Schedule a counseling session with the client and his or her physician.
3. Teach clients the importance of proper warm-up and cool-down, monitoring them for compliance. Just as the increase in exercise intensity should be gradual during onset, the cool-down should also be progressive to avoid hypotension and fainting due to vaso-vagal syncope. Making sure that clients keep walking slowly after a workout will prevent blood pooling and risk for such complications.
4. Ask symptomatic clients exhibiting irregular heart rate, chest discomfort, or sudden/ severe breathlessness to seek medical consultation before continuing their programs. Implement an emergency response in cases of collapse or other severe symptomology by calling for help as per the American Heart Association guidelines before initiating basic CPR. Heart patients often describe symptoms such as a dull ache or pressure in the chest. All of these complaints warrant a halt in exercise and immediate referral to a physician or a call to 911, even if the individual does not describe these sensations as "pain." Awareness and vigilance for these symptoms can be life-saving for helping some clients deal with denial. The exertional sudden death of marathoner Jim Fixx is a case in point.
5. Fitness professionals should also be aware of the potential cardiovascular complications of exercise, including the rare cases of sudden death during exercise. Studies in this area point to **silent congenital heart abnormalities** in the majority of cases of sudden collapse from heart arrhythmias during physical exertion. Such victims are young (13–35 years of age), and often have a thickening of the heart muscle wall called hypertrophic cardiomyopathy. Individuals with a family history of sudden death during, or even unrelated to, exercise should have medical clearance prior to undertaking a progressive exercise program. In contrast, exertional sudden deaths, especially in male clients over 40 years of age, are usually due to

underlying coronary artery disease with rupture of an often previously silent atherosclerotic plaque. Such individuals may experience sudden cardiac death as the presenting symptom from the onset of ventricular fibrillation, making defibrillation with an automated external defibrillator (AED) the first priority after initiation of cardiopulmonary resuscitation (CPR). This emphasizes the importance of appropriate screening in older patients, especially with risk factors for underlying heart disease. Clients should be continuously assessed for any changes in their physical condition. The warm-up and cool-down phases of an exercise session protect against the risk for such fatal arrhythmias. Additionally, in 2009 the U.S. Preventive Services Task Force issued guidelines recommending daily aspirin use for the primary prevention of cardiovascular events in low-risk men over 40 years of age and women over 45 years of age up to 90 years of age.(23) Fitness professionals should encourage their clients to discuss this recommendation with their physicians and be supportive of this strategy.

Basic mastery of the concepts of exercise physiology and the role of the cardiovascular system will better prepare the instructor to inform students. This, in turn, will enrich their understanding of the body's adaptation to regular exercise and the specific changes involved in promoting fitness. See references at the end of this chapter for more information on cardiovascular, and other medical, aspects of exercise that will enable fitness professionals to provide sound advice and reassurance to their clients.

Exercise-Induced Conditions

In spite of all its benefits, exercise is a stressor to the body, carrying a degree of risk. The following conditions—asthma, anaphylaxis, and hives—can all be induced by exercise in susceptible individuals.

Exercise-Induced Asthma

The process of heat and humidity exchange from the lung space to the outside air can lead to condensation of moisture around the nose and throat, constriction of the bronchial tubes, and symptoms of coughing and wheezing—the definition of exercise-induced asthma (EIA). Such individuals may have a background of allergies or be unaware of any respiratory symptoms except during exercise. Cold weather and dry air can also provoke coughing and the sensation of tightness in the central chest area. Exercise-induced asthma is similar to the bronchial response experienced in "allergic" asthmatic bronchitis, but triggered by the temperature and water exchange mechanisms rather than allergic sensitivity. Symptoms may vary from day to day, may remain stable and then improve, and may worsen during the post-exercise period.

ACTIONS

1. Clients should be encouraged to bring a metered dose aerosol inhaler to class and to use this as directed even prior to a workout. Exercise-induced asthma can be blocked and even prevented by pre-exercise inhalers used 20 to 30 minutes prior to exercise with aerosol medication as prescribed and recommended by their health care provider.

2. Persons susceptible to exercise-induced asthma should be examined, treated, and encouraged by their health care providers, to participate in full exercise activity for the benefit of physical conditioning. Lung function is maintained and preserved through such a program. In severe cases of asthma, types of exercise in high humidity environments, such as swim-

ming, may be appropriate.(10) Avoidance of air pollutants, including secondhand smoke, is essential for individuals with reactive airways disease.

Exercise-Induced Anaphylaxis

Fitness professionals should be aware of a rare, but medically significant, condition known as exercise-induced anaphylaxis. During exercise, some individuals may experience sudden facial swelling or a sense of tightness in the throat with difficulty in breathing. This reaction is similar to the type of reaction that can occur after a bee sting or penicillin exposure in a highly allergic individual. This condition may require emergency medical treatment as injection of epinephrine using a bee-sting kit prescribed by their physician. Exercise-induced anaphylaxis should be considered in any client who develops sudden difficulty breathing, especially if accompanied by facial swelling.

ACTIONS
1. Call emergency medical personnel immediately.
2. Keep client as calm as possible until help arrives.
3. If client has a bee-sting kit (epinephrine), give assistance in using it.

Exercise-Induced Hives

Fitness professionals may note that some individuals develop a blotchy red rash, sometimes with itching, at the beginning of a workout. This is called exercise-induced hives, or urticaria, and results from histamine release in the skin due to rapid superficial temperature changes. The client should be assured that this condition is harmless. Low doses of antihistamines can be helpful in diminishing symptoms as long as the drowsiness side effect is not more bothersome.

ACTIONS
1. Determine if client has had this reaction before and knows about it.
2. Reassurance, as this condition is generally harmless.

Other Medical Considerations

Smoking Cessation and Exercise

Exercise training improves the motivation for smoking cessation of becoming an ex-smoker for women participating in smoking cessation programs. Smoking and sports do not mix, including the need to decrease exposure to secondhand smoke.

Exercise and Cancer Risk

While there is a great volume of literature on the beneficial effects of exercise in the primary and secondary prevention of coronary artery disease, research is less conclusive on the relationship of exercise to prevention of cancer. Several studies have demonstrated that exercise has a protective effect against three most common cancers: (a) breast, (b) colon, and (c) prostate.(15,16) The 2006 American Cancer Society Guidelines on Nutrition and Physical Activity for cancer prevention state that adults should engage in moderate to vigorous physical activity for at least 30 minutes on 5 or more days of the week. This effect is due to the strengthening of the immune system, particularly the NK or Natural Killer cells, which are responsible for the destruction of mutated cells that lead to cancer. The guidelines also emphasize maintaining a healthy weight throughout life, eating a healthy diet with a focus on plant sources, and limiting consumption of alcoholic beverages.(17)

Exercise and Obesity

Exercise is the leading treatment modality in the effort to combat the current virtual epidemic of obesity affecting the U.S. population at all ages. Obesity increases the risk to, and exacerbates the severity of, many of the chronic diseases being treated today, such as cardiovascular disease, diabetes, and cancer.(7,18) Many studies support the therapeutic benefits of regular participation in physical activity in the prevention and control of syndrome X (also known as metabolic syndrome) and diagnosed diabetes mellitus.(1,5,7, 18)

Summary

Understanding the basic physiology of exercise and its benefits will enable fitness professionals to guide clients toward sound exercise programs to enhance their physical and emotional health. Knowledge of the potential complications of exercise assists the fitness professional in helping clients to achieve positive outcomes and enhance their overall well-being. Fitness professionals should be well-versed in AFAA's Emergency Response Plan Guidelines (see Chapter 16) and certified in basic CPR, including the use of an AED. Promoting exercise while saving lives is the fullest realization of the fitness professional's mandate.

Reference Notes

1. U.S. Department of Health and Human Services. (1996). Physical activity and health; A report of the Surgeon General. Atlanta, GA: U.S. Department of Health and Human Services, Public Health Service, CDC, National Center for Chronic Disease Prevention and Health Promotion.
2. U.S. Preventive Services Task Force. (2002). Behavioral counseling in primary care to promote physical activity: recommendations and rationale. *Guide to clinical preventive services* (3rd ed.). Periodic Updates, August. Available at http://www.preventiveservices.ahrq.gov
3. American College of Sports Medicine. (2010). *ACSM's guidelines for exercise testing and prescription* (8th ed.). Baltimore, MD: Lippincott Williams & Wilkins.
4. Haskell, W.L., Lee, I.M., Pate, R.R., et al. (2007). Physical activity and public health. Updated recommendation for adults from the American College of Sports Medicine and the American Heart Association. *Circulation*, 116; DOI: 10.1161/circulationaha.107.185649.
5. American College of Sports Medicine. (2010). *ACSM's guidelines for exercise testing and prescription* (8th ed.). Baltimore, MD: Lippincott Williams & Wilkins.
6. Barone, B.B., Wang, N.Y., Bacher, A.C., & Stewart, K.J. (2009). Decreased exercise blood pressure in older adults after exercise training: contributions of increased fitness and decreased fatness. *British Journal of Sports Medicine*, 43, 52–56.
7. American College of Sports Medicine. (2009). *Exercise management for persons with chronic diseases and disabilities* (3rd ed.). Champaign, IL: Human Kinetics.
8. Beck, B.R., & Snow, C.M. (2003). Bone health across the lifespan: Exercising our options. *Exercise and Sports Science Reviews*, 31(3), 8.
9. American College of Sports Medicine. (1996). The ACSM position stand on exercise and fluid replacement. *Medicine & Science in Sports & Exercise*, 28(1), i-vii.
10. Weiler, J.M., Bonini, S., Coifman, R., et al. (2007). American Academy of Allergy, Asthma, and Immunology Work Group Report: Exercise Induced Asthma. *Journal of Allergy & Clinical Immunology*, 119, 1349–1358.

11. Williamson, D.F., et al. (1991). Smoking cessation and severity of weight gain in a national cohort. *New England Journal of Medicine*, 324, 739–45.

12. Chinn, S., Jarvis, D., Melotti, R., et al. (2005). Smoking cessation, lung function, and weight gain: a follow-up study. *Lancet*, 5 (7–13); 365 (9471), 1600–1.

13. Daughton, D.M., et al. (1991). Effect of transdermal nicotine delivery as an adjunct to low-intervention smoking cessation therapy: A randomized, placebo-controlled, double-blind study. *Archives of Internal Medicine*, 151, 749–52.

14. Chen, Y., et al. (1991). Increased susceptibility to lung dysfunction in female smokers. *American Review of Respiratory Disease*, 143, 124–1230.

15. Courneya, K.S., & Friedenreich, C.M. (1997). Relationship between exercise pattern across the cancer experience and current quality of life in colorectal cancer survivors. *Journal of Alternative and Complimentary Medicine*, 3, 215–26.

16. Friedenreich, C.M. (2001). Physical activity and cancer prevention: From observational to intervention research. *Cancer Epidemiological Biomarkers Prevention*, 10, 287–301.

17. Kushi, L.H., Byers, T., et al. (2006). American Cancer Society Guidelines on nutrition and physical activity for cancer prevention. *A Cancer Journal for Clinicians*, 56, 254–281.

18. Ross, R., Freeman, J.A., & Janssen, I. (2000). Exercise alone is an effective strategy for reducing obesity and related comorbidities. *Exercise and Sport Sciences Reviews*, 28, 165–69.

19. American Council on Exercise. (1999). *Clinical exercise specialist manual.* San Diego, CA: American Council on Exercise.

20. Erhman, J.K., Gordon, P.M., Visich, P.S., & Keteyian, S.J. (2008). *Clinical Exercise Physiology.* Champaign, IL. Human Kinetics.

21. Maharam, L.G., Hew, T., Siegel, A.J., Adner, M., Adams, B., & Pujol, P. (2006). International marathon medical directors: Revised fluid recommendations for runners and walkers. Approved by IMMDA: 6 May, Barcelona, Spain. Available at http://www.aims-association.org/guidelines_fluid_replacement .html, accessed, 6 Dec 2006.

22. Thompson, P.D., Franklin, B.A., Balady, G.J., Blair, S.N., et al. (2007). Exercise and acute cardiovascular events placing the risks in perspective: a scientific statement from the American Heart Association Council on Nutrition, Physical Activity, and Metabolism and the Council on Clinical Cardiology. *Circulation*, 115(17), 2358–68.

23. U.S. Preventive Services Task Force. (2009). Aspirin for prevention of cardiovascular disease: U.S. Preventive Services Task Force recommendation statement. *Annuals of Internal Medicine*, 17 March, 150(6), 396–404.

14

Voice Care for Instructors

Carol Swett, MA, CCC
and
Jo-Ann Ross, MA, CCC

Focus

One of the most important musculoskeletal systems of the body, the voice, tends to be severely neglected by the fitness instructor population. Group fitness instructors depend upon their voices to provide appropriate directions and cues so that students can enjoy a smooth flow throughout their workouts. A voice that is clear, easily understood, and carries well will be the most effective for the class members and will bode well for the instructor. Research has shown, however, that group fitness instructors are a "high-risk group of professional voice users due to the exceptional demands placed on their voices" (Newman, Kersner, 1998). This is why group fitness instructors, as professional voice users, must learn how to care for and condition their voices as they would any other major muscle group.

Anatomy and Physiology of the Vocal Mechanism

Vocalization involves integration and balance of the respiratory and cardiovascular systems, as well as the spine, shoulders, neck, jaw, articulators, and the larynx, or vocal cords. The larynx, which is comprised of muscles, cartilage, and connective tissue, houses the vocal cords (Figure 14-1). These cords are a group of paired muscles that create the movement necessary for swallowing protection, respiration, assistance in muscular mechanical advantage (Valsalva maneuver), and creating voice.

To be able to use the voice, appropriate breathing must first be considered. The muscles responsible for inhaling are the diaphragm, external intercostals, sternocleidomastoid, and pectoralis major and minor. The muscles of exhalation work with the passive properties of torque, tissue elasticity, and gravity and are the rectus abdominis, transverse abdominis, and internal and external obliques.

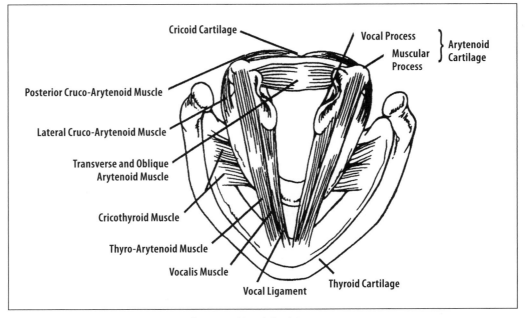

Fig. 14-1. Vocal Cord Anatomy

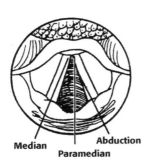

Fig. 14-2a.
Normal Larynx Phonation

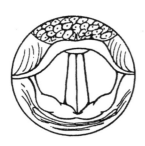

Fig. 14-2b.
Closed Vocal Cords

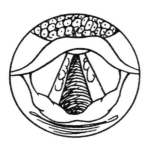

Fig. 14-3.
Vocal Nodules

During non-aerobic activities, the shoulders should not move up and down, and the upper chest should remain still. When breathing, movement is generally restricted to the abdominal area of the midsection, which moves outward and allows the body to relax and eliminate tension from the throat. The amount of time for inhalation and exhalation is about equal, except during vocalization when inhalation is rapid and exhalation is prolonged.

When working aerobically, the physiological demands change and as the exercise becomes more vigorous, the breathing rate is deeper, faster, and heavier. The vocal cords are being forced apart in order to allow more space for the increase in oxygen supply (Figure 14-2a). When the instructor voices during this time they are actually working against the body's natural response to keep an open air space.

Another way instructors work against the body's natural rhythm is when working anaerobically, during floor or isolated movements. At this time posture is key to performing exercises such as squats, lunges, push-ups, and weight training. In order to perform the exercise, contraction of the abdominals (obliques and transverse) stabilizes the core torso. This constricts the vocal airway and does not allow for deep inhalation which is required for speaking. This, in turn, produces a strain on the vocal folds which may lead to vocal injury.

Excessive vocal use, vocal abuse, or inappropriate use of the vocal mechanism may result in one or more vocal cord injuries or warning signs. Inflammation of the vocal cords during an infection, including sinus infection and even nasal allergies, may actually increase your chance of developing vocal cord damage. Injury to the vocal cords can be either traumatic or chronic depending upon the abuse that is occurring. Vocal injury can result in swelling and/or reddening of the vocal cords, laryngitis (illness-related or trauma-induced from extreme yelling or abuse), vocal nodules (Figure 14-3), and contact ulcers. Nodules are more prevalent among group exercise instructors and are characterized by calloused, benign growths on the vocal cord edges. They vary from the size of a pinhead to the size of a pea. The following warning signs and symptoms may indicate the possibility of a vocal cord injury in need of evaluation by a health care provider.

Warning signs and symptoms of vocal injury:

- Tired voice
- Feeling a lump in the throat or need to clear the throat
- Dry throat
- Sore throat
- Tightness or increased tension in throat

Warning signs and symptoms that you or others might hear:

- Hoarseness
- Loss of voice or no voice at all
- Squeaky, breathy, or rough voice
- Frequent coughing and throat clearing
- Voice not heard clearly and worsens at night

Teaching Tips

1. Relaxation—Keep the head, jaw, neck and shoulders tension-free.
2. Posture—Demonstrate abdominal exercises or push-ups without speaking if possible, then move out of that position and continue to speak while instructing.
3. Projection—Speak out, not down or up, not high or forced. Face the audience.
4. Pitch—Use a natural pitch that allows comfortable speech without effort.
5. Cueing—Incorporate gestural and visual cueing whenever possible.
6. Environment—Keep music at a moderate volume. Move around the room to accommodate all students.
7. Microphones—If a facility has one—use it! If not, insist that one be purchased. Be careful not to shout into the microphone or project unnaturally.

Summary

The voice is a muscle system that must be respected by the professional fitness instructor. Proper conditioning and using the voice correctly in class are crucial to good vocal health. If any of the warning signs listed above are experienced, a health care provider should be consulted or seek a referral to an otolaryngologist. If a vocal injury has occurred, speech or voice therapy may be recommended by a health care provider as it has proven to be effective in eliminating vocal injuries. Being aware of basic vocal functions, appropriate pitch levels, posture, and projection techniques, as well as the warning signs, will ensure a voice that is powerful, commanding, and easily understood by students.

References

1. Bernthal, J.E. (Ed.). (1997). *Articulation and Phonological Disorders.* Needham Heights, MA: Allyn & Bacon.
2. Newman, C., & Kersner, M. (1998). *Voice problems of aerobics instructors: implications for preventative training.* King George Hospital, Department of Human Communication Science, University College, Log Phon Vocol; 23; 1770180. London, UK.
3. Timmermans, B., De Bodt, M., Wuyts, F., & Van de Heyning, P. (2003). *Vocal hygiene in radio students and in radio professionals.* Logoped Phoniatr Vocol 28: 127–132.
4. Zemlin, W.R. (1998). *Speech and hearing science: Anatomy and physiology* (4th ed.). Needham Heights, MA: Allyn & Bacon.

Voice Care Guidelines

1. Stay in good health
2. Hydration
3. Voice rest and pacing
4. Avoid irritants such as smoke, smog, etc.
5. Avoid medications
6. Avoid negative vocal behaviors
7. Limit talking in noisy places
8. Learn vocal and overall relaxation
9. Focus your voice
10. Avoid certain foods that have an irritating effect
11. Warm up your voice
12. Develop good breathing habits
13. Avoid shouting or talking loudly

---

15 Safe Foundations: Shoes and Floors

Mary Yoke, MA, MM

Focus

Proper shoes, quality flooring, and safe technique are three of the most important safeguards against exercise-related injuries. In this chapter, we take a look at the physical foundations of exercise safety—the shoes you wear and the flooring on which you stand, jog, jump, dance, step, and stretch.

Shoes

Wearing the proper shoe is key for injury prevention, stability, and better performance. Below, we will review foot structure and biomechanics, shoe anatomy, fitting considerations, sport-specific applications, and injury prevention.

Foot Structure and Biomechanics

For the best fitting shoe, know your foot type. Feet are generally categorized into three basic types: (a) normal arch, (b) high arch, and (c) flat foot (no arch). To find out which type you are, take the Wet Test—simply wet one foot and stand on a surface that will show an imprint of your foot. Check your imprint to determine your foot type.

- A foot with a **normal arch** leaves an imprint that clearly shows an arch, however, the forefoot and the heel are connected by a thick band.
- A foot with a **high arch** leaves an imprint of a forefoot and a heel with little to no connection between the two.
- A **flat foot** leaves an imprint in which almost the entire bottom of the foot is in contact with the floor.

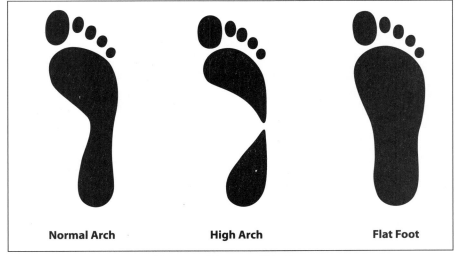

| Normal Arch | High Arch | Flat Foot |

Fig. 15-1. Diagram of Wet Test

Another strategy for identifying your foot type is to look at the bottom of your exercise shoes. A shoe that is worn down on the inside (medial) edge can indicate that you over-pronate and probably have flat feet. A shoe that is worn down on the outside (lateral) edge typically indicates over-supination, a condition often accompanied by high arches.

<table>
<tr><td>

Did you know?

Each of your feet has 26 bones, 33 joints, 107 ligaments, and 19 muscles and tendons.

</td></tr>
</table>

When walking and running normally, the foot strikes the ground with the heel and quickly distributes the force to the ball of the foot and the toes. Also, upon striking the ground, the arch of the foot is normally lifted, then immediately rolls inward and down as the weight moves to the front of the foot. This phenomenon is described as normal supination followed by normal pronation of the foot. A person who spends too much time with the arch lifted and doesn't roll inward appropriately displays over-supination. Spending too much time with the foot rolled inward and flattened is called over-pronation.

A person who excessively supinates (or, more accurately, "under-pronates") tends to have a more rigid gait, with a foot that is hypomobile and doesn't move enough to properly dissipate the stress of impact. This foot type calls for a shoe with plenty of shock absorption, cushioning, and arch support.

Those who excessively pronate often have problems with too much lower leg and foot motion, which can put abnormal stress on the joints of the foot and may lead to knee problems. This condition requires a firm, stable, control-type shoe to help prevent unnecessary movement. For those who over-pronate, motion control is more important than shock absorption for injury prevention.

To summarize, think of the two C's—cushioning and control. High arched, stiff feet need cushioning; flat, motion-prone feet need shoes that can control that motion. Average feet need a shoe in the middle, one that has both cushioning and stability features.

Common Injuries Associated with Foot Type	
High Arched, Rigid Foot	**Flat, Movable Foot**
Plantar fasciitis	Achilles tendinitis
Metatarsalgia	Plantar fasciitis
Metatarsal and tarsal stress fractures	Posterior tibialis tendinitis
Peroneal tendinitis	Patellofemoral pain
Iliotibial band syndrome	Tibial stress syndrome (shinsplints)

(Reprinted with permission from *Athletic Injuries and Rehabilitation* by Zachazewski, J.E., Magee, D.J., and Quillen, W.S. 1996. W.B. Saunders Company.)

New Trends

A new trend in athletic footwear is dorsiflexion technology; these shoes are sometimes known as negative heel shoes. According to the manufacturers of dorsiflexion footwear, wearing a shoe that places the ankle in a greater degree of dorsiflexion than when standing barefoot places the posterior muscles of the lower leg in a position of increased stretch. This is said to increase reactivity, explosive power, and improve posture and breathing. Some manufacturers claim that such shoes increase calorie expenditure.

Shoes with rocker bottoms have also been developed. These shoes literally have a sole shaped somewhat like the bottom of a rocking chair, thus providing an unstable base. This type of footwear is said to increase the activity of the lower leg muscles, and provide medical and health benefits (Nigg, B.M., et al, 2004).

Another trend is a rollbar or special plate placed in the sole under the metatarsal heads to increase and facilitate the roll of the foot, theoretically helping with push-off.

Shoe Anatomy

Finding the right shoe with the best fit is easier if you know some of the technical jargon used in shoe design.

- **Last**—a foot-shaped mold around which the shoe is built. There are three basic ways in which lasts are constructed:
  1. *Board lasted*—cardboard literally runs the length of the shoe, providing support and improving stability. This is best for those with flat, over-pronated feet.

The Life of a Shoe

How long will your shoes last? Typically, the more you perform high-impact activities in your shoes, the more quickly they will break down. For example, in running, it is estimated that 25% of shock absorption is lost after 50 miles, 33% is lost after 100–150 miles, and after 250–500 miles shoes retain less than 60% of their original ability to absorb shock. In general, high-impact shoes apparently have about a 500-mile life span, which translates roughly into 100 hours of high-/low-impact classes. Other factors that can reduce the longevity of shoes include a heavier body weight, cheap construction quality, and a rough flooring or outdoor exercise surface.

Also, beware of shoes that have been sitting on warehouse shelves for a year or more; glue and some shock absorbing materials can begin to disintegrate with age, heat, and sun. It is ideal to buy two pairs of shoes and use them on alternate days, allowing the shoes adequate time to breathe and expand between workouts.

---

2. *Slip lasted*—the upper part of the shoe is sewn together under the last, then the last is slipped out, leaving a flexible, less stable shoe with a seam running the length of the shoe (under the insole). This shoe is typically best for those with high arches.

3. *Combination lasted*—cardboard is left in the rear of the shoe for motion control and stability, while the last has been slipped out of the front of the shoe, allowing for flexibility under the ball of the foot.

In addition, lasts can have three different shapes:

1. A *straight last* is the widest last and therefore the most stable. This is appropriate for those who over-pronate.

2. A *curved last* is the thinnest last; a curved strip connects the ball of the foot to the heel. A shoe with this type of last is light and flexible, and best for those who over-supinate.

3. A *semi-curved* last is in between the straight and the curved lasts, providing both flexibility and stability. This shoe is for individuals with "normal" or "average" arches.

- **Upper**—an athletic shoe's upper is generally made of synthetic leather and mesh nylon and covers the upper part of the foot.

- **Counter**—the heel counter wraps around the back of the foot and provides motion control and stability. It should be rigid and difficult to bend or flex. Many counters have an Achilles notch that helps to prevent excessive friction on the Achilles tendon.

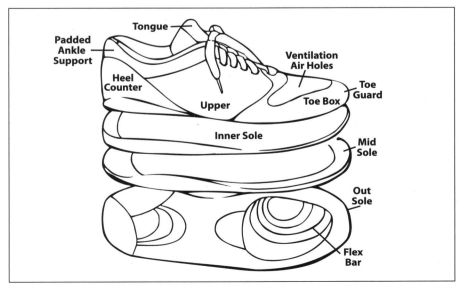

Fig. 15-2. Illustration of a basic shoe showing the features described above

- **Midsole**—the part of the shoe that provides most of the shock absorption and cushioning, depending on the targeted activity. It is usually made of EVA (ethylene vinyl acetate), or polyurethane, and may contain other shock-reducers, such as gel, air, or Hydroflow.
- **Insole**—the removable inner lining that can increase comfort, cushioning, shock absorption, and arch support.
- **Bottom sole**—the bottom (outer) sole is shaped according to the demands of the sport for which the shoe is designed. It is made of durable rubber, molded in designs that enhance traction.
- **Toe cap or box**—the front upper part of the shoe, which should be rounded with plenty of room for the toes to fully extend in proper alignment. The end of the toe box should be half an inch from the end of the big toe. Proper width and height of the toe box are important to minimize toe and bunion irritation.

In addition to the anatomical features described above, there are other important elements to consider for comfort and injury prevention:

- **Shock absorption** (more accurately described as shock dispersion) is the most important reason to wear athletic shoes. Shock dispersion and cushioning are provided by the mid-sole, bottom sole, and insole of the shoe. The mid-sole is especially affected by repetitive impact forces, and will break down over time, reducing the life of the shoe (see box above).
- **Flexibility** is important for activities such as high-/low-impact, step, and running sports with a forward/backward motion. A good shoe will bend comfortably under the metatarsal heads and allow the toes to push off easily when moving from back to front. If it does not, excessive stress may be placed on the foot and Achilles tendon. Flexible shoes are especially appropriate for those who over-supinate, whose feet tend to be more rigid.

  Test your shoe's flexibility by holding it in both hands and twisting crosswise. The stiffer the shoe, the better it will be for exercisers who over-pronate.
- **Stability**, also known as motion control, is especially important for those who over-pronate. A stable shoe limits excessive pronation and side-to-side motion. Motion control in a shoe is provided by the heel counter, which prevents excessive rear-foot movement, and by external support straps and stiff construction in the upper, which helps control the tendency of the forefoot to roll over. The need for stability in a shoe varies according to the activity or sport, which is why it's ideal to own a variety of footwear for sport-specific applications. For example, high-/low cardio and step utilize more lateral (side-to-side) and twisting movements than running, which has a front to back movement pattern. High-/low-impact choreographed classes and step thus require more stabilization in the forefoot to prevent rolling over, whereas running requires more stability in the rear foot to prevent excessive pronation during foot strike.

The Right Fit

Fit is a universal priority when exercising in athletic shoes. When buying footwear, consider the following guidelines.

1. Since most people have one foot that is larger than the other, have both feet measured and fit to the larger size.
2. Don't insist on fitting into a certain shoe size, because sizes vary among manufacturers. Also, many athletic shoes run a size or two larger than dress shoes.
3. Stand during the fitting and be sure there is about 3/8 to 1/2 inch (at least one thumb's width) between the end of your longest toe and the shoe. Shoes that are too short can cause blisters, black toe syndrome, and aggravate bunions.
4. Heels should fit with a minimal amount of slippage.
5. The ball of the foot should fit comfortably in the widest part of the toe box.
6. Try on shoes at the end of the day when feet tend to be larger.
7. Wear the socks and any orthotic devices you would normally wear while exercising.
8. Do not rely too much on "breaking in" your shoes. Properly fitting shoes should feel comfortable the moment they are put on.
9. Try replacing the shoe's insoles with over-the-counter insoles to provide extra cushioning and arch support, especially if you have high arches and/or tend to over-supinate. Extra cushioning is also needed as people age and the fat pad at the bottom of the foot thins.

Floors

Safe flooring in the group exercise room should have a smooth, non-slip surface for safe motion, as well as resilience for shock absorption. A floor that yields upon impact (vertical deformation) is important for injury prevention; in addition, a floor that feels "bouncy" and resilient can be motivating and fun for participants.

According to ACSM's Health/Fitness Facility Standards and Guidelines, group exercise rooms "should have a wood or comparable floor surface in conjunction with a subfloor system that eliminates dead spots and provides for adequate absorption. Numerous options for achieving such a level of deflection exist, including spring systems, floating floors, resilient rubber padding, and wood furring strips."

Probably the most popular type of group exercise flooring is a floating or suspension wood floor, usually made of maple or oak. The subfloor, or layer immediately under the wood, is usually a type of rubber pad that serves as a buffer zone between the exerciser and the hard bottom surface. Other options include layered padding covered with carpet or linoleum, and synthetic snap-together tiles. Unfortunately, no single floor surface appears to be ideal for all types of group exercise classes. Non-slip surfaces are very important in step classes. Use of a step on gripping carpet or treaded surface is better than on smooth wood, especially when sweat falling to the floor is an issue. On the other hand, dance-based classes require a smooth surface for sliding and turning. Sliding and shuffling-type moves on a carpeted or high traction surface may lead to tripping, resulting in twisted ankles. A deeper carpet may feel best for yoga or

Pilates-based classes, while rubber mats may be most appropriate in a room used for stationary indoor cycling.

Standards have been developed to help ensure floor safety. Many flooring manufacturers in the United States adhere to the DIN (Deutsches Institut fur Normung) standards. The DIN standards for physical activity flooring (classed as having a protective function with some sports function characteristics) state that floors should have: (a) a minimum of 53% shock absorption, (b) 2.3mm standard vertical deformation and 90% ball deflection, (c) 15% maximum deflective indentation, (d) sliding characteristics between 0.5 and 0.7, and (e) a rolling load of 337.6 lb.

Summary

Flooring is only a contributing factor to exercise safety. Shoes and safe technique must also be relied on for injury-free fitness. For instructors, exercise moderation is important to consider since overuse injuries are still common to the profession. Over a prolonged period, even the most up-to-date, high-tech flooring cannot safeguard against muscle fatigue and biomechanical imbalance, both of which can cause foot and leg injuries associated with repetitive impact. However, the importance of safe flooring cannot be disregarded. Quality flooring and shoes are the foundations of exercise safety.

References

1. American Orthopedic Foot and Ankle Society. (1998). Choosing Athletic Footwear (Patient Brochure). Seattle, WA.

2. Frey, C. (1997). "Footwear and stress structures." Clinical Sports Medicine. 16.2: 249–56.

3. McPoil, T. (2000). Athletic footwear: design, performance and selection issues. *Journal of Science and Medicine in Sport*, 3 (3): 260–267.

4. Nigg, B.M. (Ed.). (1996). *Biomechanics of running Shoes.* Champaign, IL: Human Kinetics.

5. Nigg, B.M., Ferber, R., & Gormley, T. (2002). Kinematics, kinetics, muscle activity, soft tissue vibrations and oxygen consumption for stable and unstable shoes. *Gait Posture*, 16 (1): 1–14.

6. Tharett, S.J., McInnis, K.J., & Peterson, J.A. (Eds.). (2007). *ACSM's health/fitness facility standards and guidelines* (3rd ed.). Champaign, IL: Human Kinetics.

7. Tufts University. (1998). "How to choose shoes: avoid painful foot problems by looking for the right features." Health & Nutrition Letter. 16.8: 3.

8. Zachazewski, J., Magee, D., & Quillen, W. (1996). *Athletic Injuries and Rehabilitation.* Philadelphia, PA: W. B. Saunders Co.

Marcia M. Ditmyer, PhD, MBA and Dorette Nysewander, EdD

16

Emergency Response Guidelines for the Fitness Professional

Focus

Emergency response protocols change often based on scientific research conducted by experts in the field of emergency medicine. Additionally, because training in emergency respiratory protocol techniques are linked to certification from nationally recognized organizations (e.g., the American Heart Association, the American Red Cross, and the National Safety Council) the contents of this chapter are for reference and review purposes only. However, the information contained in this chapter will give you a jump-start on any emergency situation. It contains the most up-to-date, medically reviewed first-aid and emergency response procedures that will assist in preparing fitness professionals to meet standards of competence and efficiency in the delivery of emergency services.

Overview

According to the Bureau of Labor Statistics (2009), 230 of 1,158,870 nonfatal occupational injuries and illnesses involving days away from work occurred to personal trainers and group exercise instructors in 2007. We are all urged to exercise in order to get fit, stay fit, and maintain a healthy lifestyle to avoid illnesses associated with obesity. Sports seem like a fun way of burning extra calories to lose weight. However, according to the 2000 U.S. Consumer Product Safety Commission report (CPSC), sports injuries among baby boomers increased significantly in that decade by 33% from 1991 to 1998. There were about 276,000 hospital emergency rooms which treated injuries to persons 35 to 54 years of age in 1991 compared to more than 365,000 sports injuries to persons of these ages in 1998. Baby boomers suffered more than 1 million sports injuries which cost over $18.7 billion in medical expenses in 1998. The highest numbers of sports-related injuries came from bicycling, basketball, baseball, and football, with a higher incidence of deaths associated with head injuries while riding a bicycle. Data compiled in 2006 by the U.S. Consumer Product Safety Commission's National Electronic Injury Surveillance System (NEISS) found that bicycling, basketball, baseball, and football are still among the higher incidence of injuries (Table 1). However, the popularity of All Terrain

Table 16-1. Incidence Rates of Sports/Exercise Injuries

Est. # of Injuries	Sport and Type of Injury
529,837	**Basketball** - Cut hands, sprained ankles, broken legs, eye and forehead injuries.
490,434	**Bicycling** - Feet caught in spokes, head injuries from falls, slipping while carrying bicycles, collisions with cars.
460,210	**Football** - Fractured wrists, chipped teeth, neck strains, head lacerations, dislocated hips, jammed fingers.
275,123	**ATVs, Mopeds, Minibikes** - Riders of ATVs were frequently injured when they were thrown from vehicles. There were also fractured wrists, dislocated hands, shoulder sprains, head cuts, and lumbar strains.
274,867	**Baseball, Softball** - Head injuries from bats and balls. Ankle injuries from running bases or sliding into them.
269,249	**Exercise, Exercise Equipment** - Twisted ankles and cut chins from tripping on treadmills. Head injuries from falling backward from exercise balls, ankle sprains from jumping rope.
186,544	**Soccer** - Twisted ankles or knees after falls, fractured arms during games.
164,607	**Swimming** - Head injuries from hitting the bottom of pools, and leg injuries from accidentally falling into pools.
96,119	**Skiing, Snowboarding** - Head injuries from falling, cut legs and faces, sprained knees or shoulders.
85,580	**Lacrosse, Rugby, & other Ball Games** - Head and facial cuts from getting hit by balls and sticks, injured ankles from falls.

Source: National Electronic Injury Surveillance System (NEISS, 2007).

Vehicle (ATV) use and increase in exercise habits has pulled these areas up to be among the higher incidence of injuries.

Over the past 10 years, the number of health club members 55 years of age and older has skyrocketed by 305%, and even after holding this population constant, the increase in injuries was an astounding 219% (IHRSA, 2007). However, by 2006 there was a period of slower growth across health club revenues, net membership growth; non-due revenues; and health club facility expansion. The percentage of the U.S. population over 6 years of age saw a 15% rise, with the number of youngsters between 6 and 17 years of age jumping by 58% (IHRSA, 2007). From 1990–1996, the CPSC (2000) recorded an increase of 54% in sports injury rates among people 65+ years of age and also deduced that this population may continue sports and fitness participation well into their 70's, 80's and perhaps even 90's which may lead to a greater rise in sports/fitness-related injuries.

Health club/fitness centers are unique settings. Owners are often responsible for the safety of their members, employees, and sometimes liable for those who work as independent contractors. It is necessary for fitness professionals (e.g., personal fitness trainers and group exercise instructors) to be trained in emergency response protocol techniques.

In 1970, Congress passed the Occupational Safety and Health Act (OSHA) to assure safe and healthy conditions for workers. This act covers employees, however does not cover those who are "self-employed" independent contractors, such as many group exercise instructors and personal fitness trainers. The basis of this standard requires conditions or adoption of one or more practices, methods, or processes to provide safe or healthful employment or places of employment (Occupational Safety and Health Administration, 2009).

Although independent contractors and members are not specifically covered under OSHA, member safety is paramount for all fitness professionals and a part of appropriate standards of practice. Therefore, fitness professionals should be trained in emergency response topics including the following.

- Recognizing an emergency
- Disease and injury prevention
- CPR/AED/First-Aid
- Bloodborne pathogen training
- Emergency preparedness

As part of industry practice, parameters include recognizing emergencies and making appropriate decisions for individuals in need of emergency services.

Recognizing an Emergency

The most important step in the treatment and care of an individual is the early recognition of a medical emergency. This can be summarized into four steps: (a) survey, (b) assessment, (c) prioritization, and (d) implementation or the "SAPI" approach. Training of how to quickly recognize an emergency can greatly reduce the response time, thus improving chances for survival or complete recovery.

STEP 1: SURVEY. In this step the area surrounding the scene of the incidence is briefly surveyed. The initial survey gives you an idea of the circumstances and potential condition of the individual, as well as hazards of those around the area. Keep in mind the safety of those in the surrounding areas as well as you, the responder.

STEP 2: ASSESSMENT. This step refers to a quick assessment of the individual.

Visualization—is the overall appearance of the individual assessed. Look for any sign that may indicate the individual is in trouble in addition to:
- Position of individual
- Skin color
- Bleeding
- Level of consciousness
- Pain and/or discomfort
- Distress

Critical situations—the sooner resuscitative efforts begin, the better chance of survival of the individual.
- If there is no response, or if there is an absence of breathing or pulse, the emergency medical system (EMS) needs to be activated by calling 911 and resuscitative efforts must begin immediately.
- In situations where a pulse and respiration are present, 911 still needs to be notified immediately. However, no resuscitation measures need to be instituted unless the situation changes or deteriorates.
- In situations where the individual has not lost consciousness, yet remains in distress, the responder should progress to the next step in the assessment phase—communication.

Communication—is the most important phase in assessing an individual's condition. This communication will direct the next phase of the assessment process. Open up the lines of communication with an individual by asking a few concise direct questions.
- What happened?
- How are you feeling?
- Where is the pain?
- If the individual's health history is unknown, ask if they have any medical problems you as the responder should know about.

STEP 3: PRIORITIZATION. In this step, the needs of the individual are rank ordered—with the most important first! Therefore, if an individual has fallen and sustained some musculoskeletal injuries but is unresponsive, it is more important to protect the airway and call for immediate medical help than to **worry about peripheral injuries.**

STEP 4: IMPLEMENTATION. In this last step the emergency response procedures are implemented, which will be detailed later in this chapter.

12 Common Illnesses and Injuries

In order to recognize an emergency, fitness professionals must be familiar with 12 common illnesses and injuries associated with exercise and safety in health clubs including the following.
- Allergic reactions
- Nosebleeds
- Diabetes/hypoglycemia
- Pregnacy emergencies
- Head injuries
- Respiratory emergencies
- Heart attack
- Seizures
- Heat-/cold-related emergencies
- Shock
- Musculoskeletal injuries
- Stroke

Keep in mind that this list is not inclusive. However, along with a brief definition of the illnesses/injuries will be a list of signs and symptoms and the appropriate first-aid response. This overview is not a substitute for the directions that a medical professional gives to patients.

Allergic Reactions

A small population of individuals may experience allergic reactions during exercise. These reactions are called exercise-induced anaphylaxis or (EIA). EIA typically lasts up to 4 hours, and is triggered by certain foods prior to exercise (e.g., eggs). Individuals can keep this under control by waiting a couple of hours after eating and incorporating a sufficient warm-up and cool-down within their workouts.

SIGNS AND SYMPTOMS
- Changes in skin color
- Heart palpitations
- Hives
- Wheezing (see asthma)

FIRST-AID RESPONSE
1. Generally, skin flushing and hives pose no health risk. Individuals who experience this may safely continue exercising.
2. In the event of respiratory problems or heart palpitations, suggest a medical evaluation and have the individual decrease activity until symptoms are alleviated. Within a short period of time, if symptoms are not alleviated, seek emergency medical help or activate the EMS by calling 911.
3. An individual who experiences induced asthma may have inhalant bronchodilators available.
4. Individuals that have known allergic reactions typically carry an Epi-Pen. These pens are an auto-injector with a preloaded does of 0.3mgs of epinephrine for adults. Should individuals need help, activate the EMS by calling 911.

Diabetes/Hypoglycemia

Diabetes is a disease by which the pancreas in unable to secrete sufficient insulin levels to support the uptake and utilization of glucose in the body, resulting in high blood sugar levels. It is important to know if an individual is a diabetic and if so, whether or not they are insulin dependent. Regular exercise is the most overlooked and crucial treatment for controlling diabetes. Exercise improves the body's ability to control glucose levels, helps keep the individual fit, reduces risk of cardiovascular disease, and improves circulation.

Type 1 diabetic. These are individuals whose pancreas has ceased function to the point that insulin by injection is needed for survival. It is in this population that hypoglycemic attacks (low blood sugar) can be frequent and potentially serious.

Type 2 diabetic. These are individuals whose pancreas continues to function, however, at a decreased capacity. Often, these individuals control their blood sugar levels with diet management, exercise, or oral medications that stimulate the pancreas to increase insulin secretion. There are some instances when treatment may include insulin injections when the initial course of treatment has failed. Although type 2 diabetics can suffer hypoglycemic episodes (low blood sugar), such manifestations are generally not as severe as with a type 1 diabetic, unless the type 2 diabetic is insulin dependent.

SIGNS AND SYMPTOMS
- Dizziness
- Disorientation

- Loss of motor control
- Profuse sweating
- Seizures
- Trembling
- Unconsciousness
- Weakness
- Changes in behavior such as mood, temper, confusion

FIRST-AID RESPONSE

1. If the individual can drink and swallow, offer fruit juices or non-diet soda which are high in sugar and can be absorbed quickly.
2. If the individual is becoming confused and refuses to drink, sugar packets, glucose packets, or cake icing may be placed in the gum area of the mouth. Anything with extremely high sugar content and will be absorbed quickly. Your organization may want to stock some high glucose preparations available at local pharmacies for emergency situations.
3. If the individual is becoming unresponsive, or is unresponsive, lie them down in the shock position and activate the EMS by calling 911. Do not offer anything by mouth as this may cause aspiration of the matter into the lungs and create a pulmonary problem.
4. Continue to monitor for changes in respiration and heart rate.

Head Injuries

Any type of injury to the head could potentially be serious. In a health club setting, falls and trauma due to weight room apparatus or sports equipment could cause injury to the head.

SIGNS AND SYMPTOMS

- Blood or fluid drainage from the mouth, nose, or ears
- Bumps and bruises
- Changes in level of consciousness (frequently immediate, but can be delayed)
- Headache, dizziness, or confusion
- Increased intracranial pressure may also cause the individual to vomit. Take care to protect airway.
- Lacerations or pain
- Paralyzed or dysfunctional facial muscles or other body areas
- Pupil changes
- Sleepiness
- Unconsciousness

FIRST-AID RESPONSE

1. For minor lumps to the head, apply ice until the swelling and pain subside. Any lacerations should be cleaned and dressed.
2. Since any head injury can be potentially dangerous, continue to monitor even the most minor injuries until the individual appears fully recovered. The individual should be instructed to follow-up with medical care following any head injury. Frequently, serious signs and symptoms of a head injury may manifest themselves as long as 2 weeks following the incident.

3. If the individual is unconscious, activate the EMS by calling 911, and assume there is a cervical spine injury until proven otherwise. Do not move the person and protect the cervical spine.

4. With serious head injuries, keep the individual lying flat or with head and shoulders elevated if there is no evidence of neck or back involvement. Do not raise the feet.

5. Continually check for changes in breathing patterns.

6. It is important not to give anything by mouth to these individuals since they frequently vomit.

7. Activate the EMS by calling 911.

Heart Attack

The most serious complication of cardiovascular disease is a myocardial infarction or heart attack. A heart attack is the result of a blockage of one of the arteries that supply blood to the heart muscles, preventing the delivery of an adequate oxygen supply. Decreased oxygen supply can cause the portion of cardiac muscle affected. Such changes can prevent the heart from pumping adequate amounts of blood to the rest of the system. The most serious complication of a heart attack can be arrhythmias, cardiogenic shock (total heart failure), or cardiac arrest.

SIGNS AND SYMPTOMS
- Dizziness
- Nausea
- Pain or squeezing in the middle of the chest
- Pain radiating in the arm (usually the left), jaw, or back
- Pain in the abdominal area (often mistaken for indigestion)
- Profuse sweating
- Shortness of breath
- Weakness

FIRST-AID RESPONSE
1. Anyone who has signs of a heart attack should stop activity, lie down, and get medical care at once. Blood pooling due to the cessation of exercise is not a consideration at this time.

2. Have the victim chew an aspirin (not Tylenol or Motrin products)

3. A paramedic team should be called via 911 or an established emergency-response system, or someone should take the person to the hospital immediately if such services are not available.

4. If the individual is experiencing chest pain and routinely takes nitroglycerin tablets for the pain, assist them with taking their required dose immediately. This may help to prevent some cardiac damage.

5. If the individual becomes unconscious and has no pulse and respiration, activate the EMS by calling 911 and begin CPR.

Heat- and Cold-Related Emergencies

The human body is equipped to withstand extremes of temperature, both hot and cold. However, the body temperature must remain constant for the body to work efficiently. A person can become ill from hot or cold temperatures, even if the temperature does not seem to be extreme. The degree of illness will depend on the likelihood of the following factors: (a) physical activity, (b) clothing,

(c) wind, (d) humidity, (e) working and living conditions, (f) a person's age, (g) and the state of health of that individual.

People at Risk for Heat or Cold Emergencies are those:

- older than 65 years of age and the frail elderly.
- who exercise or work strenuously outdoors.
- who have had heat-/cold-related problems in the past.
- who have cardiovascular disease or any other condition that can cause poor circulation.
- who take medication to eliminate water from the body (diuretics).
- with health problems.
- younger than 13 years of age or with smaller body mass.

HEAT-RELATED EMERGENCIES

All of these conditions are due to overexposure to heat, and all are preventable. Heat cramps are the least severe, but they can be a signal to the person that the body is being affected by the heat. Proper hydration before exercise is the best preventive measure. In 1996, ACSM issued a position stand on exercise and fluid replacement. These recommendations were intended to guide those who exercise in maintaining an optimal hydration status. It is recommended that individuals drink about 500 ml (about 17 oz) of fluid approximately 2 hours before exercise to promote adequate hydration and allow time for excretion of excess ingested water. During exercise, individuals should begin drinking early and at regular intervals to consume fluids at a rate sufficient to replace all the water lost through sweating (body weight loss), or consume the maximal amount that can be tolerated. During exercise lasting less than 1 hour there is little evidence to suggest that individuals need a carbohydrate-electrolyte drink to ensure physical performance. Therefore, it is recommended that at this level plain water is sufficient. After exercise, it is recommended to drink at least a pint of fluid for every pound of water lost during exercise.

Heat Cramps

Heat cramps are muscle spasms that are painful. It could be a warning signal or sign of a heat-related emergency. They usually occur in the legs or in the abdominal region.

FIRST-AID RESPONSE
1. Rest the individual in a cool place.
2. Give him or her cool water.
3. Do not give salt tablets or salt water to drink.

Heat Exhaustion

More severe than heat cramps and usually occurs after a long period of strenuous exercise or work in the heat and/or humidity.

SIGNS AND SYMPTOMS
- Cool, moist, pale, or red skin
- Headache or dizziness
- Nausea
- Normal or below normal body temperature
- Weakness and/or exhaustion

FIRST-AID RESPONSE
1. Activate the EMS by calling 911.

2. Get the individual out of the heat.
3. Cool the body with cool, wet cloths, such as towels.
4. Loosen all tight clothing.
5. If the individual is able to swallow, give cool water to drink (slowly).
6. Minimize shock.

Heat Stroke

The least common heat emergency, but it is the most severe. It usually occurs after the signals of heat exhaustion are ignored. In heat stroke, dangerously elevated internal temperatures cause vital body systems to fail.

SIGNS AND SYMPTOMS
*   Change in consciousness
*   Rapid, shallow breathing
*   Rapid, weak pulse
*   Red, hot, dry skin

FIRST-AID RESPONSE
1. Activate the EMS by calling 911.
2. Get the individual out of the heat.
3. Cool the body with cool, wet cloths, such as towels.
4. Loosen all tight clothing.
5. Do not give anything by mouth.
6. Minimize shock.

COLD-RELATED EMERGENCIES

Hypothermia

Hypothermia occurs when the body can no longer generate enough heat to maintain normal body temperature. It is a general cooling off of the body. The air temperature does not have to be below freezing for hypothermia to develop. Wind and humidity have some affect on the body's ability to control its temperature. Anyone who remains in cold or wet clothing for an extended period of time may develop hypothermia. Medical conditions, such as infection, diabetes, a stroke, or drinking alcohol, are other things that can affect the body's ability to maintain normal body temperature.

SIGNS AND SYMPTOMS
*   Apathy and decreased levels of consciousness
*   Numbness or glassy stare
*   Shivering (could be absent in latter stages)
*   Slow, irregular pulse
*   Pale cool skin
*   Patches of cyanosis, or blue color to lips and skin

FIRST-AID RESPONSE
1. Activate the EMS by calling 911.
2. Remove wet clothing and dry the individual.
3. Gradually warm up the body with blankets and dry clothes.
4. Move to a dry, warmer environment.
5. Do not warm individual too quickly as this could lead to heart problems.
6. Monitor vital signs and wait for the EMS.

Frostbite

Frostbite occurs when body parts (usually those furthest from the heart) are exposed to extreme cold temperatures. The air temperature, wind speed, and length of exposure are all contributing factors to frostbite. Body fluids cool and eventually freeze, destroying cells and tissues. Frostbite can cause loss of fingers, hands, arms, toes, feet, and legs.

SIGNS AND SYMPTOMS
- Lack of feeling in affected area following intense pain
- Skin that appears waxy
- Skin that is cold to the touch

FIRST-AID RESPONSE
1. Handle the area gently and with extreme care.
2. Never rub that area as it can cause further damage.
3. Gradually warm the affected area in 100–105° water.
4. Affected area should not touch side or bottom of container.
5. Keep in water until area is red and warm to the touch.
6. Bandage area with a dry, sterile dressing.
7. If the affected area is a toe or finger, gently and carefully place gauze between them.
8. Get medical attention as soon as possible.

Musculoskeletal Injuries

Developing a better understanding of the structure and function of the body's framework can help in better assessing musculoskeletal injuries and in giving the appropriate response. Musculoskeletal injuries are often painful, but they are rarely life-threatening. However, they can have serious consequences and even result in permanent disability if ignored or not cared for properly. It is important to understand the differences between various types of musculoskeletal injuries, both acute and chronic. Examples of acute trauma are sprains, strains, and fractures. Chronic injuries, if not cared for, have the potential to progress to an acute process, such as shin splints leading to stress fractures with constant overuse. At this point in time, the injury should be treated as acute.

SIGNS AND SYMPTOMS
- Abnormal lumps or deformities (usually only with fracture and/or dislocation)
- Discolored skin (will look red at first then it will look bruised)
- Inability to use or move the affected part (e.g., loss of motion or inability to lean weight)
- Numbness
- Pain, swelling (can appear rapidly, gradually, or not at all)

When you don't know how serious the injury is, treat it as if it was serious. Some signs of serious injuries include popping or snapping of the bone, numbness, tingling, or change of color in the extremities. The cause of an injury may also suggest its severity.

EMS should be called whenever:
- a fracture, dislocation, deformity, or point of tenderness over bone is suspected.
- individual is unable to move or use injured body part.
- the injury involves the head, neck, or back.

- whenever the instructor has any doubt as to the severity of the injury, or the safety of the individual.

FIRST-AID RESPONSE

The best way to deal with an injury is to take precautionary measures in the first place. But accidents do occur and by knowing what to do, you can help prevent further damage to the injured person. For most soft tissue injuries, the first-aid treatment is **R.I.C.E.—rest, ice, compression, and elevation**. This allows for a quicker recovery. If appropriate, then you should splint the wound.

Rest. Rest means restricting movement. Once pain is experienced, stop any activity. Pain is the body's way of indicating something is wrong. Splints, tape, and bandages may be necessary to help prevent damaging movements.

Ice. Applying cold compresses (ice) to soft tissue injuries reduces bleeding and swelling by narrowing blood vessels. Keep a barrier between the ice and the skin to prevent tissue damage. Ice cups, or frozen packs of peas or corn can be used for these injuries. To make an ice cup, fill a Styrofoam cup with water and keep it in the freezer. When frozen, it can be used for massaging an injury and keeping the swelling down. Apply ice for 20 minutes, then remove for 20 minutes; use this method for the first 24–48 hours.

Compression. Compression (pressure) helps reduce swelling and blood flow to the injured area. Apply pressure by wrapping the injury with an elastic (ACE) bandage. Compression should always be used while icing the injured part. These bandages should be tight, but not too tight to cut off the circulation. If fingers or toes begin to feel numb or lose color, loosen the bandage.

Elevation. Elevation reduces internal bleeding in the injured area and helps blood return to the heart more easily. To be most effective, the injured body part should be elevated higher than head or heart. Keep the injured area elevated whenever possible. Elevation can also eliminate pain by reducing the throbbing sensation caused by blood pooling at the injury site.

SPLINTING

To immobilize an extremity injury you can use a splint. There are three types of splints: (a) soft, (b) rigid, and (c) anatomic. You should splint only if the injured person needs to be moved.

The purposes of immobilizing an injury are to:
- lessen pain.
- prevent closed fractures from becoming open fractures.
- prevent further damage to soft tissues.
- reduce the possibility of loss of circulation to the injured part.
- reduce the risk of serious bleeding.

It is important to support the injured part in the position in which it was found. If the wound is open, then it should be covered with a dressing and bandage. The area below the injury site should be checked for feeling, warmth, and color. The splint should be applied to immobilize the joints or bones above and below the injured area. Once the splint is in place, recheck below the injury site for feeling, warmth, and color, and elevate the splinted part. An ice pack can be applied after the area is immobilized. The person should be encouraged to rest in the most comfortable position. If a fracture of the ankle or foot is suspected, elevate the limb but do not attempt to remove the shoe. This may contribute to further injuring the area due to manipulation.

Nosebleeds

Nosebleeds, although relatively common, can become severe and require medical attention. They can also be secondary to another disease process such as hypertension, or may be a result of internal or external trauma.

SIGN or SYMPTOM
- Spontaneous, bloody drainage from the nose

FIRST-AID RESPONSE
1. Have this individual stop activity and rest. Lean the person's head forward and apply direct pressure to the bridge area of the nose for 10 minutes or until bleeding stops.
2. To prevent re-bleeding in more severe nosebleeds, an icepack may be applied.
3. If bleeding persists despite the pressure for a prolonged period of time (15 minutes), take the individual to the hospital or urgent care center.

Pregnancy Emergencies

Prior to beginning any exercise program, a pregnant client needs medical clearance from her obstetrician. Generally, pregnancy is not a contraindication to exercise. The pregnant exerciser, however, may have unpredictable complications and may be more prone to musculoskeletal problems. Refer to AFAA's Standards and Guidelines for Prenatal Fitness and Chapter 39 for specific exercise protocols which adhere to the American College of Obstetrics and Gynecology guidelines.

SIGNS AND SYMPTOMS
- Bloody show (spotting or frank bleeding)
- Cramping (possibly severe)
- Premature contractions

FIRST-AID RESPONSE
1. Have the individual stop exercising and sit or lie down.
2. If the cramping and contractions continue, make arrangements to transport the individual to the hospital.
3. If bleeding is severe, lie the person down in the shock position with legs elevated.
4. In advanced pregnancy, do not lie the individual flat since this will limit breathing and decrease blood flow to the fetus.
5. Activate the EMS by calling 911.
6. Re-evaluate the individual frequently for changes in breathing or cardiac status.

Respiratory Emergencies

Chronic Obstructive Pulmonary Disease (COPD). COPD is a condition where the air exchange, especially an exhalation, is limited due to the constriction of the bronchial branches. This narrowing allows for the air to forcefully enter the alveoli (air sacs) under negative pressure, but decreases the speed of air exchange out of the lungs. COPD can have many causes. Smoking and environmental hazards can damage the bronchioles, narrowing the branches and decreasing air flow.

Asthma. A common type of COPD, seen more frequently in the younger population, is asthma. In the asthmatic patient, bronchiole spasms are responsible for decreasing air flow. High levels of activity can precipitate an asthma attack. In fact, some individuals suffer from exercise-induced asthma.

SIGNS AND SYMPTOMS
- Bluish tint to the nails, lips, or skin
- Shortness of breath and difficulty exhaling
- Skin color may change to a dusky hue
- Sweating and increase in heart rate
- Wheezing or a "squeaking" or "whistling" sound when exhaling

FIRST-AID RESPONSE
1. The first reaction to an individual with difficulty breathing is to stop the exercise which will decrease the oxygen demand. Have the individual sit down or lie down with their shoulders and chest elevated. It may be helpful to have them lean against a wall when seated.
2. If they have constrictive clothing, loosen or remove the constrictive pieces.
3. Many asthmatics carry bronchodilator medications for inhalation during attacks—ask if they have this medication and help them administer it.
4. Observe them frequently for improvement or deterioration. If their condition continues to worsen, activate the EMS by calling 911 or get the individual to the hospital immediately if EMS is not readily available.

Seizures

Two major signs of a serious epileptic attack are seizures and loss of consciousness. Attacks can be so mild they are not noticed by others or they may be so severe that, without medical intervention, they can be life threatening.

Most epileptic patients take medication to control attacks. The presence of epilepsy should be documented on their health history form. Seizures can also be associated with head injury, poisoning, infections, high fevers, toxemia in pregnancy, or conditions resulting in lack of oxygen supply to the brain (e.g., severe heart attack or arrest).

SIGNS AND SYMPTOMS
- Drooling
- Foaming at the mouth
- Periods of unconsciousness
- Rigid muscles
- Seizures with uncontrollable shaking, jerking motions

FIRST-AID RESPONSE
1. Activate the EMS by calling 911.
2. Do not restrain seizure individuals. Protect them from injury by moving objects away from them. Never attempt to put anything into their mouths or force anything between their teeth. Never attempt to insert fingers in their mouth.
3. When the jerking movements stop, position the individual on one side to allow for drainage from the mouth. Keep their airway open and reassess frequently to make sure they are breathing.

4. Seizure attacks are generally followed by periods of rest or sleep. Moving around can precipitate another attack. Provide for rest while immediate medical care is arranged for the individual.

Shock

Shock is a general term for the changes the body experiences with a serious injury or cardiac event. In any shock situation, blood pressure begins to drop depressing all body functions. If untreated, shock will result in death. There are three major types of shock.

Hypovolemic Shock—results from excessive loss of body fluids from hemorrhaging, profuse sweating, vomiting, or diarrhea.

Cardiogenic Shock—happens when the heart loses its ability to pump effectively. This can be as a result of a heart attack.

Anaphylactic Shock—results from a severe allergic reaction. The blood vessels lose their tone and a blood pressure cannot be maintained.

SIGNS AND SYMPTOMS
*   Anxious and fearful—feeling of impending doom
*   Cool and clammy skin
*   Dizziness, confusion, or changes in level of consciousness
*   Feeling of profound weakness
*   Heart rate and respiratory rate may be elevated
*   Numbness or tingling in the extremities

FIRST-AID RESPONSE
1. Comfort and calm the individual. Keep them lying down, comfortable, and attempt to maintain a normal body temperature.
2. If the individual is hot or in the sun, provide shade.
3. If it is cool, keep the individual warm.
4. There are a variety of positions beneficial to the shock individual that the rescuer must be knowledgeable about.

Standard Position: Keep the feet up or the injury elevated. This aids circulation back to the heart. However, do not elevate any unsplinted fractures.

Head and Shoulder Positions: If the individual has a head injury or is having trouble breathing, elevate the head and shoulders. If the problem is respiratory, elevation of head and shoulders decreases pressure on the diaphragm and allows for greater chest expansion. Head and neck should not be elevated if a neck or back injury is suspected.

Flat Position: If a back injury or fractures are suspected or if the responder is unsure of what position is correct, leave the individual lying flat.

Side-Lying Position: An individual who is bleeding from the mouth or may vomit needs to lie on one side. This prevents blood or stomach contents from flowing into the lungs and compromising breathing.

Stroke

A stroke or Cerebral Vascular Accident (CVA) is a sudden, often severe impairment of body functions brought on by a disruption of blood flow to the brain. When blood flow fails to reach parts of the brain, the affected brain cells die and leave an infracted area. The location and magnitude of the injury determines the residual damage to the individual. There are three types of strokes.

Thrombotic Stroke—is a result of the atherosclerosis process as seen in CVD. The arteries are narrowed due to plaque deposits decreasing blood flow to vital tissues.

Embolic Stroke—is caused by a blood clot (embolus) that breaks loose and travels through the vascular system until it lodges in a smaller vessel. About 20% of all strokes are embolic.

Hemorrhagic Stroke—occurs when a blood vessel in or around the brain bursts, spilling blood into the surrounding brain tissue. This can be the result of an aneurysm which is weak, a ballooning spot in a vessel, or it may be from trauma to the head.

Transient Ischemic Attack

Sometimes called a mild stroke, Transient Ischemic Attacks (TIAs) manifest themselves with the same signs and symptoms of a stroke, but to a lesser degree and for a shorter time frame. Despite the fact a person has seemingly recovered from a TIA, it is necessary for them to seek medical help. TIAs are signs of underlying pathology and can be precursors to serious strokes.

SIGNS AND SYMPTOMS

An individual experiencing a stroke may have a number of neurological changes.

- Change of mood or affect
- Confusion, disorientation to self, time, or place
- Difficulty speaking
- Difficulty swallowing
- Dizziness, loss of balance, unexplained fall
- Headache, usually sudden and severe, or an unexplained headache pattern
- Numbness, paralysis, or weakness of face, neck, or limbs occurring on one or both sides of the body
- Persistent ringing in the ears
- Sudden blurred vision or loss of vision in one or both eyes

FIRST-AID RESPONSE

1. Keep a stroke individual lying down and protected.
2. Attempt to maintain normal body temperature and activate the EMS by calling 911.
3. Do not give them anything to eat or drink.
4. If the individual is semi-conscious or unconscious, turn them to their side to prevent secretion from falling back into their lungs (aspiration). Due to the potential pressure in the brain, stroke individuals may vomit.
5. Reassess the person's respiratory status in case their condition deteriorates and begin CPR if necessary.
6. In cases of a TIA, where the individual seems to regain all faculties, protect the individual from accidents and physical exertion. Suggest follow-up medical attention. It is also recommended to notify a family member of a suspected TIA to inform them of the incident, and to insure that someone is aware of the suggestion for medical follow-up.

CPR/AED/First-Aid

The steps for performing CPR include (American Heart Association, 2005) the following.

1. **Attempt to wake individual.** Gently shake and/or rub knuckles against the individual's sternum. If the individual does not wake, activate the EMS by calling 911.
2. **Begin rescue breathing.** Open the individual's airway and check for breathing. If not breathing, give the individual a breath big enough to make the chest rise.
3. **Begin chest compressions.** Place the heel of your hand in the middle of the individual's chest. Put your other hand on top of the first with your fingers interlaced. Compress the chest about 1-1/2 to 2 inches (4–5 cm). Allow the chest to completely recoil before the next compression. Compress the chest at a rate equal to 100/minute. Perform 30 compressions at this rate.
4. **Repeat combination chest compression/rescue breaths.** Perform combination at a ratio of 30:2 for about 1 minute before rechecking for pulse. Continue until help arrives.
5. **Use of Automated External Defibrillator (AED).** If you have access to an AED, attach to the individual after approximately 1 minute of CPR (chest compressions and rescue breaths).
6. **Compression-Only CPR.** If you are not comfortable giving rescue breaths, still perform chest compressions (Bohm, Rosenqvist, Herlitz, Hollenberg, & Svensson, 2007; SOS-KANTO study group, 2007).

The most vital role of being able to intervene or save a life in the event of an emergency is to know when and how to perform CPR and First-Aid. Not every CPR class is the same. There are CPR classes for healthcare professionals as well as CPR classes for the layperson. Before you take a CPR class, make sure you select the right course for you. There are national organizations where fitness professionals can go to get their training. A requirement prior to attaining a group exercise or personal trainer certification is to have successfully completed CPR training. There are national organizations where you can complete both theoretical and practical skills for CPR. These include (but are not limited to): (a) the American Red Cross, (b) the American Heart Association, and (c) the National Safety Council. You can contact the local chapters of these organizations for more information on CPR training in your home area. It is critical to be sure to renew your CPR certification prior to its expiration date and stay current with all the changes that occur. Not only will a refresher course help in maintaining practical skills, but a valid certification could help prevent a law suit should the emergency situation turn into a legal one. It is vitally important to remember to always activate the EMS by calling 911 prior to beginning CPR. Skilled staff and early medical intervention is the only chance for the victim's survival.

Bloodborne Pathogens

In assessing if your organization is impacted by the bloodborne pathogen standard, you will need to refer to OSHA Standard 29 CFR 1910.1030 (U.S. Department of Labor, 1992). According to this standard, employers that have employees exposed to blood or other potentially infectious materials are required by OSHA to have a written Exposure Control Plan. In addition, employers will need to provide training for all employees. The OSHA Bloodborne Pathogens Standard covers all employees who could be "reasonably anticipated" as the result of performing their job duties to face contact with blood and other potentially infectious materials. OSHA has not attempted to list all occupations where exposures could occur, however, "Good Samaritan" acts such as assisting a co-worker with a nosebleed would not be considered occupational exposure. Also, increases in community acquired infections, such as MRSA (methicillin-resistant Staphylococcus aureus) the "superbug" and VRE (vancomycin-resistant enterococci), have become real infectious hazards for all.

Exposure Control Plan

The standard requires employers to have a written exposure control plan which identifies tasks and procedures, as well as job classifications, where occupational exposure to blood occurs—without regard to personal protective clothing and equipment. It must also specify procedures for evaluating circumstances surrounding exposure incidents. The plan must be easily accessible to employees and available to OSHA inspectors upon request. This written plan must be reviewed and updated, if appropriate, at least annually. If workplace changes affect the exposure control plan, it must be updated more often if necessary.

Methods of Compliance

This standard mandates universal precautions (i.e., treating bodily fluids/materials as if infectious), emphasizing engineering, and work practice controls. The standard stresses hand washing, and requires employers to provide facilities for employees to use following exposure to blood. It sets forth procedures to minimize needle sticks and/or the splashing and spraying of blood, ensure appropriate packaging of specimens, and regulated wastes. It includes proper labeling of waste that is contaminated before shipping to servicing facilities, as well. Employers must provide, at no cost, and require employees to use appropriate personal protective equipment such as gloves, gowns, masks, mouthpieces, and resuscitation bags. Employers must clean, repair, and replace these when necessary. It specifies methods for disposing of contaminated sharps (such as syringes) and sets forth standards for containers for these items and other regulated waste. Furthermore, the standard includes provisions for handling contaminated laundry to minimize exposures.

Information and Training

The standard mandates employee training within 90 days of effective date, initially upon assignment, and annually. Employees who have received appropriate training within the past year need only receive additional training in items not previously covered. The training must include making accessible a copy of the regulatory text of the standard and explanation of its contents, general discussion on bloodborne diseases and their transmission, exposure control plan, engineering and work practice controls, personal protective equipment, hepatitis B vaccine, response to emergencies involving blood, how to handle exposure incidents, the post-exposure evaluation and follow-up program, and signs/labels/color-coding. Employees must have an opportunity for Q&A during the training. The person conducting the training must be knowledgeable enough in the subject matter to sufficiently provide answers to employees.

For more information on how to prepare the exposure control plan and training program, review the OSHA Standard 29 CFR 1910.1030 (U.S. Department of Labor, 1992).

Emergency Preparedness

The OSHA guidelines regarding emergency preparedness will vary depending upon your organization type and facility size. For specific requirements it is recommended to contact your local OSHA office or www.osha.gov for customized details. If an organization has 10 or less employees the plan can be communicated orally. Otherwise a plan must be written, kept in the workplace, and viewed by all employees. In addition, employers will need to provide training for all employees (U.S. Department of Labor, 2007). Life threatening emergencies can happen anytime. Local American Red Cross Chapters can assist your organization with the appropriate Medical Emergency Response Plan, CPR/AED Standards/First-Aid Kits, Bloodborne Pathogen training, and Emergency Preparedness (American Red Cross, 2007). Provided for you is a summary and reference for each area.

Emergency Response Plan

It is important for every organization to set up an Emergency Response Plan. Each plan should include the following core elements (American Red Cross [n.d.]).

- Coordinated and practiced response plan
- Effective and efficient communication throughout the organization
- Implementation of lay rescuer/AED
- Risk reduction strategies
- Training and equipment for First-Aid/CPR

The possibility of public health emergencies arising in the United States concerns many people in the wake of recent hurricanes, tsunamis, acts of terrorism, and the threat of pandemic influenza. Though some people feel it is impossible to be prepared for unexpected events, the truth is that taking preparedness actions helps people deal with disasters of all sorts much more effectively when they do occur. It seems a daunting task to complete a written emergency response plan for use in fitness facilities. However, there are many resources that can help with this task. Understanding what should be included in the emergency response plan, such as severe weather, bomb threats, workplace violence, and so forth, is an important element. To help, the Centers for Disease Control and Prevention (CDC) (2009) and the American Red Cross (2007) have teamed up to answer common questions and provide step-by-step guidance you can take now to protect you and your loved ones

CPR/AED Standards/First-Aid Kits

Automated external defibrillator (AED) is a device that can restart a heart that has stopped beating effectively. It analyzes the heart's rhythm and, if necessary, tells the lay rescuer of your organization to deliver a shock to an individual in sudden cardiac arrest. This shock, called defibrillation, may help the heart to reestablish an effective rhythm of its own (American Red Cross, 2007).

First-aid responses previously stated should be coupled with the appropriate training and equipment strategically placed throughout your organization. OSHA standards (1910.151 and 1926.50) do not require specific first-aid kit contents, however, recommend ANSI Z308.1-2003, Minimum requirements for workplace first-aid kits. Depending upon the size of your organization, first-aid kits in compliance with this standard will provide a basic range of products to deal with most types of needs encountered including the following minimum contents.

Table 16-2.	
Item	**Min. Qty**
Absorbent compress, 32 sq. in. (81.3 sq. cm) with no side smaller than 4 in. (10 cm)	1
Adhesive bandages, 1 in. x 3 in. (2.5 cm x 7.5 cm)	16
Adhesive tape, 5 yd (457.2 cm) total	1
Antiseptic, 0.5g (0.14 fl oz) applications	10
Burn treatment, 0.5 g (0.14 fl oz) applications	6
Medical exam gloves	2 pair
Sterile pads, 3 in. x 3 in. (7.5 x 7.5 cm)	4
Triangular bandage, 40 in. x 40 in. x 56 in. (101 cm x 101 cm x 142 cm)	1
Optional items and sizes should be added to the basic contents listed above to augment a first-aid kit, based on the specific hazards existing in a particular work environment.	
Bandage compress 2 in. x 2 in.	4
3 in. x 3 in.	2
4 in. x 4 in.	1
Eye covering with means of attachment	1
Eye wash – 1 fl oz (30 ml)	1
Cold pack – 4 in. x 5 in.	1
Roller bandage 2 in. (5 cm)	2
4 in. (10 cm)	1
NOTE: A CPR barrier is also recommended, but not required. (Minnesota Department of Labor, 2003).	

Summary

In summary, your organization can never be too safe. Appropriate employee training, equipment, and protocols should be continually inspected and practiced to ensure the safety of all individuals.

References

1. American College of Sports Medicine. (2010). *ACSM's guidelines for exercise testing and prescription* (8th ed.). Philadelphia, PA: Lippincott Williams & Wilkins.

2. American Heart Association. (2005). American heart association guidelines for cardiopulmonary resuscitation and emergency cardiovascular care. *Circulation*, 112 (24 Suppl), IV1-IV203.

3. American Red Cross. (2007a). *First-Aid/CPR/AED for the workplace participant's workbook.* Washington, DC: The American National Red Cross.

4. American Red Cross. (2007b). *American red cross first-aid and preparedness booklet.* Washington, DC: The American National Red Cross.

5. American Red Cross. (n.d.). *Emergency management guide for business and industry.* Retrieved April 25, 2009, from http://www.redcross.org/services/disaster/beprepared

7. Bohm K., Rosenqvist, M., Herlitz, J., Hollenberg, J., & Svensson L. (2007). Survival is similar after standard treatment and chest compression only in out-of-hospital bystander cardiopulmonary resuscitation. *Circulation*, 116(25), 2908–2912.

8. Bureau of Labor Statistics, U.S. Department of Labor. (2009). Fitness workers in *Occupational outlook handbook*, (2008-09 ed.). Retrieved April 25, 2009, from http://www.bls.gov/oco/ocos296.htm

9. Centers for Disease Control and Prevention. (2009). *Emergency preparedness and response.* Retrieved April 25, 2009, from http://emergency.cdc.gov/

10. International Health and Racquet Sports Association. (2007). *Profiles of success*, 2006. Boston, MA: International Health and Racquet Sports Association.

11. Minnesota Department of Labor, Occupational Safety and Health Division. (2003). *Contents of first-aid kit*. Retrieved April 25, 2009, from http://www.doli.state.mn.us/pdf/fact_firstaid.pdf

12. Occupational Safety and Health Administration. (1970). *Occupational safety and health (osh) act of 1970*. Washington, DC: United States Department of Labor. Retrieved April 25, 2009, from http://www.osha.gov/pls/oshaweb/owadisp.show_document?p_id=2743&p_table=OSHACT

13. SOS-KANTO study group. (2007). Cardiopulmonary resuscitation by bystanders with chest compression only: An observational study. *Lancet*, 369, 920–926.

14. U.S. Consumer Product Safety Commission. (2000). Baby boomers sports injuries, in *Consumer Product Safety Review*, 4(4), 3-4.

15. U.S. Consumer Product Safety Commission's (CPSC) National Electronic Injury Surveillance System (NEISS). (2007). Retrieved April 25, 2009, from http://www.cpsc.gov/LIBRARY/neiss.html

16. U.S. Department of Labor, Occupational Safety and Health Administration. (1992). OSHA's bloodborne pathogen standard, 29 CFR 1910.1030. Retrieved April 25, 2009, from http://www.osha.gov/pls/oshaweb/owadisp.show_document?p_table=STANDARDS&pid=1005

17. U.S. Department of Labor, Occupational Safety and Health Administration. (2007). Emergency response and preparedness - 72:51735-51743. Retrieved April 25, 2009, from http://www.osha.gov/pls/oshaweb/owadisp.show_document?p_table=FEDERAL_REGISTER&p_id=19915

Latest updates from the American Heart Association

Based on the 2010 American Heart Association Guidelines for Cardiopulmonary Resuscitation and Emergency Cardiovascular Care, Supplement to *Circulation*, the following summarizes the revised steps for **adult** CPR to be given by a **nonprofessional rescuer (general public)**.

1. Make sure the scene is safe.
2. Shake the victim's shoulders and shout to see if he/her responds.
3. If the victim does not respond and the victim is not breathing or not breathing normally, yell for someone to call 9-1-1 and get an AED, if available.
   a. If you are alone, call 9-1-1 and get an AED if available. Follow the AED's voice prompt.
   b. If no AED is available, immediately start CPR, beginning with compressions.
4. **Compressions:** Push hard and fast on the center of the chest 30 times, at a rate of at least 100 compressions a minute. Push down at least 2 inches with each compression. If you have not been trained in CPR, continue to give compressions until an AED arrives or trained help takes over.
5. **Airway:** If you have been trained in CPR, continue CPR by opening the airway with a head tilt-chin lift.
6. **Breathing:** Pinch the victim's nose closed. Take a normal breath and cover the victim's mouth with your mouth, creating an airtight seal. Give 2 breaths (1 second each). Watch for the chest to rise as you give each breath.
7. Keep giving sets of 30 compressions and 2 breaths until the AED arrives or trained help takes over.

New AHA Slogan: CPR is as easy as **C-A-B**:

Compressions	**A**irway	**B**reathing
Push hard and fast in the center of the victim's chest	Tilt the victim's head back and lift the chin to open the airway	Give mouth-to-mouth rescue breathing

Part 5

How to Teach—Basics

Basic Exercise Standards and Guidelines

Instructor Training and the Importance of Continuing Education

Instructor Motivation and Adherence: Getting Them & Keeping Them

Monitoring Exercise Intensity

Building Traditional Group Exercise Choreography

Training for Flexibility

Balance and Coordination: Key Components to Overall Fitness

17 Basic Exercise Standards and Guidelines

AFAA Education
Advisory Board

I. Introduction

Introduced in 1983, the Aerobics and Fitness Association of America's (AFAA's) *Basic Exercise Standards and Guidelines* were the first nationally developed standardized guidelines available to fitness professionals to assist them in providing exercise leadership to clients. This revised edition of the guidelines reflects an ongoing process of research, critique, and consensus by a multidisciplinary team of fitness industry experts and organizations. These standards and guidelines apply to adults: (a) without known physiological, biomechanical, or medical conditions that would in any way restrict their exercise activities, and/or (b) adults who have been cleared by their health care provider to exercise. However, the application of these standards and guidelines to the delivery of service is dependent upon the application of individualized professional judgment. It may also be appropriate in the application of independent professional judgment to adapt these guidelines for special populations (i.e., individuals with medical conditions or elite athletes). Please refer to AFAA's *Exercise Standards & Guidelines Reference Manual* for specialty recommendations. And, although these *Basic Exercise Standards and Guidelines* emphasize the group exercise setting, many of the principles are applicable for the personal fitness trainer working with individual clients. For more in-depth study, fitness professionals who are also involved in personal training should refer to AFAA's *Personal Fitness Training: Theory & Practice.*

II. General Principles of Exercise Training

A. The FITT Principle: Training Variables

Exercise programs will provide optimal results with minimal risk of injury when developed appropriately. Training variables, such as F̲requency, I̲ntensity, T̲ime, and T̲ype, must be considered when designing an exercise program.

- Frequency refers to the number of exercise sessions per week.
- Intensity refers to the difficulty of an exercise or exercise session.
- Time refers to the duration or length of each exercise session.
- Type refers to the mode of activity performed.

It should be recognized that training variables are interrelated, and therefore, each variable may influence the other exercise variables. A significant increase in exercise intensity, for example, will likely result in a decreased duration of that exercise session. Changes in the mode or type of exercise performed may also affect the other training variables. For example, a runner may find that he/she cannot perform the same exercise duration when cycling as when running because the training stresses are applied differently to the body.

B. The Principle of Overload

To achieve desired training improvements or effect, the relevant body system must be overloaded beyond its normal level or present capacities. When the body is stressed in this manner, it then responds by adapting so that its capacity increases. The physiological changes that occur in the body as a result of exercise overload are referred to as a training effect. A training effect will occur if the exercise is sufficient and appropriate in frequency, intensity, and time for a given type of exercise. The principle of overload applies to all types of physical conditioning. Fitness programs that lack overload and/or variation will serve to maintain, but not improve, one's existing level of fitness.

C. The Principle of Progression

For continued improvements in fitness, an exercise program should provide gradual increases or progressions in frequency, intensity, time, and/or type of exercise. Proper progression includes a systematic change in overload over time, designed to maximize fitness gains while keeping the risk of over-training and related injuries low. For program progressions allow for the initial conditioning phase to last 4–6 weeks, improvement phase 4–5 months, and maintenance thereafter. Recommended progressions will vary depending on the participant's age, physical limitations, and fitness level.

D. The Principle of Specificity: SAID

Specificity of training is also referred to as the SAID principle: Specific Adaptation to Imposed Demands. The body will adapt to the type of physiological stresses placed on it. In order to improve in a particular area of fitness or sport, the precise movement or movement pattern should be rehearsed. For example, to become a better hurdler one must jump hurdles. The principle of specificity also applies to the training variables (frequency, intensity, time, and type). For example, to be successful, a marathon runner must include distance running in his/her training program. Cycling would not suffice as his/her main training type. In addition to movement patterns and training variables, the challenge to the physiological systems needs to be specific to the activity performed. For example, the capacities of the aerobic athlete (e.g., runner, cyclist, swimmer) have minimal transference to anaerobic performance (sprinting or power weight lifting) and vice versa.

E. The Principle of Reversibility

If one's training workload is discontinued or decreased, detraining in performance will occur. Cardiorespiratory fitness generally appears to decrease after only 2 or 3 weeks without training. Muscular fitness (strength and/or endurance) generally appears to decrease after 2–3 months without training.

F. The Principle of Overtraining

The body needs time to recover and the musculoskeletal system needs time to rebuild from the stress of vigorous exercise. When the training variables utilized do not allow sufficient recovery, overtraining of the body can occur. Overtraining can also occur when training volume and/or intensity are too high or too rapidly increased.

III. Health- and Skill-Related Physical Fitness Components

A complete physical fitness program should seek to improve and then maintain each of the common components of health and fitness, used herein to bring about well-being.

A. Health-Related Components

1. **Cardiorespiratory Fitness**

   Cardiorespiratory fitness (aerobic fitness) can be defined as the ability of the body to take in, transport, and utilize oxygen. It involves the capacity of the heart and lungs to exchange and deliver oxygen to working muscles during sustained motion.

2. **Muscular Strength and Endurance**

   Muscular strength is defined as the amount of weight (maximal force) that can be lifted one time by a particular muscle group, whereas muscular endurance is the ability of a muscle group to lift a submaximal (lesser) weight many times. Muscular endurance also refers to the ability of a muscle group to hold (stabilize) a fixed or isometric contraction for an extended period of time.

3. **Flexibility**

   Flexibility (mobility) is commonly defined as muscle suppleness as well as the range of motion available at a joint(s). Adequate mobility also implies that the muscles are able to elongate to accommodate the full range of motion required by the joint.

4. **Body Composition**

   Body composition refers to the absolute and relative amounts of the structural components of the body—fat, fluid, muscle/tissue, and bone. Body composition assessments generally focus on body fat since excessive amounts may increase the risk of disease. Maintaining an appropriate level of body fat is essential for good health and may lower the risk of heart disease, diabetes, and some cancers.

B. Skill-Related Components

Skill-related components of physical fitness may be targeted to achieve improvement in sports, work, or daily life performance as well as help certain individuals avoid serious injury.

1. Agility—ability to change the body's position and direction with quickness and accuracy.

2. Balance—ability to maintain equilibrium (or certain posture) while moving or stationary.

3. Coordination—ability of the body to utilize the senses and body parts in a harmonious relationship to perform a task smoothly and with accuracy.

4. Power—ability or rate at which one can exert strength to perform work quickly.

5. Reaction time—the time required to initiate a response to a given stimulus.

6. Speed—ability to move the entire body quickly.

IV. Health and Fitness Training Recommendations

A. Health Benefits versus Enhanced Fitness Benefits

In 1996, the *U.S. Surgeon General's Report on Physical Activity and Health* was a call to encourage more Americans to become active. The report states that by becoming moderately active, Americans can lower their risk of premature death and the development of chronic illnesses, such as heart disease, hypertension, and diabetes. Among its major findings were the following points.

- People who are usually inactive can improve their health and well-being by becoming even moderately active on a regular basis.
- Physical activity does not need to be strenuous to achieve health benefits.
- Enhanced fitness or physiological changes occur when the amount (frequency, intensity, and time) of the activity is increased. All American adults should accumulate 30 minutes of moderate physical activity equivalent to brisk walking on most, if not all, days of the week.

In 2008, the U.S. Department of Health and Human Services (USDHHS) introduced the *Physical Activity Guidelines for Americans* which reinforced the 1996 Surgeon General's Report. The key guidelines for adults are as follows.

1. All adults should avoid inactivity. Some physical activity is better than none, and adults who participate in any amount of physical activity gain some health benefits.

2. For substantial health benefits, adults should perform at least 2 hours and 30 minutes (150 minutes) a week of moderate-intensity (e.g., brisk walking) aerobic physical activity, or 1 hour and 15 minutes (75 minutes) a week of vigorous-intensity (e.g., running) aerobic physical activity, or an equivalent of a combination of moderate- and vigorous-intensity aerobic physical activity. Aerobic activity should be performed in episodes of at least 10 minutes, and preferably, it should be spread throughout the week.

3. For additional and more extensive health benefits, adults should perform 300 minutes (5 hours) a week of moderate-intensity aerobic physical activity, or 150 minutes a week of vigorous-intensity aerobic physical activity, or an equivalent combination of moderate- and vigorous-intensity activity. Additional health benefits are gained by engaging in physical activity beyond this amount.

4. Adults should also perform moderate- or high-intensity muscle-strengthening activities, and involve all major muscle groups on 2 or more days a week since these activities provide additional health benefits.

B. AFAA Fitness Training Recommendations

AFAA supports the guidelines from the American College of Sports Medicine (ACSM) for maximum health and fitness benefits with regard to training recommendations. AFAA also recognizes that the treatment of health conditions, as opposed to the maintenance or enhancement of wellness, should be determined and managed by a licensed health care provider rather than fitness professionals.

AFAA FITT-at-a-Glance

	Cardiorespiratory Fitness	**Muscular Strength and Endurance**	**Flexibility**
Frequency	3–5 days per week * For promoting and maintaining health: 5 days of moderate intensity, or 3 days of vigorous intensity, or a combination of moderate and vigorous intensity 4–5 days per week, along with regular daily activities of living.	Minimum of 2–3 non-consecutive days per week for each major muscle group (arms, shoulders, chest, abdomen, back, hips, and legs); vary exercise selection regularly for maximum results. * Individuals who are new to strength training should begin with 1 set of separate exercises targeting each of the major muscle groups and add additional sets or exercises only after adaptation to the current program has occurred.	Minimum of 2–3 days (ideally 5–7 days) per week for each major muscle and tendon group with special attention to those joints and body segments with a reduced range of motion.
Intensity/Volume	HR_{max}: 64–94% HRR: 40–85% RPE: 6–20 scale: 12–14 (moderate to somewhat hard); 15–16 (hard) or 10-point scale: 4–6 for moderate and 7–8 for vigorous **Volume:** ≥ 1,000 kcal per week (2,000–4,000 may be optimal) • Moderate = 40% to < 60% HRR (or VO_2R) * that noticeably increases HR and breathing • Vigorous = ≥ 60% to 85% HRR (or VO_2R) that results in substantial increases in HR and breathing * Percent VO_2R is determined through clinical laboratory data.	To the point of muscle fatigue while maintaining proper form; typically 8–25 repetitions, 1–4 sets, depending if focus is strength or endurance.	To the end of range of motion, to the point of tightness, without discomfort performing 1–4 repetitions*. * Reference is to statically held stretches.
Time	20–60 minutes of continuous or intermittent (10-minute bouts accumulated throughout the day) aerobic activity * For promoting and maintaining health: 30 minutes of moderate intensity or 20–25 minutes of vigorous intensity.	20–60 minutes (time of sessions may vary based on training protocol).	15–60 seconds (per each static stretch). The amount of time spent on flexibility training will be dependent upon the focus and goals of the class. Time may vary from 5–10 minutes to an entire 60-minute class.
Type	An activity that is continuous, rhythmic, and utilizes the large muscle groups (e.g., dancing, walking, hiking, running, jogging, cycling, swimming, stair climbing, inline skating, cross-country skiing, stepping, choreographed cardio kickboxing).	Any activity that creates overload to the musculoskeletal system in the form of external, gravitational, or isometric resistance (e.g., progressive weight training, calisthenics, elastic tubing, stabilization exercises); multi-joint exercises that involve more than one muscle group are recommended to enhance the functional carryover.	Activity that focuses on elongating muscles and moves joints safely through a full range of motion (e.g., yoga, stretch class, cool-down periods).

NOTE: Physical activity (PA) should be preceded by a licensed health care provider examination and clearance for high-risk participants as defined by ACSM and those of moderate risk who wish to participate in vigorous PA. Low-risk participants may pursue a PA program without prior medical exam and those at moderate risk may pursue a moderate-intensity PA program without an exam. Medical clearance should be provided for children, adolescents, or young adults about to enter competitive athletics or vigorous exercise programs.

C. Prevalence of Obesity

It is well established that excessive body fat increases the risks of heart disease, high blood pressure, type 2 diabetes, some forms of cancer, low-back pain, and other musculoskeletal problems. In 2009, approximately two-thirds of American adults were classified as overweight representing a body mass index (BMI) of ≥ 25, and about 32% of adults classified as obese (BMI ≥ 30). The group exercise setting may lend itself to an educational opportunity regarding body composition and weight management. Class participants can receive their BMI estimations by logging onto http://www.cdc.gov/healthyweight/assessing/bmi/.

V. Professional Responsibilities and Concerns

A. Professional Responsibilities

1. **Personal Liability Coverage**

   Since laws vary widely from state to state, it is advisable for instructors to investigate specific legal requirements that are applicable to their particular state. It is recommended that instructors carry comprehensive liability insurance that includes personal injury liability, general liability, and professional liability coverage applicable to their delivery of actual services.

2. **Training and Certification**

   Fitness instructors should complete a training and certification program that incorporates both theoretical knowledge and practical application.

3. **CPR/AED and First-Aid Training**

   Fitness instructors should maintain current nationally and/or internationally recognized adult-level CPR and AED certifications. It is recommended that instructors also receive training in a nationally and/or internationally recognized standard level first-aid course. (For more information, go to www.afaa.com.)

4. **Facility Pre-Exercise Participation Screening**

   A written procedure should be used by the fitness facility regarding pre-participation screening. The Physical Activity Readiness Questionnaire (PAR-Q) is recommended by ACSM as the minimal standard for use by entry-level participants in a moderate-intensity exercise program.

5. **Medical Clearance and Pre-Exercise Testing**

   It is recommended that instructors follow the ACSM guidelines regarding appropriate medical clearance and pre-exercise testing before participation is allowed.

   ACSM (2010) revised their recommendations to the following.
   - High-risk participants to have a medical exam, medical clearance, and exercise testing before participating in moderate to vigorous exercise. High risk is defined as men and women of any age with one or more of the major cardiovascular, pulmonary, or metabolic disease signs/symptoms or diagnosed with cardiovascular, pulmonary, or metabolic disease.
   - Moderate-risk participants to have a medical exam and clearance before participating in vigorous exercise. Moderate risk is defined as men and women with ≥ 2 atherosclerotic cardiovascular disease (CVD) risk factors*, but without symptoms.

- Low-risk participants in most instances do not require a medical clearance before participating in moderate to vigorous exercise. Low risk is defined as men and women who are without symptoms and have ≤ 1 CVD risk factor.*

  Risk factors include: age, family history, cigarette smoking, hypertension, unhealthy cholesterol levels, prediabetes, obesity, and sedentary lifestyle.

6. **Environmental Monitoring**

   Fitness instructors should check for obvious hazards (e.g., debris, uneven or wet floor surfaces, broken equipment, lighting, room temperature) prior to and throughout an exercise class. When possible, the instructor should try to remedy the hazard. In some cases when hazards cannot be corrected, those hazards need to be reported to management and to participants so they are warned of the hazard. If a warning will not suffice, such as with equipment in need of repair that remains unrepaired, it needs to be removed from service.

7. **Emergency Response Plan**

   All emergencies need to be handled in a professional manner, keeping in mind the best interest of the person needing attention, while ensuring the safety of others. It is recommended that all facilities establish and implement a written emergency response plan. Fitness instructors should have the knowledge to recognize that an emergency exists and to take appropriate action. Such plans should be at least periodically rehearsed and practiced. Some authorities recommend rehearsals at least four times per year. The steps that should be followed in an emergency include the following.
   - Survey the scene.
   - Assess the person in need of attention.
   - Call 911 (or the designated emergency response number).
   - Provide appropriate care until emergency medical services (EMS) arrives.

B. Instructional Concerns

1. **Exercise Danger Signs**

   If any one of the following signs are observed or if the participant complains of any of the following symptoms, the participant should stop vigorous exercise immediately and the fitness instructor should assess and implement the need for emergency response procedures.
   - Nausea and/or vomiting
   - Dizziness, lightheadedness, or unusual fatigue
   - Tightness or pain in the chest, neck, arms, jaw, or other bodily areas connoting a potential cardiac problem
   - Loss of muscle control, staggering
   - Severe breathlessness (gasping) with inability to recover
   - Allergic reactions (e.g., rash, hives, anaphylactic shock)
   - Blurred vision
   - Acute illness
   - Mental confusion
   - Cyanosis (bluish coloring of skin)
   - Acute musculoskeletal injury

2. **Signs for Exercise Modification**

   If any of the following signs are observed or the participant complains of any of the following, he or she should be encouraged to modify or discontinue exercise until the signs disappear. When required, an emergency plan should be implemented.
   - Labored breathing
   - Excessive heart rate elevation
   - Evidence of strain, holding breath, or unusual redness
   - Musculoskeletal pain
   - Lack of proper body control

3. **Effects of Drugs and/or Medications**

   Fitness instructors need to be aware that certain prescriptions, as well as nonprescription medications, such as antihistamines and antibiotics, may elicit side effects during exercise similar to those listed under "Exercise Danger Signs" above. Some medications can alter heart rate response (e.g., beta-blockers). Individuals on medications should consult their physicians about possible side effects before beginning an exercise program.

4. **Symptoms of Overtraining**

   Fitness instructors and participants should be aware of the following symptoms of overtraining.
   - Fatigue
   - Anemia
   - Amenorrhea
   - Overuse or stress-related injuries
   - Increased resting heart rate
   - Slower recovery of heart rate
   - Decrease in strength performance
   - Constant muscle or joint soreness on effort or motion, leaning toward pain

5. **Avoiding Overtraining**

   Fitness instructors should recommend (and themselves follow) these suggestions for avoiding overtraining.
   - Vary class type and intensity to alter localized stresses (step aerobics, low-impact, cycling, pilates, yoga).
   - Limit the number of high-impact or advanced level classes (no more than 8–12 per week and no more than 2 per day).
   - Always perform an adequate warm-up and cool-down.
   - Limit amount of active demonstration by verbal cueing and use of instructor assistants.
   - Decrease teaching schedule, as needed, when medical conditions or burnout warrant.
   - Ingest a nutritious diet with adequate total calories, carbohydrates, protein, and water.
   - Be aware of, and correct, muscle imbalances.

6. **Hydration and Rehydration**

   Participants should be advised to hydrate before, during, and after exercise, when appropriate based on individual needs, in order to replenish necessary body fluids and to maintain electrolyte balance. Generally, participants should drink approximately 8–12 oz of fluid shortly before exercise. However, due to the differences in "sweat rates" between individuals and the variation in physical activity, sports, and environmental conditions, it is difficult to assess the actual water and electrolyte losses in a given setting. Therefore, a "one size fits all" recommendation would not be appropriate. In 2007, *ACSM's Position Stand on Exercise and Fluid Replacement* was revised and suggests the following.

- Participants should monitor their hydration status by taking regular urine and body weight measurements before and after exercise. Check for color and quantity of urine (should be clear and plentiful).
- Body weight changes can reflect sweat losses during exercise, and can be used to calculate individual fluid replacement needs for specific exercise and environmental conditions. For every pound of weight lost, drink 2 cups of fluid.

Prior to Exercise
- Pre-hydrating with beverages, if determined to be required, should be performed over a period of at least several hours before exercise to allow for fluid absorption and urine output to return toward normal levels.
- Consuming beverages with sodium and/or salted snacks or small meals with beverages can help stimulate thirst and retain needed fluids.

During Exercise
- To prevent hypo-hydration, individuals should develop customized fluid replacement programs that prevent excessive weight loss over the course of the activity (i.e., keeping losses of body weight to <2% from the time of exercise start). The routine measurement of pre- and post-exercise body weights is recommended for determining sweat rates and individualized fluid replacement programs.
- Consuming beverages containing electrolytes and carbohydrates can help maintain fluid-electrolyte balance and exercise performance. Whether to use water or an electrolyte drink to replace vital body fluids is dependent on the type and intensity/duration of the exercise.

After Exercise
- Electrolyte deficits should be replenished. The rate of rehydration should be based on the amount of bodily electrolyte fluid loss. If there is time, consumption of normal meals and beverages is adequate to restore normal water body content.

7. **Attire**

Fitness instructors should wear and recommend appropriate clothing and footwear for the type of activity performed during class. This would include, but is not limited to, the following.
- Fabrics that breathe, rather than those that retain body heat
- Comfortable clothing that doesn't hinder movement
- Shoes with proper design, support, and cushioning

8. **Instructor Etiquette**

Fitness instructors need to act as role models for their participants, and should always conduct themselves in a courteous and professional manner. Professional work habits include, but are not limited to, the following. Instructors should:

- arrive on time, fully prepared to teach class;
- introduce themselves to new class participants;
- be positive when addressing problem situations;
- dress neatly and appropriately in a manner that is non-intimidating to participants;
- communicate with, and/or correct, participants in an appropriate manner, taking care not to offend or embarrass them with either their choice of words, voice tone, "spotting technique," or body language;
- be sensitive to the needs and requests of the class participants when it comes to music selection, volume, and pitch; and
- make themselves available for questions before and/or after class.

9. **Class Level**

When deciding on an appropriate class level (or intensity), many factors should be considered, including class size and differences in participant skill and fitness level. One recommended approach is to teach at an intermediate level, and explain and/or demonstrate to the class how to modify the choreography to achieve both more and less intense variations. However, since beginners tend to follow the instructor's movements, instructors may need to frequently go back and forth between beginner and more advanced versions.

10. **Music Usage, Selection, and Speed**

AFAA recommends a music selection that is appropriate to the chosen activity. Different modalities will require different beats per minute (bpm) in order to accommodate each participant's lever length (arms, legs, and torso). It is important to monitor the group to make sure that participants are able to safely complete a full range of motion for the chosen exercises without excessive momentum. If they are unable to perform safely, then instructors need to adjust the tempo/pitch or choose more appropriate music (including ethnic or highly-skilled dance styles).

Example bpm recommendations include the following.

- Warm-up: 120–134 bpm
- Low- and high-impact cardio: 130–155 bpm
- Cardio kickboxing: 125–135 bpm (up to 140 bpm for skilled participants)
- Step aerobics: 118–128 bpm (up to 128–135 bpm for advanced, highly-skilled participants)
- Muscle sculpting: under 130 bpm (unless movements are half-tempo)
- Flexibility training: under 100 bpm

11. **Breathing as Applied to the Workout**

Breathing should follow a consistent rhythmic pattern throughout exercise. The level of activity will dictate rate and depth of ventilation. In general, inhale and exhale through the nose and mouth in a relaxed fashion. However, some forms of exercise (e.g., yoga), may use different breathing techniques.

- When performing cardiorespiratory movements, breathing can act as an indicator of exercise intensity (e.g., implementing the "talk test"), allowing adjustment of exertion level.
- When performing a strength training movement, exhale during the exertion or hardest phase of the exercise.
- When performing flexibility training movements, breathe calmly, easing into the stretch to help lessen a desire to hold the breath.
- Holding the breath while exercising may induce the Valsalva maneuver (i.e., the glottis closes and creates an unequal pressure in the chest cavity, which may cause a rise in blood pressure).
- Hyperventilating or breathing too hard while exercising can irritate the nasal passages as well as cause lightheadedness.

VI. Exercise Evaluation and the AFAA 5 Questions™

A. Exercise Evaluation

Individuals in a fitness class usually have diverse characteristics and goals. Therefore, more conservative guidelines are recommended than might be otherwise indicated when working one-on-one or with a specialized population, such as elite athletes (e.g., gymnastics, track and field). During exercise evaluation there needs to be a continuum by which instructors in a group setting can evaluate an exercise from two viewpoints—effectiveness (benefits) and potential risk (injury quotient) for the potential participant. With this perspective in mind, AFAA has created the AFAA 5 Questions.

B. AFAA 5 Questions™

1. **What is the purpose of this exercise?**
   Consider: muscular strength or endurance, cardiorespiratory conditioning, flexibility, warm-up or activity preparation, skill development, and stress reduction

2. **Are you doing that effectively?**
   Consider: proper range, speed, or body position against gravity

3. **Does the exercise create any safety concerns?**
   Consider: potential stress areas, environmental concerns, or movement control

4. **Can you maintain proper alignment and form for the duration of the exercise?**
   Consider: form, alignment, or stabilization

5. **For whom is the exercise appropriate or inappropriate?**
   Consider: risk-to-benefit ratio; whether the participant is at a beginner, intermediate, or advanced level of fitness; and any limitations reported by the participant

High Risk **Appropriate Modification**   **High Risk** **Appropriate Modification**

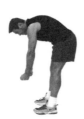 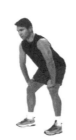

1. Sustained unsupported
   forward spinal flexion

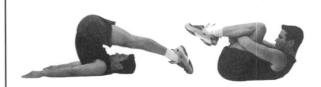

6. Full plough

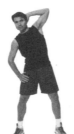

2. Sustained unsupported
   lateral spinal flexion

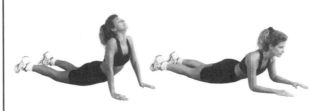

7. Full cobra

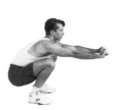 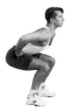

3. Repetitive or weighted
   deep knee bends

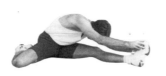

8. Hurdler's stretch

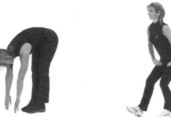

4. Bouncy (ballistic)
   toe touches

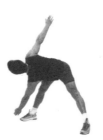

9. Windmills: a rapid side-to-
   side movement that combines
   spinal flexion and rotation

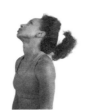 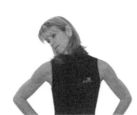

5. Rapid head circles

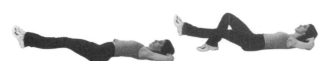

10. Supine double straight leg lifts
    without spinal stabilization

High Risk   Appropriate Modification   **High Risk   Appropriate Modification**

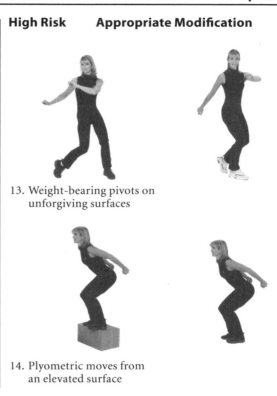

11. Prone combination double leg/double arm lifts

12. Painful, forced splits

13. Weight-bearing pivots on unforgiving surfaces

14. Plyometric moves from an elevated surface

The following is a list of some exercises that AFAA does not recommend in a general fitness class due to their high risk-to-benefit ratio on the exercise continuum. Some of the following exercises are commonly performed in other disciplines or practices where they should only be used with proper progression, training, alignment, and supervision. In many cases, these exercises can be modified to lessen their potential risk (areas of stress/concern are listed in parentheses). It is important to note that these other exercises, done with and without equipment, should not be carried out. Such determinations need to be based upon the application of individual professional judgment.

1. Sustained unsupported forward spinal flexion (spinal ligaments)

2. Sustained unsupported lateral spinal flexion (spinal ligaments)

3. Repetitive or weighted deep knee bends (knee ligaments)

4. Bouncy (ballistic) toe touches (back, hamstrings, and calves)

5. Rapid head circles (cervical spine)

6. Full plough (cervical spine)

7. Full cobra (lumbar spine)

8. Hurdler's stretch (medial knee ligament)

9. Windmills: a rapid side-to-side movement that combines spinal flexion and rotation (lumbar spine)

10. Supine double straight leg lifts without spinal stabilization (lumbar spine)

11. Prone combination double leg/double arm lifts (lumbar spine)

12. Painful, forced splits (ligaments in hip and knee joints, groin area)

13. Weight-bearing pivots on unforgiving surfaces (ankles and knees)

14. Plyometric moves from an elevated surface (compression concerns)

C. Body Alignment

Fitness instructors should monitor participants' body alignment throughout each section of class. There are a number of basic exercise positions to consider: standing, lunge, bent-over, seated, supine (lying on your back), prone (lying on your front), side-lying, and kneeling, as well as alignment in movement. The following are key points instructors should keep in mind when evaluating and cueing for exercise body alignment. The standing alignment below has a complete head to toe description. The other positions described will only include specific alignment cues unique to those postures.

1. **Correct standing alignment**
   - Feet are positioned a comfortable distance, about shoulder-width, apart (a little wider for greater stability).
   - Toes point in the same direction as the knees.
   - Legs may be straight or bent, without hyperextending (locking) the knees.
   - Pelvis is neither tipped forward (anterior tilt) nor tucked under (posterior tilt), but is in neutral alignment.
   - Abdominal muscles are engaged (isometrically contracted) and rib cage is lifted.
   - Entire spinal column is in ideal alignment from neck (cervical spine) to pelvis (which means that the four natural curves of the vertebral column are in a balanced relationship to each other; no one curve is excessive).
   - Shoulder blades are slightly down, neither rounded forward nor excessively pulled back.
   - Head should be held high with the ears in line with the shoulders.
   - From a side view, there should be a straight, vertical line from the head to the feet indicating anterior/posterior balance.

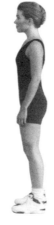
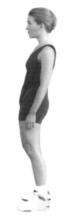
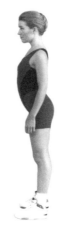

Correct standing alignment

Incorrect standing alignment (posterior pelvic tilt)

Incorrect standing alignment (anterior pelvic tilt)

2. **Correct alignment for squats (parallel and plié) and lunge (staggered) stances**
   - Toes and knees point in the same direction.
   - Knees do not extend past the toes.
   - Hips are at or above the height of the knees.
   - Hips and shoulders are kept squared to the front.
   - Abdominal muscles are engaged to support the spine in neutral posture.
   - Shoulders are kept down away from ears.

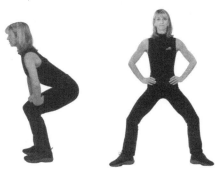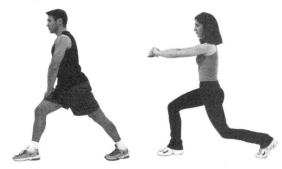

Correct alignment for squats   Correct alignment for lunges

3. **Correct bent-over alignment**
   - The bent-over position may be performed by flexing at the hips or spine.
   - When flexing from the hips, engage the back and abdominal muscles to support the torso in neutral. If additional support is needed, use one or both hands on the thigh(s), floor, or other stable surface (e.g., chair, pole, or wall).
   - When flexing from the spine (rounding the back), one or both hands should be placed on the thighs, ankles, floor, or other stable surface or object. The additional support is required because in the forward spinal flexed position, the abdominal and back muscles are not effectively co-contracting to stabilize the torso. Since the spinal extensors are not adequately contracting, there is increased stress to the ligaments and other soft tissue surrounding the vertebrae.

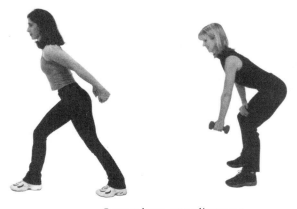

Correct bent-over alignment

4. **Correct seated alignment**
    - Maintain the spine in neutral alignment, with upper body weight directed onto the sitting bones (ischial tuberosities).
    - Knees are bent at a 90° angle (if on a chair) or held straight, slightly bent, or folded (if seated on the floor) to facilitate a neutral spine.
    - Shoulders are down, scapulae neutral, neck relaxed.
    - Toes and knees should point in the same direction to avoid ligament and knee stress.

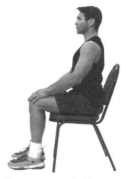 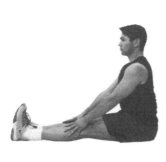 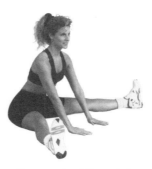 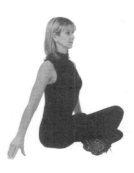

Correct seated alignment   Correct long seated alignment   Correct straddle seated alignment   Correct cross-legged seated alignment

5. **Correct supine alignment**
    - Lie on back and maintain a neutral spine by engaging the abdominal muscles and placing the pelvis in neutral.
    - Some participants will need to keep one or both knees bent with feet flat on the floor in order to maintain a neutral spine.

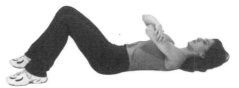

Correct supine alignment

6. **Correct prone alignment**
    - Lie down with face looking down or turned to one side (head may be placed on forearms).
    - Maintain a neutral pelvis and spine by engaging the back and abdominal muscles.

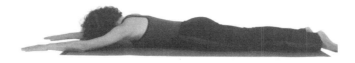

Correct prone alignment

7. **Correct side-lying alignment**
   - Stack hips and shoulders to maintain a square alignment.
   - Use top arm in a support position by placing the hand on the floor in front of the body.
   - Rest the head on the bottom arm to keep the neck in neutral alignment, or support an elevated torso position on the elbow (if in an elevated position, place the elbow directly under the shoulder).
   - If in an elevated position, keep the spine in a straight line rather than allowing the torso to slouch.
   - Knees and hips can be extended or flexed (the flexed position will allow for greater stability).

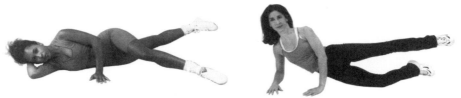

Correct side-lying alignment

8. **Correct kneeling alignment**
   - Kneeling positions may be performed full-kneeling on two knees with torso upright or half-kneeling on one knee with other leg in a 90° forward support position.
   - Kneel on one knee with the other foot in front, placed far enough away that the front knee is bent at no more than a right angle (90°).
   - Remain upright or hinged at the hips (even if one leg is extended), keeping the spine as neutral as possible.
   - Abdominal and back muscles should be engaged.
   - Shoulders should be down, with neck in neutral alignment.

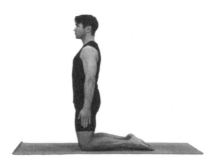   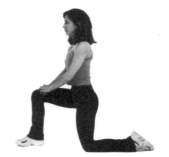

Correct full-kneeling alignment   Correct half-kneeling alignment

9. **Correct hands (or elbows) and knees alignment**
   - Place the hands or elbows on the floor directly under the shoulders.
   - Kneel with knees directly under the hips.
   - Keep shoulders and hips square.
   - Keep the neck in neutral alignment.
   - Engage the abdominal muscles to maintain neutral spinal alignment (avoid arching the low back).

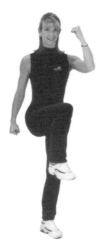

Correct alignment while moving

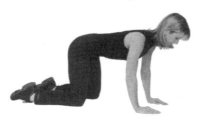

Correct hands and knees alignment

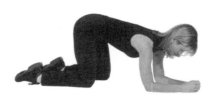

Correct elbows and knees alignment

10. **Correct alignment while moving**
   - Maintain all of the above mentioned points as they apply to the execution of an exercise or the body in movement.
   - Alignment will vary according to the specific requirements of the desired exercise or movement.
   - Participants should control their range of motion in order to maintain posture and alignment throughout all movements.

VII. Group Exercise Class Format

The format/design of a class should reflect sound application of the principles of training so that fitness gains are fostered while injury risks are kept at a minimum. Depending upon the class type and objectives, the format will vary. However, AFAA does recommend that every class include the following components.
   - Pre-class announcements
   - A warm-up/activity preparation period
   - Body of the workout (e.g., cardio, strength, flexibility training)
   - Post-exercise relaxation, stretching, and/or cool-down

VIII. Class Components

A. Pre-Class Announcements

The fitness instructor should introduce himself or herself and announce the type, level, and format of the class. He/she should ask if there are any new participants and remind them to work at their own level. Let participants know what type of intensity monitoring will be utilized and be sure they are familiar with it.

B. Warm-Up

1. **Definition, Purpose, and Duration**

   Definition

   A warm-up is the preparation period for a specific workout.

   Purpose

   The warm-up should increase core temperature as well as prepare the muscles and joints for movements that will follow. This can be accomplished by combining limbering and movement rehearsal, and/or light preparatory stretches when appropriate. A proper warm-up should prepare the body for vigorous exercise and may reduce the risk of injury.

Duration

The duration of the warm-up will be dependent on the length and type of class, as well as fitness level and age of the participant. A typical warm-up period for a group exercise class is 8–12 minutes. However, it may vary (e.g., 5–10 minutes) depending on the type of exercise and class design. Keep in mind that in a cardio workout, there may not be a clear-cut demarcation between the warm-up and cardio sections.

2. **Common Warm-Up Methods**

Movement Rehearsal

Movement rehearsal involves performing lighter or less intense versions of movements or patterns that will be used in the workout to follow (e.g., low kicks prior to a vigorous kickboxing segment, marching prior to higher impact jogging, or performing resistive movements without weights prior to the weighted segment). The goal is to increase the blood flow and core temperature as well as facilitate performance and coordination.

Limbering Movements

Limbering movements are smooth, moderately-paced, non-weighted, full-range movements that increase joint mobility and core temperature (sometimes referred to as "dynamic stretching"). Examples would include shoulder circles, overhead arm reaches, side-to-side lunges, and other fluid movements. In some cases, there will be a similarity between limbering and movement rehearsal.

Preparatory Stretching

Preparatory stretches are gentle stretches (held for less than 15 seconds, typically 8–16 beats of music). These stretches are designed to ease the muscles through a range of motion to ensure proper movement mechanics rather than increase isolated muscle flexibility. Over the years, controversy has arisen within the fitness industry regarding whether or not to include stretching within the warm-up. Until further research is compiled, AFAA's stance is that light, preparatory stretching is optional based on the needs of the participants, activity, or environment, while more intense or longer-held stretches (> 15 seconds) should not be included as part of a warm-up, but rather during the post-workout flexibility section.

NOTE: AFAA recommends the use of an appropriate combination of the above mentioned methods, taking into consideration those muscles that are commonly tight and need special attention for the intended workout, fitness level of participants, time of day, environmental temperature, and so forth.

3. **Special Considerations**

Intensity and Impact

It is important to keep the participants below their training heart rate range during a warm-up. Movements should be low intensity and build gradually. Movements or repetitions that lead to muscle fatigue are inappropriate. High-impact movements that travel laterally should be avoided until the ankles and feet are sufficiently warmed up (usually 3–4 minutes).

Speed and Control

Movements and stretches performed too rapidly or without control can become ballistic (bouncy or jerky with momentum). This type of movement may induce the stretch reflex (i.e., muscle contracts against the stretch in a protective manner) and may increase the risk of injury. Therefore, it should be avoided.

Range of Motion (ROM)

When beginning a warm-up, start with moderate ROM movements and slowly build to a greater ROM as the body warms up. Although some participants may be flexible enough to omit statically-held stretches, instructors should keep in mind that others in a group may benefit from gentle static stretching.

Sequence

Follow any order, making sure to include all major muscle groups. Warming up from either head to toes, or vice versa, is an easy way to avoid omitting any muscle groups.

Spinal Issues

Make sure to prepare the spine with controlled movements in all functional ranges (including flexion, extension, rotation, and lateral flexion). Participants who have a history of low-back injuries should perform the single-plane movements of back flexion and extension prior to rotation and/or lateral flexion of the spine. Avoid sustained, unsupported forward or laterally flexed positions of the spine (rounding the back or side bending), as over-stretching of the ligaments in the lower back may occur. Support the torso by placing hands on the thighs, depending upon individual flexibility level.

4. **Sample Exercises**

Common warm-up movements for the upper body
   - Movement Rehearsal or Limbering: alternating rear shoulder circles, non-weighted front and rear flys
   - Optional Preparatory Stretches: chest and anterior deltoid stretch

Common warm-up movements for the middle body
   - Movement Rehearsal or Limbering: overhead reaches, light-range alternating punches
   - Optional Preparatory Stretches: supported spinal forward and lateral flexion

Common warm-up movements for the lower body
   - Movement Rehearsal or Limbering: marching in place, step touch, knee lifts
   - Optional Preparatory Stretches: standing calf, standing hip flexor

Sample Warm-Up Movements

Movement Rehearsal and Limbering

Preparatory Stretches

C. Cardiorespiratory Training

1. Definition, Purpose, and Duration

Definition

The cardiorespiratory section of class utilizes continuous and rhythmical aerobic activities that target the large muscles of the body to create an increased demand for oxygen over an extended period of time. Modalities include, but are not limited to, walking, hiking, stepping, high/low-impact aerobics, stationary cycling, inline skating, and cardio kickboxing.

Purpose

Cardiorespiratory training exercises improve the heart, circulatory, and pulmonary systems. This can be accomplished by utilizing a variety of training methods that target cardiorespiratory endurance (e.g., continuous, interval, and circuit training).

Duration

The duration will vary depending on the class format and level, but will typically last 20–45 minutes in a 60-minute class (or several short bouts of 10 minutes each in a circuit format).

2. Methods of Cardiorespiratory Training

Continuous or Steady-State Training

Cardio exercises are performed in such a way that the intensity gradually increases, is held at steady state for the majority of the workout, and then gradually decreases. Choreography is developed in such a way that intensity fluctuations are minimized in an attempt to keep the heart rate at a certain level within the training (target) heart rate range (THRR). If plotted on paper, the intensity of continuous steady-state training would depict a flat top bell curve.

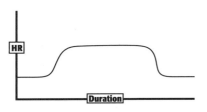

Bell Curve Graph (Steady State)

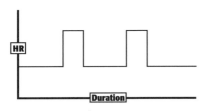

Interval Training Graph

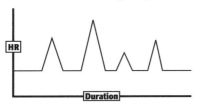

Intermittent Training Graph

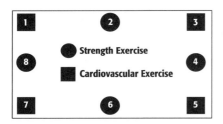

Circuit Training Diagram

Interval Training

Interval training is characterized by timed bouts of higher-intensity work followed by periods of lower-intensity active recovery. During the work phase, participants perform movements that may take them to anaerobic levels (above their aerobic THRR), or to the high end of their aerobic range. During the active recovery, participants work at or below the low end of their aerobic THRR. The work and recovery phases are performed in a timed ratio, for example 1:3 (30 seconds of work followed by a 90-second recovery).

Intermittent Training

This training method is also known as variable intensity training or spontaneous training. It is a less structured form of interval training with randomly interspersed peak movements followed by lower-intensity movements.

Circuit Training

Circuit training involves timed bouts of activities/exercises performed in a station-to-station, or sequential, manner. A class can perform a circuit in a stationary position with all participants performing the same activity simultaneously, or with participants moving around the room from station to station performing different exercises. These activities can be designed to improve cardiorespiratory endurance, muscular strength, or a combination of both. A greater cardiorespiratory benefit will occur if all the activities or stations are cardiorespiratory in nature.

NOTE: AFAA recommends the use of any or all of the aforementioned cardiorespiratory training techniques. If higher-intensity interval training is used, participants should be advised to limit or space workout times to allow for adequate recovery.

3. **Special Considerations**

Monitoring Intensity

AFAA recommends monitoring intensity approximately every 10–15 minutes during the activity, as well as at the completion of the post-aerobic cool-down. A variety of methods, such as pulse check, rating of perceived exertion, talk test, or a heart rate monitoring device, can be used effectively, as long as proper monitoring techniques have been taught.

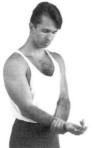

Heart rate
wrap around method

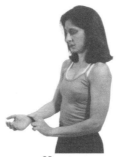

Heart rate
finger tip method

Cross-Training

Participants and fitness instructors should cross-train by varying the modalities of their cardiorespiratory activities to help decrease biomechanical stress, avoid mental burnout, and increase adherence.

Intensity Issues

Instructors should offer a variety of intensity options/modifications for movements to allow participants to stay within their proper training range. Commonly used options include the following.

- Adding or eliminating dynamic arm movements
- Adding or eliminating impact or propulsion
- Increasing or decreasing the range of a movement
- Increasing or decreasing the speed of a movement
- Making a pattern of movements that may be either more or less intricate
- Substituting moves (e.g., marching rather than jogging)

It is recommended that individuals who are moderately to highly de-conditioned start with intensities that are slightly lower (e.g., 64–74% of HR_{max} or 40–55% of HRR/VO_2R), remain in a comfort zone (around "moderate" on RPE scale), and gradually increase over time.

Music Speed

If using music with choreography, AFAA recommends music speeds that will allow the arms and legs to move throughout their full range of motion with control while maintaining proper form and alignment. (See section V.B.10.)

Range of Motion

Participants should control their range of motion in order to maintain posture and alignment throughout all movements. The movement in the limbs needs to match the ability to stabilize the core of the body (e.g., avoid kicking so high that the back cannot remain upright, but flexes to compensate). When performing certain moves, participants must be sure to complete a full range of motion (e.g., when performing impact moves, with the exception of lunges or repeating lunges, bring the heels to the floor on each landing).

Repetitive Stress Issues

To help prevent repetitive stress injuries, avoid extended periods of consecutive movements, such as hops, kicks, jumps, or punches. For example, use a variety of high-, low-, and mid-range elevation of the arms to avoid stressing the shoulders and avoid hopping on one leg for more than eight consecutive counts.

Cardiorespiratory Cool-Down (Post-Aerobic)

At the end of the cardiorespiratory segment, AFAA recommends performing 3–5 minutes of lower-intensity rhythmic activity. An appropriately designed cool-down will help participants avoid blood pooling in the extremities as well as aid them in a gradual heart rate recovery. Fitness instructors may also want to include some upright static stretches to regain the range of motion and flexibility in muscles that have been shortened during the workout.

4.   Sample Cardio Movements

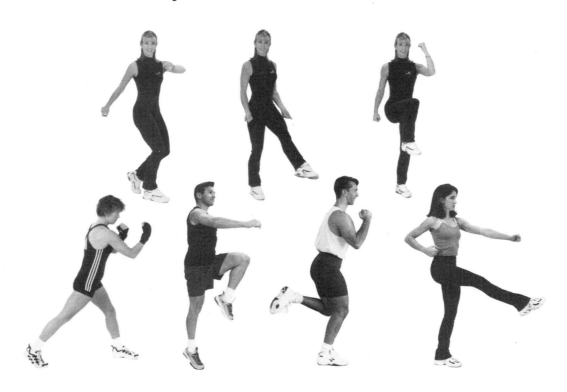

D.   Muscular Strength and Endurance Training

1.   Definition, Purpose, and Duration

Definition

Muscular strength and endurance training involves working individual or groups of muscles against a resistance to the point of muscle fatigue. Different forms of resistance can be used, such as dumbbells, weighted bars and balls, resistance tubes, or body weight. Example workouts include calisthenics/floor work, body sculpting, or circuit training.

Purpose

Both muscular strength and muscular endurance are important for overall health. Benefits include an improved ability to perform everyday activities, increased muscle mass, increased metabolism, stronger bones, decreased risk of injury, improved posture and symmetry, and improved athletic performance.

Duration

The time required for muscular training varies depending on the type and format of the class. A typical strength workout lasts between 45 and 60 minutes, including the warm-up and flexibility work. If the strength training is only a portion of the workout, it may only last 15–20 minutes. In the latter case, fewer muscle groups may be targeted (e.g., upper body and abdominals only).

2. **Common Methods of Muscular Strength and Endurance Training**

In a group exercise setting, exercises will involve either concentric, eccentric, or isometric muscular contractions.

-   Concentric Muscular Contraction: A concentric contraction occurs when tension generated by the muscle is sufficient to overcome a resistance, and moves (at a joint) a body segment of one attachment toward the segment of its other attachment (e.g., the upward or shortening phase of a biceps curl).

-   Eccentric Muscular Contraction: An eccentric contraction occurs when a muscle slowly lowers a resistance (lengthening phase) as it returns from its shortened phase to normal resting length.

-   Isometric Muscular Contraction: An isometric contraction describes a static (held) position in which tension is developed in the muscle, but the muscle length and joint angle do not change.

NOTE: The following methods and exercises use one or both types of muscle contraction(s).

Muscle Isolation (Prime Movement)

Isolation exercises are used to target a specific muscle group by utilizing the primary movement (joint action) of that particular muscle. Examples include biceps curls, calf raises, and deltoid raises.

Multi-Joint/Multi-Muscle

As the name implies, multi-joint exercises involve more than one joint and target several muscle groups in the same exercise. In a squat, for example, movement occurs at several joints (hip, knee, and ankle) and many muscles (quadriceps, gluteal muscles, and hamstrings) are targeted simultaneously.

Torso Stabilization

Commonly referred to as torso, core, or spinal stabilization, these exercises will enhance the ability to maintain proper spinal alignment and posture. The primary focus of these exercises is to keep the axial skeleton (torso) stable, whether in a held position against gravity (e.g., modified V-sit) or resisting the movement of an extremity (e.g., supine alternating toe taps, with low back held in neutral). To be executed correctly, the abdominal and back muscles must work together in a co-contracting isometric manner.

Functional Training

Functional training describes exercises that replicate movements commonly used in activities of daily living. A narrow stance squat, for example, duplicates the action of getting in and out of a chair. In many cases (e.g., the squat), functional exercises are not always separate or distinct from multi-muscle /multi-joint or stabilization exercises.

NOTE: AFAA recommends that a combination of the aforementioned training techniques be used in most fitness programs. Each technique challenges the body differently and offers distinct training benefits. The key to exercise selection is based on the participants' goals, their ability to maintain proper form and alignment, and the amount of available training time.

3.   **Special Considerations**

Muscle Balance

Muscle balance is achieved when muscles on all sides of a joint are properly trained for proper posture, body mechanics, and injury prevention. Thus, for every primary muscle worked (agonist), the opposing muscle group (antagonist) should also be worked. It is important to note that although both agonist and antagonist muscles should be trained, not all muscles have the equal capacity of their opposers (e.g., calves and anterior tibialis).

It is important for the instructor to be familiar with the most common muscle imbalances so that class time is used wisely. In general, weak, loose muscles (thoracic and upper back) need to be strengthened or tightened, and excessively tight muscles (chest and anterior deltoids) need to be stretched or lengthened.

Range of Motion

Isotonic exercises should be taken through a full ROM. This will allow the muscle to function at its best throughout its usable range, as well as to maintain adequate joint mobility. Care should be taken not to overload a muscle past its ability to control the movement. Control is often compromised when working at either end of the range of motion—the beginning and end of the motion are often weaker than mid-range.

Speed and Control

Muscle conditioning exercises should be performed at slow-to-moderate speeds that allow full range of motion and concentrated work in proper alignment. Performing an exercise too quickly often relies on momentum; this is both less effective and more likely to lead to joint or muscle injury.

Intensity

Train a muscle or muscle group to the point of muscle fatigue. Adjust the resistance so that the muscle is fatigued within a reasonable number of repetitions (generally 8 to 15). In group exercise, adjustments of training variables, such as the number of repetitions (up to 25), sets (1–4), or sequencing, may be necessary if the equipment does not offer sufficient resistance.

Torso Stabilization Exercises

If inadequate abdominal strength is present, certain torso stabilization exercises may place inappropriate stress on the spine. In a group exercise setting, extreme care should be used and sufficient modifications properly cued to accommodate individual needs with these torso stabilizing exercises. Properly performed stabilization exercises can be a positive complement to traditional isotonic forms of abdominal training (e.g., crunches and curls). Both methods may be included in a complete training program.

Resistance Equipment Techniques

Participants should not use external resistance (e.g., weights or resistance tubing) until they can perform the given exercises with proper alignment and technique without resistance. When all the repetitions can be completed comfortably with proper form, the amount of resistance should be gradually increased in order to continue to overload the muscles and stimulate improvement. Some general points to keep in mind when cueing exercises that use resistance equipment are as follows.

- Keep the hands relatively relaxed. Avoid a tightly clenched fist; this can potentially cause blood pressure elevation.

- Maintain a neutral wrist. Avoid flexing or extending the wrists while gripping weights, bands, or tubes. Excessive repetitive wrist flexion or extension can increase the risk of carpal tunnel syndrome and tennis elbow.

- Teach participants to bend over and pick up their equipment properly for low-back pain prevention. One hand is on the thigh for support, while the other hand picks up the weight or tubing. For picking up heavier items, use correct squatting technique and a two-handed lift.

- For exercises that are not equipment-based, position the muscle so that it is directly opposed by gravity for the most effective and time-efficient work.

- When using elastic resistance, it is important to control the eccentric, or return, phase of the exercise; "rebounding," or suddenly returning to the starting position without control, can cause injury. Additionally, for healthy joint mechanics, the instructor needs to be attentive to utilizing tubing only when there is correct line of pull.

Muscle Conditioning Exercises in the Water

Water exercise differs from land exercise in several important ways. Instead of gravity constantly exerting a downward force (as on land), there is the upward force of buoyancy in the water. In addition, muscle actions are different; all actions in the water are concentric (shortening), whereas on land the actions are both concentric and eccentric (lengthening). Because of these differences, instructors may need additional training or experience in working in water.

4. **Sample Exercises**

The following chart is a compilation of a variety of common exercises. The exercises listed are organized into several approaches to exercise selection. It may also be used as a reference chart to primary muscles and their joint actions.

Table 17-1

Body Part/ Muscle	Prime Movement (joint action that isolates targeted muscle)	Exercise Variations are Based on Body Position (appropriate in a group exercise class with gravity, weights, or tubing for resistance)	Exercises Single-joint	Exercises Multi-joint	Exercises Stabilization
Shoulders/ deltoids	Shoulder flexion, extension, abduction, horizontal abduction	**Standing:** Raises, upright rows, overhead presses **Seated:** High rows with elastic tubing, overhead presses **Prone:** Push-ups **Supine:** Dips **Bent over:** Posterior raises	Anterior, lateral and posterior raises, rotation	Push-ups and upright rows	Planks, hovers (down position of push-up)
Front of upper arm/biceps	Elbow flexion	**Standing:** Variety of curls **Seated:** Lat pull-downs and seated rows, variety of curls and rows	Curls	Pull-ups and rows	Bent arm hangs
Back of upper arm/triceps	Elbow extension	**Standing:** Wall push-ups, overhead extensions **Seated:** Dips, overhead extensions **Prone:** Push-ups **Supine:** Presses **Bent over:** Kickbacks	Kickbacks	Dips, push-ups, presses	Planks
Muscles of the lower arm/a variety of small flexor and extensor groups	Wrist and finger flexion, extension, forearm supination and pronation, wrist abduction and adduction	**Standing and Seated:** Variety of flexion and extension exercises	Wrist curls and extensions, wrist abduction and adduction	Rotation curls	Weight-bearing or weight-holding positions with wrist in neutral alignment
Chest/pectorals	Horizontal shoulder flexion/adduction, and medial rotation of the arm	**Prone:** Push-ups **Supine:** Flys, chest presses, pull-overs	Flys	Bench presses, push-ups	Basic planks and hovers
Upper mid-back: trapezius and rhomboids	Scapular elevation, adduction/retraction	**Standing:** Shrugs, upright rows **Seated:** Rows (with tube), overhead presses **Prone:** Reverse flys **Bent over:** Rows and reverse flys	Straight arm scapular retraction	Rows and overhead presses	Reverse planks
Mid-back: latissimus dorsi	Shoulder joint adduction and extension	**Standing:** Pull-downs (with tube) **Seated:** Pull-downs and rows (with tube) **Supine:** Pull-overs **Bent over:** Rows		Rows and pull-ups	Bent arm hangs and side planks
Anterior torso/ rectus abdominis, obliques	Spinal flexion, lateral flexion and rotation	**Seated:** V-sits **Supine:** Curls (all variations) **Hands and knees:** Pelvic tilts **Side-lying:** Lateral flexion		Curls, reverse curls, rotation curls	V-sits, supine leg presses, basic planks, and hovers, exercises performed in non-supported hip flexion
Posterior torso/erector spinae	Spinal extension	**Seated:** V-sits **Prone:** Leg and arm lifts **Hands and knees:** Opposite arm and leg lifts		Prone or on hands and knees: opposite arm and leg lifts	V-sits, reverse planks, exercises performed in non-supported hip flexion
Buttocks/glutei	Hip extension and external rotation	**Standing:** Rear leg lifts, lunges and squats **Prone:** Rear leg lifts **Supine:** Hip lifts **Hands and knees:** Rear leg lifts	Rear leg lifts	Lunges and squats	Standing balance work, reverse planks

Body Part/ Muscle	Prime Movement (joint action that isolates targeted muscle)	Exercise Variations are Based on Body Position (appropriate in a group exercise class with gravity, weights or tubing for resistance)	Exercises Single-joint	Exercises Multi-joint	Exercises Stabilization
Anterior thigh/ iliopsoas, quadriceps	Hip flexion and knee extension	**Standing:** Front leg or knee lifts, lunges and squats **Seated:** Knee extensions and single straight leg raises **Supine:** Knee extensions and single straight leg lifts	Knee extensions, single straight leg raises	Lunges and squats	Standing balance work, wall sits
Posterior thigh/ hamstrings	Knee flexion and hip extension	**Standing:** Hamstring curls, lunges and squats **Prone:** Rear leg lifts and hamstring curls **Supine:** Hip lifts **Hands and knees:** Rear leg lifts and hamstring curls	Hamstring curls and rear leg lifts	Lunges and squats	Standing balance work, reverse planks
Outer thigh/ gluteus medius and tensor fasciae latae	Hip abduction	**Standing:** Abduction leg lifts, single leg squats **Supine:** Hip abduction **Side-lying:** Abduction leg lifts	Abduction side leg lifts		Single leg squats, single leg balance work, side planks
Inner thigh/ hip adductors	Hip adduction	**Standing:** Adduction leg lifts, single leg squats **Supine:** Hip abduction **Side-lying:** Adduction leg lifts	Adduction leg lifts	Plié squats with drag	Single leg squats, single leg balance work
Anterior lower leg/tibialis	Dorsi flexion	**Standing:** Toe raises **Seated:** Ankle flexion	Toe raises		Walking on heels
Posterior lower leg/ gastrocnemius, soleus	Plantar flexion	**Standing:** Heel raises **Seated:** Plantar flexion (with tubing)	Heel raises	Jumps	Walking or balance work on toes

Sample Muscular Strength and Endurance Exercises

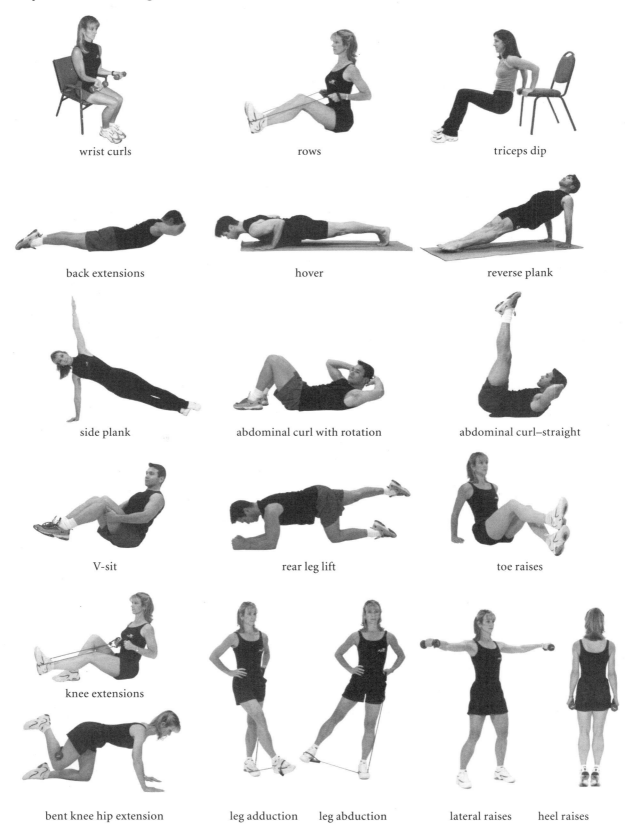

wrist curls

rows

triceps dip

back extensions

hover

reverse plank

side plank

abdominal curl with rotation

abdominal curl–straight

V-sit

rear leg lift

toe raises

knee extensions

bent knee hip extension

leg adduction

leg abduction

lateral raises

heel raises

E. **Flexibility Training**

1. **Definition, Purpose, and Duration**

Definition

Flexibility training focuses on joint mobility and muscle suppleness, muscle flexibility, and the reduction of muscular tension. When performed as a segment of a class, it usually takes place in conjunction with a post-aerobic cool-down, or the final relaxation segment. Some common flexibility-based classes include fitness stretching and yoga. Some classes, such as yoga, promote a blend or combination of muscular strength and flexibility.

Purpose

Flexibility training improves joint mobility. Having adequate and balanced flexibility may decrease the risk of potential injury and may enhance physical performance.

Duration

The amount of time spent focusing on flexibility training will be dependent upon the focus and goals of the class. The time allotment may vary from as few as 5–10 minutes (near the end of a cardiorespiratory training session) to an entire 60-minute stretching class.

2. **Common Methods of Stretching**

Static Stretches

Static stretching involves placing the targeted muscle or muscles in a position of elongation and holding that position. Individuals are recommended to perform 1–4 repetitions for each stretch holding for 15–60 seconds. In a group exercise setting 1 repetition may be appropriate, due to time allocation, to target all the major muscle and tendon groups.

Dynamic Stretching/Full Range of Motion

Dynamic stretching involves stretching with movement through a full range of motion. These stretches can range in intensity from a controlled, limbering movement to a ballistic, forceful one. For the purposes of group exercise, the focus should be on multiple repetitions of a controlled movement, ideally contracting the antagonistic muscle while slowly moving through the end range of motion.

Proprioceptive Neuromuscular Facilitation (PNF) Stretches

PNF stretches involve an active contraction of the muscle prior to the stretch (often referred to as the contract/release method). PNF stretching has been shown to be as effective or more effective than static stretching. To properly perform most PNF stretches, outside assistance is needed. Some stretches can be achieved with the use of a towel or stretching strap, but in most cases a trained assistant or physical therapist is needed. For this reason, PNF stretching is not often used in the group exercise environment.

3. **Special Considerations**

Intensity

Stretch to the end of the range of motion or to the point of tension. Never stretch past the point of discomfort or to the point of pain, which may result in microscopic tears in the stretching muscle.

Speed and Control

Dynamic stretches, when performed too forcefully or quickly, become ballistic. This type of movement may induce the stretch reflex mechanism that shortens rather than lengthens the muscle to be stretched. In addition, ballistic stretches increase the risk of injury and should be avoided for the general fitness population. However, ballistic stretching may be more appropriate for individuals who are participating in sports involving ballistic movements.

Range of Motion

Stretch a muscle through its available range of motion. Stretching beyond the muscle's current range of motion can result in injury to the connective tissue and supporting structures.

Body Temperature

Ideally, there should be a noticeable increase in muscle or body core temperature, whether induced by previously performed exercises or external factors (e.g., clothing or room temperature), prior to performing flexibility work.

4. **Sample Exercises**

Common Upper Body Stretches
*   Pectorals/Anterior Deltoids
    Level I: Standing—hands behind head
    Level II: Seated—hands behind back
*   Upper Back/Mid-Trapezius/Rhomboids/Posterior Deltoids
    Level I: Standing—upper back stretch
    Level II: Seated—hug knees
*   Triceps
    Level I: Standing—support hand is in front of body
    Level II: Seated—hand behind head
*   Neck
    Level I: Standing—ear to shoulder
    Level II: Seated—ear to shoulder, opposite arm extended down

Common Middle Body Stretches
*   Low Back
    Level I: Standing—spinal flexion with hands supporting
    Level II: All-fours position—cat stretch
*   Latissimus Dorsi
    Level I: Standing—one arm overhead
    Level II: Kneeling—extended seal
*   Obliques
    Level I: Standing—single arm overhead reach
    Level II: Supine—spinal rotation
*   Rectus Abdominis
    Level I: Standing—both arms overhead reach
    Level II: Prone—modified cobra

Common Lower Body Stretches
*   Hamstrings
    Level I: Standing—single leg sit back
    Level II: Supine—single leg lift
*   Quadriceps
    Level I: Standing—modified lunge
    Level II: Standing—bent knee hand holds foot

- Hip Abductors
  Level I: Standing—leg crosses behind
  Level II: Seated—bent knee cross
- Hip Adductors
  Level I: Standing—side lunge
  Level II: Seated—bent knee butterfly

Sample Flexibility Exercises

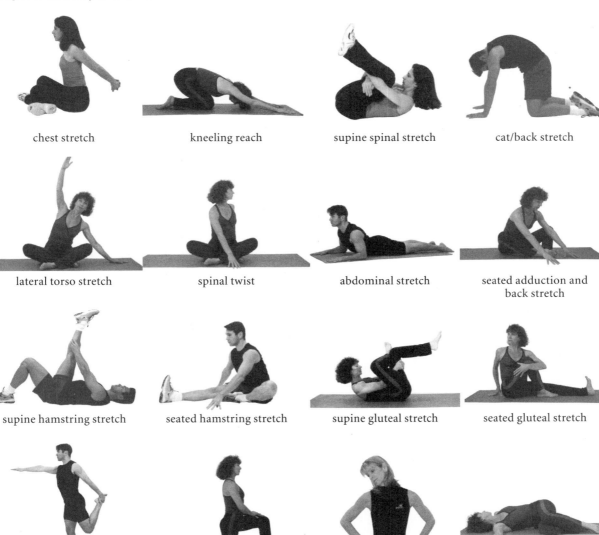

chest stretch

kneeling reach

supine spinal stretch

cat/back stretch

lateral torso stretch

spinal twist

abdominal stretch

seated adduction and
back stretch

supine hamstring stretch

seated hamstring stretch

supine gluteal stretch

seated gluteal stretch

standing hip flexor and
quadriceps stretch

kneeling hip flexor and
quadriceps stretch

neck stretch

supine twist

F. **Final Class Segment**

1. **Definition, Purpose, and Duration**

   Definition

   The final class segment is the closure of a workout, in which instructors can include stretching and/or other relaxation and stress reducing techniques.

   Purpose

   The final class segment is designed to promote mind-body awareness and facilitate the relaxation response, a state in which the heart rate and blood pressure are decreased, muscles relax, and physiological stress is reduced. It is an optimal time for participant education. It also provides a sense of completion.

   Duration

   The time allotment for the final segment of the class will vary depending on the instructor's class design, typically 5–10 minutes.

2. **Common Relaxation Methods**

   Physical Focus

   This method focuses on the participants' bodily systems and sensations in an attempt to increase relaxation. This can be done through a variety of methods using careful verbal cueing and/or calm, peaceful music.

   Mental/Abstract Focus

   This method uses the participants' imagination in order to create a greater sense of relaxation.

   Combination Focus

   It is common for instructors to combine both the physical and mental focuses in order to see even greater relaxation responses than either method might produce on its own.

3. **Special Considerations**

   Heart Rate Monitoring

   It is a good idea to take a post-exercise heart rate or exertion check at the end of class. Participants should notice that their heart rates have returned back, or near, to their pre-exercise heart rates. This final heart rate can help participants increase their appreciation of relaxation for stress management.

   Saunas and Hot Tubs

   Saunas, hot tubs, steam rooms, and the like are problematic for some individuals if they have not sufficiently cooled down after exercising and for others with adverse health conditions. If core temperature is still elevated post-exercise, taking the body into a hot environment can increase the risk of a heat-related disorder. Heart rate can be an indicator of increased internal temperature and potential heat stress, especially if the post-exercise heart rate is greater than 110 bpm.

   Method Selection

   When choosing an appropriate final class segment method, be sensitive to language that might make participants uncomfortable. For example, some attendees aren't comfortable with spiritual comments or affirmations in the exercise setting.

4. **Sample Exercises**
   Breathing (Physical Focus)

   Diaphragmatic breathing is used to decrease stress and tension and to enhance the relaxation response. In a proper diaphragmatic breath, cue students to lower the diaphragm on the inhale, causing air to flow into the lungs. The deeper the inhale, the more the diaphragm drops, causing the abdominals to be displaced outward—the abdomen relaxes out. On the exhale, cue them to allow air to flow up and out of the lungs, the diaphragm rises, and the abdominals relax back in. This type of breathing is physiologically correct, usually very relaxing, and is a valuable stress reduction technique. This is the most basic breathing technique used by fitness instructors, although there are many other choices.

   Breathing (Combined Focus)

   "Lie on your back in a comfortable position, legs relaxed and slightly apart, arms a little distance away from the body, palms facing the ceiling, eyes closed. Allow your abdomen to rise and fall as you slowly and rhythmically breathe. Think of filling a balloon all the way to the bottom with each breath. Let each breath become slower and slower, taking the deepest, most relaxing breaths of your day. Imagine that fresh, healing oxygen is rushing in to nourish every cell on each inhale. Imagine that stale, tired air is carrying out unnecessary tension on each exhale."

   The Contract and Relax Method (Physical Focus)

   This method is also known as the progressive relaxation technique. It is used to help increase body awareness and release muscular tension. Cue participants to selectively contract and release muscle groups one by one, allowing their bodies to enter into a state of deepened relaxation. As a result, participants become more aware of the difference between the feeling of tension and the feeling of relaxation.

   Visualization (Mental Focus)

   Visualization, or guided imagery, techniques are often used for stress management and as an aid to relaxation. Suggest peaceful images, eliciting sights, sounds, smells, and sensations that mentally transport participants to a more relaxing environment, facilitating the relaxation response.

Exercise Guidelines and Protocol

Fitness instructors have access to a variety of resources that focus on exercise design and implementation. Understanding the nature of scientific writing, as well as the research and publication process, is important in determining the accuracy and validity of the source.

Peer-reviewed journals. Generally, when one speaks of "research" or "research articles," he or she is referring specifically to articles that are published in peer-reviewed or refereed journals. Articles submitted for publication in these journals are generally descriptions of the laboratory experiment results, clinical trials, reviews of previous studies, or meta-analyses (i.e., a technique for evaluating a number of studies and drawing new conclusions based upon existing data). The editorial boards of these journals are experts in their fields, and evaluate an article based of its own merit (such as sound study design and appropriate data analysis), in addition to the context of other research in a given subject area. The peer-reviewed journals are useful in identifying or analyzing new or evolving areas of thought in a particular discipline.

Articles in non-refereed journals (such as those found in consumer magazines), as well as newspaper and television stories, are sources of information for both fitness professionals and the general public. Although magazines and newspapers have editorial staffs to ensure that the information they publish is accurate, they do not have the access to expert opinion of the peer-reviewed journals, nor do they review articles in the same way. Articles in these sources tend to cover broader topics, are more often based on opinion or casual observation than scientific study, and may be influenced by commercial interests. While they can provide the fitness professional with valuable insights (especially about consumer attitudes and fitness), they are typically a good starting point for further inquiry rather than an end point in themselves.

Textbooks. For instructors seeking to build a general knowledge base (such as basic anatomy or biomechanics), a textbook or reference book may be a better source. College-level textbooks provide a balanced discussion of a given topic and will highlight areas of controversy. While textbooks bring together diverse points of view and provide consensus, they might not be as "up-to-date" as journal articles (check the copyright date).

Web-based resources. The Internet has opened the door to a multitude of resources for fitness instructors from peered-reviewed journal articles, to online courses, to educational handouts for participants, and more. However, the challenge is to locate credible sites. Look for online research articles and supportive data from acclaimed industry associations and organizations, for example: (a) American College of Sports Medicine (www.acsm.org), (b) Centers for Disease Control and Prevention (www.cdc.gov), (c) National Institute on Health (www.nih.gov and http://medlineplus.gov), and (d) U.S. Department of Health and Human Services (www.usdhh.gov). Fitness instructors can locate information addressing exercise physiology, anatomy and kinesiology, exercise programming and technique, nutrition, injury prevention, wellness, and more. Many of the sites are free to users or may require a membership fee.

References

1. Albano, C., & Terbizan, D.J. (2001). Heart rate and RPE differences between aerobic dance and cardio-kickboxing. Abstract. *Medicine & Science in Sports & Exercise*, 33(5), S604.

2. Alter, M.J. (2004). *The science of flexibility* (3rd ed.). Champaign, IL: Human Kinetics.

3. American College of Sports Medicine. (2007). *ACSM's health/fitness facility standards and guidelines* (3rd ed.). Champaign, IL: Human Kinetics.

4. American College of Sports Medicine. (2007). ACSM's position stand on exercise and fluid replacement. *Medicine & Science in Sports & Exercise*, 39(2), 377–390.

5. American College of Sports Medicine. (2009). *ACSM's exercise management for persons with chronic diseases and disabilities* (3rd ed.). Champaign, IL: Human Kinetics.

6. American College of Sports Medicine. (2010). *ACSM's resource manual for guidelines for exercise testing and prescription* (6th ed.). Baltimore, MD: Lippincott Williams & Wilkins.

7. American College of Sports Medicine. (2010). *ACSM's guidelines for exercise testing and prescription* (8th ed.). Baltimore, MD: Lippincott Williams & Wilkins.

8. Baechle, T., & Earle, T. (2003). *Essentials of strength training and conditioning* (3rd ed.). Champaign, IL: Human Kinetics.

9. Baker, A. (1998). *Bicycling medicine: Cycling nutrition, physiology, and injury prevention and treatment for riders of all levels.* New York, NY: Fireside.

10. Bell, J., & Bassey, E. (1994). High and low-impact aerobic dance heart rate and VO_2 responses. *European Journal of Applied Physiology*, 68, 20–24.

11. Bellinger, B., St. Clair, G.A., Oelofse, A., & Lambert, M. (1997). Energy expenditure of a noncontact boxing training session compared with submaximal treadmill running. *Medicine & Science in Sports & Exercise*, 29(12), 1653–1656.

12. Berñando, L.M. (2007). The effectiveness of Pilates training in healthy adults: An appraisal of the research literature. *Journal of Bodywork Movement Therapies*, 11(2), 106–110.

13. Berry, M.J., Cline, C.C., Berry, C.B., & Davis, M.A. (1992). A comparison between two forms of aerobic dance and treadmill running. *Medicine & Science in Sports & Exercise*, 24(8), 946–951.

14. Bijlani, R.L., Vempati, R.P., Yadav, R.K., Ray, R.B., Gupta, V., Sharma, R., Mehta, N., & Mahapatra, S.C. (2005). A brief but comprehensive lifestyle education program based on yoga reduces risk factors for cardiovascular disease and diabetes mellitus. *Journal of Alternative & Complementary Medicine*, 11(2), 267–274.

15. Bissonnette, D., Guzman, N., McMillan, L., Catalano, S., Giroux, M., Greenlaw, K., Vivolo, S., Otto, R.M., & Wygand, J. (1994). The energy requirements of karate aerobic exercise versus low impact aerobic dance. *Medicine & Science in Sports & Exercise*, 26(5), S58.

16. Brown, P., & O'Neill, M. (1990). A retrospective survey of the incidence and pattern of aerobics-related injuries in Victoria, 1987-1988. *Australian Journal of Science and Medicine in Sport*, 22(3), 77–81.

17. Bushman, B. (2002). Female athlete triad: Education is key. *ACSM's Certified News*, 12(2), June. Retrieved May 1, 2009, from http://www.acsm.org

18. Church, T.S., Earnest, C.P., Skinner, J.S., & Blair, S.N. (2007). Effects of different doses of physical activity on cardiorespiratory fitness among sedentary, overweight or obese postmenopausal women with elevated blood pressure: A randomized controlled trial. *Journal of American Medical Association*, May, 297, 2081–2091.

19. Clapp, J., & Little, K. (1994). The physiological response of instructors and participants to three aerobics regimens. *Medicine & Science in Sports & Exercise*, 26(8), 1041–1046.

20. Davis, M., & Bahamonde, R.E. (2000). A survey of shoes and injury characteristics of aerobic instructors. *Medicine & Science in Sports & Exercise*, 32(5), S1520.

21. DeVreede, P., Samson, M., & VanMeeteren, N. (2005). Functional-task exercise vs. resistance strength exercise to improve daily tasks in older women: A randomized controlled trial. *Journal of American Geriatrics Society*, 53, 2–10.

22. Dowdy, D.B., Cureton, K.J., Duval, H.P., & Ouzts, H.G. (1985). Effects of aerobic dance on physical work capacity, cardiovascular function and body composition of middle-aged women. *Research Quarterly for Exercise and Sports*. 56(3), 227–233.

23. Dwyer, J. (1995). Effect of perceived choice of music on exercise intrinsic motivation. *Heath Values*, 19(2), 18–26.

24. Eickhoff-Shemek, J.M., & Selde, S. (2006). Evaluating group exercise leader performance. *ACSM Health & Fitness Journal*, 10(1), 20–23.

25. Eickhoff-Shemek, J.M., Herbert, D.L., & Connaughton, D.P. (2008). *Risk management for health/fitness professionals: Legal issues and strategies.* Baltimore, MD: Lippincott Williams & Wilkins.

26. Funk, D.C., Swank, A.M., Mikla, B.M., Fagan, T.A., & Farr, B.K. (2003). Impact on prior exercise on hamstring flexibility: A comparison of Proprioceptive neuromuscular facilitation and static stretching. *Journal of Strength & Conditioning Research*, 17, 489–492.

27. Gotchalk, L., Berger, R., & Kraemer, W. (2004). Cardiovascular responses to a high-volume continuous circuit training protocol. *Journal of Strength & Conditioning Research*, 18(4), 760–764.

28. Grant, S., Davidson, W., Aitchison, T., & Wilson, J. (1998). A comparison of physiological responses and rating of perceive exertion between high-impact and low-impact aerobic dance sessions. *European Journal of Applied Physiology and Occupational Physiology*, 78(4), 324–332.

29. Grier, T.D., Lloyd, L.K., Walker, J.L., & Murray, T.D. (2001). Metabolic cost of aerobic dance bench stepping at varying cadences and bench heights. Abstract. *Medicine & Science in Sports & Exercise*, 33(5), S123.

30. Hamilton, N., Weimer, W., & Luttgens, K. (2008). *Kinesiology: Scientific basis of human motion* (11th ed.). Boston, MA: McGraw-Hill.

31. Herbert, D.L., & Herbert, W.G. (2002). *Legal aspects of preventive, rehabilitative, and recreational exercise programs* (4th ed.). Canton, OH: PRC Publishing.

32. Hoffman, S. (2009). *Introduction to kinesiology: Studying physical activity.* Champaign, IL: Human Kinetics.

33. Hostler, D., Schwirian, C.I., Hagerman, R.S., Staron, G., Campos, K., Toma, M.T., & Hagerman, G. (1999). Skeletal muscle adaptations in elastic resistance-trained young men and women. *Medicine & Science in Sports & Exercise*, 31(5), S1632.

34. Kravitz, L. (1994). The effects of music on exercise. *IDEA Today*, October, 55–63.

35. Kravitz, L., Greene, L., & Wongsathikun, J. (2000). The physiological responses to kickboxing exercise. Abstract. *Medicine & Science in Sports & Exercise*, 35(5), S148.

36. McCord, P., Nichols, J., & Patterson, P. (1989). The effect of low impact dance training on aerobic capacity, submaximal heart rates and body composition of college-aged females. *The Journal of Sports Medicine and Physical Fitness*, 29(2), 184–189.

37. McGill, S.M. (2007). *Low back disorders: Evidence-based prevention and rehabilitation* (2nd ed.). Champaign, IL: Human Kinetics.

38. McGinnis, P.M. (2005). *Biomechanics of sport and exercise.* Champaign, IL: Human Kinetics.

39. McMillan, D.J., Moore, J.H., Hatler, B.S., & Taylor, D.C. (2006). Dynamic vs. static-stretching warm up: The effect on power and agility performance. *Journal of Strength & Conditioning Research*, 20, 492–499.

40. Olson, M., Williford, H., Blessing, D., & Greathouse, R. (1991). The cardiovascular and metabolic effects of bench-stepping exercise in females. *Medicine & Science in Sports & Exercise*, 23(4), S27.

41. Requa, R.K., & Garrick, J.G. (1993). Injuries in various forms of aerobic dance. *Medicine & Science in Sports & Exercise*, 25(5), S270.

42. Ricard, M., & Veatch, S. (1990). Comparison of impact forces in high and low impact aerobic dance movements. *International Journal of Sports Biomechanics*, 6, 67–77.

43. Solomon, R.L., Solomon, J., & Cerny-Minton, S. (2005). *Preventing dance injuries*. Champaign, IL: Human Kinetics.

44. Thrash, L.E., & Anderson, J.J. (2000). The female athlete triad: nutrition, menstrual disturbances, and low bone mass. *Nutrition Today*, 35(5), 168–174.

45. U.S. Department of Health and Human Services. (2008). *2008 physical activity guidelines for Americans*. Washington, DC: Office of Disease Prevention and Health Promotion (U0036)/http://www.health.gov/paguidelines

46. Wilmore, J.H., Costill, D., & Kenney, W.L. (2008). *Physiology of sport and exercise* (4th ed.). Champaign, IL: Human Kinetics.

47. Wolfe, B.L., Lemura, L.M., & Cole, P.J. (2004). Quantitative analysis of single vs. multiple-set programs in resistance training. *Journal of Strength & Conditioning Research*, 18(1), 35–47.

Instructor Training and the Importance of Continuing Education

Nancy Gillette, MA

18

Focus

There are dozens of ways in which future instructors receive training. Some programs meet national standards—others miss the mark entirely. How can instructors evaluate various training programs? What should they include? How important is it that they adhere to nationally accepted standards? Once the training is completed, how important is continuing education while working in the field?

Background

Until about 1983, fitness instructor training was haphazard at best. No educational organizations or training associations existed purely for the benefit of the instructor and his/her training in the exercise field. Generally, an instructor entered the field as a star student filling in for an absent instructor, mimicking the exercises and style of the absentee instructor, obtaining what is referred to as "on the job non-training." Many found themselves with new part-time jobs. The only prerequisites for being an instructor in those days were a pair of athletic shoes, leotard and tights, and an audio music tape.

The field of aerobics and fitness has matured substantially since then. Now there are a variety of training options open for the instructor or would-be-instructor.

One of the major accomplishments within the exercise field in the past 20 years has been the creation of training and certifying organizations. The accumulation of research and data on which to base standards, guidelines, and proper content of such trainings has served to put credibility and substance into these groups' criteria and curricula.

However, because the exercise arena is still maturing in terms of substantiated evidence and information relating to fitness, new studies are coming out that don't always comply with what was always thought to be "true" within the art and science of exercise. Because of conflicting or new information that disproves old studies and theories within the fitness field, selecting a club, organization, or individual to act as a trainer for instructors can be a difficult decision to make.

The training group or individual should be as up-to-date on the latest research as possible. This isn't easy because information is constantly changing or being upgraded. A trainer should ideally be linked into a larger research or educational organization, for it's relatively impossible for one person to stay abreast of all that is happening within the exercise arena, no matter how conscientious he or she is.

How to Select a Training Organization or Professional Trainer

When selecting a training organization, an instructor or would-be-instructor needs to evaluate the credentials and certifications offered by several different groups and ask some questions. How long have they been in business? What are their reputations? Do they offer continuing education? Are they nationally accredited? Are their "graduates" satisfied with the training they received? Will you have to travel to another city for the training sessions? What expenses will be incurred for the training? How many hours or days are included in the program? Is the certification a test of both theory and practical knowledge? Is the course offered online? What will you receive upon completion of their program? Will you be certified? Are their various certificates recognized locally, regionally, nationally, or internationally?

Participants looking for an individual professional trainer might ask some of the same questions above concerning a trainer's certification. They should also ask: How long has he/she been training professionally? Who trained him or her? What is his or her reputation (ask for references)? Has he or she kept up-to-date with continuing education? There are many factors to consider.

Content of Instructor Training

The content of an instructor's training program will determine the future quality of that instructor-to-be. Both theory and its practical application within the class setting should be taught in conjunction with practical "how to's" of creating, instructing, and demonstrating an appropriate fitness class.

The following should be included in a solid, complete training program:

Basic theory
- anatomy and kinesiology
- physiology
- nutrition
- injury prevention
- cardiorespiratory considerations

Practical application of theory
- class format
- risk factor assessment
- first-aid and CPR
- medical responsibilities/emergency situations
- exercise selection
    - level of class skill
    - special population needs
    - local trends—cycle/spin, yoga, Pilates, mind/body, muscle pump, jump rope, cardio intervals/cross-training, power step, cardio combat, latest street dances, super sculpt, light start, sports conditioning, core strength, balance, functional strength, posture perfect, tai chi, world beat, kickboxing, boot camp, flexible strength, etc.
- cueing—alignment, safety, anticipatory
- choreography
- exercise evaluation
- transitions
- attire/shoes
- music selection—beats per minute guidelines
- professional conduct
- voice projection and protection—using a microphone
- relating to and motivating your students
- continuing education—post-training

> *Any training program that does not include these components will leave gaps in an individual's skill or knowledge level, and will result in either ineffectual or unsafe teaching techniques.*

Which to Choose?

Individual Professional Trainer

An individual professional trainer who is well known in the field of exercise and has an outstanding reputation as being up-to-date, as well as personable and skilled in one-to-one training, can be an excellent choice. Often clubs will hire instructors solely on the basis of having been trained by a certain individual because the club then knows what to expect regarding the quality and style of the new instructor. This is especially true in smaller cities throughout the United States where a trainer with a good local reputation has made a name for himself or herself. The drawback in selecting an individual, rather than an organization, is that the person may be teaching outdated information or even incorrect information that could cause the instructor to injure a student, or even be sued and lose that lawsuit due to negligence or poor training.

Health Club Training

Many instructors-to-be select local training within a chain of clubs in their area. The advantage to this approach is that the club usually has instructor positions available for those who attend their trainings. Also, if an instructor wants to teach at more than one club (or later is relocated to a different city), it is convenient if the clubs are all owned or operated by the same individual or group.

Training Organization

One of the advantages of selecting a training organization, rather than an individual who owns his or her own training business, is the combined expertise and information the group shares among its members or partners. This is especially true if there is a board of advisors, an educational base to the organization, a newsletter or magazine for updating information to those who belong, or a research and data collection department within the organization that will dispense the latest information to the trainers.

Another advantage is the networking opportunities that are available to relocate to another city, state, or country. Locating open positions and having certification or a training certificate from a well-established and respected organization can be an entree into a new locale or business. Having those credentials, or a resume that mentions a training organization by name, can ensure one's level of expertise as an instructor particularly for those who have no previous knowledge of that instructor.

Importance of Being Certified

Most health clubs or fitness studios require some sort of certification from their instructors prior to being hired. In addition to wanting to ensure the expertise and quality of an instructor, owners/managers are also concerned with lawsuits and the club's reputation. For these reasons, an instructor who has certification from a training organization that requires both practical as well as theoretical knowledge assures the club/studio of the safety and effectiveness of the instructor's class formatting and instruction, both of which sometimes come under scrutiny during lawsuits from clients/students when an injury occurs.

Importance of Continuing Education

The majority of certifying bodies require instructors to attend and complete a certain number of Continuing Education hours of study in order to keep their certifications current. Even if no such requirement exists, it is still prudent to continue to educate oneself in the fitness field in order to maintain one's professionalism and to stay abreast of the latest research trends.

Some groups or colleges offer on-site courses to attend. Many book or DVD home self-study courses are also available. Since the Internet has entered the world of education, some fitness education organizations can now offer study units by completing online courses, complete with interactive quizzes and final examination. A few such educational resources (e.g., AFAA Distance Education Center courses) even offer interactive study groups, reachable faculty, video conferencing, and more. These opportunities will continue to expand as the technology is invented to accommodate the unique visual requirements of fitness learning.

Summary

When selecting a training organization or continuing education provider, look for quality of instruction, a good track record and reputation, and a complete curriculum, including both practical application as well as theoretical knowledge on a broad range of exercise and physiology subjects. Seek out a training program that provides instructors with a certification and future support, not just a temporary job. Be sure that the continuing education provider has a history of offering a variety of curricula that will adequately prepare an instructor for continued excellence in the latest fitness trends and techniques.

When selecting an individual trainer, determine if he or she was certified by a reputable training organization, has a strong reputation for staying up-to-date, and has a personality and teaching style that can motivate and encourage exercise adherence for students.

Recommended Reading

1. Caldwell, B.J. (1993). *The return to the mentor: Strategies for workplace learning.* London, England: Falmer Press..
2. Collins, N.H. (1983). *Professional women and their mentors.* Englewood Cliffs, NJ: Prentice-Hall.
3. Daloz, L.A. (1990). *Effective teaching and mentoring.* San Francisco, CA: Jossey-Bass.
4. Gross, R. (1990). *Peak learning.* Los Angeles, CA: Jeremy P. Tarcher.
5. Jensen, E.P. (2008). *Brain-based learning: The new paradigm of teaching.* Thousand Oaks, CA: Corwin Press.
6. Kiewra, K.A., & Dubois, N.F. (1997). *Learning to learn: Making the transition from student to lifelong learner.* Boston, MA: Allyn & Bacon.
7. Leonard, G. (1991). *Mastery—The keys to long-term success and fulfillment.* New York, NY: Dutton Books.
8. Orlick, T. (2007). *In pursuit of excellence.* Champaign, IL: Human Kinetics.
9. Palmer, P.J. (1998). *The courage to teach: A guide for reflection and renewal.* San Francisco, CA: Jossey-Bass Publishers.
10. Powers, B., & Rothwell, W.J. (2007). *Instructor excellence: Mastering the delivery of training.* San Francisco, CA: Pfeiffer.
11. Silberman, M. (1996). *Active learning: 101 strategies to teach any subject.* Boston, MA: Allyn & Bacon.

19 Motivation & Adherence: Getting Them & Keeping Them!

Ken Alan, BS and
Diana McNab, MEd

Focus

How do I motivate people to exercise? How do I get a person to try my class? What can be done to keep them coming back? Is there something I should do so they don't drop out? How do I keep some fitness fanatics from over-exercising? These are essential questions to ask a certified fitness instructor. There has been a long running debate whether fitness instructors can actually motivate someone to exercise. Interestingly, many exercisers think they can, as suggested by these statements about different fitness instructors:

"The way she yells and doesn't let us slack off—she is the most motivating instructor I've ever had."

"She is so caring and nice, never yells or screams—she is the most motivating instructor I've had."

"She explains the exercises well. I've learned a lot—she is the most motivating instructor I've ever had."

"She hardly talks. The class starts, the music rocks, she cues us, we follow—she is so motivating, the best instructor I've had."

As these comments illustrate, the perception of a "motivating" instructor is as individual as the participants in a class. It is helpful to remember in any discussion about motivation and adherence, there are multiple perspectives—the participant's, the instructor's, and an overall global perspective.

This chapter looks at the dynamic relationship between a fitness instructor and participants. It will provide an overview of the concepts of motivation, adherence, and determinants of exercise behavior. This chapter will examine the characteristics of people who attend or might attend classes, and develop strategies to promote adherence. After discussing teaching philosophy, through your readings, you will delve into instructional techniques, communication skills, and leadership principles that increase the motivational atmosphere of your class. The end result will have people saying, *"You are the most motivating instructor I've ever had!"*

Motivating the Masses

Knowledge in the physiological sciences is your foundation to develop and implement fitness programs. You must then take your knowledge and transform it into a delicious, irresistible buffet of exercise options to wet the appetite of the people in your community. It's a matter of motivating the masses.

Motivation to exercise is easy when you like to exercise and/or like its benefits. Yet, a lot of people do not like to exercise. The numbers say so. A landmark publication from the United States Department of Health & Human Services, Physical Activity & Health: A Report of the Surgeon General (Pate et al., 1995; USDHHS, 1996) revealed the following.

- Only an estimated 15% of Americans are currently physically active enough to derive substantial health benefits from that activity.
- 60% of the population is not getting a minimum amount of recommended physical activity.
- About 25% lead a sedentary lifestyle.

- Around 50% of people who start an exercise program drop out within 6 months.

Similar statistics may be common in other industrialized countries. With numbers like these, you have formidable challenges yet simultaneously, you have a very real opportunity to start turning these numbers around.

It is rewarding when you are able to get a person hooked on exercise, and group exercise can be the hook that captures them. A group exercise class is a markedly different experience from solo exercise. Working out in a group offers participants your leadership and expertise. You also have the dynamics of group cohesion and social camaraderie. Rapport starts to build and relationships evolve which create a community—a sense of belonging—and this can be a positive influence for establishing a regular exercise habit (Carron et al., 1996).

Adherence and Compliance

Adherence to exercise is an active, voluntary, and long-term involvement while compliance refers to a mandatory action. If participants have to exercise, they comply by coming to class. If participants choose to exercise, they adhere by attending class. Exercise adherence is not simple—it is a complex issue. There are multiple variables that act as determinants of exercise behavior:

- Environmental conditions
    - Is the location convenient, safe, and welcoming? The farther away a person lives/works from where a class is held, the more likely of not staying with the program.
    - Floor, ventilation, acoustics, and equipment need to be conducive for exercise.
- Cultural values
    - Exercise may not be widely accepted as appropriate in different cultures.
    - Societal norms change at different rates—it used to be "unfeminine" for women to sweat or to be physically active.
- Demographics
    - Socioeconomic status is an indicator of exercise adherence.
    - Higher income individuals are more likely to exercise.
    - More educated individuals are more apt to adhere to an exercise program.
- Health/medical status
    - Injuries can limit or restrict physical activity.
    - Obesity, cardiovascular disease, or medical conditions affect the type of exercise safely tolerated.
- Psychological status
    - Body image can both positively and negatively impact exercise adherence.
    - If you feel you have no control of your own health (locus of control: a person's belief about what causes the good or bad results in his or her life), it is extra challenging to stick with an exercise program.
    - Self-motivated individuals are prone to adhere to exercise.
- Support network
    - Support from family/friends increase adherence rates.
    - Rewards help to motivate some individuals to exercise.
    - An exercise buddy can be beneficial; you have an unofficial commitment to each other to keep consistent with the program.

– A written contract with yourself is (surprisingly) effective in helping to stay engaged in exercise.
- Barriers
  - Lack of time
  - Activity history
  - Previous negative exercise experiences
  - Current daily physical activity
  - Lack of knowledge about benefits of exercise
  - No interest in improving health or fitness level

Studies in the psychology of exercise have yet to precisely predict or explain exercise adherence with the reproducibility required to design fail-proof action plans to change physical activity patterns. As research continues in this area, we can further refine and develop interventions to target the varying determinants, needs, and issues encountered with getting people physically active (Dishman, 1994). We can however, explore motivation concepts and strategies that enhance exercise adherence for various population segments.

Population Types

People are classified into three general categories in terms of physical activity.
- Athletic/very active individuals
- Weekend warriors/"on-again/off again" exercisers
- Mostly sedentary/inactive individuals

The group exercise domain further divides the population into four sub-groups.
- Type A. Advanced
- Type B. Intermediate
- Type C. Beginner
- Type D. Everybody else

The Advanced Participant (Type A)

Type A are the most committed and fit individuals in an exercise class. They intend on maintaining a high level of fitness and like to be pushed. If a class description/name has "extreme" in it, they are there. Passionate for intense workouts, they look forward to challenging exercises and choreography. They bring boundless enthusiasm and energy to group exercise. Many attend a fitness class every day. Some take two classes back-to-back or return for another workout later in the day. They often become attached to one instructor, tweaking schedules to attend their favorite instructor's class. These people keep you on your toes expecting creative, stimulating, and intense training regimens.

Common classroom traits include:
- positioning themselves in the front of the room (especially rooms with mirrors).
- territorial; standing in the same spot in every class.
- distressed if someone is standing in their usual place.
- requests louder music volume.
- prompts you to "pitch up the tempo."
- disappointed with substitute instructors.

Two of the most significant Type A characteristics for instructors to be aware of are the following.
- *May be willing to risk injury to work at very high levels of intensity.*
- *May be in the class for competitive reasons.*

Exercise Addicts

Some Type A individuals, unintentionally, love exercise too much. Their passion turns into an addiction and can impact other aspects of their life. Many are working out—often in a compulsive way—to avoid the negative consequences of being overweight and out of shape. Obsessive exercisers sometimes have food issues and exhibit disordered eating patterns in their quest to achieve their ideal body. For women, these behaviors can result in amenorrhea. If left unchecked, it leads to a higher risk of osteoporosis among other health problems. This sequence of events is referred to as the female triad (Hobart & Smucker, 2000).

A female participant who thinks she is always too fat or never thin enough may have a poor body image of herself. Men are also susceptible to body image problems (Beals, 2003). Muscle dysmorphia or the "Adonis complex" refers to men who believe they never have enough muscle size or their body fat level is never low enough. For women and men body image issues can fuel over-exercising. It can also be triggered by something that is out-of-control in a person's life. Exercise becomes a way of dealing with emotional or psychological stress. Type A exercisers may have similar traits to Type A personalities: (a) hard-driven, (b) success-oriented, (c) self-motivated, (d) hurried, (e) short-tempered, and (f) perfectionist tendencies. This carries over into fitness. Over-training signs include:

- dull pain or chronic aches in the lower extremities;
- unexpected drop in performance;
- mood disturbances (e.g., anxiety, depression, anger);
- general fatigue; and
- changes in sleep pattern.

Action Plan

Scheduling

> Type A exercisers often participate in high-impact workouts every day. A number of studies show [lower body] injury rates are substantially greater in high-impact activity compared to low-impact activities (Mutoh et al., 1988; Brown & O'Neill, 1990). Exercise mode plays a crucial role in injury prevention. It is the musculoskeletal system, not the cardiorespiratory system, which incurs injuries from high-impact activities. Alternating low-impact with high-impact workouts reduces accumulative trauma and the opportunity to develop overuse injuries. A variety of workouts (e.g., step training, kickboxing, cycling) provide different mechanical stresses to the body while allowing high-intensity options for advanced training. Additionally, strength training is critical for lowering injury risk from high-impact exercise. You (or your fitness director) can also address the issue by scheduling or offering high-impact programs no more than 3 days per week instead of on a daily basis.

Orientation

Type A enthusiasts become territorial when selecting a spot, so your role as motivator and teacher is to acknowledge their desire to be close to the front or to you, but to also respect the needs of the group. Remember, your participants' first priority is to feel good. A few tactful adjustments could be in order, along with a friendly suggestion to certain aggressive individuals. You can periodically reverse the class orientation, where the back of the room becomes the front. There may be a few disgruntled persons initially, but it usually dissipates and participant positioning becomes more equitable in the class.

Boredom

Many Type A's find one type of exercise or class becomes their favorite workout and often their only form of exercise. This can lead to an impending problem—boredom. This occurs in recreational activities as well as fitness classes, where an individual participates in one activity exclusively until any enjoyment or pleasure from it has vanished. In time they abandon the activity altogether. Cross-training through a variety of programs and activities is fundamental for minimizing boredom. Group exercise was at a time just one type of class: high-impact aerobics. That was it. With dozens of class formats today, there is no reason not to participate in different workouts.

Creating Unwanted Competition

In general, instructors should strive to have participants feel they are not in competition with others in class. This not only keeps egos in check, but also minimizes temptation for a person to do something beyond what is safe for him or her. You facilitate this when you are sensitive to the least flexible participant or the individual using the least amount of resistance and match that individual in range of motion or amount of resistance. As an example, if you are stretching in a range of motion greater than anyone in class, you may be creating competition, even if you say, "We're non-competitive. It doesn't matter how far anyone stretches except yourself." Be aware of these situations—they occur frequently. The workout is for your participants, not yourself. Your job is to ensure each person is in their appropriate range of motion, not for you to be in your greatest range of motion. Make sure your physical performance and demonstration complement and promote a non-competitive ideology.

Creating Competition

Interestingly, some Type A's become inspired by competing with other people in class. Competition is a motivator, which is why you will see them:
- aspire to kick highest in kickboxing.
- boast of the puddle underneath their bike in a cycling class.
- exhibit phenomenal flexibility in yoga.

Recognize when you can use a competitive spirit to advance group camaraderie. The desire to compete is fuel for some boot-camp and sports-oriented programs. There is a place for competing, provided it is applied in a fun or playful context. Instructors of cycling classes will pit riders against riders, or half of the class against the other half of class. Participants can get inspired when competition is used to engage everyone in the class rather than to just determine who are the winners and losers.

Overzealous Type A's should be encouraged to reassess their reasons for working out as frequently/intensely as they do. Fat loss? Stress reduction? Competitive drive? Fitness advertisements often emphasize cosmetic exercise benefits, such as firmer thighs or chiseled abs. While this is important to some individuals, it has little to do with function, health, or wellness unless sporting a six-pack truly improves one's self-esteem. Fitness professionals have an obligation to meet the fitness goals of all participants, including Type A. Strike a balance between appearance, function, and fitness-for-health goals. It is wonderful to have a body that looks great. It is even more wonderful to have a body that feels and functions great.

The Exercise-For-Life Participant (Type B)

Type B do not feel pressured to push themselves to the max, since the higher the intensity of exercise, the higher the dropout rate (Dishman, 1988). Comparing Types A and B, Type B may exercise as much as a Type A, but they exercise at more moderate intensity levels. This group prospers nicely with three to four workouts weekly rather than daily workouts. They rotate between low-impact and high-impact workouts, whereas Type A favors high-impact workouts. Type B understands that staying well-hydrated pays off and good workout shoes are worth the investment. They listen to their body and choose to exercise, whereas Type A has to exercise. They are sensible, not compulsive about fitness and have embraced it without compromising other aspects of life. They see the big picture and are in it for the long-haul. Type A generally think about the short-term outcomes.

Incentives are not typically needed for Type B to adhere to exercise. Motivation for Type B is sustained through feedback, support, recognition, and encouragement. For them, exercise itself is rewarding. The intrinsic satisfaction and sense of well-being from working out maintain the drive and desire to stay active. Provide general and specific feedback and positive reinforcement to support their consistent efforts. Feedback is information you give participants about the quality of their performance or a task (Wlodkowski, 1984). Even if you do not have a chance to talk to a participant after class, you can still text, phone, or email him or her. Examples of appropriate feedback may include the following.

- General feedback: "Your alignment is looking good. Keep it up."
- Specific feedback: "Your alignment for lunges is looking good. Keep it up."
- General compliment: "You did great in class today."
- Specific compliment: "You nailed the lunge series today. Great job."
- Recognition: "Your posture has improved since joining our class."
- Acknowledgement: "Just wanted you to know it's a pleasure to have you in class. Your energy is great."

Tangible rewards or awards for adopting healthful behaviors can also be reinforcing (Wagman, 1997). Class members enjoy such tokens as the following.

- T-shirt: "ACHE member - Ali's Cardio Health & Exercise"
- Ribbon: "1-Year ACHE Member"
- Commemorative certificate: "ACHE - Official Member"

Ultimately, a pat-on-the-back and smile from you is often enough to recognize consistent efforts.

The Novice/Beginner Participant (Type C)

A majority of exercise classes are on-going, meaning people have attended for varying amounts of time. It can be intimidating for an inactive person to go to a class where everyone seems to know what to do. When people make the choice to try your class, it is important to put yourself in their shoes. Remember what it is like to be a beginner. An empathetic attitude and genuine desire for them to have a successful experience is really what a novice participant wants from an instructor.

Action Plan

New participants need to feel welcomed, accepted, and most of all, they need to feel comfortable. Courtesy, sensitivity, and appropriate guidance are required to make a person comfortable in class. Techniques to facilitate this include the following.

1. **An Enthusiastic, Warm Welcome**

   Introduce yourself. Thank the person for joining your class today.

2. **Take Interest**

   Make sure the individual has been properly screened prior to exercise. Refer "at risk" persons to their physician for clearance. Do a brief verbal screening before class. Three questions to ask:

   a. "Have you been working out?" If yes, ask about their program (to determine fitness experience).

   b. "Do you have any knee problems, back problems, anything like that I should know about?"

   c. "When was the last time you had a medical check-up?" Continue with:
      - "How is your heart?"
      - "How is your blood pressure?"
      - Are you taking any medications that might affect exercise?"

3. **Appropriate Guidance**

   Provide specific guidance based upon the response you receive to the above questions. "Take it easy, listen to your body, and work at your own level" is general not specific guidance, it is somewhat nebulous, and it is by and large forgotten once the class begins. Depending on the information you have obtained, specific guidance might be, "Thank-you for the information. In today's class, I'm going to suggest what you should do, what not to do, when to slow down or speed up, what level to work at, when to stop and just watch and when to join in again, because I want to make sure you can walk tomorrow. I don't want you to be too sore or uncomfortable. If anything starts to hurt you, stop doing it. Pain is your body's signal something is wrong. The workout is for you, so do what feels right to you. It might take a few workouts to figure out what's going on. If you get lost or become unsure of anything—no problem. Just observe. As we go along, I'll monitor you often by asking, "How does this feel?" Okay? Nice to have you with us today."

4. **Clear Expectations**

   Describe the workout and what to expect. No one should be in the dark.

5. **Observe and Assist**

   Before the class begins, inform new participants that you may suggest alternative movements when you believe it is in their best interest. This sets the stage for any modifications you give and you reduce the likelihood they will feel singled out or are intimidated. Scan your room constantly and when needed, you can confidently provide modifications knowing you prepared individuals in advanced for it.

6. **Use Terminology to Support Your Efforts**

   When giving modifications or variations, the "beginner" label is not well-accepted by all. Eliminate implications inherent with "beginner, intermediate, advanced" by using terms like "Level 1, 2, 3" or "Option A, B, C" (Vogel, 2009).

7. **Everyone Marches to a Different Drummer**

   If exercise is paced to music, expect some participants to be rhythmically-challenged. Moving to a beat is hard for certain individuals. With having to listen, watch, process, and follow you, some people will not hear the rhythm or beat. Matching the music cadence should not be a priority and emphasizing it creates unneeded stress. Use the music's energy and tempo, but understand some people will move at their own pace. Cycling, circuit, boot camp, and water exercise are workouts where movements may not be synchronized to music.

8. **De-emphasize Transitions**

   Changing movements when you cue to change is far less critical for novice exercisers than it is for experienced participants. Cue for all transitions, but when a person does not change at the right time, let it be. The fact that a person is moving at all is more important than whether he or she transitions with the rest of the class. Allow beginners to be beginners!

9. **Corrections**

   If a participant is exercising improperly so as to risk acute injury, you need to give a correction. If a person's technique or form is not injurious but could be improved to enhance the effectiveness of an exercise, it is optional rather than mandatory to give the correction. Too many corrections can lead to "information overload." The result is frequently a poorer, not better performance and more anxious participants (Price, 2002). Save corrections for when they are most needed rather than every time you see an opportunity for improvement. Always follow any correction or modification you give with a compliment or acknowledgement. This reinforces the appropriate technique and leaves participants feeling positive about themselves (Wagman, 1997).

10. **Practice What You Preach**

    Offer modifications whenever possible for new individuals. Then, continue performing the modification yourself. By doing so, you make it "okay" to work at a lower intensity/complexity level. This is important, as novices often attempt the hardest level of an exercise even if it is inappropriate for them (Vogel, 2009). They tend to emulate you—you are the role model. If you exercise intensely, they want to do the same. Avoid confusing messages where you say it is fine to "take it easy" while you continue doing advanced or intense movements.

11. **Position for Success**

    Place new participants where they can easily hear and see you. This is essential to be able to follow you. Positioning them together is also beneficial. They can work at the same relative fitness level as a group, rather than individually scattered around the room "sticking out" from the majority. Additionally, it is easier for you to give instructions when they are together rather than randomly positioned in your room.

12. **Think Positive**

    The times new participants most need positive feedback are as follows.

    a. Upon a well-executed task or effort
    b. After you give a correction, modification, or assistance
    c. Immediately post-workout

    Frequently, novices judge their performance based upon unrealistic expectations. Some people think they should have mastered the program in the first class. When those expectations are not realized, discouragement sets in and increases the likelihood of dropping out. Acknowledge their problems or concerns, and respond to any negative self-statements in a positive tone. For example:

    • Comment: "I'm so inflexible. I couldn't even touch my toes."

Response: "Not a problem. I did not expect you to touch your toes. It takes a while before you can do that."

- Comment: "I was mixed-up and couldn't figure out what you were doing."
  Response: "I understand how you feel. Just march-in-place and observe any difficult movements a few times—you'll learn it much faster that way."

- Comment: "I couldn't keep up; I had to stop."
  Response: "That is a prerequisite for taking this class—if you could do it all, you would be teaching it! Seriously, each week you will be able to do a bit more as your cardiovascular fitness improves."

Discuss and determine realistic goals, and give copious amounts of positive feedback when a person is first beginning a program.

13. **Report Cards**

Design a monthly report card for newer participants similar to school report cards that a parent or guardian had to sign. Subject areas might be cardiovascular training, flexibility, strength, and attitude. For a fun twist, request a child's (or spouse/friend) signature before returning the card to you. Though novel, around the seventh month when you no longer give it out, participants ask, "Where's my report card?"

14. **Vary it Slowly**

Make sure participants feel successful in an existing exercise before you vary it (Larkin, 2008). Variety is an important element of instruction for Type A and B. Too much variety for Type C leads to frustration as people never feel confident with the exercise, routine, or program.

15. **As a Fitness Professional**

Your enthusiasm for your participants' progress and desire to see them excel is often stronger than a person's ability to perform a movement correctly or successfully complete a set of exercises. There is an inference that a beginner level is less prestigious than an advanced level. Perhaps unconsciously, we do everything possible to move them up to an intermediate level quickly, as if there is something wrong with being a beginner. Beginners need to be made to feel "okay" and that they are one of the "good guys" just like more experienced and fit participants. Beginners should be celebrated even more so than advanced exercisers. It takes courage, determination, and discipline to join an exercise class. If they have the fortitude to do that, think of what you can do to turn them into regular participants. Their first experience in your class is critical. They are either turned on or turned off to exercise, and if it is the latter, you may not have a second chance. Most of the attention, the accolades, and the glory is bestowed upon the Type A, the physically elite, and the top athletes, deservingly so—they have earned it. Yet, it is Type C who is the real hero. Be there for them.

Follow-Up

Post-workout follow-up is essential for encouraging adherence until exercise becomes intrinsically rewarding. Be interested in the outcome and response of new participants (Damush et al., 2005). Participants receiving follow-up calls adhere better to health behavior changes. After a person has taken your class, find out how he or she feels about the program. It takes less than a minute to

---

Teaching Tip

Generally, participants create horizontal levels in a class, with advanced participants in front, intermediates behind them, and beginners in the back of the room. Instead, divide your class into vertical sections by placing advanced participants on the left, intermediates in the center, and beginners on the right. People feed off the energy of other people. High-intensity exercisers like to be next to others working at their level. Lower-intensity exercisers prefer to be near others working at their level. Positioning new participants together so they can see and hear helps ensure they have a positive exercise experience. It makes your job easier, too. You give instructions to new exercisers together in a group instead of scattered around the room.

contact the participant to ensure he or she is not too sore from the workout. People appreciate the personal follow-up. It makes them feel special that you cared enough to contact them. Your interest in the well-being of everyone who takes your class influences participant adherence. Fitness professionals are incredibly important providers of emotional support, particularly for female exercisers (Kravitz, 2009).

Reward the Process

Three tips to promote adherence are as follows.

- Document and track participation.
- Perform periodic fitness assessments to determine program effectiveness and to update fitness goals.
- Recognize behavioral changes as well as fitness improvements.

It is important to acknowledge healthy behaviors to counter any disappointment when new exercisers have not met their goals like "losing 10 pounds in 2 weeks." People will drop out because results do not come quickly enough. It can take months to obtain significant, measurable changes in various fitness parameters. Since we lose about 50% of exercisers within 6 months into a program, it makes sense to give them positive feedback in every workout. Positive reinforcement is critical through the cognitive phase when exercise may not be so enjoyable or rewarding (Hoffman and Jones, 2002).

Everybody Else! (Type D)

The majority of people in our communities can exercise, but for one reason or another, choose not to be physically active. Interestingly, studies do not show any relationship between physical activity and other health or change behaviors (Dishman, 1988). For example, educational campaigns have been effective in changing people's diet and smoking habits, but they have had no effect on exercise and physical activity habits. Data from surveys (both inactive and active populations) that ask, "Why not more exercise?" also suggest lack of time, willpower, and apathy.

Non-exercisers also wonder how well they would fit into a structured fitness program. Some classes have a strong "age" association; where people believe only a certain age group will fit in. For example, water fitness and tai chi are for older people, or kickboxing and indoor cycling are for younger people. Some activities require minimal coordination such as walking, while other activities demand substantial coordination like dance-based exercise. Age, skill, coordination, and/or a sense of belonging can be barriers to exercise.

	ACTIVE	INACTIVE
No time	51%	42%
No willpower	14%	18%
Don't feel like it	7%	13%

The Future: Tackling Barriers to Exercise

Exercise requires much more time and energy than other health-related activities. Some sectors of the health club industry promote the appearance benefits of exercise as a reason to get physically active. The medical community promotes the physiological benefits of exercise. The wellness community promotes the psychological, spiritual, and mental benefits from exercise (Sonstoem, 1984). Instructors need to understand all of these benefits and then step out of the box to help individuals understand how exercise will benefit them.

Make an effort to reach out to people even when they are not attending your program. If a person tells you she does not have time for exercise, be empathetic. Although you could hint she develop better time management skills, a better response is showing her how to incorporate more activity into her day, for example, using stairs instead of escalators, stretching during television commercials, or walking an extra block to increase energy expenditure. When she is ready for more formal exercise, the advice you provided paves the way for her to return to you.

Three-minute stretch breaks at worksite locations offer a convenient opportunity to exercise. At only 3 minutes duration, most anyone could do it successfully. Perform it a few times a day; you would accumulate about 10 minutes of activity—a great beginning for inactive individuals. Think of the number of people who could participate in a 3-minute exercise break who would not consider a full hour class.

Shorter workouts attract those stressed for time. Thirty-minute classes back-to-back appeal to more people than one 60-minute class, offering consumers two choices instead of one longer option. Thirty minutes is becoming the most popular class length as it better fits the schedule of today's consumers (Lofshult, 2002). Just as important are the psychological aspects. More people are capable of exercising for 30 minutes compared to 60 minutes. It is better to have a person leave a 30-minute class thinking, "I did it all!" compared to leaving a 60-minute class thinking, "This was way too much for me." Also keep in mind the intensity factor. As intensity increases, so does the drop-out rate. The picture is clear—shorter, less intense exercise attracts more people.

To catch the attention of men, focus on muscle strength and endurance using resistant equipment. Strength training is attractive and less threatening for men than a choreographic-driven workout. If your objective is a well-rounded fitness class, gradually add cardiovascular and flexibility training, but only after they have experienced success through strength-oriented programming. When ready to introduce aerobic training, 32-count combination choreography is generally not as popular with men as sports and athletic drills or martial arts-based movements.

For older populations, music can mean success or calamity. It appears the songs you enjoyed in your formative years are the songs that become life-long favorites. If you liked Benny Goodman and Duke Ellington as you were growing up, it will be a favorite for senior exercise. Were Frank Sinatra and Ella Fitzgerald on the airwaves in your teenage years? You will like working out to them, too. If you grew up in the 1950s and 1960s, Elvis, the Beatles, and Aretha Franklin are on your hit list. Did you grow up to Madonna or Rhianna? Hold onto those CDs; it will be your senior music a few decades from now.

Perhaps more than any other age group, older adults benefit from group cohesion and the socialization that evolves in an exercise class. People have a need for affiliation. This need is one of life's great motivators and can be met in a class. We are social beings who thrive on acceptance, approval, and appreciation. Meeting people with similar interests is a strong bond and belonging to that group can add significant self-esteem to our lives. Once a feeling of acceptance has been established, we are willing to take risks and challenge our comfort zone. We need to feel secure to do this, and a great exercise instructor can make this possible by mingling with participants and showing true empathy and concern. This behavior is contagious, and serves to unify the group and create a class that, through affiliation, is self-stimulating and self-motivating. Both functional and psychological improvements can occur as a result of being engaged in group exercise classes (Grant et al., 2004).

If possible, keep chairs nearby. If someone is unable to stand for an extended period, many exercises can be modified to seated positions. Inactive people feel more comfortable and confident knowing they can sit if necessary, and chairs add a measure of safety for those with balance problems. Individualize routines and exercises. You can say, for example, "There are 18 people in class today. It is perfectly fine to see 18 different variations of this movement." Fit the difficulty level of the class to the ability of the participants. Be willing to create and adjust as the needs change within your class.

In the United States, teenagers often have a rebellious spirit. They do not necessarily want to do the same workout that their parents do. To target adolescents, you need to get on their level. Use the music they like, even if you do not care for it. Have them create or show you a dance move, and make it a part of the workout. Have participants pair up or form small groups; let them select a song, and have them design an exercise routine for it. When ready, have them lead the others in their routine. It is an effective way to raise enthusiasm and motivation, and watch how supportive they become of each other. The class should feel less like exercise and more like a good-time party—something they usually find more engaging than formal exercise.

Contemporary Christian music is an antidote for those who find some Top 40 music explicit or offensive. An oldies-but-goodies workout or a cardio-swing class could attract people who prefer those music styles. Latin music will appeal to those inspired by its distinct, energetic rhythms.

Be tuned in to potential participants. Step workouts with user-friendly choreography are the ticket for those who tried step training, and quietly exited confused and dumbfounded. They reached their target training zone; unfortunately it was likely from the stress of trying to figure out the combinations rather than from actually working out. Outdoor workouts utilize the local environment and surroundings in creative, fun ways. You can start in the exercise room, move outdoors, and return to your room to end class back in a controlled environment. Participants welcome an opportunity to exercise in beautiful weather.

Find out what a person is passionate about. Inquire about what gives a person great pride and satisfaction. What elicits a smile from their face and brings a twinkle to their eye? Exercise should leave you with that seem feeling of pride and satisfaction. If it does not, you haven't had the right exercise experience. It may take time to modify the exercise program so that it is the right fit for an individual.

Taking the Right Approach

No matter what population you are trying to reach, behavior-oriented interventions appear to be more effective for increasing physical activity levels than cognitive approaches (attempting to change knowledge, beliefs, or attitudes). Just telling people that exercise is good and it will improve health will rarely motivate anyone to action (Conn, 2008). What works is providing individuals with simple, action-oriented strategies to increase their activity level. For example, tracking exercise over time through a log or diary increases awareness and provides motivation for improvement. Wearing a pedometer is a way to track activity, and can provide a lot of inspiration to become more active. Recommend that people schedule exercise in their appointment books. Just by putting it down in writing makes people commit to the behavior. Prompt them to set their workout clothes and shoes out the night before. Ask how they can reward themselves if they accomplish the goal. People may feel overwhelmed by the thought of exercise and think they have to work out for 60 minutes at a time. Give people the license to start. Start with 5 minutes. That will provide a sense of accomplishment which is crucial when implementing a new behavior. They have the rest of their lives to work up to 60 minutes of exercise!

Teaching Style

No matter what type of exercise you teach, there are three basic styles of instruction, and each one affects participants differently. The command style gives the instructor full responsibility for everything from music to choreography to room temperature. He or she comes with a single game plan and follows it through, no matter what. This is a common, entry-level teaching style. The class may feel comfortable in the instructor's hands, but there seems to be a lack of spontaneity and individual attention because the instructor actually distances himself or herself from the class. It becomes "the instructor" and "the participants," with no real empathy for what each person is going through. New instructors use this style because they need to make it through the class without distraction. As a new instructor, you may have some anxiousness teaching your first classes. You hardly can pay attention to anyone because you are thinking about what you are going to do next. You are deciding how to cue the next movement and when to end the current exercise. You are determining if you are on the right beat and count. In essence, you want to complete the class without making any major errors.

Your confidence grows with practice and experience. Each class becomes easier to teach. As your instruction improves, your personality begins to come through. Teaching becomes less nerve-wracking and your self-assurance takes off. Eventually, teaching class will feel second nature to you. This allows you to pay more attention to the class. As you become more comfortable in your teacher mode, you become more comfortable interacting with participants. Interpersonal interaction is what teaching is really all about. Without it, an exercise class would not be much different than working out to a DVD.

The submissive style of teaching has no real game plan or has vague class goals. There is a lack of organization. The instructor decides to wing it and everyone can just follow along. You are never sure if even the instructor knows what is coming up next. This leaves the class feeling tentative, insecure, and unmotivated. Once a person has lost faith and trust in the instructor, it is only a matter of time before he or she drops out. An unprepared instructor is an unprofessional instructor, and is his or her own worst enemy. An awesome physique, great looks, impressive athleticism or dance skills do not overcome an unprofessional approach to teaching.

The cooperative style combines the best of all worlds: it is organized yet not totally authoritarian. The instructor is creative, open to changes and suggestions, and involved in the flow of the class. He or she "sees" the needs of the class unfolding. The participant feels a sense of belonging in this atmosphere, and has confidence the instructor is competent and will keep an eye out on everyone. The goal of good teaching is to encourage independence and self-growth. We want participants to incorporate what we teach them into their lives. We aspire to be real change agents who believe that our participants are more important than the workout. Helping people develop healthy lifestyles is a long-term objective, and this can be done through subtle teaching skills, discussed later in the chapter. The underlying message is that you, the instructor, care for them as human beings, and accept and trust them. This climate will allow growth to occur. Remember that each person in your class comes to you with his or her own agenda, and your job is to acknowledge all your participants the way they are, thus creating an opportunity for them to change in an atmosphere of unconditional acceptance.

Teaching Philosophy: Motivation

Motivation is a set of reasons that prompts a person to engage in a specific behavior (Weinberg, 2008). What can you do to help people develop motivation for exercise? Start by determining your teaching philosophy. A philosophy consists of beliefs or principles that serve as guides to action. These principles help you address participant concerns, problems, or difficulties; however, a philosophy is of little use unless you own it and practice it. Consider the following.

- What is your philosophy of teaching and how is it incorporated into your classes?
- Do participants come first?
- What is your role in their fitness development?
- Are you an educator, motivator, and communicator in the area of health and fitness, keeping up with and developing your skills, strategies, and techniques?
- Are you interested more in your own fitness and advancement than your classes?

A teaching philosophy should be centered on the participant. They must come first. You are not only a teacher, but also a guide and coach. It is more than just follow-the-leader. You educate people about how exercise can make them feel and function better, and how to care for their bodies. This teaching format is both physical and intellectual, and encourages participants to consciously take control and ownership of their fitness and health. Credibility and accountability are what people are seeking today. You must be willing to grow, learn, and share insights with your class. Knowledge is power—when you know how to use it.

A teaching philosophy should also center on motivation. The best motivation comes from within, or intrinsically. When individuals first begin to exercise, they may not feel good after working out due to any number of reasons; over-exertion, under-exertion, too challenging, too easy, and so forth. Intrinsic motivation is created, develops, and emerges when you begin to feel better after a workout compared to how you felt before a workout. When you experience exercise that makes you feel better, you begin to look forward to your workout. The workout itself becomes enjoyable. It is internally, or intrinsically, rewarding (Wankel et al., 1985). An important element of "enjoyable" is fun; are you able to bring a sense of fun and playfulness to exercise? Or has the workout become just that—work.

Intrinsically motivated people are pursuing the "pleasure principle" and have discovered the joy of movement. They strive to be competent. They take pleasure in feeling successful after mastering a task. These people (many are Type A and B) work hard and are an instructor's dream. In order to reinforce this type of motivation, share your enthusiasm for fitness and provide involvement for everyone. Educate your class about the processes taking place during exercise, since the more understanding you have about why you are doing something, your desire to continue is increased. Socializing is a great intrinsic motivator.

People like to exercise in a group because they derive a nurturing satisfaction and a feeling of belonging from interacting with others in class (Kennedy-Armbruster & Yoke, 2009). The friendships that develop and the support we get from new "exercise friends" provide a wonderful form of inspiration and acceptance. Create a warm and supportive environment, reward personal achievements (e.g., attendance, goals), emphasize moderation and variety, and acknowledge healthy behaviors and efforts. You can further enhance a feeling of well-being with a smile, a gentle touch, and by having a genuine interest in each participant.

Another way to reach participants is through direct motivation. This occurs when you appeal to a person's pride in the hope that he or she will work harder and more consistently to obtain the results wanted. Providing positive comments, praise, and suggestions helps to accomplish this. Establishing progressive goals keeps people on track. Keep asking them, "What is your fitness goal now?" and make them accountable for the answers. Know the values of your participants and respect them. People will respond to a caring, competent instructor who makes the effort to know each individual in the group.

People who adhere to an exercise program usually have a strong internal locus of control, knowing they are responsible for their lives and the choices they make. Skill-oriented individuals are drawn to new steps and choreography. Socially motivated people come for the interpersonal connections, and end-result participants just want to shape up. People are there for many reasons, so you want to keep all possibilities open for everyone.

True motivation comes from meeting your participants' needs, and addressing this issue adds an important dimension to any philosophy of teaching. People attempt to satisfy their needs according to a system of priorities (Maslow, 1962). These needs can be divided into two categories: (a) deficiency needs, such as hunger, thirst, safety, and security, and (b) growth needs, such as love, self-esteem, and self-actualization. Deficiency needs have the highest priority. According to Maslow, once a need is met or satisfied, it is no longer a need and that person can move up the hierarchy to the next one.

Following Maslow's theory, it would be interesting to put each participant into their respective needs category. Exercise enthusiasts are usually exercising for fun, which meets their need for stimulation and excitement. They also want to be with people to satisfy social needs. And finally, they want to demonstrate competence and feel worthy.

Since people have a basic need for stimulation, they seek an optimum level of arousal. An ideal state of arousal is called "flow," in which you are totally absorbed in your activity, feeling very much in control and the experience is pleasurable. There is also an endorphin release in flow state that enhances an exerciser's sense of well-being. As an instructor, it is very much within your control to set up a stimulating and energizing class. The exercise floor brings people together from varied backgrounds and experiences working for a common goal—to improve one's health and fitness. By the end of class, they also find they can manage stress better, mood and attitude have improved, and they feel better about themselves. The magic of the exercise floor is that it reduces and elevates everyone to the same level—a common denominator that becomes a special place, an almost sacred space, for physical, mental, and spiritual growth.

Make the workout floor a special place and people will be drawn to it. Here is a recipe for creating a special place, for setting up a motivating, stimulating, energizing environment, and for getting your class into a flow state. While many of the ingredients are common sense, make sure they become common practice.

Pre-Class Procedures

1. **Arrive early.**
   This allows time to organize equipment, prepare the workout room (e.g., temperature, ventilation, lighting, etc.) and screen new participants. It is the prime opportunity for talking, interacting, and building rapport with participants.

2. **Be prepared.**
   Have your music ready. Have back-up music in case your first source does not work. As a fitness professional, dress one level up from the general demeanor of participants. Keep a towel handy and be aware of personal hygiene. Have water ready and drink during class—it is good for your voice and to role model hydration. Keep candy or another source of sugar nearby (for people experiencing low blood sugar). Be familiar with building exits and emergency procedures. Keep a first-aid kit and phone nearby.

3. **Meet and greet.**
   Welcome each participant as they enter your room—a key reason for arriving early. People like to be recognized. You want to say hello to them before they say hello to you.

4. **Who are they?**
   Learn at least one name per class until you learn all names. Knowing someone's name makes it easier for you to converse with the individual, and it makes her or him feel important.

5. **Make new participants your priority.**
   Perform a brief verbal screening with a new participant even when a written exercise/health questionnaire has been completed. It shows you are truly interested in him or her. Give appropriate guidance based upon the information you obtain.

Ready to Begin

1. **Introduce yourself.**
   If you think some people may not know your name, introduce yourself to the class ("My name is Chris for those I haven't met").

2. **Position to please.**
   Adjust positions so it is comfortable for everyone. Participants tend to stand close together. Spread them out when crowded so no one will hit or bump into another person. In small classes, people tend to distance themselves from you. Bring them closer toward you so you may appropriately instruct for the group size. Otherwise, you have to project like the room was filled to capacity, and that feels awkward if it is only partially filled.

3. **New participants arriving late.**
   Obtain the bottom-line exercise information about those who arrive late. A fitness professional would not let a new person exercise in class without knowing if he or she has been physically active. It is too late to wait until after class to find out this information.

4. **Express gratitude.**
   Find a way to say, "Thank-you for being here" at the beginning of the class. Making the effort and showing up deserves an acknowledgement.

5. **Qualify your re-asking of names.**

   If there are participants whose names you have forgotten, you can ask repeatedly when you qualify yourself… "What's your name again? It takes me a while to remember, please don't mind if I ask you a few more times."

Class Strategies

1. **Size it up.**

   There is safety in numbers. The more people in your class, the more comfortable they are to respond to your questions, cheers, and prompts. It makes a big class fun to teach. Small classes are fun to teach as well, when you take advantage of the class size. Break in a new combination or routine in a small class. It is better to find the problems in it with a small group rather than a roomful of people. Try out a new choreographic style or new music. Individually assist people you don't normally have an opportunity to help. There may be enough space to do exercises utilizing the wall. Try out partner exercises. Most of all, by the end of class know everyone's name, know what other workouts they do besides yours, and find out who is a native of the area if you do not already know this information. Participants should feel like they had a semi-personal training session with you by the end of class. It is how a small class becomes a bigger class.

2. **Maintain eye contact.**

   Scan the room constantly. You will know if you are maintaining eye contact by watching a videotape of yourself teaching a class. Play it back without sound. Are you looking at your leg or looking at their legs during leg exercises? It is second-guessing motivation and assistance if you do not know what is actually going on in your class.

3. **Stay real.**

   An easy way to do this is to ask at least one non-fitness related question during the class, such as, "What did you think of yesterday's weather?" This shows you are still a person, not just "the exercise expert." People enjoy periodic non-exercise related conversation. It helps them connect to you and builds rapport.

4. **Ask open-ended questions.**

   If you ask your class a question and nobody responds, it is because everyone thinks someone else will answer so they keep quiet. You also could have asked a close-ended question, meaning people can respond with a nod of the head—they don't have to say anything. Ask questions that require more than a "yes" or "no" answer. This creates a dialogue. If you have done all the talking, it is a monologue. Teaching is communication. Communication is a two-way exchange—a dialogue—not a monologue. Example: instead of "Did you have a good week-end?" ask, "What did you do this weekend?" Listen to an audio recording of yourself teaching class. If participants have said nothing other than "yes," "no," or let out a whoop or a groan, you asked close-ended questions resulting in a monologue.

5. **Talk to everybody.**

   Have at least one verbal communication with each person in every class. It could be hello, goodbye, a correction, or a compliment. What matters most is by the end of class, everyone can say to him/herself, "The instructor talked to me today." Avoid talking to just your favorite participants. Everyone deserves your attention. Treat everybody like a somebody.

6. **Be interested.**

Discover something new about a participant in each session. Examples: "Melissa, I've never asked if this exercise bothers your knees"; "Tom, are you from here originally?" This shows interest in your participants as people. It is invaluable in making everyone feel important.

7. **Change your position.**

Those standing in back of you see you differently than those standing sideways to you. Changing which direction you face allows everyone to see you from different perspectives when looking at you for visual cues. If you have a platform or stage, use it for visibility when the number of people warrants its use. Otherwise, you want to be on the floor with participants as much as possible. Being elevated on a platform can be somewhat distancing. Among the top complaints revealed in a magazine poll on health clubs was: "Instructors who look at themselves in the mirror instead of the students." You need to be able to face your participants often, whether or not there are mirrors in the room. When you face the class, you must mirror them. This means you cue the opposite direction or opposite limb of what you are doing. For example, if you say, "Grapevine right" while facing participants, perform your grapevine to your left to move in the same direction as the class. Practice mirroring, as it is an essential skill for a smooth-flowing class and it is frequently a source of cueing errors. Position yourself in the center of the room for supine and prone exercises (e.g., push-ups, crunches). More people can see you in the center of the room than when you are at the front. Be at, or return to, the front of the room for front-facing exercises.

8. **Walk the talk.**

It is good to move about the room, but have a reason to do so. Moving around nebulously or with a blank face does not accomplish much. It can in fact, make participants anxious because they know you form an opinion about their performance. Be sensitive to this. Participants become uncomfortable wondering what you are thinking. Diffuse any anxiety by communicating verbally or non-verbally to each person you pass. You cannot assume they can read your mind.

9. **Talk the walk.**

Be willing, able, and comfortable to cue exercise sequences without physically performing them. Great teachers are able to have their class execute exercises by delivering clear, concise, and properly timed cues. Make an audio recording of your class. Determine if someone could follow your program from your instructions. The best teachers, coaches, and trainers do not do everything they ask of their athletes. Their job is to bring out the best in people they work with. This is your job, too. Adept verbal skills offer precise directions to successfully perform an exercise task. One major benefit: you can teach more classes without over-taxing yourself.

10. **Choose your words carefully.**

You disempowered your messages when you use "we," "us," "our," "let's," and "those." For more effective communication, use "I," "my," "you," and "your." Example: replace, "Let's feel those core muscles work" with, "I want you to feel your core muscles work."

11. **Teach positively.**

    Ask for what you want, rather than what you do not want. Each time you say "don't," someone might perceive it as if he or she is doing something wrong. Eliminate the word "don't" and replace it with any of the following: "avoid," "rather than," "are you," "be aware of," "I want you to," "I'd like you to," or "please think about." You will get your message across and maintain a positive class environment.

12. **Accentuate the positive.**

    Catch people doing things right. Be sincere as people can read artificial compliments.

13. **Smile.**

14. **Smile more.**

    Especially during aerobic activity. Review a videotape of yourself teaching a class. Notice your expression; will it say, "She is having a great time. She loves what she does."? While there are appropriate times for a serious tone, you can usually lighten up during cardiovascular training.

15. **Avoid asking for smiles.**

    It rarely improves the mood of a group. If you have to ask participants to smile, you haven't given them anything to smile about. Establish an upbeat atmosphere through interpersonal interaction with participants. Then you can avoid having to say, "Come on, smile—let's have fun!" It should already be enjoyable. They should already be having fun.

16. **Are we having fun yet?**

    A noble goal is to have each participant smile at least once during class. You enhance adherence when your class is safe, effective, fun, and enjoyable. You do not have to be a comedian to make people smile. Share a human-interest story, or something about yourself.

17. **Give thanks.**

    At the end of class, thank people for their attendance. It is personal, polite, and professional.

18. **Follow-up.**

    Communicate (by phone, fax, email, or text) to individuals who leave class early. People appreciate receiving a message from you. Example: "You left early. I wanted to tell you that your endurance has improved substantially. See you Monday, and have a great weekend."

Post-Workout Procedures

1. **Single them out.**

    Be available after class to answer questions and make people feel as if they truly count. Listening skills are probably one of teaching's greatest motivators. How you attend to participants will determine whether or not they feel good and come back to your class. Give individual positive feedback to as many people as you can. Individual compliments are more effective than group compliments.

2. **Return engagement.**

    As participants leave, ask when they will be returning. It creates an informal commitment to return, and can improve adherence. When debating on attending your class, a participant will remember what he or she said to you.

3. **Leave participants on the high note.**

   It is always nice when participants think highly of you as a fitness professional. When you receive a compliment, you can amiably accept it. Then, respond with a positive statement about the participant. As an example, if someone says she really enjoys your class, let her know you really enjoy having her in class.

4. **Re-order.**

   Consider building variety into a class by changing the exercise order. For example, if on Monday you performed core exercises followed by lower body exercises, reverse the order on Wednesday. The simple change in order can spike up new enthusiasm and energy.

5. **Group cohesion.**

   People gravitate to group fitness because it is a group of people exercising together rather than working out by oneself. Group cohesion is developed before and after class through interaction with participants (Vrazel et al., 2008). It is nurtured during the workout, and participants give signals when they need interaction if you know what to look for. When participants begin talking during class, it is a signal they want to talk and connect to each other. Although you may feel it is discourteous or disruptive, it is really an indication there has not been an opportunity in class to interact with others. This is the time for you to be creative and flexible. Go with it instead of against it. You can allow opportunities to talk without it being disruptive to others. Insert a sequence where participants do not have to look at you in order to do the task. Walking or running in a big circle, spontaneous circuit stations around the room, or partner exercises are examples where people can talk and exercise simultaneously. An instructor who can allow interaction amongst participants while maintaining control of the class is an instructor who becomes very popular. Being able to connect to other people builds group camaraderie which reaps many social, emotional, and psychological health benefits.

6. **Educate.**

   Provide at least one piece of health/fitness news or information in every class. It could be anything from technique to tai-chi to healthy teas. Some instructors find participants will come by just for the "tip of the day."
   There are participants who exercise to look better, yet remind your class that exercise makes you feel and function better. Eventually, that becomes as important as or more important than appearance.

7. **Be a student.**

   Participants like to see instructors taking a class. Periodically, attend a class your participants may go to. You get new ideas and become familiar with another instructor's teaching style and format, which is invaluable for substituting in the future. Offer to give the instructor constructive feedback and ask the same of him or her. Consider who is a good match for you as a team-teacher, and eventually provide participants with a special team-taught class. Team-teaching can be quite fun for everyone, including you.

8. **Provide balanced feedback.**

   Always follow any correction or assistance you give with a compliment or positive feedback. No matter how kindly you assist or help an individual, a person may interpret the correction in a negative way, like he or she is incapable of following directions or is inept. A positive statement balances your feedback.

9.   **Solicit ideas.**
Cooperatively evolve your class, and ask for suggestions to involve participants in the workout. People like to share and contribute ideas and they take a more vested interest in the workout when you use one of their suggestions (e.g., music, exercise, equipment, etc.)

10. **Keep a positive attitude.**
It always starts with you. You can look at teaching as either a job or an opportunity. You have to leave any personal baggage at the door because for the next hour, it is not about you. It is not about your body, your fitness level, nor your athletic abilities. It's about them—the individuals who have entrusted you with their bodies. It's about making them feel better about themselves which in turn, makes them feel better about the world around them. On a 1-10 scale, if someone was a "2" at the beginning of class, by the end of class the number is a "5." If "6" is the walk-in rating, you have moved it to "9" upon departure. It does not take weeks or months to derive benefits. Every class is a chance to make an immediate impact. It's about transforming people's attitude about physical activity—the right exercise will make you feel better than you were. What a wonderful opportunity, indeed.

Summary

We can conclude that a physically active lifestyle is opposite of a sedentary lifestyle. There is no doubt people avoid exercise. Exercise is often challenged by competing activities, whether it is work, family, the Internet, or it may be unrealistic goals or previous negative experiences. In a society that expects instant gratification, benefits of exercise take too long, resulting in an overly ambitious attempt to make up for years of inactivity in 1 week. The soreness alone is enough to discourage regular participation. Sedentary people may simply have a fear of failure. Nobody wants to participate in something at which they fail. People want to do things they are successful at doing. This, then, is your challenge—to instruct, coach, motivate, educate, and lead exercise sessions that give people built-in opportunities for success rather than failure.

The choice of an appropriate teaching style coupled with finely-tuned communication skills can make becoming a true motivator possible. Once you have developed an inspirational teaching philosophy, what remains is the task of getting your message across in an efficient, professional, positive, and caring manner. Motivation comes from within and is transmitted to others. It is actually the transfer of energy from one person to the next, and you, as instructor, are the vehicle facilitating this transfer. Great teaching is about empowering others to set goals and take risks, and then guiding them in their efforts. A true sign of teaching success is a philosophy of selflessness: "I am here for you physically, mentally, and spiritually. I unconditionally accept your presence in class. Please watch me, listen to me, and follow my actions. Let's hold hands and walk the path together." Teach exercise classes that not only benefit already active individuals, but also seduce, entice, and meet the physical, emotional, and spiritual needs of the inactive person, so they too can embrace exercise and its glorious benefits the way you have embraced it.

References

1. Beals, K. (2003). Mirror mirror on the wall, who is the most muscular one of all? *ACSM Health & Fitness Journal* March: 6-11.

2. Benyo, R. (1990). *The exercise fix.* Champaign, IL: Human Kinetics.

3. Brown, P., & O'Neill, M. (1990). A retrospective survey of the incidence and pattern of aerobics related injuries in Victoria. *Australian Journal of Science Medicine and Sport* 22(3): 77–81.

4. Carron, A., Widmeyer, W., & Mack, D. (1996). Social influence and exercise: a meta-analysis. *Journal of Sport and Exercise Psychology,* 18: 1–16.

5. Conn, V. (2008). Behavior strategies motivate people to move. *Patient Education and Counseling,* 70(2), 157; University of Missouri July 23.

6. Damash, T., Perkins, S., Mikesky, A., et al. (2005). Motivational factors influencing older adults diagnosed with knee osteoarthritis to join and maintain an exercise program. *Journal of Aging and Physical Activity,* 13(1): 45–60.

7. de Jong, A. (1999). Motivate participants to focus on long-range goals. *ACSM Health & Fitness Journal,* 3.2: 37–38.

8. Dishman, R. (1988). *Exercise adherence: its impact on public health.* Champaign, IL: Human Kinetics.

9. Dishman, R. (1994). *Advances in exercise adherence.* Champaign, IL: Human Kinetics.

10. Gavin, J., & Gavin, G. (1995). *Psychology for health fitness professionals.* Champaign, IL: Human Kinetics.

11. Gerson, R. (1999). *Members for life.* Champaign, IL: Human Kinetics.

12. Grant, S., Todd, K., Aitchison, N., Kelly, P., & Stodart, D. (2004). The effects of a 12 week group exercise program on physiological and psychological variables and function in overweight women. *Public Health* 118(1): 31–42.

13. Hobart, J., & Smucker, D. (2000). The female athlete triad. *American Family Physician,* June 1. 3357–3366.

14. Hoffman, J., & Jones, K. (2002). Reducing attrition from exercise: practical tips from research. *ACSM Health & Fitness Journal,* (6)2: 7–10.

15. Kennedy-Arnbruster, C., & Yoke, M. (2009). *Methods of Group Exercise Instruction.* Champaign, IL: Human Kinetics.

16. Kravitz, L. (2009). Women's health research update. *IDEA Fitness Journal* May: 26–33.

17. Larkin, M. (2008). Move—surefire ways to motivate and inspire older adults to be active. *The Journal on Active Aging* 7(3): 78–84.

18. Lofshult, D. (2002). Group fitness trend watch. *IDEA Health and Fitness Source,* July: 69–76.

19. Maslow, A.H. (1962). *Toward a Psychology of Being.* New York, NY: Van Nostrand.

20. Mutoh, Y., Sawai, S., Takanashi, Y., & Skurko, L. (1988). Aerobic dance injuries among instructors and students. *Physician and Sports Medicine* 16(12): 81–86.

21. Pate, R.R., Pratt S., Blair, S., Haskell, W., Macera, C., Bouchard, C., Duchner, D., Ettinger, W., Heath, G., & King, A. (1995). Physical activity and public health: A recommendation from the Centers for Disease Control and Prevention and the American College of Sports Medicine. *Journal of the American Medical Association* 273(5): 402–407.

22. Peeke, P. (2007). *Fit to Live.* New York, NY: Rodale.

23. Price, J. (2002). Taking a leap of faith: provide a platform your senior clients can use to confidently spring through exercise anxieties. *IDEA Personal Trainer,* 13: 14–20.

24. Roberts, G. (1992). *Motivation in sport and exercise.* Champaign, IL: Human Kinetics.

25. Smith, D.H., & Theberge, N. (1987). *Why people recreate.* Champaign, IL: Life Enhancement Publications.

26. Sonstoem, R. (1984). Exercise and self-esteem. *Exercise and Sport Sciences Review,* 12: 100–130.

27. U.S. Department of Health and Human Services. (1996). *Physical activity and health: A report of the Surgeon General.* Atlanta, GA: U.S. Department of Health and Human Services, Centers for Disease Control and Prevention, National Center for Chronic Disease Prevention and Health Promotion.

28. Vogel, A. (2009). Get up to speed with group. *IDEA Fitness Journal,* February: 46–53.

29. Vrazel, J., Saunders, R., & Wilcox, S. (2008). An overview and proposed framework of social-environmental influences on physical activity behavior of women. *American Journal of Health Promotion,* 23(1): 2–12.

30. Wagman, D. (1997). Remotivating the motivated. *Strength and Conditioning Journal,* (19) 4: 60–66.

31. Wankel, L. (1985). Personal and situational factors affecting exercise involvement: The importance of enjoyment. *Research Quarterly for Exercise and Sport,* 56: 275–282.

32. Weinberg, R. (2008). Does imagery work? Effects on performance and mental skills. *Journal of Imagery Research in Sport and Physical Activity,* 3(1): 1–21.

33. Wlodkowski, R. (1984). *Enhancing Adult Motivation to Learn.* San Francisco, CA: Jossey-Bass.

20

Monitoring Exercise Intensity

Gregory Welch, MS

Focus

Cardiorespiratory exercise is the method by which we are able to improve our aerobic capacity. Aerobic capacity is the determining factor in sustaining both the duration and intensity of the exercise. Thus, the benefit of training the cardiorespiratory system is to enable more oxygen to be delivered and ultimately consumed by the body, allowing the activity to continue. It is important for the fitness professional to understand and be able to monitor cardiorespiratory exercise in order to determine that it is safe as well as effective in improving aerobic capacity.

The most important application for the fitness professional to monitor cardiorespiratory activity is with submaximal exercise, in the group exercise setting. Maximal exercise monitoring is done primarily in the clinical setting, with an expanded set of objectives, and is not applicable to this writing. Personal fitness trainers must also monitor their client's aerobic work. However, they have the clear advantage of knowledge gained through pre-exercise screening and assessment information. They will utilize the same monitoring protocols yet, unlike group instruction, are able to focus on the specific needs of the individual within a predetermined time frame and a calculated protocol of progression.

There are, however, significant challenges when monitoring the cardiorespiratory response to exercise in a group atmosphere. In any given class, group exercise instructors must deal with a large range of age, number of participants, and varying levels of physical conditioning. Furthermore, they do not have the luxury of pre-exercise screening and classes are likely ongoing so the continuity of progression is virtually non-existent. Therefore, a monitoring protocol must be in place to control the exercise environment for the benefit of the entire class.

Monitoring By Heart Rate

A linear relationship exists between heart rate and oxygen uptake. At the onset of exercise there is an increase in heart rate. As the intensity increases, more oxygen is required causing the heart rate to increase as well. Because of this relationship, heart rate is often considered as an effective monitoring tool for cardiorespiratory exercise. However, to best to use this tool, we must understand how to establish safe parameters of the heart rate as well as the intensity necessary for establishing cardiorespiratory fitness.

Calculating Heart Rate Parameters

In order to establish safe and effective heart rate parameters, it is necessary to first determine the maximum heart rate (HR_{max}). The most accurate way is to directly measure the HR_{max} with an electrocardiogram (EKG) monitoring device during a graded exercise test. Due to the impracticality of this procedure, another method is to estimate HR_{max} by using the prediction equation of "220 - age." This formula was introduced as far back as the 1930s, and has been widely accepted by the health and fitness community. While simple to use, the American College of Sports Medicine (ACSM) recognizes the high degree of variability with this method stating, for example, that it underestimates HR_{max} for both sexes younger than 40 years of age and overestimates HR_{max} for both sexes older than 40 years of age. Therefore, in the 8th edition of ACSM's Guidelines for Exercise Testing and Prescription (2010), the work of Gellish et al. (2007) is offered with the formula $HR_{max} = 206.9 - (0.67 \times age)$ as the most accurate.

Similar to the historical formula for estimating HR_{max}, utilizing the training heart rate range (THRR) has been the benchmark by which fitness professionals have guided their clients and classes to establish the training effect. For many years, ACSM has recommended that healthy adults work within an intensity range of 55–90% of maximum heart rate for developing and maintaining cardiorespiratory fitness. However, the new parameters have been adjusted to 64–94% HR_{max} (ACSM, 2010). THRR is calculated as $HR_{max} \times$ desired low/high percentage. See Table 20-1.

By estimating the maximum heart rate, establishing a training range is simply a matter of manipulating the desired percentage of the estimated maximum heart rate. The following examples in Table 20-1 will first calculate the THRR by the historical formula and then by the Gellish et al. (2007) formula for the benefit of comparison.

Table 20-1.

Example: Determine the training heart rate range of 64–94% for a 55-year-old male.

Historical Formula: Estimated (HR_{max}) = 220 - age
 HR_{max} = 220 - 55 (age) = 165 beats per minute (bpm)
 HR64% = 64% x 165 = 106 bpm
 HR94% = 94% x 165 = 155 bpm
 Training HR range (THRR) = 106–155 bpm

Gellish Formula: Estimated (HRmax) = 206.9 - (0.67 x age)
 HR_{max} = 206.9 - (0.67 x 55) = 170
 HR64% = 64% x 170 = 109 bpm
 HR94% = 94% x 170 = 160 bpm
 Training HR range (THRR) = 109–160 bpm

Another method for calculating the training heart rate range is known as the Karvonen or heart rate reserve method (HRR). This technique factors in resting heart rate, reflects the percentage of the heart rate from rest to maximum, and provides similar intensities as equivalent values of percentages of oxygen uptake reserve (VO_2R). The VO_2R is the range of oxygen consumption (VO_2) from rest to maximum. The ACSM cites the work of Swain and Leutholtz (1997) which determined that HRR and VO_2R reflect the rate of energy expenditure during physical activity more accurately than the other exercise intensity prescription methods.

> **Table 20-2.**
>
> **Example:** Determine the training heart rate range of 40–85% for a 55-year-old male with a resting heart rate of 58 bpm. Both formulas for estimating HR_{max} will be worked.
>
> **The Heart Rate Reserve Method (Karvonen Formula)**
> $(HR_{max} - HR_{rest})$ x % desired low/high intensity + resting HR
> $HR_{max} = 220 - 55 = 165$ bpm
> $HR_{reserve} = 165 - 58 = 107$ bpm
> $HR_{40\% \ HRR} = (40\% \times 107) + 58 = 101$ bpm
> $HR_{85\% \ HRR} = (85\% \times 107) + 58 = 149$ bpm
> Training HR range (THRR) = 101–149 bpm
>
> **The Heart Rate Reserve Method (Gellish Formula for HR_{max})**
> $HR_{max} = 206.9 - (0.67 \times 55) = 170$ bpm
> $HR_{reserve} = 170 - 58 = 112$ bpm
> $HR_{40\% \ HRR} = (40\% \times 112) + 58 = 103$ bpm
> $HR_{85\% \ HRR} = (85\% \times 112) + 58 = 153$ bpm
> Training HR range (THRR) = 103–153 bpm

Heart Rate Monitoring Method

AFAA recommends that the group exercise instructor guide the participants to take a pulse count or rating of perceived exertion (RPE) at three different times during a class.

1. Five minutes after the beginning of aerobic work to determine if the participants are working within their training heart rate range.
2. At the completion of the most intense aerobic work to see if participants have maintained aerobic training level.
3. At the completion of post-aerobic cool-down to determine if participants have sufficiently recovered from aerobic work.

NOTE: If taking HR at these three times is not feasible, then a pulse check or RPE should be taken at the completion of the most intense cardiovascular work rather than not at all. Alternative methods such as the talk test or heart rate monitors may be used.

The instructor should indicate in advance when the pulse or RPE is to be taken. The following steps illustrate AFAA's recommended method of pulse taking.

- Locate the radial artery (AFAA preferred site) pulse within 2 to 4 seconds and find the beat of the heart.
- Begin with the count of "1" and continue counting the beats for 10 seconds.
- Multiply by 6 to determine exercise working heart rate.
- It is important to continue moving the feet while taking the pulse in order to prevent lightheadedness or blood pooling in the extremities (especially individuals who are less fit or who may be taking antihypertension medication).

Heart Rate Monitoring Method

Recovery heart rate reflects the speed at which heart rate returns to pre-exercise level, and is an indicator of whether or not the cool-down period was sufficient. It is also an indicator of improvements in fitness because, as cardiorespiratory fitness improves, the speed at which the heart rate recovers also improves. After 5 minutes, the heart rate should be less than 55% of the estimated HR_{max}.

The Problems of Heart Rate Monitoring

Understandably, a great deal of emphasis is placed on heart rate monitoring. Given their relatively linear relationship to work intensity, heart rate measures are a useful guide to experiencing the training benefits of exercise. There are, however, some drawbacks in acquiring heart rate values that fitness professionals should know so as to keep the limitations in perspective.

As stated previously, ACSM recognizes a "high degree of variability" when estimating the maximum heart rate by the historical formula of 220 - age. Even though a new formula has been introduced to be more accurate, it is still an estimation. Additionally, there is no distinction between men and women in any heart rate formula when it is clearly known that, on average, a female's heart rate is higher than a male's.

With regard to taking heart rates during exercise, the method of palpating heart rates is flawed. The reason for this is because of the time it takes to actually complete the process. For example, after the instructor announces to the class to find a pulse, it takes 5–7 seconds for the entire class to do so, and another 3–5 seconds for the instructor to have everyone begin together. The heart rate began to drop the moment the exercise was reduced to enable the heart rate reading. By the time another 10 seconds is added for the actual reading, the true exercise value of the reading has diminished.

Of course, it should be said that with the advancement of technology, the optimal way to monitor heart rate during exercise is with a wireless telemetry device (heart rate monitor). Only then can a true real time reading be taken with "at-a-glance" convenience. They are very accurate, inexpensive, and mobile, nevertheless, the fact of the matter is that they are rarely seen on a regular basis.

Rating of Perceived Exertion (RPE)

In the early 1950s, Gunnar Borg developed the rating of perceived exertion (RPE) scale to subjectively measure an individual's effort during exercise. The original scale is a 15-point system that begins at 6 and ends at 20. A more recent, simplified scale begins at 0 and progresses to 10 (Table 20-3). The terminology used with the revised scale is believed to be better understood by the participant. When using the 15-point scale, values of 12 to 13 (light to somewhat hard), and 16 (hard) correspond to 50–74% (average of 60%), and 85% of heart rate reserve, respectively (ACSM). The respective values on the 10-point scale are 4–6 and 7–8.

Perceived exertion is simply how hard each exercising individual feels they are actually working. Regardless of the pace of the group, the participants can self-evaluate and adjust the workload specific to how they feel. This serves as a two-fold benefit in that it enables the exercising individual ultimate control over the exercise intensity and reduces the potential liability of the group instructor. The only downside to effectively using the RPE scale is not teaching it properly to the participants. Keeping in mind the teaching nature of the group exercise instructor, however, it is likely to be accomplished if covered as often as palpating heart rates. Additionally, an RPE chart should be visible to the participant in every group exercise room or studio.

The RPE scale is considered a reliable guide as it has a strong linear relationship to heart rate. Although RPE has been considered an alternative to heart rate, both are uniquely valuable and should be used together. It is common to see charts on the walls of group exercise facilities that provide an at-a-glance view of where their heart rate should be according to their age. The

RPE chart is equally, if not more, important and should be placed next to the heart rate chart.

Table 20-3 Rating of Perceived Exertion Scales			
15-Point RPE Scale (6–20 Scale)		**Revised 10-Point RPE Scale**	
Rating	Description	Rating	Description
6		0	Nothing
7	Very, very light	0.5	Very, very light, just noticeable
8		1	Very light
9	Very light	2	Light (weak)
10		3	Moderate
11	Fairly light	4	Somewhat hard
12		5	Heavy (strong)
13	Somewhat hard	6	
14		7	Very heavy (strong)
15	Hard	8	
16		9	
17	Very hard	10	Very, very heavy (almost max)
18			
19	Very, very hard		
20			

Reprinted with permission from "Psychological Bases of Physical Exertion" by Gunnar Borg, 1982, *Medicine & Science in Sports & Exercise.* 14 (377-381).

The Talk Test

The talk test is another tool used to evaluate an individual during cardiorespiratory exercise. The ability to engage in conversation during exercise represents work at or near a steady rate. When oxygen supply meets demand, a person is able to breathe rhythmically and comfortably. If the work encroaches upon anaerobic metabolism, respirations increase due to an elevation in lactic acid production and the ability to talk diminishes. The talk test has been criticized to be safe "to a fault" because it can actually keep a person that could otherwise handle more intense work from doing so because the priority is slanted to the ability to talk.

The Dyspnea Scale

This method uses a subjective scale to represent how participants perceive their relative difficulty in terms of breathing (dyspnea refers to shortness of breath/difficulty breathing).

+1   Mild and noticeable to participant, but not to an observer
+2   Mild, with some difficulty noticeable to an observer
+3   Moderate difficulty, but participant can continue to exercise
+4   Severe difficulty, and the participant must stop exercising at that level

This scale is helpful for participants who have pulmonary conditions (such as asthma or emphysema) or who feel limited because of breathing difficulties. The scale should be used in conjunction with RPE and HR, and participants should reduce intensity when their breathing becomes more labored (+3). Participants with breathing difficulties should consult with their primary care physician regarding their exercise goals and methods.

Summary

There are few others in the fitness industry that face such a high degree of responsibility as does the group exercise instructor. The multifaceted nature of the "group" dictates that they are nomadic, diverse in their ability, and span a wide range of biomechanical as well as physiological capability. Furthermore, there is minimal opportunity for advanced wellness information or the continuity of progression. The instructor's goal is to provide a choreographed workout, teaching some while leading all, through issues of timing, cueing, transitions, technique, pace, and rhythm. Additionally, and even more importantly, the group exercise instructor ensures that the participant encounters a positive and fun experience while simultaneously meeting the ultimate objective of cardiovascular improvement.

With that said, the goal of this chapter was to provide an overview of the tools, such as estimated heart rate formulas, rating of perceived exertion, and the talk test, to monitor cardiorespiratory response to exercise such that the objective can be met safely as well as effectively. However, the calculations to determine various heart rate ranges are, at best, estimates of where each participant is physiologically. Short of actual wireless telemetry, the more important tool therefore, is probably the rate of perceived exertion (RPE). The underestimated value of the RPE, while only a perception, is that it is the "participant's" perception of how hard they are working. This not only shifts the responsibility of the intensity to the participant, but also empowers the individual to help control their movements accordingly.

References

1. American College of Sports Medicine. (1998). Position stand: The recommended quantity and quality of exercise for developing and maintaining cardiorespiratory and muscular fitness, and flexibility in healthy adults. *Medicine & Science in Sports & Exercise*, 30, 975–991.

2. American College of Sports Medicine (2006). *ACSM's guidelines for exercise testing and prescription* (7th ed.). Baltimore, MD: Lippincott Williams & Wilkins.

3. American College of Sports Medicine. (2010). *ACSM's guidelines for exercise testing and prescription* (8th ed.). Baltimore, MD: Lippincott Williams & Wilkins.

4. Borg, G.A. (1982). Psychophysical bases of physical exertion. *Medicine & Science in Sports & Exercise*, 14(5), 377-381.

5. Gellish, R.L., Goslin, B.R., Olson, R.E., McDonald, A., Russi, G.D., & Moudgil, V.K. (2007). Estimating maximum heart rate from age: Is it a linear relationship? *Medicine & Science in Sports & Exercise*, 39(5), 821.

6. Noble, B.J., Borg, G.A., Jacobs, I., et al. (1983). A category-ratio perceived exertion scale: Relationship to blood and muscle lactates and heart rate. *Medicine & Science in Sports & Exercise*, 15, 523–528.

7. Pollack, M.L., & Wilmore, J.E. (1990). *Exercise in health and disease: Evaluation and prescription for prevention and rehabilitation* (2nd ed.). Philadelphia, PA: Lea & Febiger.

8. Robertson, R.J., & Noble, B.J. (1997). Perception of physical exertion: Methods, mediators, and applications. *Exercise and Sports Science Reviews*, 25, 407–452.

21 Building Traditional Group Exercise Choreography

Lynne G. Brick, BSN

Focus

Traditional group exercise choreography is the coordination of music and movement through time and space. It is designed, developed, and created using methods similar to those in traditional dance choreography. Regardless of your professional fitness teaching level of experience or ability, it is essential for you to know and understand the basic principles of choreography. This chapter offers principles and techniques designed to help you, the instructor, develop an endless number of traditional "free-style" movements for your class participants. These techniques can help your participants feel emotionally connected to your class, and therefore help you to consistently deliver a "world class" experience, every class! As a bonus, your participants will want to keep coming back for more of your classes!

Trends

At least 30 years ago, participants world-wide enjoyed Jacki Sorensen's Aerobic Dance and Judi Sheppard Missett's Jazzercise, Inc. These programs were choreographed from the first inhale to the last exhale. Every move was set to the music. It seems we have come "full circle." In the past 5 years or so, a number of choreographed branded programs have emerged that are also traditional in nature. Les Mills International programs, such as BodyAttack™, BodyStep™, BodyVive™, or Body Training Systems programs, such as Group Step™, and Group Active™, and Zumba™, have created loyal fans. Why? The choreographed moves "fit" the musical phrasing, the musical section, and the musical style. Participants and instructors have become fans of choreographed programs all over again. However, that is not the focus of this chapter. While traditional "free-style" moves are not set to the music, you are encouraged to create a connection between your music and your moves. This will help you consistently deliver "world class" classes. The first step is to understand how music is written.

Music Basics

Music is most often written in 4/4 time. In other words, there are 4 beats or musical accents per musical measure. These 4 musical beats are grouped together in sets of 8 to create a musical phrase consisting of 32 beats. Musical phrases are linked together to create musical sections.

Music usually follows a logical sequence of musical sections. Typically a song starts with an introduction, followed by the first verse, then the chorus, followed by the second verse, repeating the chorus again, followed by a musical interlude (instrumental) or a bridge, finally repeating the chorus again until the song fades. The chorus is dynamic and often contains the title or the "hook" of the song as part of the lyrics. The verse, chorus, or variations of either may be repeated.

These musical sections can occur in a variety of sequences. For example, the chorus may be the first section you hear, followed by an instrumental section. Each song has unique characteristics. For dramatic effect, music may have pauses or breaks in the sound, but the beat of the music continues. It is important for instructors to know their music so they can anticipate creative musical variations.

Professionally designed audio tapes, compact discs, or digital downloads can be purchased through professional fitness music companies. These companies compose, create, and design music specific to group exercise and the fitness industry. The music is blended from one song to another to create an environment of continuous, nonstop music, which is the perfect accompaniment for the moves that you choose to use. Professionally produced music is:

1. designed so that the musical phrasing consists of 8 sets of 4, or 32 beats of music;
2. legally approved by performing rights music companies, such as ASCAP, BMI, or SESAC;
3. designed with the instructor in mind, deleting bridges (extra beats that connect one musical section to another) and adding musical cues to help the instructor clearly hear the musical phrasing.

Interpretation of the music used helps you to create a fun, "world class" experience for your participants. Incorporate a variety of musical selections or styles, such as Latin, Rock, Top-40, or Old School, to add variety to your classes, and to keep participants inspired, content, and consistently present. Music is one of the motivators to help your participants to move!

Movement Basics

In traditional dance, movements and movement patterns, with the following characteristics, are artistically developed.

1. Movement patterns have a simple theme. Unrelated movements or themes are saved for other dance pieces.
2. Movement patterns are consistent.
3. Once a movement pattern is established, it is repeated throughout the dance piece. Either the movement is identical when repeated or just the movement qualities (i.e., elements of variation, such as movement intensity, rhythm, tempo) are repeated.
4. Movement patterns are designed in a "bite-size" step-by-step method.
5. All dance movements have the following elements: (a) design, (b) dynamics, (c) rhythm, and (d) motivation.

Remember these elements for developing traditional dance choreography as you review the basics of aerobic fitness choreography.

It is essential to understand the basic foundation of group exercise choreography before you start to creatively develop and design new choreography. The basics of aerobic fitness choreography are divided into **lower body movements** (depending upon degree of impact of the foot on the floor) and **upper body movements**.

Lower body movements are divided into four impact categories: (a) non-impact, (b) low-impact, (c) moderate-impact, and (d) high-impact.

Low-impact aerobics (LIA) is identified as keeping at least one foot on or as close to the floor as possible. For example, a **Grapevine** can be done in any of the following intensity options:

1. Step right, cross back left, step right, tap left toe. Step left, cross back right, step left, tap right toe. The dynamics of the height of the body remain the same while doing the three steps and the tap of the toe.
2. Knees bent, body low: step right, cross back left, step right, straighten the body as you tap your left toe. Knees bent, body low: step left, cross back right, step left, straighten the body as you tap your right toe. There is a dynamic difference in the height of the body while stepping as compared to tapping the toe.

3. Knees bent, body low: step right, cross back left, step right, hop as you bring your feet together. Knees bent, body low: step left, cross back right, step left, hop as you bring your feet together. This is the highest intensity level which is referred to as a single-impact action. In other words, out of four counts, three counts are low-impact and one of the counts is high-impact.

Moderate-impact aerobics (MIA) is characterized by both feet staying on the floor, but the feet roll through a toe-ball-heel action every time. The body bobs up and down similar to high-impact activity due to the heel lifting up and down. There are fewer impact forces to the feet because the whole foot is not leaving the floor. This is similar to **non-impact aerobics (NIA)** where upper body arm movements, along with active thigh movements, are employed to elevate heart rate while the feet remain in contact with the floor at all times. (NOTE: The term non-impact is also used to describe other cardiorespiratory training modalities, such as swimming and cycling, where there is no foot strike.)

High-impact aerobics (HIA) is characterized by both feet leaving the floor alternately or at the same time. The impact forces on the foot are high and, when executed continuously for extended periods of time, can potentially cause physical injury.

The following basic movements are the simplest forms of impact, which constitute the basic foundation of aerobic fitness choreography:

NIA	LIA	MIA	HIA
Biking/Spinning	March	Skip	Jog
Swimming (laps)	Step touch	Twist	Jump
Squats	Touch step	Plié/Relevé (up on toes)	Hop
Lunges	Squat/Plié	Knee lifts with heel lifts	Jack
Seated/Chair aerobics	Step touch while raising up on toes	Any move between LIA and HIA	Splits/Scissors
			Pendulum

Note that most of these movements are bilateral (i.e., involving both sides of the body) and/or single count moves. For example, a knee lift is not a basic move. It is a 2-count march that takes the leg through a higher plane of space. Also, a lateral lunge is a touch step with a spatial plane variation that turns the body to alternately face the side walls. These basic moves, regardless of what form of impact you are teaching, are the moves that identify the beginning of a movement combination and *lay the foundation for building, creating, and designing your movement choreography.*

Six of the above basic moves are ideal for transitioning. These basic moves are called **neutral** moves because both feet are on the floor and the weight of the body is centered. Any movement can follow these moves. Neutral moves are:

Squat/Plié	Twist
Plié/Relevé	Jump
Skip	Jack

Upper body movements can be divided into basic movement types as well.
- **Push/Abduction**: moves away from the center of the body.
- **Pull/Adduction**: moves in toward the center of the body.
- **Rotation (Internal or External)**: twisting of the arms from the shoulder.
- **Circle**: forms a circular design.

- **Isolations**: moves only one part of the upper body at a time (e.g., shoulders or ribs).

Every move you create, teach, and execute in aerobic fitness is the coordination of lower body moves with upper body moves. Let's put these basic movements together. You can choose one of the lower body basic moves to coordinate with any of the upper body basic moves.

Lower Body	with	Upper Body
March		Bilateral Chest Press
Touch-Step (Rear Lunge)		Posterior Deltoid Raises
Skip		Small Arm Circles At Chest Level
Splits		Bilateral Lat Pull-Down
Twist		Alternate Arms Push-Up
Jacks		Abduction (Lateral Deltoid Raises)
Step-Touch		Alternate Isolated Shoulder Circles

The following are factors that may influence your effectiveness to teach basic movements. It's important that you understand:

1. your comfort level of executing, coaching, and cueing basic movements.
2. your ability to communicate and teach basic movements, starting with lower body movements, gradually adding upper body movements.
3. your participants' ages.
4. your participants' level of coordination.
5. your participants' level of experience.
6. if your participants have particular risks to develop injuries.
7. for whom the movement is **F.O.R.** This acronym refers to your participants' **Frame Of Reference**. While you teach, try to have an "out-of-body" experience. You should see yourself teaching, and see yourself taking your class at the same time. Perceive your ability to teach your choreography the same way as your participants perceive your ability to teach and create a "world class" experience.

Now you have laid the foundation and are ready to progress to create a movement combination. From this point, in order to build, develop, or change the move you have taught, it is necessary to know and understand coaching/cueing techniques, the primary factors of smooth transitioning, and the key elements of variation.

Cueing/Coaching Techniques

The following examples of cueing techniques will help you effectively communicate to your participants.

1. **Footwork**: refers to which foot you want them to move, right or left.
2. **Directional**: refers to the direction you want people to travel (e.g., diagonal right front, half turn around, diagonal left rear, half turn around).
3. **Rhythmic**: refers to the rhythm of the movement (e.g., slow-slow-quick-quick-quick-quick; single-single-double; 1-2-3, 1-2-3; step-ball-change, step-ball-change).
4. **Numerical**: refers to the number of repetitions you want participants to execute, or the number of repetitions they have left. For transitioning purposes, avoid saying the number "1." If you take the time to say the number "1," you will not have the time to tell them what you want them to do next. Your numerical countdown cueing should be this rhythm: "4-3-2-change." Also note that you should always count down for

transitioning purposes, never up. Why? When we count down, we never say 4-3-2-1-0-(-1)-(-2). They know once you get to one, the next beat of the music should be the next move. Counting up, on the other hand, has no finish or stopping point.

5. **Step**: refers to the name of the step. "Pony," "Chassé-Ball-Change," and "Cha-Cha-Cha" are all examples of step cueing.

6. **Alignment**: refers to body posture and placement throughout the entire class, not just during the muscle conditioning portions of class. For example, knees over toes, abs braced.

7. **Verbal and Nonverbal**: refers to the "7-38-55" Rule of Communication. 7% of what you communicate consists of the words that you say; 38% of what you communicate is the way that you say those words; 55% of what you communicate is your body language. Never underestimate the power of communicating through your bodily gestures and posture. Let's face it. You may teach the most fabulous combinations, but if you don't believe in yourself or project a positive image, your class will not believe in you either!

8. **Visual**: refers to cueing that is communicated through hand gestures and sign language. In other words, hand gestures indicate if the participants should move forward, back, right, or left, start from the top of the movement sequence or numerically prepare the class for the next move. These are just a few examples of visual cueing. Make up your own and use what is best for you and, most importantly, what is best for your participants to follow you.

9. **Functionality**: Functionality refers to how you parallel the movement your participants execute in class to activities of daily living, such as picking up grocery bags, reaching to the top cabinet of the kitchen shelf, or pressing off the arm rests of an easy chair.

10. **Conspicuous**: Conspicuous Cueing is the combination of all nine cueing/coaching techniques to help your class be a "world class" experience.

Transitioning Techniques

Smooth Transitioning

Transitioning from one move to the next or from your right foot to your left foot is an important component for effective classes.

Effective transitioning techniques assure the following.

1. Smoothness of class flow from one movement to another.
2. Effectiveness of your ability to teach. When moves smoothly flow from one to another, there are no "speed bumps" or stopping of movement sequencing.
3. Safety in movement execution. You literally help people prevent from tripping over their own two feet!
4. Ability of your participants to follow you.
5. Control of all of the participants simultaneously.
6. Class experience is excellent.
7. Participant success and satisfaction is high!

There are three **primary factors that facilitate smooth transitioning**.

1. Change one thing at a time.
2. Begin your next movement where your original movement ends.
3. Use Conspicuous Cueing.

Sample Transitioning Aerobic Moves
1. Hamstring/knees: single – single – double
2. 4 repeater knees
3. Neutral moves
4. 3 sets of any move (e.g., grapevine x 3, 1 "V" step)
5. Step – hop – step – step
6. Hold (e.g., step – knee counts 1 & 2, & hold counts 3 & 4)

Sample Transitioning Step Moves
1. Single knee, hamstring, abductor, or glute (buttocks)
2. Repeater moves (x3)
3. Neutral moves (e.g., jack, press-up, squat, jump, etc.)
4. "L" step
5. Cha-cha-cha
6. Turn step/chassé turn

Elements of Variation

The elements of variation are the tools to help you to change, design, or develop exciting and creative movements from your basic movement. Elements of variation will also help you to transition smoothly from one movement to the next. These elements are also known as the secondary factors that facilitate smooth transitioning.

Rhythm

Rhythm is measured motion with regular recurrence of elements or features, such as the beat of the music. The rhythm of movement is executed to every beat or in between every beat of the music. Half time, single time, double time, triple time, as well as syncopation are all examples of rhythm. Syncopation incorporates the "and" beat of the music. The following is an example of syncopation:

Move	Counts
Step-touch x 4 repetitions (R-L-R-L)	Counts 1 through 8
In order to syncopate the rhythm, complete 3 step-touches (right, left, right).	Counts 1 through 6
Hold the tap of the third step-touch (left foot).	Count 7
Then lift your left foot, follow with your right foot as you do the last step-touch to the left.	Counts "and" 8

Most traditional aerobic fitness classes use music that is grouped in phrases of 32 beats. Therefore, the movements you choose should correspond to the same type of musical phrasing. The first movement count should begin at the same time as the first musical count. Count "1" of the music should be count "1" of the movement. In addition, the accents that you choose to use, such as claps, snaps, or touches, should correspond with the musical accents or the "up" beat of the music. This occurs on *counts 2, 4, 6, and 8*. This will help your class feel more motivated because the "up" beat of the music is a more driving beat.

The rhythm of movement can be varied regardless of the rhythm of the music through sound, look, and feel. *Claps, vocalizations, and stomps* are examples of rhythmic sound variations. Play around with the many ways to vary sound. For example, with a grapevine right and left (movement counts 1–8), traditionally, you clap on counts 4 and 8. You can vary the rhythm by clapping on counts 1 and 5.

Adding or subtracting movement repetitions changes the look of the movement (e.g., the syncopation example above or single, single, double). Movements rhythmically feel different from one another when dynamics (e.g., strong vs. soft; staccato/short vs. lyrical/long) and other movement qualities are used (e.g., swinging, suspending, vibrating, sustaining, collapsing, and percussive).

Additionally, rhythmic variations can help to stylize your movements, especially when you are using music with a Latin beat.

Intensity

The degree of physical, emotional, and psychological energy exerted to execute movements defines the concept of intensity. *Basically, the closer the feet and hands are to the ground, the less intense the movement. The farther the feet and hands are away from the ground, the more intense the movement.* Also, if movements are long lever and are executed from the trunk (shoulders and hips), the intensity will increase. If movements are short lever and are executed from the knee or elbow joint, the intensity will decrease.

If your participants are under a great deal of emotional stress, the intensity level may be greater than or less than normal exertion, depending on each individual's coping capabilities.

Psychologically, the intensity may also vary due to the participant's level of coordination and kinesthetic awareness. He/she may feel frustrated if movements that you choose are too complex or too difficult to execute. The intensity level drops significantly when this occurs.

Suggested rules of thumb are as follows.

1. Offer *varied intensity options* so participants can choose which level is best for them.
   Option 1: Least intense
   Option 2: Intermediate intensity
   Option 3: Highest intensity
2. Be sure that all movements are *broken down into "bite size" pieces.* Begin with basic movements, then gradually add one element of variation at a time, regardless of your participants' experience or ability. This is the "Part-to-Whole" Method of teaching.
3. Have your *participants leave every class that you teach feeling "successful."* In other words, they should feel as if they can do all of the movements you ask them to do. This does not mean that they have to look like you as they exercise, but the "Part-to-Whole" Method of teaching each move will enable your participants to feel more successful each step of the way.
4. *Alternate higher intensity moves with lower intensity moves* so that your participants can expend calories more efficiently.

Direction

The direction is the floor pattern over which the whole body travels. Think of the aerobic studio floor as a big stage. Then divide the stage into lines on which your participants can travel. Forward and back, side to side, diagonal, up and down, lines, small circles, large circles, and any combination of these are all examples of directional moves.

Particular movements are done most effectively in one direction. Jacks, skips, and hops are usually most effective in a backward direction. The same movement can be done facing a different direction and can be perceived as a different movement.

Simple directional changes are a great way to add variety without creating too much complexity. It is important to cue your directional changes clearly and well enough in advance so that your participants will not be confused. Give your participants landmarks to focus their eyes on or to move toward. For example, "face the front or the North Pole," or "face the back, the South Pole."

Symmetry

Symmetry refers to the similarity of form or arrangement on either side of a dividing line or plane of the body. In other words, symmetrical movement is bilateral movement. Novice or beginner participants feel best executing a symmetrical move because it is more balanced, more controlled, and easier to perform. An example of a typical symmetrical movement is to do lateral arm raises as the feet do jumping jacks or touch-step.

For your participants who really enjoy a challenge, offer a variety of different types of movements. Asymmetrical moves, in which one side of the body does one thing and the other side of the body does something else, are a great way to challenge participants. For example, as the lower body does grapevine right and left, the right arm can push and pull when traveling right and both arms circle when traveling left. This not only offers variety to break up the monotony of doing the same moves all of the time, but also may help to alter intensity level.

Spatial

The planes of space are as follows.
1. **Frontal** = movements that are side to side or along the frontal plane (e.g., Lateral Raise or Side Lunges)
2. **Transverse** = movements on a diagonal or rotational (e.g., "Wood Chop")
3. **Sagittal** = movements that move forward and back, through the midline of the body (e.g., Biceps Curls or Forward Lunges)

Basically they are vertical (up and down), horizontal (side to side), and diagonal (up on one side and down on the other). When you put your movements together, try to focus on all the parts of the body that are attached to the trunk, which have unlimited planes of space to use.

In other words, with directional variations, the whole body moves. Spatial variations, however, refer to the planes of space in which the extremities, all joints, and the head can move. In addition, these planes of space can form specific, creative body designs as discussed later in this chapter under "The Link Method with a Theme."

Style

Style refers to the amount of individual *personality,* or "*attitude,*" that each participant applies while executing moves. Traditional HIA, MIA, or LIA may not require a particular style. Funk, step, Latin, or dynamic stretching classes are best when participants add their own individual flair to the movements.

All of these elements of variation will help to create an endless variety of movements and movement styles. It is important to remember: *there is safety with*

Choose a variety of music styles. Encourage your participants to stylize their movements to the music.

variety. In other words, the more you mix and match different types of movements, the more the safety factors increase due to altering impact stress factors to the feet and to the joints. For example:

Teach These Moves in One Combination		
Right foot forward and back x 2 (Mamba)	Arms alternately pump	Counts 1–8
Jack x 2	Arms symmetrically lift laterally	Counts 9–12
Plié/Relevé x 2	Arms symmetrically press up	Counts 13–16

Reverse all with the left foot leading. Use the 32-count total for the entire combination. As an advanced option, the second plié/relevé can be one power jump.

As you can see, this combination uses all types of impact forces on the foot (LIA, MIA, HIA, and power) and a variety of spatial upper body moves so as not to stress the shoulder joint.

The Link Method

Now you are ready to put movements together. In order to do this, try using the Link Method which is the *Part-to-Whole Method* of teaching. The Part-to-Whole Method is a teaching tool that has been used by educators for quite some time. Educators found that people learn complex skills more easily when the "parts" of the "whole" skill are broken down and taught one step at a time, then linked together to make up the whole skill. This is also commonly referred to as the add-on method.

Start by teaching a basic lower body move. Then add a basic upper body move. You now have a choice of three options, as outlined below.

1. Keep your movement a simple movement, that is, a movement with consistent spatial patterning.
2. You can change the lower body by using only one element of variation, and/or change the upper body by using only one element of variation. This will transform your original move to a new move.
3. You can combine the option-one movement with option-two movement to make a complex movement: two or more simple moves that involve multiple elements of variation. Establish a pattern of movement repetitions (e.g., step-touch 4, march 8). Then you can make your movements travel (see boxes that follow).

Visually, the Link Method looks like this:
Teach Movement A using the Part-to-Whole Method of teaching.
Teach Movement B using the Part-to-Whole Method of teaching.
Repeat "whole" Movement A; repeat "whole" Movement B.
Teach Movement C using the Part-to-Whole Method of teaching.
Repeat "whole" Movement A, "whole" Movement B, "whole" Movement C.
Teach Movement D using the Part-to-Whole Method of teaching. Repeat "whole" Movement A, "whole" B, "whole" C, and "whole" D.

The Link Method requires that each simple and complex movement is taught using the Part-to-Whole Method. A new movement or a *new element of variation is not added to the move until the participants feel comfortable executing the present move.* This process is repeated for each new movement that you intend to teach. Each "whole" movement is linked together with the previous "whole" movements that you have already taught.

| \multicolumn{5}{c}{**Steps to Create a Traditional Aerobic Combination with the Link Method**} |

Steps to Create a Traditional Aerobic Combination with the Link Method				
RL = Right Lead S = Single O-T-S = On the Spot D = Double		LL = Left Lead F = Forward B = Backward		
	Musical Counts	**Lower Body then add**		**Upper Body**
Step 1	(1–16 cts.)	RL Step touch O-T-S* x 8		Shoulder abduction x 4
		Abduct + add Clap x 4		
Step 2 (Cut reps in half)	(17–32 cts.)	March O-T-S X 16		Alternate punch-up x 16
Step 3	(16 cts.)	RL Step touch x 4 O-T-S		Abduct + Clap x 4 Alternate punch-up x 8
		March x 8 O-T-S		
Step 4 (Add travel)	(16 cts.)	RL Step touch x 4 travel F		Abduct + Clap x 4
		March back x 8		Alternate punch-up x 8
Step 5 (Add direction)	(16 cts.)	RL Step touch x 4 travel F		Abduct + Clap x 4
		March around in semi-circle x 8		Alternate punch-up x 8
Step 6	(16 cts.)	Repeat until participants feel comfortable		
Step 7	(16–32 cts.)	RL Hamstring curls O-T-S		Low row (pull elbows back)
Step 8	(32 cts.)	RL Hamstring curls S-S-D*		Low row x 4
		LL Hamstring curls S-S-D*		Low row x 4
		Repeat		
Step 9 (Add spatial variation)	(64 cts.)	RL Hamstring curls S-S-D		Low row x 4
		LL Mamba x 2		Overhead raise x 2
		LL Hamstring curls S-S-D		Low row x 4
		RL Mamba x 2		Overhead raise x 2
Step 10	(64 cts.)	Repeat until participants feel comfortable		
Step 11	(32 + 32 cts.)	LINK ALL together:		
		RL Step touch x 4 travel F		Abduct + Clap x 4
		March in semi-circle x 8		Alternate punch-up x 8
		RL Hamstring curls S-S-D		Low row x 4
		LL Mamba x 2		Overhead raise x 2
		Reverse all LL		
32 counts of movement to music RL PLUS 32 counts of movement to music LL EQUAL 64 counts of Movement to Music!				

	Steps to Create a Traditional Step Combination with the Link Method		
	Musical Counts	**Lower Body** then add	**Upper Body**
Step 1	(32 cts.)	RL Basic x 4	Low row x 8
	(32 cts)	LL Basic x 4	Low row x 8
Step 2	(16 cts.)	RL Basic x 2,	Low row x 4
		"V" step x 2	Alt. arm, reach high to make letter "V", then return to hip x 2
	(16 cts.)	Reverse all LL	
Step 3	(16 cts)	RL Single knee & freeze	Punch R arm up
		Hold x 3 cts.	Hold Punch
		LL March x 4 on the floor	Pump arms F & B
		LL Single knee & freeze	Punch L arm up
		Hold x 3 cts.	Hold Punch
		RL March x 4 on the floor	Pump arms F & B
		Repeat until participants feel comfortable with rhythm of the movement	
Step 4	(32 cts.)	Link together:	
		RL Basic x 2	Low row x 4
		"V" step x 2	Alt. arm reach up to "V" x 2
		RL Single knee & freeze (hold 3 cts.)	Punch R arm up x 1
		LL March on the floor x 4	
		LL Basic x 2	Hands on Hips
	(32 cts.)	LL Reverse all	
Step 5	(32 cts.)	RL Repeat all	
		delete: 2 Basics at end	
		add: 2 Alternate gluts	Reach forward x 2
	(32 cts.)	LL Reverse all	
Step 6	(64 cts.)	Link ALL together:	
		RL Basic x 2	Low row X 4
		"V" step x 2	Alt. arm reach up to "V" x 2
		RL Single knee & freeze	Punch R arm up x 1
		LL March on the floor x 4	Pump arms F & B
		LL Alternate glut x 2	Reach forward x 2
		LL Reverse all	
32 counts of movement to music RL PLUS 32 counts of movement to music LL			

Additional Link Method Principles

1. Take your time teaching each of the parts of your movements.
2. Make each of your movements consistent, whether they are simple or complex, each time that you repeat them.
3. Know your music.
4. Limit the number of simple "part" moves that comprise a complex movement to four.
5. Let the style of the music dictate the style of movements that you choose.
6. Remember, teaching group exercise choreoghraphy (aerobics) is the coordination of music and movement through time and space. Relax, take your time, enjoy, and have fun! Then your participants will have fun, too!

The Link Method is designed to help you to teach and create movements, from the "parts" to the "whole," that transition smoothly from one to another, even if you are creating your combinations on-the-spot. But, what do you do when you make up a fabulous "whole" combination when you are in a creative mood (e.g., in the car, the bathtub, or just before you fall asleep)? How do you break this combination down so that you can teach each "part?" The following are recommended steps to identify each of the "parts" so that you can create your "whole."

1. Determine how many simple or basic lower and upper body moves exist in the combination.
2. Identify the first basic lower body move.
3. Identify any elements of variation that are necessary to change the basic lower body move.
4. Add the basic upper body move.
5. Identify any elements of variation for the upper body move.
6. When you have completed the breakdown of the first part of the combination, identify the key components to transition from the first lower body basic move to the second lower body basic move.
7. Identify the key components of transition from the first upper body basic move to the second upper body basic move.
8. Link together the first lower and upper body moves with the second lower and upper body moves.
9. Repeat this process for the remaining identified basic moves.
10. Practice the best ways to break down your combination. Remember that a combination can be successfully broken down several ways. Choose the best way to break your combination down so that it is easiest for you to teach and coach, and more importantly, so that your participants can enjoy their experience and have success!

The Link Method with a Theme

The **Link Method with a Theme** focuses on movements and variations that have common traits. This is not musical or holiday themed choreography, but movements and designs the *body can make in the planes of space as well as in directional floor patterning.* Focus on creating your Link Method with a Theme based on directional, rhythmic, spatial/planal, and symmetrical elements of variation.

Here is a sample Link Method with a Theme of "Up and Down."

Musical Counts	Lower Body	Upper Body
Movement A: 16 counts	March forward x 4 March O-T-S x 4 (up and down dynamics) Repeat all back and O-T-S	Punch down x 4 Punch up and down x 2 Repeat
Movement B: 16 counts	Alternate knee lifts (MIA) x 8	Alt. biceps curls x 8
Movement C: 16 counts	R knee up, walk x 3 Repeat L-R-L	Press up and lower with curved arms
Movement D: 16 counts	Plié/Relevé x 8	Overhead press x 8
* O-T-S — On the Spot		

The Link Method with a Theme is really an enjoyable way to design and create non-traditional types of movements for your classes. You may find that you are most creative with the body or floor pattern designs when you can visualize your "whole" combinations. Below is another example of sample movement combinations for the Link Method with an **Asymmetrical Theme**.

Musical Counts	Lower Body	Upper Body
Movement A: 16 counts	RL Step touch x 8* (cross R foot back behind)	L arm reaches up on diagonal R arm reaches down across body with LL*
Movement B: 16 counts	Zigzag: RL 3 steps F on R diagonal, hop;	R arm reaches laterally on R diagonal, clap.
	LL 3 steps forward on L diagonal, hop;	Arms alternately punch up, L arm reaches laterally on L diagonal
	Reverse traveling back	L arm reaches laterally on L diagonal, clap
Movement C: 16 counts	RL Step-L knee lift; L step-ball-change x 4	R arm punches up. R arm punches across lateral R side of the body
Movement D: 16 counts	RL Grapevine x 1 Twist O-T-S x 4 cts. Grapevine, Jack x 2 Reverse all LL	Shoulder shrug x 2 Twist upper torso x 4LL Shoulder shrug x 2, Big arm circles x 2
* RL — Right Lead LL — Left Lead O-T-S — On the Spot		

The Building Block Method

The Building Block Method is an effective free-form style of teaching. This method is an "add on" technique in which a new basic "whole" move is added on one at a time. All movements are basic "whole" moves, so there are no "parts" to teach, and they are added on after a patterning of previously sequenced moves are done. The key element is to consistently add on the new move every time you direct your participants to the same location (e.g., one side of the room or one wall to face). They will anticipate your cues for the new move once this pattern is established. Visually, the Building Block Method looks like this:

Movement A:	Jog (arms reach and clap)
Movement A + B:	Jog (arms reach and clap) + Skip (circle arms low)
Movement A + B + C:	Jog (arms reach and clap) + Skip (circle arms low) + Alternate knee lifts (bilateral biceps curls)
Movement A + B + C + D:	Jog (arms reach and clap) + Skip (circle arms low) + Alternate knee lifts (bilateral biceps curls) + Splits (alternate arm reach forward in opposition).

Basic "whole" moves usually have the following characteristics.

1. **Symmetrical**—Symmetrical moves are easy to cue and teach. Both sides of the body mirror one another.
2. **Balanced**—The arms move in opposition to the foot that is leading. The left arm reaches forward as the right foot steps forward, the right arm reaches forward as the left foot steps forward. An example is the HIA splits as the arms alternately reach forward in opposition.
3. **Centered**—All movements start from the center of the body, which is located in the center of the chest for men and in the center of the upper pelvic region for women. Centering refers to proper posture and alignment with a "pulled up" and controlled feeling. Some centered movements are both symmetrical and balanced. An example of a

centered move is the relevé/plié as the arms reach up and down. Often, participants will flop their upper body and their feet around as they do this move. Teach control and focus on the movement as it extends from the center of the body. As an option, one of the Building Blocks you have sequenced together can be a "whole" movement combination in a series of movements you are linking together.

The California Style

The California Style of teaching refers to directional variations as well as floor patterning. This technique is called the "California Style" because in the mid 1980s, classes were often very full and held in small studios. In order to break up the monotony created by facing the same wall all of the time, the class turned to face different directions or different walls as the same movements were repeated. Through the participants' perception, the movements were not boring even though they were identical with each directional change.

Today, this concept still works quite well, but the moves take on any directional change. Here are just a few examples:

1. Jog 8 to the right front diagonal, 2 alternate knee lifts on-the-spot, skip 4 counts, and turn around to face the left rear diagonal.
2. Walk forward x 3 and jump, walk back x 3 and jump moving toward each diagonal corner.
3. Divide your class into six lines. Give each of the lines a different move to perform. After several reps, have your participants power walk or jog forward and circle around within their line to face front. Then reassign each line a new move. (You can even use this technique as a circuit for muscle conditioning.)
4. Jack 4, kick 4, twist 8, jog 8 facing each wall.

The California Style helps to motivate your participants, and gives you a technique with which to try out your favorite moves with directional changes.

Summary

The Link Method, the Link Method with a Theme, the Building Block Method, and the "California Style" are tools you can use to help create and build choreography for your traditional aerobic dance and step classes. These are just a few of many different methods of putting music together with movement through time and space.

The principles and techniques of creating and teaching group exercise class choreography may seem overwhelming. However, the more you practice these step-by-step approaches, the more comfortable you will feel, and the more success you will experience as a teacher. You may have heard that practice makes perfect. Correction! Perfect practice makes perfect! In other words, practice your moves, your cueing, and your coaching as if you are teaching in front of a live class. Then practice again and again and again until you feel you can deliver a "world class" experience. By the way, even if you are a "seasoned" instructor, you should continue to practice, practice, practice. You will know when you are successful by the number of participants you retain and attract to take your classes!

The more teaching experience you have, the more you can identify your own movement and teaching style and personality. You will discover the specific movement and teaching styles which will naturally "click" with your own personality.

Building your group exercise class choreography and perfecting your teaching skills will help you to be the best instructor that you can be!

Recommended Reading

1.　Bray, S.R., Millen, J.A., Eidsness, J., & Leuzinger, C. The effects of leadership style and exercise program choreography on enjoyment and intentions to exercise. In *Psychology of Sport & Exercise*. Abstract. Retrieved May 6, 2009, from http://www.cababstractsplus.org/abstracts/Abstract.aspx? AcNo=20053099845

22 *Training for Flexibility*

Judy Gantz, MA, CMA

Focus

Flexibility is a basic fitness component. From the Latin flectere—to bend, training for flexibility requires moving in the full range of motion of our joint anatomy. Developing a healthy range of stretch allows us to "bend" and move with greater ease, and keeps muscles supple and responsive to the demands of jobs performed at a computer desk, along with daily activities and exercise. Training for flexibility requires us to move the most active joints of the spine, hips, shoulders, ankles, and feet in a balanced range of motion. The spine bends forward, backwards, laterally, and rotates right to left. Stretching techniques of yoga and dance are useful to move in all directions, as well as limbering moves associated with these and other forms of martial arts and exercise. For a healthy approach to flexibility extreme stretches are not always needed, but applying principles of general "fitness flexibility" is very important to every exercise population.

Stretching and Flexibility

Stretching with good biomechanics (posture and body alignment) provides most people with an overall feeling of lessening muscle tension and loosening joint movement. How you stretch is very important to fitness. Stretching in excess can make the connective tissue surrounding joints too "loose" and this can lead to injuries. First, determine what type of flexibility is needed; are you training to be a yoga or dance performer? Do you participate in sports requiring high degrees of joint range (long strides, high kicks)? What are the demands of your lifestyle?

There are two definitions of flexibility.

- **Static flexibility**: the capacity to move a joint throughout its full range of motion (ROM) and hold the position. For example, when a yoga teacher lifts their leg behind their head and keeps it there for 1 minute.
- **Dynamic flexibility**: having responsive muscles that are conditioned for their elastic properties in order to move a joint throughout full ROM at varying speeds with varying forces. For example, when a dancer does a high kick to fast music.

Both types of flexibility require training. Static flexibility is achieved by slowly taking a stretch into a position and holding that position for at least 10–30 seconds. This is very common in many forms of yoga. Holding a position while you feel a stretch in the torso or leg gradually allows muscle contraction to release and connective tissue to become more pliable. Static flexibility is very useful to increase relaxation, and can be a gentle approach to gaining flexibility for someone who may be very "tight" and new to flexibility training. Dynamic flexibility is conditioning that allows someone to perform movements of the spine or hip using speed and force, such as a high leg kick in dance. Training needs to start with slow, limbering moves that gradually build up to greater force and speed. In most dance aerobic classes you will see the warm-up using "limbering" moves to increase circulation and gain dynamic range of motion. Starting a dance class with slow-range-of-motion actions is a great way to prepare and condition for dynamic flexibility.

When teaching either type of flexibility, it is important to evaluate the movement goals of clients or participants. Anyone involved with activities demanding high degrees of flexibility moving fast and strong, wants to include dynamic stretching into the workout. If you are training a professional dancer, be aware that some dance styles can result in overstretching. If your hip joint has to increase to 180°, you will be overstretching that joint to achieve an aesthetic goal. Since overstretching is linked to injuries, be careful not to demand the same flexibility training with general fitness flexibility. Stretching moderately and following kinesiological guidelines will bring positive long-lasting flexibility gains. When it comes to flexibility, more is not always better!

Flexibility Benefits

There are many benefits attributed to stretching: (a) improved movement function, (b) reduced muscle tension, (c) enhanced relaxation, (d) improved posture and coordination, (e) reduced stiffness, and (f) delay of the physical deterioration associated with aging. Most of these benefits are reported from clinical and empirical findings because science is still studying the various effects of stretching. The notion that stretching before exercising can prevent injuries is surrounded by controversy. On the other hand, medical science is supporting the benefits of stretching as it relates to stress reduction. Kinesiologically, there is large agreement that safe stretching improves movement function. Increasing flexibility improves the range of motion available to our joints, and reduces muscle stiffness and tension. A common compensation for tight calf muscles is to allow the foot to roll in (pronate). Foot pronation places undesired stresses on the foot, ankle, and knee. Excessive pronation can contribute to such common injuries as shin splints, Achilles tendinitis, and knee cap problems (e.g., patello femoral arthralgia or patellar tendinitis).

Most experts favor stretching as a means of reducing muscle tension. Holding less tension in the muscles makes the body feel more relaxed. Incorporating visualization and breathing techniques while stretching can promote relaxation and alter neurological responses to stress.

Regular stretching can improve posture and enhance coordination, limbering the body for easier movement. Connective tissue is entwined with muscle tissue, yet these tissue types are different in structure and function. Connective tissue is NOT elastic; it binds and supports muscles tissue, but also creates cross-links from collagen fibers which inhibit motion in areas of the body that lack movement. When we stretch and extend our joints these cross-links are broken down which allows greater muscle stretch. A flexible muscle is believed to provide less internal resistance to stretch, potentially enhancing speed and efficiency during performance.

Some of the characteristics of aging, such as stiffness and reduced activity, are countered by stretching. Flexibility training conditions the elastic properties in muscle tissue and breaks down cross-links. Although the fastest growing age group in America is over 65, there are few studies on the effects of stretching on the older adult. To date, we know stretching increases flexibility at any age, but we do not know how much change is possible when one starts stretching as an older adult. A limber body at 70 years of age is not the same as a limber body at 7 years of age.

Research studies are not conclusive as to how stretching prevents injuries. Some evidence reveals that adequate flexibility may prevent injuries associated with activities that move the joints beyond normal range of motion at rapid speeds. In power lifting or dancing, flexibility is crucial to the movement demands of these activities. Flexibility-induced performance enhancement may also result from increased musculotendinous compliance facilitating the use of elastic strain energy. This may at least partially explain why athletes state they feel they can throw harder and faster with increased flexibility.

There are multiple benefits to stretching, but some are questionable benefits. Fortunately, science is continuing to study and research the factors that influence flexibility. Understanding these factors sheds light on how to evaluate and design effective stretch programs.

Factors That Influence Flexibility

Many factors determine and influence our flexibility, including the following.
- Genetic bony and connective tissue structure
- Tight or loose ligaments
- Muscular fascial sheath, joint capsule
- Connective tissue structures
- Stress and muscular tension
- Injury, pregnancy, age

The first factor, genetic bony structure, is something we cannot alter. The shape and size of our bones and the type of connective tissue we have is mainly determined by our genetic inheritance, that is, the structure we are born with.

Knowing the natural limitations of our anatomical structure allows us to stretch safely. Every joint in the body has a different range of motion (ROM) dictated by shape, size, and how the bones fit together. Different body types are built with varying degrees of joint range. For example, the pelvis and hip joints are often shaped differently in men and women. A wider pelvis allows for greater turn-out in the hip. Consequently, the range of motion at the joint is greater. If an individual is born with the anatomical disposition for greater external hip rotation, they will be able to develop a larger "stretch" at that joint. Each joint can have variations in structure that enhance or limit flexibility. Although generally, everyone has the same basic joint design, these differences result in variations of mobility or stability.

Joints and Stability

The major joints responsible for movement are classified as nonaxial, uniaxial, biaxial, and triaxial. The most stable joint types are uniaxial (move in one plane), such as the elbow which flexes and extends. Joints that move in two (biaxial) or three (triaxial) planes, such as the knee (flexion, extension with some rotation) and the hip (flexion, extension; abduction, adduction; rotation) respectively, are more mobile and rely to a greater degree on the surrounding connective tissues (ligaments, fascia, tendons) and muscles for support. It is difficult to overstretch a uniaxial joint because the bony design limits the movement in only one direction, and often there is a natural feel for where the stretch will stop. However, when stretching a triaxial joint, such as the hip or shoulder, there is a greater range of motion at the joint allowing more freedom when stretching. It is important not to overstretch the joints, which produce most of our human action.

The second influence on our flexibility is the quality of connective tissues: (a) ligaments, (b) fascial sheath, (c) joint capsule, and (d) the musculotendinous unit. Although muscles have the greatest elastic properties, the fascial sheath covering muscle is composed of connective tissue that is rather non-elastic.

Muscle tissue can stretch and return to its original shape and size, whereas connective tissue (CT) remains extended once it is stretched. The role of CT is to bind and hold things together, as in the case of ligaments binding bone to bone. Each type of CT has varying degrees of elasticity. If our ligaments have a higher proportion of elastic fibers, it makes us appear "naturally flexible." The quality of elasticity in the connective tissues (ligaments, fascia, and the musculotendinous unit) has a tremendous influence on why some people appear "naturally" limber.

Ligament Laxity

The condition of ligament laxity results from being born with ligaments that have a higher degree of elastic properties. Ligaments attach bone to bone, providing joint stability through tensile strength. Tensile strength is the ability to withstand being pulled or drawn apart. A joint with ligament laxity is more mobile and can extend further. The term "double jointed" is often used to describe ligament laxity because of the extreme positions that can be manipulated and held, forcing joints beyond their normal range. People with ligament laxity can be more prone to injury if they do not have adequate strength to support their joints. Stretching with this condition is considered safe if the body is well-positioned in each stretch, and there is a balance of strength to flexibility. Moving a joint beyond the limit to which it can be actively controlled is a set-up for injury.

Affects of Stress

Stress that is carried as muscular tension keep muscles in a shortened, contracted state. When muscles relax, tension is released. High levels of muscular tension tend to decrease sensory awareness and can contribute to an elevation in blood pressure. Habitually tense muscles tend to cut off blood circulation. Reduced blood supply results in a lack of oxygen and essential nutrients, and causes toxic waste products to accumulate in the cells, leading to fatigue and pain.

Many scientists believe emotional tension and muscular tension are related. According to some researchers, ailments from emotional tension include headaches, joint and muscle pain, even stomach ulcers. Chronic muscle tension (called contracture) causes a muscle to be continually in a shortened state, resulting in tightness and reduced strength.

Flexibility and Pregnancy

Pregnancy, injury, and age all influence the quality of our flexibility. During pregnancy, the hormone relaxin causes ligaments and connective structures to increase in their elastic properties. Although it can be helpful for some women to stretch, caution should be followed not to overstretch areas of the pelvis. When seated with soles of the feet together, pregnant women should avoid pushing down and out on the inside of the knees. Following this precaution prevents unintentional injury of the softened cartilage and supportive tissues of the pelvic and hip joint.

Injury

Musculoskeletal injury interferes with the functioning of our soft tissues. Often an injury, such as a sprained ankle, results in reduced range of motion. This is because there is a build-up of scar tissue function resulting from connective tissue repairing itself. Stretching can enhance or hinder an injury; therefore, secure medical evaluation and advice before attempting any rigorous flexibility program.

Aging

The relationship between age and flexibility is still being researched. One thing science does agree upon is that as we age, connective tissue (CT), which is made up primarily of collagen fibers, forms cross-links in areas that have restricted motion. Age is often associated with a sedentary lifestyle. The older and less active an individual is, the more rapidly these cross-links build up and limit the motion of muscles and joints. If the joints are not extended through various ranges, collagen cross-links are laid down in the tissues making our bodies feel stiff and less flexible. Stretching breaks down cross-links and research suggests that regular stretching/mobilization can decrease cross-link build-up.

Physiology of Stretching

Muscles are made up of a series of larger to smaller bundles encased in multiple layers of connective tissue. Every small muscle fiber is surrounded by a sheath called the endomysium. These small fibers are organized into bundles, called fasciculi, which are surrounded by a sheath called perimysium. The whole muscle is made up of fasciculi bundles that are held together by a connective tissue sheath, the epimysium. To initiate movement, the force of a muscle contraction is transmitted from the smaller fibers through the connective tissues to the bones. The endo, peri, and epimysium coverings form the fascial sheath and become the attachment of tendon to bone. This fascial sheath offers the greatest resistance to stretch. When we stretch, we must stretch muscle and fascia together. Fascia becomes more pliable when it is warm. Physiologically, long-lasting changes in flexibility are more easily accomplished when stretching is performed with an elevated body temperature.

The interplay of the nervous system and the muscular system produces movement through muscles shortening and lengthening. The mechanism responsible for muscles shortening or contracting is located in the small units of a single muscle fiber, the sarcomere. The sarcomere is composed of thin and thick filaments called actin and myosin. When an impulse is generated by the nervous system, it triggers the actin and myosin causing the two filaments to pull closer together. This is the "contractile mechanism" or "contractile theory" of how muscles change length.

Muscles are protected by neurological commands carried out by reflexes. A reflex is a response that bypasses the brain and is transmitted directly from muscles to the spinal cord and back to the muscles. Embedded in the musculo-tendinous unit are two intrinsic receptors, the muscle spindle and the Golgi tendon organ (GTO). The function of these receptors is to detect when a muscle has been extended or stretched and to respond by cueing the muscle to contract or release. Anytime a muscle is stretched, a signal is sent to contract that same muscle. This reaction is called the stretch reflex.

The muscle spindle lies parallel and between the contractile fibers in muscles. It is a very small receptor responsible for activating the stretch reflex. The spindle is sensitive to length changes (tonic response) in a muscle (such as when we stretch) and responds to the rate or speed (phasic response) at which the change in length occurs. Most spindles have two types of intervention. Primary afferent fiber (Type I) responds to the speed of a stretch. The faster you stretch, the greater the response. Stretching with fast, bouncing movements will cause the monosynaptic stretch reflex to fire and immediately send a signal to the muscle being stretched to contract (and relax the opposing muscles). The secondary fibers (Type II) conduct impulses at a slower rate. They respond to the final stretch length and act to relax the prime muscle, thus facilitating the stretch. For example, when a stretch is done slowly, these Type II fibers become active. Stretching slowly and holding the stretch allows the muscle spindles to reset (to become sensitive at a longer length) and shuts off the stretch reflex signal causing muscle contraction. Resetting a spindle allows a muscle to be stretched further before it fires.

The GTO is located at the musculotendinous junction. This receptor is a protective device detecting changes in muscle tension and length. The GTO responds by inhibiting muscle contraction; for example, when the elbow is extended and excessive loads are placed on the joint area, the GTO will respond by signaling muscles to release, thereby causing the elbow to flex or bend.

Knowing the physiology of muscle composition and nerve receptors is the basis for understanding the pros and cons of different stretching techniques.

Techniques of Stretching

The physiological aspects of muscles, connective tissue, and the stretch reflex have influenced the controversy as to what stretching methods are the safest and most effective.

There are three major stretching techniques:

1. **Dynamic–Phasic–Ballistic**: A high-force, short duration method relying on speed and body weight to stretch the muscle. The speed used in this method causes the stretch reflex to be activated very quickly. Two opposing forces act on the muscle group: (a) the force generated from the fast stretch attempting to lengthen the muscle, and (b) the reflexive contraction of that same group. Using fast bouncing, rhythmic motion, especially if there is a high degree of force, can be, and is often, associated with greater muscle soreness. "Pulsing" is also included in this category.

2. **Static**: This is the most popular form of stretching. A static stretch is slow and held in a terminal position from 10–30 seconds in order to increase motion at a particular joint. This is the technique used in yoga. Holding the stretch allows the muscle spindle to rest, and the initial muscle contraction triggered by the stretch reflex to diminish. The static position promotes long-term changes in passive flexibility because it is low force and long duration. This method is considered very safe and will not cause undue muscle soreness.

3. **PNF (Proprioceptive Neuromuscular Facilitation)**: PNF is a form of static stretching. This is a method of stretching that originated from physical therapy as a clinical technique. Generally requiring a partner (although a wall or bar can be used for some positions) this method involves a series of steps alternating contraction, relaxation, and movement of specific muscle groups. The steps are as follows:

   1. Put the muscle group in an elongated position.
   2. Gradually contract the stretched muscle group isometrically (without moving the joint) until near maximum effort.
   3. Hold the contraction 6–10 seconds.
   4. Relax the contracting muscles.

Contract concentrically the opposing muscle group, extending the stretch (the partner can aid this stretch with gentle pressure to move the limb). Repeat the above process three to four more times to fully stretch the muscle groups.

Why PNF is effective is not totally clear. Physiologically, this technique takes full advantage of the muscle spindle, stretch reflex and GTO responses along with reciprocal inhibition. The one drawback to PNF is the need for a partner. PNF does not lend itself to a class situation but is very useful in one-to-one training.

Increasing Flexibility

Long-term changes in flexibility are not well documented, but most experts agree that permanent muscle changes are possible when tissue temperature is elevated and low force, long duration is applied. Studies have shown that raising the temperature of a tendon increases the amount of permanent length change. The viso-elastic properties of all connective tissues make them more pliable when warm. For this reason, warming up before you stretch should make stretching more productive and possibly safer.

Using stretch techniques that limit the involvement of the stretch reflex appear to reduce stretching soreness. To increase flexibility, hold stretches for 10–30 seconds and move in and out of the stretch positions slowly.

The greatest resistance to stretch is provided by the fascial sheath that covers the muscle. For this reason, it is important to feel the sensation of stretch in the center portion of the muscle. If the stretch pulls on the attachment sites, such as the base of the kneecap (attachment of the patella ligament to the tibial tuberosity), undue strain can be placed on the ligaments. Concentrate on extending the muscles in positions that do not put stress in a joint or on the attachment points where ligaments are connected to bones.

Summary

Stretching is a natural activity, but effective and safe conditioning for flexibility requires an understanding of kinesiological principles. As with all fitness components, flexibility is developed by following a consistent program. Structuring a regular time to stretch helps to maintain regularity. Because stretching is a time to slow down, it can be a time to increase body awareness and reduce stress. As the body becomes more supple, moving with greater range of motion will make all other exercising easier and more enjoyable.

Stretching Guidelines

To ensure quality training for flexibility remember the following.

1. Use stretch positions that are safe for the joints. Be aware of body alignment while stretching.
2. Stretch until a feeling of mild tension, but not terrible pain, is perceived in the muscle. Monitor the pulling sensation in the belly of the muscle. Avoid discomfort around the ligaments of the joints.
3. Hold the stretches 10–30 seconds. Avoid bouncing and pulsing because they can elicit the stretch reflex.
4. Breathe slowly without breath holding and with concentration. Create a relaxed mental state, and stretch in a comfortable environment.
5. Stretch when the body is warm. The best results occur when muscles are warmed up. Consider jogging, marching in place, or stationary cycling for 5–10 minutes until "a sweat is broken" before doing a stretch routine. Also stretch at the end of an exercise program.
6. Keep the program simple, regular, painless, and soothing. Incorporate stretching into an exercise program at least 3 days or up to 7 days per week.

References

1. Alter, M. (1996). *Science of Flexibility*. Champaign, IL: Human Kinetics.

2. American College of Sports Medicine. (2010). *ACSM's guidelines for exercise testing and prescription* (8th ed.). Baltimore, MD: Lippincott Williams & Wilkins.

3. Buroker, K., & Schwane, J. (1989). Does postexercise static stretching alleviate delayed muscle soreness? T*he Physician and Sportsmedicine*, 17: 6.

4. Clippinger, K. (2007). *Dance anatomy and kinesiology*. Champaign. IL: Human Kinetics.

5. Clippinger-Robertson, K. (1987). Flexibility for Aerobics and Fitness. Seattle Sports Medicine Seminar.

6. Cornelius, W. (1990). Modified PNF stretching: improvement in hip flexion." *National Strength and Conditioning Association Journal NSCA*, 12 44–46.

7. Dumas, G.A., Adams, M.A., & Dolan, P. (1998). Pregnancy-related changes in hip and trunk flexibility: A pilot study. Presented at the North American Congress on Biomechanics, Waterloo, Ontario, Canada,

8. Etnyre, B., & Lee, E. (1988). Chronic and acute flexibility of men and women using three different stretching techniques. *Research Quarterly for Exercise and Sport*, 59.3: 222–228.

9. Fasen, J.M., O'Connor, A.M., Schwartz, S.L., Watson, J.O., Plastaras, C.T., Garvan, C.W., Bulcao, C., Johnson, S.C., & Akuthota, V. (2009). A randomized controlled trial of hamstring stretching: Comparison of four techniques. *Journal of Strength & Conditioning Research*, 23(2):660–667, March.

10. Guissard, N., & Duchateau, J. (2006). Neural Aspects of Muscle Stretching. *Exercise & Sport Sciences Reviews*, 34(4):154–158, October.

11. Hortobagyi, T., et al. (1985). Effects of intense 'stretching' flexibility training on the mechanical profile of the knee extensors and on the range of motion of the hip joint. *International Journal of Sports Medicine*, 6 317–321.

12. Hough, P.A., Ross, E.Z., & Howatson, G. (2009). Effects of dynamic and static stretching on vertical jump performance and electromyographic activity. *Journal of Strength & Conditioning Research*, 23(2):507–512, March.

13. Layne, V.A., & Fitzpatrick, J.J. (2008). Stretching midlife maladies away: A guide for women. *Nurse Practitioner*, 33(12):33–38, December.

14. Luttgens, K., & Hamilton, N. (1997). *Kinesiology: Scientific Basis of Human Motion* (9th ed.). Boston, MA: McGraw-Hill,

15. McAtee, R.E., & Charland, J. (1999). *Facilitated stretching*. Champaign, IL: Human Kinetics.

16. Perez, M., & Fumasoli, S. (1984). Benefit of proprioceptive neuromuscular facilitation on the joint mobility of youth-aged female gymnasts with correlations for rehabilitation. *American Corrective Therapy Journal*, 38(6), 142–146.

17. Roundtable. (1984). Flexibility. *National Strength and Conditioning Association Journal*, (August/September): 10–73.

18. Ryan, A.J., & Stephens, R.E. (1988). *The dancer's complete guide to healthcare and a long career*. Chicago, IL: Bonus.

19. Shellock, F.G., & Prentice, W.E. (1985). Warming-up and stretching for improved performance and prevention of sports-related injuries." *Sports Medicine*, 2 267–278.

20. Wilson, G., et al. (1992). Shorten cycle performance enhancement through flexibility training. *Medicine & Science in Sports & Exercise*, 24 116–123.

21. Wilson, G., Elliot, B.C., & Wood, G.A. (1991). Optional stiffness of the series elastic component in a stretch-shorten cycle activity. *Journal of Applied Physiology*, 70, 825–833.

23 Balance and Coordination: Key Components to Overall Fitness

Judy Gantz, MA, CMA

Focus

The group exercise class is full of bodies bobbing up and down. Across the room, an exerciser is moving with grace and precision while another participant is struggling with what foot to use and over what direction to go. What accounts for the dramatic difference in movement? The precise and controlled mover has mastered coordination, the component that is often underplayed and overlooked in fitness programs.

Training for strength or aerobic endurance requires moving in patterns that use specific amounts of speed and force. The ability to move with accurate form, fluidity, balance, and control is determined by our coordination. When coordination is poor, joint alignment suffers and a multitude of strains and tears can occur. To avoid injury, one must exercise with biomechanical precision. For this reason, coordination is actually the foundation for all other fitness components.

Responding Neuromuscularly

Human movement takes place only as a result of neuromuscular activity. The simple action of taking a step involves a series of neuromuscular commands. Muscles are programmed to work in concert, creating primary joint actions while simultaneously calling into play muscles to stabilize, neutralize, and extend in their opposite directions. Although we often think of "working the hamstrings," the brain does not perceive single muscle commands. Bending the knee involves a series of neuromuscular changes that are learned, practiced, and remembered in sequences and patterns.

When we exercise, our movements are learned as sequences of action. Holding a barbell and squatting up and down is not only developing strength, but programming the nervous system in a particular coordination pattern. Any error in our coordination produces faulty alignment, better known as improper technique. Moving with improper technique offsets bony articulation and places undue stress on the soft tissues, cartilage, and muscles surrounding the joints. Our soft tissues—ligaments, fascia, tendons—were not designed to withstand high degrees of compressive forces. It is our bones and, to a degree, cartilage that have the capacity to withstand impactive loads. For this reason, having poor coordination (especially when moving strenuously) can contribute to injury.

Well-coordinated movement is characterized by minimal expenditure of energy, while simultaneously producing force and applying it in the most advantageous direction. In teaching group exercise classes, how often have you given students corrections to keep their lower backs from hyperextending when executing a routine? When lifting weights, people also need careful instruction in how to maintain form and avoid awkward positions that will stress the spine, knees, or shoulders. Once we have mastered coordination and movement efficiency, our actions look controlled and graceful. For some this comes naturally; for others it is a fitness component that must be learned, cultivated, and practiced.

Fitness instructors can play an important role in helping an exerciser move with greater precision. The attention an instructor gives to correcting body position in any exercise activity is the first step in teaching coordination.

> *Coordination =*
>
> *Correct form and technique =*
>
> *Efficient movement*

Proprioceptive Feedback

Developing coordination demands learning how to sense and feel how the body moves through space. The "movement sense" or kinesthetic perception involves proprioceptive feedback, which tells us where the joints are positioned and how muscles exert effort. The kinesthetic and proprioceptive mechanisms rely on an ebb and flow of information between the sensory and motor neurons of the nervous system.

Kinesthetic Knowledge

Our sensory system detects movement information and sends this to the nervous system for processing. Sensory feedback detects errors in coordination, for example, when someone feels his or her lower back hyperextending during an exercise. The response from the sensory information comes from the motor neurons which produce muscle action and movement. The motor system processes the response of how to correct those errors, and feeds into our "kinesthetic knowledge," educating the neuromuscular system for error correction. The interplay of how the sensory and motor responses are organized varies the degree of force, timing, and muscular control.

Coordination has been defined by medical expert Hans Kraus as the "well-timed and well-balanced functioning together of several muscles in a single movement." Coordination requires training the neuromuscular system through repetition and feedback so the chosen movement activity becomes efficient.

Efficient movement is impossible without the smooth function of the nervous system. In any movement, all the systems of the body are brought into play and work through the nervous system to produce balance, timing, and muscular control.

Elements of Coordination

The three main elements of coordination are as follows.
- **Balance Control**—The ability to adjust the center of gravity effectively to any base, stationary, or moving.
- **Timing Control**—Setting and following the rhythm of a motion.
- **Muscular Control**—The ability to relax and keep muscles un-contracted if they are not needed for the execution of a movement.

Developing balance, timing, and muscular control is a complex learning process. When you are teaching adults, remember to provide:
1) awareness and conscious attention to various movement patterns;
2) feedback and instruction to gain kinesthetic skills in error detection and error correction; and
3) successful practice to establish new and accurate coordination patterns.

Learning to move in new ways is a complicated phenomenon. All elements of coordination work together, but for purpose of explanation, each area will be looked at individually. Suggestions will be given about how to incorporate coordination principles into teaching practices and warm-up routines.

Balance Control

Developing a kinesthetic sense for balance requires learning how to shift weight. Weight shifting is the ability to mobilize the center of weight (located in the pelvis in an upright position), for the purpose of changing spatial directions or levels. Weight shifting informs the mover what foot is bearing the body's weight. Many students who feel clumsy in aerobic dance lack the kinesthetic perception of knowing how, where, or when to shift their weight. Mastering balance control makes picking up exercise combinations much easier.

The following methods will assist in teaching the skill of weight shifting.

1. Begin by having participants focus awareness on the pelvis. The pelvis is the center of weight when standing and transfers weight through the legs, feet, and ground surface.

2. Slowly transfer or shift weight from right foot to left foot in directions of front-back, side-side, and diagonals front and back. Give feedback if the weight shifting is occurring with proper alignment through the spine, hips, knees, and ankles.

3. Design routines that shift weight through space on two feet and in various directions. Include moves that shift from two feet to one and hold balance on one leg.

4. Observe how participants perceive the accuracy of their movement. Do they know when and how the weight is shifting? Can they self-correct, or do they still need more feedback from the instructor? Observe and ask questions of your participants. Give them feedback.

Timing Control

All movement takes place in time with specific rhythmic structures. How quickly you shift weight or the timing used to move up and down from a step is timing control.

The following methods will assist you in teaching the skill of timing.

- Clap the rhythm while standing in place. (This is similar to what some instructors do as a lead-in to warm-up.) Add clapping and step-together in a slow weight-shift pattern. Establish that the participant can hear and perform the clap with accuracy.

- Start with moves that are slow and even. Add speed and rhythmic complexity to increase skill level. Ask the participants to count and observe if their tempo speeds up or slows down drastically.

- Move the whole body in one rhythm. Do not split up body parts, such as having the feet do one rhythm and the arms another.

- Observe how participants perceive the accuracy of their timing. Do they know when to initiate a move? Can they self-correct their timing to match the instructor's or do they still need more feedback and assistance?

Muscular Control

Coordinated moves always look effortless, even when they're not. The ability to engage just the right amount of muscular effort comes with fine-tuning motion in every practice. When extra muscles are contracted or hold tension without purpose, our coordination is impaired and we look tight or awkward. Learning how to relax unnecessary muscle tension is a very important aspect of coordination.

Muscle control also involves executing actions that integrate the body parts. When our trunk (spine and pelvis) and limbs (arms and legs) move as a whole, every part looks connected and the flow of motion produces fluidity and precision. Many deep muscles connect the limbs to the spine, and most often the spine is either the stabilizer or initiator of the movement. When an exerciser lifts a weight overhead, the spine stabilizes the work of the arms. In a pitcher's throw, the spine and pelvis give mobilizing power and thrust to the arm.

The following methods will assist in teaching muscular control.

- Demonstrate how to initiate a move, emphasizing where the movement starts in the body and what areas stabilize. For example, when a person presses a weight overhead, the spine stays held in upright alignment, while the arms lift and push upwards.
- Make corrections when extra muscle tension is used during an action. Give clear instructions to move or relax a joint area, such as, "Move the shoulders up when the weight is lifted." Telling a participant not to use a single muscle, such as the trapezius, is not as useful as identifying the specific body areas, such as the shoulder area. Check to be sure the feedback is understood by watching the participant execute an action without instructions. It can be helpful to use various methods of feedback, such as touch (kinesthetic), verbal instructions (auditory), or a mirror (visual).
- Teach exercises that use the whole body in one action, then trade off with exercises that isolate body parts. For example, lead a warm-up that reaches high with the arms, torso, and legs; alternate with smaller, isolating actions for the shoulders, hips, or trunk.
- For the participant who carries a great deal of tension, or may have difficulty with overall sequencing of movement, additional relaxation exercises and somatic therapy techniques, such as Bartenieff Fundamentals, Feldenkrais, Alexander, Body/Mind Centering, or stretching and yoga, will assist in developing the kinesthetic sense to identify muscle tension and learn how to release it.

Summary

Many skillful movement and fitness professionals already teach coordination principles when they correct exercise form. The growth of the somatic movement field (e.g., Bartenieff Fundamentals, Feldenkrais, Alexander, Body/Mind Centering, etc.) offers more in depth learning of developmental movement patterns, body connectedness, and kinesthetic awareness. Incorporating somatic principles into fitness training will build greater movement awareness and coordination. As with all fitness elements, every person has genetic gifts that seem to enable them to excel in strength, aerobic endurance, flexibility, or coordination. The challenge for a group exercise instructor or personal fitness trainer is to create balanced programs that work all areas of fitness development for the beginner to the advanced participant or client. Each type of exercise—especially those associated with sport and dance—should provide knowledge of how to master correct form and movement efficiency while improving physical conditioning. Every fitness program stands to benefit from including instruction in coordination.

References

1. Allison, N. (Ed.). (1999). *The illustrated encyclopedia of body-mind disciplines.* New York, NY: Rosen Publishing Group.
2. Bartenieff, I. (1980). *Body movement: Coping with the environment.* New York, NY: Gordon & Breach.
3. Barker, S. (1981). *The alexander technique.* New York, NY: Beaufort Books, Inc.
4. Cohen, B.B. (1993). *Sensing, feeling, and action.* Northampton, MA: Contact Editions.
5. Eddy, M. (1991). An overview of the science and somatics of dance. *Kinesiology and Medicine for Dance,* 14(1), 20-28.

6. Gantz, J. (1998). Science and health-therapeutic practices; Section VIII in *International encyclopedia of dance*. New York, NY: Oxford University Press.

7. Hackney, P. (1998). *Making connections: Total body integration through Bartenieff fundamentals*. Amsterdam: Gordon and Breach.

8. Latash, M.L. (1998). *Progress in motor control*. Champaign, IL: Human Kinetics.

9. Latash, M.L., & Zatsiorsky, V.M. (2001). *Classics in movement science*. Champaign, IL: Human Kinetics.

10. Schmidt, R.A., & Wrisberg, C.A. (1999). *Motor learning and performance*. Champaign, IL: Human Kinetics.

Part 6

Fitness: Theory & Practice

How to Teach— Multitraining™

Aquatic Exercise

Cardio Kickboxing

Circuit and Interval Training

Indoor Cycling

Resistance Training in the Group Exercise Setting: Utilizing Free Weights, Resistance Tubing, and/or Body Weight Exercises

Mat Science: An Integration of Basic Conditioning, Dance, Pilates, and Yoga Activities

Sports Conditioning

Step Training

24 *Aquatic Exercise*

Mary E. Sanders, PhD

Focus

A collective "ahhh" emerges from the group of women who step slowly into the pool. Laughter, light conversation, and vigorous yet nimble movements create an experience of shared joy.

Together, they've discovered a private liquid weight room that offers natural support for freedom of movement. The resistive and supportive environment also provides a time-efficient exercise modality for cardio-resistance training with the fear of falling washed away.

Health Trends

Current public health trends, such as rising obesity rates, coupled with an aging population and climbing health care costs signal a call to new action. We all know that exercise is essential, but some people may have chronic or age-related conditions that limit their ability to perform physical activity on land.

Barriers to exercise include fear of falling, pain, discomfort, and not being fit enough to participate.(1) Aquatic exercise has shown promise as an effective, comfortable, and safe option for people who are unable to perform traditional physical activity.(2) Water's natural resistance and buoyancy allow people with physical limitations to take charge of their own health by adopting exercise as medicine.

Water Exercise Solutions for Health

More scientific research is needed, but there is already promising evidence that supports aquatic exercise for health. The comfort, safety, and effectiveness of water can help people overcome some barriers so they feel confident to use exercise as medicine for both treatment and prevention of a variety of conditions. The following studies show the value of aquatic exercise in key areas.

Weight management. The properties of water make it a safe, effective environment in which to build muscular endurance and expend kilocalories for energy. By minimizing the pounding impact of gravity against the joints, water provides a more comfortable setting for vigorous exercise. This makes the aquatic workout an excellent option for many older adults, including those focused on weight loss or maintenance.

In the water, the cost of energy rises as the speed of movement increases, making water exercise an efficient mode for spending stored energy. For example, running in shallow water at maximal effort can burn an estimated 17 kcal per minute.(3) To sustain this level of intensity for a longer period, one must develop muscular endurance. Short running bouts added to water programs increase the kcal cost of any workout, while muscular endurance gradually improves.

In one study, healthy older women (average age 66.4) performed shallow water exercises at intensity levels recommended by the American College of Sports Medicine (ACSM), and achieved positive training results for cardiorespiratory conditioning and weight management.(4)

In another study, researchers combined diet plus water exercise and land-based walking for a weight loss program. Forty-four obese, sedentary women with a BMI of 34.9, (mean age 40), were randomly assigned to an aquatic exercise and walking on land combination group or a land walking only group for 16 weeks. In the combination group, total body weight, cardiorespiratory fitness, flexibility,

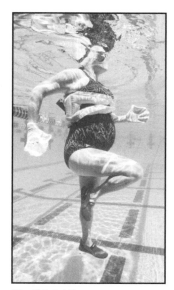

Fig. 24-1. Water accommodates individual differences. Here, a pregnant marathon runner continues her training without impact.

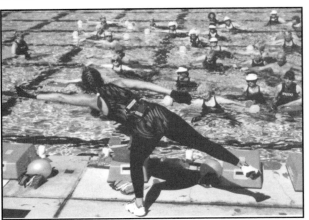

Fig. 24-2. Increased Range Without Fear of Falling—Golden Waves Participants (Reno, Nevada)

strength, and health-related quality of life significantly improved over time similar to the land-only walking group. Slightly greater non-significant losses in body weight, improvements in flexibility, greater attendance rates, and significantly greater enjoyment scores were reported for the combination group.(5)

This suggests that aquatic exercise in combination with walking can serve as an alternative to walking alone for women during periods of weight loss, and leads to improved functional status.

Deep water running using a buoyancy device for support may provide an effective and comfortable alternative to land-based walking or running. It is a non-impact option for vigorous exercise that contributes to total exercise energy expenditure for weight management, cardiorespiratory conditioning, and muscular endurance all during one session. Estimated kcal expenditure for deep water jogging ranges from 8–16 kcal/minute based on intensity.(6) This range compares to running on land at a pace of 8–11 minutes per mile.

Healthy hearts and bodies. Aquatic immersion decreases circulatory resistance and improves heart contraction efficiency. Patients participating in aquatic exercise were found to have significantly improved muscle function and exercise capacity while reporting nearly a 40% improvement in quality of life.(7)

In one study, older adults (60 to 75 years of age, average age 68) experienced a 6% improvement in back extension strength by performing self-paced, vigorous shallow water exercise that included walking backwards for 60 minutes per session, 3 days per week for 12 weeks.(8)

Additionally, the subjects improved significantly in cardiorespiratory endurance and body composition, muscle power for knee extension/flexion, vertical jumping, and side-step agility.

In other research, a 16-week U.S. pilot study included women (60 to 89 years of age) who self-selected to an aquatic exercise group or a control group. Replicated in Japan, women (50 to 80 years of age) volunteered to participate in an ongoing community-based program, self-selecting to attend 1, 2, or 3 days a week. In the United States, the exercise group improved sit-to-stand performance by 31% and walking speed by 16%, while the control group did not change significantly. In Japan, sit-to-stand improved by 22% after 52 weeks of training and walking speed improved by 9% after 40 weeks of training. Neither group reported any injuries.(9)

The Unique Benefits of Water

According to Carol Kennedy-Armbruster, lecturer and former program director of fitness and wellness at Indiana University, "Water should be regarded as any other resistance device. To not include water as part of the training program means that you're leaving out a piece of equipment important as a training choice."(10) At Indiana University, learning how water fits into a resistance progression program is part of the training for all personal fitness trainers. Along with bands, balls, machines, and weights, water should be considered as part of the exercise repertoire of every trainer. Let's examine some of water's unique benefits in this regard.

- **Lifetime Skills**

  Water provides a private and safe multi-dimensional environment, in which lifetime exercise skills (e.g., walking) are developed and can be performed as your body changes over time. Swimming skills are not necessary with vertical water exercise, but participants will need to learn how to coordinate arms and legs to work effectively through water's resistance and buoyancy.

- **Buoyancy**

  Buoyancy encourages freedom of movement, without the fear of falling down. Participants practice large ranges of motion and challenge both balance and recovery-to-stand skills with ease and support (Figure 24-2). Higher intensity jump training, especially for athletes, can be performed in water with lower risk of injury.(11)

  Due to buoyancy, impact can be personally adjusted from about 50% of body weight at waist depth to zero in deep water, making the exercises comfortable (Figure 24-1). Beginning exercisers, participants with balance problems, or those who need to limit impact can easily adjust intensity according to personal need by working in shallow (navel to nipple depth), transitional (shoulder depth), or deep water (fully suspended without feet touching the bottom).

- **Hydrostatic Pressure**

  Hydrostatic pressure pushes against the chest and body. This helps strengthen the breathing system, and as a result, breathing on land becomes easier.(12) Hydrostatic pressure aids venous circulation and contributes to reduction in edema or swelling, and is especially helpful for prenatal participants.

- **Functional Rehabilitation**

  Aquatic therapy has been documented to be beneficial for functional rehabilitation resulting from injury or disease.(13) However, if rehabilitation is required, the services of physical or occupational therapists or other health care providers will be necessary to design specific progressions so that participants continue their exercise program using the gentle buoyancy of water to modify, protect, and help heal the affected area.

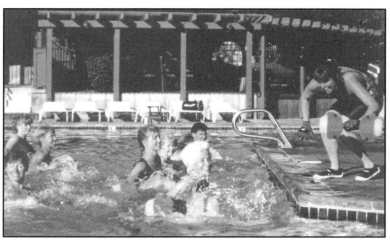

Fig. 24-3. Participants of all ages and fitness levels can participate in a class together, individually modifying intensity as needed.

- **On-Demand Resisted Movement**

  Liquid resistance surrounds the body during water-based exercise, providing on-demand work in many planes of movement, overloading and mimicking real life movements. The resistance of movement performed at an average speed in water is estimated to be approximately 12 to 15 times that of air-based exercise, given that water is about 800 times more dense than air.(14) Since all movements can be resisted in the water, muscular conditioning can be completed in a time efficient program. For example, biceps and triceps can be overloaded concentrically during the same exercise. Group resistance training

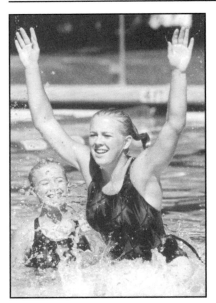

Fig. 24-4. Sports—Volley Jump

is popular, and the "liquid weight machine" of water, along with a variety of equipment for overload, allows participants to individualize resistance work while exercising in a group.

• **Time Efficient, Integrated Cardiorespiratory Resistance Training**
Integrated cardiorespiratory and strength classes are a top fitness trend. Water provides an opportunity for time efficient training during a single session with crossover training. For example, muscular conditioning exercises for the upper body can be designed to use the lower body vigorously enough to contribute to cardiorespiratory work.

• **Water Power**
The harder and faster you push through water, the greater the resistance is against the body. Because speed is used to increase resistance, water is also an effective modality for power training. Important power muscles used during walking, such as the gastrocnemius, were shown to have greater activity during water walking when compared to walking on land at the same speed.(15)

• **Individualized Progressive Training**
Intensity progressions are individual, and intensity is regulated "on demand" using variations in speed, surface area, equipment, and water currents. Group exercise resistance classes can be "individualized" in the pool by allowing participants to choose their own equipment, regulate their own speed (by not working on the beat of the music), and by working either in a stationary or traveling mode (Figure 24-3).

• **Compound Movement Patterns**
Compound patterns, such as lifting a load while jogging, can be safely overloaded at slower speeds (1/2 to 1/3 compared to land) for training proper biomechanics during functional living patterns (e.g., walking, gripping/releasing, and balancing all at the same time).

• **Intensity and Volume Without Risks**
By using buoyancy and resistance, participants may be able to pace themselves as they gradually increase the volume and intensity of training, while working more comfortably with less impact and without increasing risk of orthopedic injury.

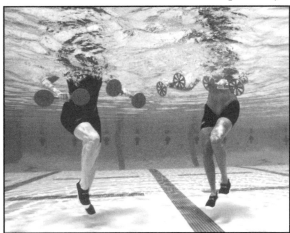

Fig. 24-5. Fitness paddles can be used at different settings. Closed for high intensity; open for lower intensity.

• **Core Time**
Water currents work constantly against the body while immersed in water to continuously challenge the trunk core muscles to maintain proper alignment, stop, start, and change directions during a movement. The abdominals work throughout the class, functionally…vertically!

• **Purposeful Play**
People of many ages, fitness levels, and abilities can put water resistance and buoyancy to work, mimicking fun sports drills. Water's buoyancy allows participants to pretend they are skiing moguls by lifting both legs off the bottom, or playing volleyball by running, scooping arms under for a serve, and then jumping for a block! In addition, water minimizes impact while slowing movement speed to check form and provides overload through the entire pattern of movement (Figure 24-4).

- **Posture, Posture, Posture**
  Water's buoyancy and currents stimulate the postural muscles constantly as participants try to maintain balance, stabilize, and change positions. Moving the body from horizontal to vertical provides unique trunk work that may translate to postural control, balance improvement, and movement corrections on the land.

Effective Water Design

Instructors and personal fitness trainers must understand the difference between land and water with regard to exercise design. For example, on land, gravity and an iron dumbbell provide concentric muscular work during a standing biceps curl, while in the water, the same movement, performed slowly with a buoyant dumbbell, works the triceps group eccentrically! Understanding water's influence on the body is essential in designing effective target training in a liquid environment.

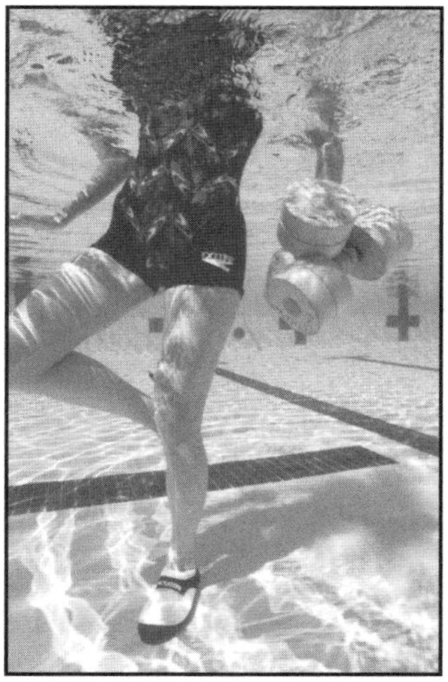

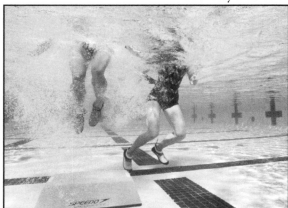

Fig. 24-6. Standing with Foam Dumbbells—Buoyancy-resisted Triceps Press and Balance Work

Pool Supervision

The YMCA of the USA recommends having an appropriate number of lifeguards on duty during any activity in the pool area. During a water fitness class, it would be the sole duty of the lifeguard to supervise participants; a water exercise instructor, even if certified as a lifeguard, should not assume both duties. As an instructor, be sure to comply with the regulations in your area concerning pool safety standards and required supervision during your activity classes.(6)

Choosing a Water Depth

Participants can work in three depths of water: (a) shallow (navel to nipple), (b) transitional (nipple to top of the shoulder), and (c) deep (any depth at which the feet cannot touch bottom). The depth you choose depends on your facility, the objective of the workout, equipment availability, the skill level of your participants, and their body composition. Each person responds differently to water based on body composition and body fat deposition. Teach proper neutral stance (ears, shoulders, and hips lined up) and remind participants frequently to correct alignment as needed, since buoyancy pushes and pulls on the body. Additionally, participant comfort and safety is essential! Basic safety skills, such as recovering from a fall to a stand in shallow water or moving from horizontal to a vertical position in deep water, must be mastered for safety and confidence!

A person who needs to reduce impact (perhaps due to an injury) may want to work out in deep water using a buoyancy belt for support. On the other hand, a participant who wants to improve a functional skill, such as speed walking, would most likely choose shallow water, which more closely mimics land activity. Each water depth requires unique exercises designed specifically for that depth.

Water Temperature

The temperature of the water will dictate exercise design. Cardiovascular work cannot be safely performed in water that is too warm, while gentle range of motion work

Fig. 24-7. Jumping on Step

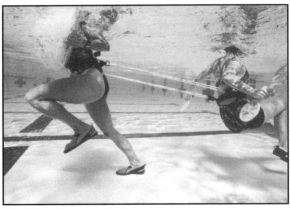

Fig. 24-8. Tethers—Pulling Partner

would be uncomfortable for participants when the water is cold. Thermal regulation must be considered during your exercise and program design. For example, in warm water, low-intensity exercises with frequent water breaks may be appropriate. When the water is cool, having clients jog during upper body muscular work may help keep them warm. An appropriate water temperature for most fitness classes is 83–86° F (29–30° C), with 84° F (29° C) as an approximate neutral temperature at which most people can balance heat loss with heat production during exercise for comfort.(17)

Individualized Intensity Regulation

Participants need to develop skills to help them feel the water and discover their own resistance levels by practicing movements through progressions. Speed, surface area, water's currents, and buoyancy are used to target both work and rest. Research indicates that since water is resistive, interval training may create the most effective cardiorespiratory workout.(18,19) Equipment can be used to target appropriate muscular overload, and different devices may be needed for different muscle groups. For example, webbed gloves may be sufficient overload for triceps work, while the biceps may require the larger surface area of a fitness paddle (Figure 24-5).

Equipment Applications

In the water, iron weights are replaced by foam dumbbells and some gravity-based tools, where poundage is replaced by resistance and gravity. Instructors need to understand the purpose of the equipment, and how it affects both exercise design and safety skills for participants. Each tool offers its own unique program.

Surface area equipment provides resistance in all directions through the water, and along with speed, can dramatically affect overload. Examples of such equipment include (a) webbed gloves, (b) fins, (c) non-buoyant dumbbells, and (d) parachutes.

Buoyancy equipment enhances the buoyancy of the limbs or body and includes buoyancy dumbbells, belts, and noodles. The body and/or limbs are assisted upward while movements downward are resisted (the opposite effect of gravity on land) (Figure 24-6).

Buoyancy/surface area combination tools are bulky enough to provide effective surface area drag, and include kickboards (held sideways), buoyant dumbbells, and ankle cuffs. Resistance can now be experienced in both upward and downward directions in relation to the water's surface.

Gravity-based equipment, such as the aquatic step, enhances gravitational load on the lower body. Participants experience more gravity overload while working on top of the step in the shallower water (with buoyancy effect decreased). Jumping movements can be performed faster off the top of the step, creating greater drag resistance against the body, and participants can land

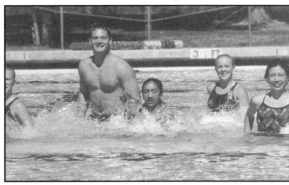

Fig. 24-9. Jogging to Warm Up the Body

either on top of the step for high-intensity work or away from the step (in the deeper water) for lower-intensity drills (Figure 24-7).

Tubing, tethers, and DynaBands are elastic equipment that can be added to increase eccentric work, to further challenge the core stabilizers, and to create fun and safe tether-together team drills, especially popular for sports cross-training (Figure 24-8).

Designing Water Exercises for Health

All movements should be designed with regard to the water's effects of buoyancy and resistance acting on the body. With that in mind, we can think of the pool as a liquid weight machine that provides resistance in most directions. Buoyancy assists movement upward and supports the body. Progressive exercises can be designed by making small variations in movement speed and range of motion, by working in either a stationary or traveling mode, and finally by adding equipment to increase overload. Participants can choose to work anywhere within the progression that fits their fitness level. Below are some sample shallow water exercises and their progression.

Conditioning Segment with Warm-Up

- Buoyancy and Cardiorespiratory Warm-Up (Figure 24-9)
  Review personal skills, such as sculling and recovery to a stand. Cue a basic move, such as jogging, to warm up the body, gradually increasing heart rate, and adjust the body to buoyancy.
  Progression: Begin jogging slowly and gradually increase the range of motion of the legs, then the speed, and finally travel through the water for the highest intensity. Check intensity using the talk test (i.e., being able to speak an entire sentence without gasping) and rate of perceived exertion.

- Cardiorespiratory Endurance (Figure 24-10)
  Cardiorespiratory endurance exercises focus on working the large muscles of the lower body. A simple basic move, such as a scissors or cross-country ski, can be varied by changing the "working positions" of the body vertically.
  Progression: Arms and legs work in opposition for balance. Intensity can be changed by choosing a working position of level 1: neutral (feet tap and slide along the pool bottom for support, chest and arms are submerged); level 2: rebound (push forcefully off the pool floor for a jumping-type movement); and level 3: suspended (feet never touch the bottom, mimicking deep water work). Monitor intensity by using the talk test and perceived exertion.

- Muscular Endurance (Figure 24-11)
  Participants may choose to use various surface area equipment to provide the right amount of overload for them. Remember—the larger the piece, the greater the resistance. ACSM guidelines recommend 8–15 repetitions for each major muscle group.(15)
  Progression: Stabilize in a lunge and slowly practice full range of motion, targeting the rotator cuff. Check for

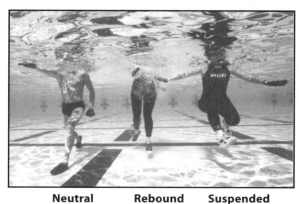

Neutral   Rebound   Suspended

Fig. 24-10. Cardiorespiratory—Scissors Demonstrated in Three Working Positions

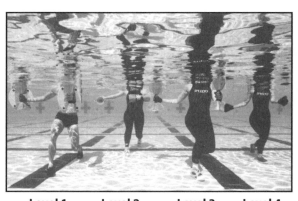

Level 1   Level 2   Level 3   Level 4

Fig. 24-11. Muscular Endurance—Underwater Rotator Cuff Exercise

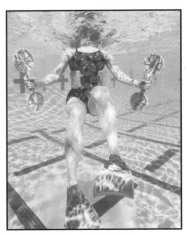

Fig. 24-12. Deep Water Cardiorespiratory and Resistance Using Paddles and Fins

proper alignment (ears and shoulders lined up, shoulders down and back, wrist in line with the forearm). Add force through the movement, increase the force, and travel backward to increase intensity again. Jog for warmth and release your grip on equipment between sets.

- Cardiorespiratory/Resistance Combination (Figure 24-12)
  Cardiorespiratory and resistance work can be targeted in water by combining high-intensity leg and upper body exercises.
  Progression: Stabilize seated position, by cueing tight abdominals, shoulders down and back, and chest up. Slowly practice fin kicking and then add the arm work for the upper back (arms move from front to the side and allow the currents to float the arms back to the front for a passive recovery). Increase intensity by kicking harder, traveling with greater speed, and by pushing faster during arm work.

- Functional Training for ADL
  Participants can improve gripping and releasing, walking and balancing by performing exercises that target multiple tasks.
  Progression: Grip and release a small sponge ball while walking forward and backwards. Increase difficulty by working the squeeze/release as the arms change positions, from overhead to under the water to diagonals, and increase the size of the stride and the speed of the walk as you change directions (forward and backwards, then on diagonals and sideways).

- Sports-Based Team Training (Figure 24-13)
  Team training is fun and effective for participants who like competition and partner work. Tethered together, each of two partners alternates between being the runner (dragging his or her partner as resistance equipment) for cardiorespiratory work, and being the "human parachute," opening and closing arms and legs for hip adductor and pectoral muscle endurance work.
  Progression: Runner runs faster, then zig zags the pattern, while the "human parachute" can spread the fingers of the webbed gloves, and open the arms and legs more fully and close them more forcefully.

- Warm-Down (Water Cool-Down) and Flexibility: Buoyancy Assisted Stretching (Figure 24-14)
  Buoyant dumbbells help assist a chest and shoulder stretch, and support the body to allow the legs to work a bicycle pattern, keeping participants warm.
  Progression: Open the arms wider, bicycle faster to increase the effects of water currents that enlarge the range of motion of the arms.

Designing a Class

Basic class formats are similar to those designed on land. Participants should understand the objective of the set and be allowed to use progressions to regulate intensity. A sample framework could include an orientation to water, safety and basic skills review, followed by a thermal and cardiorespiratory warm-up. The conditioning segment can alternate cardiorespiratory and muscular endurance sets (circuit style), or as continuous segments of each (but remember to use intervals throughout to provide rest). Additional sets can be included that target sports or functional ADL drills (sit to stand, stair climbing), dynamic

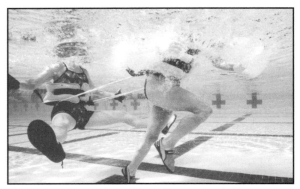

Fig. 24-13. Sports-Based Team Training with Human Parachute and Tethers

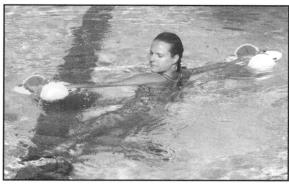

Fig. 24-14. Buoyancy Stretching Using Buoyancy Dumbbells and Cycling

flexibility patterns (reaching, leaping), or a fun play set (choreography, noodle tug of war). A warm-down completes the class to prepare participants for land.

Build an Amphibious Team!

A combination of land and water programs targeting health objectives can provide a lifetime of balanced exercise options. Market your water and land programs together as healthy lifestyle activities that complement each other. Cross-train yourself professionally by learning to teach both land and water classes effectively, and understand the benefits of each mode, helping participants develop a balanced exercise program.

New Waves

New developments offer more opportunities and accessibility to aquatic exercise. Pools with smaller footprints use a smaller space at a reasonable cost. These small pools that accommodate one to eight people can include in-floor treadmills to adjust speed, adjustable water depth with zero-depth entry, multi-directional jets for functional overload resistance and massage, and underwater cameras that allow trainers to view underwater body mechanics from the deck. Small pools can broaden the variety of training options available for a more diverse population.

Trainers can integrate water exercise into an overall program that addresses safety and individual needs.

Water-based exercises can safely provide training choices for people who need to work at a lower intensity and/or impact than land exercise, or those who are at high risk of falling.

Programs that encourage people to go at their own pace and those that provide safe and effective protocols based on current scientific evidence hold the most promise. Trends in aquatic exercise options broaden the opportunities for seniors to make lifestyle changes using exercise as medicine.

Summary

Explore the benefits of water by expanding your instructor training to include the pool. Data was analyzed for 10,518 women and 35,185 men, 20–88 years of age who participated in activities at the Cooper Institute Clinic, Dallas, Texas. Investigators learned that long time runners and swimmers have similar health benefits over time. These health benefits were found to be greater even when compared to people who chose walking as their primary lifetime activity.[20] Discover with your participants how to add variety to their training by broadening their exercise choices. Learn how to use the technical water environment, and then share the skills for a lifetime of purposeful activity, health, and fun!

Water Fitness Training Resources

ACSM (American College of Sports Medicine): (317) 637-9200; www.acsm.org

AEA (Aquatic Exercise Association): (888) AEA-WAVE; aeawave.com

AFAA Japan: 81-3-5915-1701; afaa.com

Aqua Fitness Home Study (AFAA): (800) 446-2322; afaa.com

National Swimming Pool Foundation, www.nspf.org

IDEA Health & Fitness Association: (800) 999-IDEA; IDEAfit.com

International Council on Active Aging, and the Journal on Active Aging, www.icaa.cc

International Journal of Aquatic Research and Education, www.HunamnKinetics.com/IJARE

YMCA of the USA: (800) 872-9622; ymca.net

Reference Notes

1. Peterson, J. (2006). 10 (Lame) reasons people commonly give for not exercising. ACSM's *Health & Fitness Journal*, 10(1), 44.

2. Sanders, M., & Maloney-Hills, C. (1998). Aquatic exercise for better living on land. *ACSM's Health & Fitness Journal*, 2(3), 16–23.

3. McArdle, W., Katch, R., & Katch, V. (1991). *Exercise Physiology, Energy, Nutrition and Human Performance* (3rd ed.). Pennsylvania, PA: Lea & Febiger.

4. D'Acquisto, L.J., D'Acquisto, D.M., & Renne, D. (2000). Metabolic and cardiovascular responses in older women during shallow-water exercise. *Journal of Strength and Conditioning Research*, 15(1),12–19.

5. Nagle, E.F., Robertson, R.J., Jakicic, J.J., Otto, A.D., Ranalli, J.R., & Chiapetta, L.B. (2007). Effects of aquatic exercise and walking in sedentary obese women undergoing a behavioral weight-loss intervention. *International Journal of Aquatic Research and Education*, 1, 43–56.

6. Sanders, M. (Ed.). (2000).YMCA, Water Fitness for Health. Champaign, IL: Human Kinetics. Retrieved June 26, 2007, from http://www.dswfitness.com

7. Becker, B. (2007). Healing waters. *Aquatics International*, 19(6),27–32.

8. Takeshima N., Rogers, M.E., Wantanebe, E., Brechue, W.F., Okada, A., Yamada, T., Islam, M.M., & Hayano, J. (2003). Water-based exercise improves health-related aspects of fitness in older women. *Medicine & Science in Sports & Exercise*, 33(3), 544–551.

9. Sanders M.E., Constantino, N.E., Hsieh, J.J., & Rogers, M.E. (2007). Water-based exercise: Transfer of benefits to land for older women in the USA and Japan. *Medicine & Science in Sports & Exercise*, 39(5), Supplement, Abstract E-36.

10. Kennedy-Armbruster, C.A. (2009). Train the trainer. Presented at *ACSM Health & Fitness Summit*, March 27, 2009, Atlanta, GA.

11. Whitehill, J., Constantino, N.L., & Sanders, M.E. (2008). *Cardiorespiratory and body composition responses to a water exercise program for athletes.* ACSM Southwest conference, November 20, 2008, Las Vegas, NV.

12. Becker, B., & Cole, A. (Eds.). (1997). *Comprehensive aquatic therapy.* Newton, MA: Butterworth-Heinemann.

13. Koury, J. (1996). *Aquatic therapy programming guidelines for orthopedic rehabilitation.* Champaign, IL: Human Kinetics.

14. DiPrampero, P.E. (1998). The energy cost of human locomotion on land and in water. *International Journal of Sports Medicine*, 7(2), 55–72.

15. Masumoto, K., & Mercer, J. (2008). Biomechanics of human locomotion in water: An electromyogrpahic analysis. *Exercise and Sport Sciences Reviews*, 36(3), 160–169.

16. Michaud, T., et al. (1995a). Comparative exercise responses of deep-water and treadmill running. *Journal of Strength and Conditioning*, 9(2), 104–109.

17. Sanders, M.E. (2008). Splash! Cultivating a water exercise program for healthy activity using an evaluation approach. Part 1. *Journal on Active Aging*, 7(1), 56–64.

18. Michaud, T., et al. (1995b). Aquarunning and gains in cardiorespiratory fitness. *Journal of Strength and Conditioning*, 9(2), 78–84.

19. Quinn, T., Sedory, D., & Fisher, B. (1994). Physiological effects of deep water running following a land-based training program. *Research Quarterly for Exercise and Sport*, 65, 386–389.

20. Chase, N.L., Sui, X., & Blair, S.N. (2008). Comparison of the health aspects of swimming with other types of physical activity and sedentary lifestyle habits. *International Journal of Aquatic Research and Education*, 2, 151–161.

Photo Credit: Tracy Frankel, Courtesy of WaterFit.com and the YMCA of the USA.

Jill Boyer-Holland and
Linda Romaine, MS,
MBA

25 *Cardio Kickboxing*

Focus

Cardio kickboxing classes, which are based on the movements of technical boxing and tae kwon do, are designed to provide cross-training benefits for consumers within the framework of a general health and fitness program. It is important to keep in mind that your participants are not professional fighters, and that physical limitations vary from person to person. For this reason, many classic self-defense movements will need to be altered for safety and alignment.

Cardio kickboxing is a cardiorespiratory conditioning class, and therefore should include a warm-up consisting of a combination of rhythmic limbering, rehearsal movements, and/or light preparatory stretches when appropriate. Emphasis on preparation of the upper body is necessary due to heavy involvement of the arms, chest, shoulders, and back throughout the punching sequences. This includes warming up and stretching the low back thoroughly in all its ranges of motion. Adequate preparation of the lower body is equally important, as the execution of kicks requires ample flexibility while maintaining proper alignment.

All movements originate from the **ready position**. The stance can face forward or slightly to the side with one foot back (staggered position). In either stance, the feet should be far enough apart to allow for isolated torso movement. Another important consideration is proper hip-knee-toe alignment. In a hip-width stance, most participants will be stable and comfortable with parallel feet; with wider stances, hips and feet should turn out slightly to avoid knee torque. Foot placement, regardless of stance, should resemble the posture commonly used for squats with the knees slightly bent, abdominals contracted, shoulders slightly protracted, elbows bent, arms close to the body, and fists about chin level.

"Bob and weave" or "slipping" movements are lateral torso isolations performed alone or in conjunction with dynamic squats. The addition of these exercises will strengthen quadriceps and buttocks muscles, and improve the ability of the erector spinae, internal and external obliques, and abdominal muscles to stabilize the torso.

Safety and alignment requirements should follow AFAA's *Basic Exercise Standards and Guidelines* (see Chapter 17) with fighting stances modified to accommodate proper hip, knee, and toe alignment. Participants should be spaced far enough apart to allow for full- range-of-motion movements without the danger of accidental contact with other participants or equipment. Cueing is similar to other group exercise classes, but greater emphasis should be placed on the proper execution of movements.

Recommended music speed is 125–135 beats per minute (bpm). This slower speed will ensure enough time to execute all movements through entire range of motion.

Footwork varies from class to class. Many aerobic favorites, such as grapevines, step touches, shuffles, and twists, can be incorporated in the workout to create variety. Three basic class formats are defined below.

1. **Drill Style**—characterized by many repetitions of the same movement sequence; not necessarily in the "combination" or "block" style. This is similar to calisthenics or military style aerobic classes.

2. **Combination Style Choreography**—movements are sequenced in repeatable patterns that follow the phrase of the music.
3. **Freestyle**—can vary from instructor to instructor. Partner drills, group formations, and circuit stations utilizing equipment are common.

The step can be incorporated in kickboxing class, but it is important to remember that step guidelines must be considered in addition to the guidelines discussed in this chapter.

The four basic punches are:

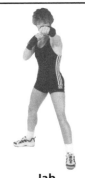
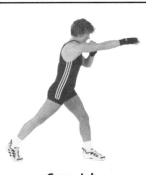
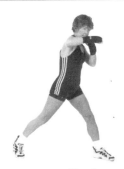
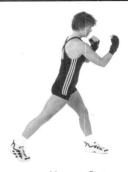

Jab	**Cross Jab**	**Hook**	**Upper Cut**
A straight punch to the front. Wrist pronates down; the torso may or may not rotate. Target point is the upper body or head.	Same as jab, but punch crosses the midline of body, causing the hip, knee, and toe to turn as a unit with the heel elevated. Target point is the upper body or head.	From starting position, abduct the elbow keeping the arm bent at a 90° angle; palm may face down or towards the body. Rotate the torso, hip, knee, and toe as a unit toward the midline with the heel elevated. The rotation of the body will bring the arm around. Punch through your target. Return the elbow to ready position prior to turning the body back to a centered position. Target point is the upper body or head.	Keeping the arm bent at the elbow (90°) and the wrist supinated so that palm is facing the body, hyperextend the shoulder so that the punch arm moves behind the body. Rotate the trunk and tilt the pelvis while flexing the shoulder. Rotate the torso, hip, knee, and toe as a unit toward the midline with the heel elevated. Target point is the ribs or chin.

NOTE: Because the arms are held in the ready position at all times to allow for rapid return, the pressor response may be a concern for some individuals, causing a rise in heart rate that overestimates oxygen consumption.

All kicks contain four phases: (a) chamber, (b) strike, (c) re-chamber, and (d) return. It is important to re-chamber the leg quickly in all kicks to avoid knee injury.

The four basic kicks are:

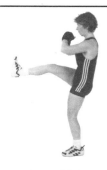 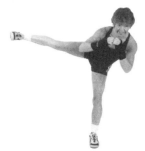 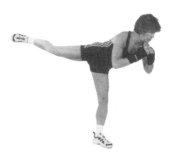 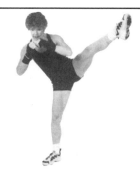

Front Kick	**Side Kick**	**Back Kick**	**Roundhouse Kick**
Flex the hip with the knee bent. Extend the knee once the leg is lifted. Kick is delivered in a thrusting motion. Point of contact is the ball of the foot; target is the opponent's knee or torso.	Abduct the leg with the knee bent. When the leg reaches hip height, extend the knee. Point of contact is the forefoot; target is the opponent's ankles, knees, or torso.	Flexing forward from the hip, rotate the hip laterally and extend at the knee in a thrusting manner. Point of contact is the heel; target is the opponent's ankles, knees, or torso.	With hips open, abduct the kicking leg with the knee bent and pointed toward the target. The knee then extends forward in a slashing movement. Point of contact is the forefoot; target is the opponent's ankle, knee, or upper body including the head. The name "roundhouse" comes from the movements that precede the kick, not from hip movement performed during the kick.

NOTE: During all kicks, the abdominals act as a stabilizer keeping the back in alignment and the pelvis neutral. Participants must have the strength to maintain torso stabilization throughout the workout. Once the kick is landed, the leg is retracted immediately and returned to the ready position. Avoid high kicks that distort proper posture and alignment.

Rate of perceived exertion or the talk test might be a better indicator of exertion level as heart rate can vary greatly depending on class type. All kicks and punches should be stopped at 99% of extension and returned by an active contraction of the antagonist muscle, thus reducing the possibility of injuries due to hyperextension.

Post aerobic cool-down can be followed by isolated conditioning exercises. End of class stretches should target all major muscle groups.

Regardless of the format or style, cardio kickboxing can be a valuable addition to any fitness program as long as safety and form are a priority.

References

1. Aerobics and Fitness Association of America. (2010). *Kickboxing: A manual for instructors.* Sherman Oaks, CA: Aerobics and Fitness Association of America.
2. Boyer, J. (1999). *Boxing basics* course outline, AFAA authorized CEU program.
3. Dopps, B. (1999). Kickboxing explodes in health clubs. *ACE Certified News.* 5(2), 2–3.
4. Dyonn, C. (1999). Triple threat course outline, AFAA authorized CEU program.
5. Kravitz, L. (1999). Fight to be fit. *Ace Fitness Matters.* 5(1), 6–7.
6. Hamilton, N, Weimer, W., & Luttgens, K. (2008). *Kinesiology: Scientific basis of human motion* (11th ed.). Boston, MA: McGraw-Hill.

26 Circuit and Interval Training

Tere Filer, MS, MPH
and Troy DeMond, MA

Focus

Two popular aerobic cross-training methods are: (a) circuit training, and (b) interval training. They are often used by individuals in the maintenance phase of conditioning who want variety in their workouts in order to prevent boredom and injury due to overuse. However, they both offer other benefits and advantages to athletes and special populations.

An advantage they both share is time-efficiency. The duration of a typical circuit or interval workout is 20–30 minutes, not including warm-up and cool-down. Another similarity is the way they use both aerobic and anaerobic metabolic pathways to provide the energy for muscle work. This chapter will explore the principles and methods of designing effective group exercise programs using circuit and interval training.

What is Circuit Training?

Circuit training (CT) is considered one of the basic systems of weight training. It is an efficient and challenging form of conditioning that works well for developing muscular strength and endurance, cardiovascular endurance, stability, balance, and coordination. Typical weight training workouts are conducted in what is called a priority system, which involves working one muscle group or performing one type of exercise to completion and then going on to the next exercise and so on. By contrast, CT involves repeating exercises and muscle group work through a series of stations.

Originally, CT was developed by R.E. Morgan and G.T. Anderson in 1953 at the University of Leeds in England. The term "circuit" refers to a number of exercises arranged consecutively where a participant moves from one station to the next with little (15–30 seconds) or no rest in between each station. The goal is to perform 8 to 20 repetitions at each station using a resistance of about 40–60% of one-repetition maximum (1RM). Each circuit is separated by a longer rest period (approximately 1–3 minutes). A circuit may use exercise machines, hand-held weights, elastic resistance, stability balls, BOSU, calisthenics, or any combination. It is important to design the circuit so that the principal muscles used alternate from station to station to prevent individual muscle fatigue and maintain a consistent heart rate intensity.

For many years, CT was used in schools and athletic facilities to accommodate large volumes of participants in the shortest amount of time with a limited variety of equipment. In fact, expensive equipment or large, bulky machines are not necessary to perform an effective workout. Body weight exercises, such as push-ups, squats, and lunges, are excellent exercises to include in a circuit. CT provides the flexibility of modifying each station to the needs and limitations of the participant's fitness level and space available. From beginner to advanced, CT is considered one of the most efficient modes of accomplishing a complete workout in a short period of time.

Numerous studies have been conducted to compare the effects of circuit weight training on cardiovascular fitness and the cardiovascular disease (CVD) risk factors. Studies evaluating circuit weight training show an average improvement in VO_{2max} of 6%. This compares to an average improvement in VO_{2max} of 18% during typical steady state aerobic activities, such as running, cycling, or

Goals of CT

1. Improved cardiovascular fitness
2. Improved muscle strength and endurance
3. Reduced body fat levels
4. Increased flexibility and injury prevention
5. Improved glucose tolerance and insulin sensitivity
6. Improved serum lipid levels (e.g., total cholesterol, total cholesterol/HDL, and LDL/HDL ratios)
7. Improved self-esteem and emotional fitness

jogging. It may be concluded from this information that circuit weight training should not be the only method used when one of your goals is to improve your cardiovascular fitness. Circuit weight training will, however, sufficiently maintain cardiovascular fitness. To better understand the role of CT in your fitness program, it is important to describe the actual format of a typical circuit weight training workout and some of the variations that could be applied.

Circuit Training (CT) for General Fitness

CT can be completed two to four times per week. As with resistance training, there should be 48 hours between sessions that work the same muscle groups. The following 10 exercises: leg press, bench press, leg curl, lat pull-down, arm curl, seated press, triceps push-down, upright row, leg extension, and seated high row, use all the major muscles in the upper and lower body and would provide a complete whole-body resistance training workout.

For general fitness, a resistance should be chosen that allows the station to be completed for the prescribed period of time (45–90 seconds). Resistance may also be applied by using body weight exercises, free weights, medicine balls, and elastic tubing. Progression can come through either increasing the station time or decreasing the rest intervals. Implement only one change at a time however. A total of one to three circuits is typical with a rest period of 1–3 minutes between each circuit.

This type of circuit can also be used by athletes during closed or off-season training. Two or three circuit resistance training sessions can be interspersed with two to three cross-training cardiovascular workouts. Routines can be developed purely for strength development, for improving endurance, or some combination of the two.

When designing a circuit, each station should work a different muscle or group of muscles so that the overall energy output can be maintained throughout the session. Since each station is performed with maximal effort in a very short period of time, the major energy system being used for this format is the anaerobic glycolytic pathway. The major energy source being utilized is muscle glycogen or stored carbohydrates. The energy cost for a 20-minute circuit workout has been shown to average approximately 200 kcal (less for women than for men). It is an excellent means of burning calories, but stored fat does not play a significant role. Because many exercisers have a concern for weight control, the circuit may take on a variety of changes that will affect the energy pathways utilized as well as the energy sources.

Super Circuits

Super circuit formats include a cardiovascular-type of station incorporated within the circuit of weight training exercises. Equipment, such as a stationary bicycle, stair climber, treadmill, rowing machine, or stepping platform, may be used or the participant may choose to jog in place, jump rope, perform calisthenics (e.g., jumping jacks, high kicks) as the aerobic component. As long as the overall intensity of the workout is maintained, the resulting cardiovascular improvement will be accomplished. By altering the time sequence, the energy pathways utilized will also allow for increased usage of stored fat as an energy source. A common pattern used would be 1 minute of muscle conditioning activity followed by 2–3 minutes of cardiovascular activity. With careful planning, this format could be adapted to a group exercise class.

Peripheral Heart Action System

Peripheral heart action system is a training session divided into several sequences of exercises. A sequence is a group of exercises, each for a different muscle group. The number of repetitions per set of each exercise may vary, but usually 8 to 12 repetitions is the norm. An exercise may combine several muscles or muscle groups or may isolate only one. All of the exercises in the sequence are repeated three times in a circuit fashion before moving on to the next sequence, which will involve doing different exercises for the same muscles. The number of sequences may vary from four to six per session.

The goal of the peripheral heart action system is to keep blood moving from one body part to the next. It is an extremely fatiguing program if a major goal of your workout is to increase cardiovascular endurance. The short rest periods and maintenance of a relatively high heart rate make this program very similar to normal circuit weight training. A cardiovascular station could also be incorporated between the exercise sequences. There is no specified time interval for the exercise sequence as long as the rest periods between exercises are kept short. The following shows a sample four-sequence peripheral heart action session.

Summary—CT

In today's fast-paced society, time efficiency is an important consideration when choosing a workout. CT has always been considered one of the best ways to see good cardiovascular and muscle strengthening results in a shorter exercise time. More dedicated exercisers also recognize the benefit of variety. Whether in a group exercise classroom or in the weight room, you can design a fun, intense, and motivating circuit workout. Be creative by using hand-held weights, balls, tubing, bands, or partner resistance. You may want to set up stations around the room, or if there is enough equipment for each participant, everyone can work simultaneously doing the same exercise. Decide what muscle groups you wish to work and what exercises will best accomplish the goals. Check form and alignment, and practice the exercises without weights or resistance before starting.

Some instructors who teach CT at clubs have a dedicated room with a variety of equipment permanently installed at strategic stations. However, you can also transform any room into a circuit training class using portable equipment. Instructors can develop a loyal following by providing participants with an extremely time-efficient workout that addresses muscular conditioning along with cardiorespiratory training.

Remember, CT is done quickly. In order to achieve the strength training and cardiovascular benefits, the rest periods are kept brief. Emphasize posture, full range of motion, and control through muscle resistance. CT can be an exciting addition to your present workout schedule, especially if you are interested in the benefits of cross-training.

What is Interval Training?

Interval training (IT) combines high- and low-intensity intervals in a single workout. By incorporating IT into their existing exercise programs, group exercise instructors can discover an effective means for training both aerobic and anaerobic systems. Participants can maximize desired fitness results through this unique approach.

Working Aerobic and Anaerobic Systems

The ultimate goal of IT is to push both the aerobic and anaerobic systems to their maximum limits. Alternating brief periods of high-intensity work with low-intensity recovery periods (commonly referred to as the intervals) results in overloading both energy systems. It is important to understand that during steady state exercise, sufficient oxygen is supplied to, and utilized by, the working muscles. Hence, there is a balance between oxygen available for the body's use and the intensity level of the activity.

However, as the exercise intensity is increased to the point that oxygen demands can no longer be met, anaerobic metabolism contributes to the energy requirements of the activity. An example of this would be a sprinter running a fast 440-yard dash and then "actively" recovering with a slow run. Or, a group exercise participant might perform a series of high-intensity power moves for 3 minutes followed by 1 minute of body conditioning work combined with low-intensity squats. Continually incorporating this type of work/rest program into any existing aerobic (cardio) training program will enable your students to reap the many benefits of IT.

Why IT Works

Unlike a program that strictly trains the aerobic system, IT allows your participants to train both the aerobic and anaerobic systems. The greatest concentration for increased oxygen and carbon dioxide exchange occurs during the high-intensity portions. It is at this level of intensity that the accumulation of lactic acid tends to be the greatest. This continual build-up of lactic acid will eventually hinder muscular contraction and overall physical performance. However, by decreasing the intensity for a brief period of time, active recovery can occur because the body's ability to utilize oxygen and deliver nutrients to the working muscles is then increased.

During this decreased intensity portion, the incorporation of hand-held weights, elastic bands or tubing, medicine balls, BOSU, or even calisthenics are excellent ways for your participants to increase muscular strength and endurance and to help eliminate toxic by-products, such as lactic acid. Hence, the participant pushes to an anaerobic training state, promotes muscular strength and endurance while actively recovering, and still remains in an aerobic training state. It is crucial to remember this important point: the participant remains in an aerobic training state if—and only if—the heart rate stays above the training threshold. If the heart rate drops below this level during the active recovery period, the aerobic training state is not maintained.

Making IT Work

Frequency

Research indicates that significant physiological improvements occur if IT is implemented two to three times per week. However, this will vary depending on the present fitness level of your participants and the exercise goals. For example, an individual concerned with improving his/her general fitness level will reap minimal "interval" benefits by participating in IT only one time per week.

A highly trained athlete will gain significant "interval" improvements by participating more times per week. However, as an effective instructor, you must remember that IT can be very stressful at any level of participation. Therefore, be aware of the possibilities of overtraining-related injuries and monitor your programming accordingly. Providing your participants with a safe and effective workout scenario is your number one priority.

Work/Active Recovery Ratio

The work interval is known as the high-intensity portion of the workout. The active recovery interval consists of low-intensity movement. Both combine to make up what is called a cycle. Generally, the number of cycles in a workout is once again dependent on your participants' current fitness levels and exercise goals.

Intensity

> **HR at Low Intensity**
>
> During active recovery periods, the optimal intensity is 55% age-predicted maximum heart rate (HR_{max}). Do not let the heart rate drop below this level. Not only does this level maintain blood perfusion through the heart and liver to facilitate the removal of lactic acid, but it also allows for optimal muscular strength and endurance work through movements that are slow, controlled, and isolated.

In attempting to increase the exercise intensity to an anaerobic threshold for a brief period, have your participants select an intensity of 85% age-predicted maximum heart rate (HR_{max}). However, it is important to assess individual fitness levels when determining intensity levels. An extremely fit student might reach an anaerobic training state at 90% HR_{max}, whereas an individual new to exercise might reach this state at 70% HR_{max}. Without metabolic testing, it is virtually impossible to determine at exactly what heart rate intensity level an individual will reach the anaerobic training state. Therefore, inform your participants that there are other indicators that the an anaerobic training state is near, such as (a) dramatic increases in heart rate, (b) increases in breathing depth and frequency, (c) possible hyperventilation, and (d) muscle fatigue. Participants can also monitor their intensity levels using the 10-point Rating of Perceived Exertion (RPE) scale. According to the 2010 ACSM guidelines, moderate intensity represents a RPE of 5–6 with noticeable increases in heart rate and breathing while a RPE of 7–8 with much higher increases in heart rate and breathing represents vigorous intensity. Remember, safety is the first concern, and for many, prolonged exercise at high-intensity levels is very demanding and may be potentially dangerous.

Work-To-Recovery Ratio

How long your participants exercise with high-intensity movement and recover with low-intensity body conditioning segments is dependent upon their exercise goals, present fitness level, and the primary energy system (aerobic vs. anaerobic) they want to train. Let's examine two extreme examples of interval workouts. First, a track athlete is likely to work with intervals of a one-to-one ratio—sprint for 1 minute and actively recover for the next. Or, another athlete might do what's known as "mile repeaters"—running a "hard" mile, followed by an "easy" mile.

Conversely, a long distance person will work with intervals of a two-to-one ratio—recovering only half the time he/she works. Remember, the long distance runner's goal is to push hard for longer periods of time than the track athlete (who needs short bursts). That is why it is critical for the effective instructor to tailor the interval workouts to the goal of the participant, if at all possible.

Taking IT to the Class

Begin your class with a 10-minute warm-up that will prep the joints, begin to increase core body temperature, and prepare it for more strenuous exercise. Design the warm-up so that the heart rate begins to reach 50–60% HR_{max} near the end of the warm-up period.

Once this is accomplished, the interval segment begins. Each interval is 4 minutes in duration and consists of 3 minutes of high-intensity power moves, jumping jacks, knee lifts, and plyometrics, immediately followed by 1 minute of

Table 26-1. The Interval Training Workout

Rhythmical warm-up/stretch	10 min
Interval Training (6 sets of 4-minute cycles) 3 minutes of high-intensity activity 1 minute of body training	24 min
Post-interval cool-down	5 min
Abdominal work	10 min
Super stretch	5 min

active recovery body conditioning. During the 3-minute high-intensity period, encourage your participants to work at 80–94% HR_{max}.

Three minutes is an optimal time because those participants who are extremely fit may challenge themselves for the entire time, or newcomers to this type of training may be encouraged to stay "more aerobic," working up to 94% HR_{max} in the latter portion of the cycle. A music fade for 5 seconds is essential between work and recovery periods. It cues your participants that change is about to occur. Then, the active recovery portion begins incorporating hand-held weights, elastic bands or tubing, BOSU, medicine balls, or even simple calisthenics to promote body conditioning. During this period, your participants' exercise intensity should be decreased to 55% HR_{max}. This is the optimal intensity for increasing blood perfusion and removing lactic acid while remaining in an aerobic training state. This 3-minute/1-minute format should be followed for 6 sets, completing the interval period in 24 minutes.

A post-aerobic cool-down, in which the movement lowers the heart rate to below 55% HR_{max}, should follow the interval segment. A 10-minute abdominal section to isolate eccentric (lengthening) contractions follows the cool-down, and a super stretch completes your participants' workout.

Now that you have a basic understanding of the physiological responses of IT and a general format of implementation, following several guidelines will allow you to make your participants' first interval class a success. First, while making your interval music, include a 5-second music fade between each work and recovery period. As mentioned earlier, this cues participants that change is about to occur and is also a great place to begin a heart rate check if needed. It also serves to educate the participants as to how their bodies are responding to the varying intensities. Most industry music companies have also designed interval music for purchase, should you choose not to develop you own.

Several ideal upper/lower body combo conditioning moves make the interval class format a success during active recovery periods, and promote muscular strength and endurance.

- Shoulder press with hand-held dumbbells/side lunges
- Upright row with elastic tubing/squat
- Lateral twist with medicine ball/front lunges
- Biceps curls with hand-held dumbbells/front lunge to BOSU
- Triceps press with elastic tubing/split lunge squat

These combinations of upper and lower body movements provide total body conditioning while the body actively recovers from each work segment.

Music

Beats per minute (bpm) during the high-intensity portion should be from approximately 150–160 bpm. Music for the active recovery periods should be 120 bpm. This allows for muscle isolation.

Summary—IT

Remember, IT is peaks and valleys in exercise intensity. IT not only improves all three energy systems, but also helps promote muscular strength and endurance. If you want to maximize student results and literally provide them with the key to achieving success in any personal fitness program—try IT.

References

1. American College of Sports Medicine. (2010). *ACSM's resource manual for guidelines for exercise testing and prescription* (6th ed.). Baltimore, MD: Lippincott Williams & Wilkins.

2. American College of Sports Medicine. (2010). *ACSM's guidelines for exercise testing and prescription* (8th ed.). Baltimore, MD: Lippincott Williams & Wilkins.

3. Bechham, S.G., & Earnest, C.P. (2000). Metabolic cost of free weight circuit weight training. *Journal of Sports Medicine and Physical Fitness*, June, 40(2), 118–25.

4. Coyle, E.F. (2005). Very intense exercise-training is extremely potent and time efficient: A reminder. *Journal of Applied Physiology*, 98(6):1983–1984.

5. Daussin, F.N., Zoll, J., Dufour, S.P., Ponsot, E., Lonsdorfer-Wolf, E., Doutreleau, S., Mettauer, B., Piquard, F., Geny, B., & Richard, R. (2008). Effect of interval versus continuous training on cardiorespiratory and mitochondrial functions: Relationship to aerobic performance improvements in sedentary subjects. *American Journal of Physiology: Regulatory, Integrative, Comparative Physiology*, July, 295(1), R264–272.

6. Fleck, S.J., & Kraemer, W.J. (2004). *Designing resistance training programs* (2nd ed.). Champaign, IL: Human Kinetics.

7. Garhammer, J. (1987). *Strength training: Your ultimate weight conditioning program.* New York, NY: Time, Inc.

8. Gastin, P.B. (2001). Energy system interaction and relative contribution during maximal exercise. *Sports Medicine*, 31(10), 725–41.

9. Gibala, M.J., & McGee, S.L. (2008). Metabolic adaptations to short-term high-intensity interval training: A little pain for a lot of gain? *Exercise Sport & Science Review*, 36(2), 58–63.

10. Gibala, M.J., Little, J.P., van Essen, M., Wilkin, G.P., Burgomaster, K.A., Safdar, A., Raha, S., & Tarnopolsky, M.A. (2006). Short-term sprint interval versus traditional endurance training: Similar initial adaptations in human skeletal muscle and exercise performance. *Journal of Physiology*, 9 (15), 575(Pt 3), 901–11.

11. Gotshalk, L.A., Berger, R.A., & Kraemer, W.J. (2006). Cardiovascular responses to a high-volume continuous circuit resistance training protocol. *Journal of Strength and Conditioning Research*, 18(4), 60–764.

12. Haltom, R.W., Kraemer, R.R., Sloan, R.A., Hebert, E.P., Frank, K., & Tryniecki, J.L. (1999). Circuit weight training and its effects on excess postexercise oxygen consumption. *Medicine & Science in Sports & Exercise*, 31(11), 1613–1618.

13. Howley, E.T., & Franks, B.D. (2003). *Health fitness instructor's handbook.* Champaign, IL: Human Kinetics.

14. Kravitz, L. (1996). The fitness professional's complete guide to circuits and intervals. *IDEA Today*, 14(1), 32–43.

15. MacDougall, D., & Sale, D. (1981). Continuous vs. interval training: A review for the athlete and the coach. *Canadian Journal of Applied Sport Science*, 6, 93–97.

16. Mayo Clinic (2008). Interval training: Can it boost your calorie-burning power? *Mayo Foundation for Medical Education and Research (MFMER).* Retrieved March 15, 2009, from http://www.mayoclinic.com/health/interval-training/SM00110

17. McArdle, W.D., Katch, F.I., & Katch, V.L. (2001). *Exercise physiology: Energy, nutrition and human performance* (5th ed.). Baltimore, MD: Lippincott Williams &Wilkins.

18. National Strength and Conditioning Association. (2004). *NSCA's essentials of personal training.* Champaign, IL. Human Kinetics.

19. Pearl, B., & Morgan, G.T. (1986). *Getting stronger.* New York, NY: Random House, Inc.

20. Pollock, M.L., Gaesser, G.A., Butcher, J.D., Despres, J.P., Dishman, R.K., Franklin, B.A., & Ewing Garber, C. (1998). The recommended quantity and quality of exercise for developing and maintaining cardiorespiratory and muscular fitness, and flexibility in healthy adults. *Medicine & Science in Sports & Exercise,* 30(6), 975–991.

21. Stone, M., & O'Bryant, H. (1987). *Weight training: A scientific approach.* Edina, MN: Burgess International Group, Inc.

22. Talanian, J.L., Galloway, S.D., Heigenhauser, G.J., Bonen, A., & Spriet, L.L. (2007). Two weeks of high-intensity aerobic interval training increases the capacity for fat oxidation during exercise in women. *Journal of Applied Physiology,* 102(4), 1439–1447.

23. Yoke, M. (2006). *Personal fitness training: Theory & practice* (Laura A. Gladwin, Ed.). Sherman Oaks, CA; Aerobics and Fitness Association of America.

27 *Indoor Cycling*

Joelle Mancuso

Focus

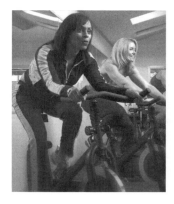

For many years, riding a stationary bike was reserved for cyclists trying to maintain fitness during the off-season or for non-cyclists who were limited to a rather boring session on a stationary cycle at the gym. In 1989, an ultra endurance athlete named Johnny G. changed the way the world would view stationary cycling by bringing his athletic training techniques onto the stationary bike and into a group setting with the SPINNING® program. The creation of the Spinning program began a new group fitness category called indoor cycling.

Indoor cycling has gained mass popularity by appealing to all ages and levels of fitness within a non-impact, non-competitive environment. The lack of complicated choreography and the ability to individually control intensity attracts individuals that have previously found traditional aerobic classes too technical and strenuous. Indoor cycling also allows for competitive athletes, fitness enthusiasts, seniors, and special populations to ride next to each other while obtaining their personal fitness and training goals.

Another unique component of indoor cycling is the use of mind-body techniques to enhance the mental aspect of training. Athletes have used mental training for many years to improve performance, but this is the first time that the average person has been exposed to the benefits of connecting the mind with the body while training. Indoor cycling participants are guided through visualizations that help promote relaxation and focus that either transport the rider onto the road or allow for a better awareness of their physical form.

Benefits of Indoor Cycling

- Strengthens heart and lungs
- Increases muscle tone in lower body
- Decreases stress and anxiety levels, better sleep
- Increases bone density
- Improves cholesterol and triglyceride levels
- Increases energy levels
- Fat loss
- Easy to learn
- Highly individualized (train at your own pace)

Becoming a Participant

The first step when beginning any new program is to find a facility with certified indoor cycling instructors. Certified instructors are trained to give you special assistance prior to class so that your first experience is safe and fun. Arrive early before class to introduce yourself to the instructor so that he/she may familiarize you with the bike and your individual set-up. There are several different models of group exercise bikes on the market and each has unique components.

Participating in an indoor cycling class is easy and requires only a minimal amount of gear. A pair of padded bike shorts, a pair of stiff-soled shoes, a towel, and a water bottle are the only equipment one needs to begin riding. A heart rate monitor, for gauging energy output, may become an important piece of equipment as you begin formulating a personal training program. Classes are typically

40–60 minutes long, but a 30-minute beginning ride may be an option at some facilities. Depending on the room set-up, the instructor will either speak to you from headphones or over a loud speaker system.

Stationary bikes are equipped with a resistance knob or lever that allows you to control the workload and exercise intensity. Turning the resistance up or down enables you to simulate hilly or flat terrain. Having this ability to control the resistance gives you the ultimate choice in how easy or difficult you want the "road" to be. In addition, because you're on your own piece of equipment (the bike), you can remain involved in class even if you're not riding at the same intensity as other riders. It is not uncommon to see a conditioned athlete next to a newcomer with neither rider feeling held back or intimidated.

Learning how to ride properly involves perfecting a few simple sitting and standing movements on the bike. Whether sitting or standing, the hands should remain light on the handlebars so that the shoulders and elbows are relaxed. Gripping or putting too much body weight onto the handlebars produces wasted movement that can develop into stress and tension in the upper body muscles.

Sitting in the saddle is the most common riding position because it offers the most efficient body posture for riding. New riders may find that the forward torso lean required for this position is difficult if the stabilizing muscles in the torso are weak. New riders are encouraged to take breaks by sitting up in the saddle to rest lower back muscles. As you become stronger, this position becomes much easier. Start slow. When you first try to stand out of the saddle, add enough resistance to the flywheel so that your pedal stroke is stable and controlled. Be sure to slow down your pedal stroke before attempting to come out of the saddle. Your body weight should remain over the pedals with the tip of the saddle lightly brushing against the back of your legs. As you become more proficient at standing movements, you will be able to relax the upper body, and your leg muscles will be able to resist fatigue. Expect some discomfort at first, as your body gets used to the seat and the movements out of the saddle. Typically, new riders need to participate in two to three indoor cycling rides per week for a few weeks before becoming comfortable on the bike. Due to the highly motivating nature of indoor cycling, it is not uncommon for new riders to overexert themselves so keep an easy pace until you become conditioned.

Becoming an Instructor

Designing an indoor cycling class is very different from creating a typical group exercise class. It is not uncommon to see riders performing different movements and pedaling at different cadences in the same class. This concept comes from road cycling, where a pack of cyclists are rarely in the same "gear" or in the same riding position as they ride down the road together.

Every ride will include a warm-up and cool-down, but the training section of the routine will be determined by the goals you set for your class as well as the individual goals of each participant. For example, you may plan on a flat, fast ride, but a new participant may need to modify the resistance and the speed to fit his or her fitness level. Be aware that it is quite easy to raise heart rates during an indoor cycling class. Riders should be encouraged to control their exercise intensity by using a heart rate monitor. A heart rate monitor can provide instant feedback for the rider, and can be used to determine whether he/she should work harder or easier.

When introducing varying road situations, be sure that there are smooth transitions between movements and changing terrain. Instead of splicing the classes into music sections, design the class to feel like a seamless piece of road. Be cognizant of the intensity progression during class, and make adjustments based on your participants' needs.

Choosing music for your ride can be the most satisfying, as well as the most challenging, part of creating a class. Unlike other types of group exercise, cycling allows greater freedom when choosing music because the absence of routines or choreography allows the instructor to use music in non-traditional ways. For example, instructors familiar with a beats-per-minute format can now choose music for its ability to elicit emotion, feeling, or simply to provide an appropriate backdrop (like a soundtrack to a movie) for the goal of your ride.

The Mental Component

The mental component allows instructors to introduce visualization and focusing techniques commonly used by athletes. The use of these mental training techniques allows the rider to become more aware of physical performance and the connection with their working body parts. Through this enhanced awareness, the participant is able to perform more efficiently and reach desired goals sooner.

There is tremendous power in visualization. Instructors learn how to use breathing, music, mental focus, and muscular focus to enhance performance. Visualization involves "seeing in your mind's eye" the action you wish to accomplish and seeing yourself being successful.

Coaching Techniques

Getting to know your participants will help you decide what coaching techniques to use. As the physical challenges increase, mental strength and conditioning become increasingly important factors in the body's ability to manage the greater demands. How you motivate your participants will determine their enjoyment and success with indoor cycling. Some coaching techniques include teaching off the bike, counting, sharpening focus, using positive affirmations, and setting goals.

Teaching Off the Bike
The indoor cycling environment allows instructors the ability to teach off the bike and work one-on-one with participants. Teaching off the bike allows you to assist new participants with form and relaxation. If someone is having difficulty with a movement, you can gently guide him or her into the right position. Walking around also gives you the perfect opportunity to check participants' heart rates and exertion levels, and prescribe adjustments if needed. Spending personal time with each rider will create a relationship that will allow you to be more effective. When teaching from the ground, make sure you are offering specific instructions instead of just "cheering" participants on.

Counting
Counting is a simple, yet powerful, tool for motivating your participants. By giving a goal of a specific amount of work or a specific amount of time, you create something tangible for your participants to achieve. For example, set a fixed time to start and finish a series of intervals by saying to your participants, "We are going to increase our heart rates by 20 beats within the next 2 minutes." Keep in mind that this technique can be overused. The emphasis should be on enjoying the process of the training session rather than accumulating a certain number of repetitions.

Sharpening Focus

Teaching focus-sharpening techniques will give your participants the ability to engage their minds quicker, which allows them to make the powerful mental connection during classes. The technique of sharpening focus involves giving specific instructions to your participants to focus intently on one thing. The focus can be applied to their breathing, the instruments in the music, an object or point in the room, or their working muscles. As they become proficient at finding their focus, their training sessions will become more relaxing and effective.

Positive Affirmations

Participants take most of their feedback from the instructor. Using positive affirmation during the ride will motivate and encourage riders during challenging sections of class. Make a list of 10 specific words or phrases that you think will motivate your students, and then learn to verbalize these suggestions in sync with the progression of the class. Some powerful and suggestive words and phrases may include "relax," "commitment," "happiness," "I am strong," and "I am focused." Make an effort to express positive affirmations with real meaning behind them, and make them specific to the class objectives. Merely repeating suggestive words without any emotion or specificity will diminish their impact.

Goal Setting

Another powerful coaching tool is goal setting. Goal setting encourages persistence and effort, provides a short-term reward, and gives participants the feeling that they are moving in a desired direction. Goal setting can be worked into many situations, and can be set by either you or the participant. For example, if you have new participants who need to develop a fitness base, encourage them to train in their aerobic base building zone (65–80% HR_{max} or 50–70% HRR) for the first 6–8 weeks. One of the benefits of the indoor cycling environment is working with participants to attain personal objectives while in a group setting.

Making the Decision

Indoor cycling offers something for everyone. Whether you are a group exercise instructor, personal fitness trainer, fitness director, club owner, or cycling enthusiast, getting involved in this dynamic form of exercise is as easy as riding a bike! If you want to become a certified instructor, the first step is to contact one of the many certifying agencies to find the indoor cycling program that is best for you and your goals as a fitness professional. Every program has its unique characteristics as well as certification requirements. The following is a list of indoor cycling certification programs:

The Spinning® Program   (800) 847-SPIN
Cycle Reebok™   (800) REEBOK-1
Keiser Power Pace™   (800) 888-7009

References

1. Aerobics and Fitness Association. (2004). *Indoor cycling workshop outline.* Sherman Oaks, CA: Aerobics and Fitness Association of America.
2. Mylrea, M. (2006). *Mindy Mylrea's super cycle (indoor cycle workout).* Retrieved April 20, 2009, at http://www.amazon.com
3. For information on AFAA's Indoor Cycling workshop, go to www.afaa.com.

Susan O. Cooper, MA
and Kathy Stevens, MA

28

Resistance Training in the Group Exercise Setting:
Utilizing Free Weights, Resistance Tubing, and/or Body Weight Exercises

Focus

This chapter will help you create and instruct well-designed resistance training workouts that address muscular strength and/or endurance. Muscle strengthening classes continue to be a very popular item on today's group exercise schedules. They go by many names from the traditional "body sculpt" or "muscle conditioning" to more creative titles like "power pump," "reps and sets," 'iron yoga," and more. In the group exercise setting, workouts may combine multiple fitness components in one "mixed" format, such as a step and sculpt class or cardio/strength circuit, or dedicate the entire class to strength training. These classes will typically use free weights, resistance tubes, and body weight exercises. They can last anywhere from 30–90 minutes.

Benefits and Training Effects of Muscular Fitness

Muscular strength and endurance, also known as muscular fitness, are components of fitness (along with cardiorespiratory fitness, flexibility, and appropriate body composition) that are important for overall health and well-being. As we go about our daily activities, muscular strength and endurance play a crucial role in how well our physical bodies meet a variety of demands and resist injury.

There are a number of documented benefits (Williams et al., 2007; Pollock et al., 2000) that can result from resistance training, such as the following.

- Increased physical capacity to perform the activities of daily living.
- Increased bone density and the strength of connective tissue.
- Increased fat free mass resulting in decreased sarcopenia (gradual loss of lean tissue with age).
- Improved motor performance.
- Decreased risk of injury.
- Enhanced feeling of well-being and self-confidence.
- Overall improvement in quality of life.

Understanding the training effects related to a strength program will help you develop effective resistance training classes. There are five basic training effects (Yoke, 2006). Muscular:

1. strength
2. endurance
3. power
4. stability
5. hypertrophy

Muscular strength is defined as the maximum force a muscle or muscle group can generate at one time.

Muscular endurance is the capacity to sustain repeated muscle actions, as in push-ups or sit-ups, or to sustain fixed, static muscle actions for an extended period of time.

Muscle power is the explosive aspect of strength, and is the product of strength and speed of movement. Power = (force x distance)/time. Power is especially important for improved athletic performance.

Muscle stability refers to the ability of a muscle or muscle group to stabilize a joint and maintain its position without movement, in other words, to be able to perform a sustained isometric, or held, contraction.

Muscle hypertrophy refers to an increase in the muscle fiber size, specifically in an increased cross-sectional area resulting from increased myofibrils.

To accomplish these training effects you will perform your classes using a sequence of exercise *reps* and *sets*. A rep refers to the completion of a single exercise movement from start to finish. A set is a series of reps performed together prior to a rest or break. The amount of resistance used is often referred to as the *load*. *Volume* is a weight training concept defined as the total number of repetitions performed multiplied by the total amount of resistance used during a single training session (ACSM, 2006). In other words reps x load = volume. Volume can be varied by changing the number of repetitions, the number of sets, the number of exercises performed, or the amount of weight used.

Amount of Resistance vs. Repetition

In the early days of group exercise smaller 2–3 pound weights and tubing were the primary tools used. Many reps and sets were performed limiting the results to greater muscular endurance. Today, we see more programs including heavier bars and dumbbells in the group exercise classes to adequately challenge participants' interest in greater strength gains.

The amount of resistance used and the number of repetitions completed dictate the type of results that can be expected from a resistance training program. Light resistance with a high amount of repetitions will primarily lead to gains in muscular endurance (e.g., 12–20 reps). To obtain a larger muscle mass and muscular strength gains, heavier weights with fewer repetitions must be included (e.g., 6–8 reps). This presents several challenges to consider when instructing in the group exercise environment. It is not always possible to have enough equipment to offer adequate resistance for all participants (in particular if working towards muscular strength gains). Additionally each participant may be limited to one or two different resistance loads making it difficult to properly challenge each muscle group. The load they choose may be perfect of a stronger muscle group like the latisimus dorsi, but too heavy for a smaller group such as the deltoids. It will be important for the instructor to sequence exercises in a way that allows the students to reach fatigue in a reasonable amount of repetitions and readily switch loads and/or make adjustments for larger (stronger) verses smaller (weaker) muscle groups. This will be further discussed in the sections on *training intensity, exercise sequencing,* and *exercise order*.

Guidelines for Muscular Strength and Endurance Programming

The American College of Sports Medicine recommends the following guidelines for resistance training for the average healthy adult (ACSM, 2010).

- Perform one set of each exercise to the point of fatigue, while maintaining good form.
- Most people should complete 8–12 repetitions for each exercise, although a range of repetitions within 3–20 (e.g., 6–8, 8–10, 12–15) may also be appropriate. (For group exercise, AFAA recommends a range between 8–25 repetitions depending on whether the focus is muscular strength or endurance.)
- Perform both the concentric and eccentric phases of the exercises in a controlled manner (~2 to 4 sec concentric, ~2 to 4 sec eccentric).
- Exercise each muscle group 2 to 3 non-consecutive days per week, and, if possible, perform a different exercise for the muscle group every two to three sessions.
- Perform a minimum of 8–10 exercises that condition the major muscle groups, with a primary goal of developing total body strength and endurance in a relatively time-efficient manner.

Physiology of Muscular Strength and Endurance

For a better understanding of the physiology of human muscle, refer to Chapter 7, "The Musculoskeletal System: Structure, Function, and Exercise Application." Learning how a muscle works will help instructors receive a better understanding of how to sequence or progress a resistance training class.

Neuromuscular Facilitation and "Muscle Memory"

Performing a muscle contraction with correct form and maximal fiber recruitment is a learned process. Muscle contractions are actually controlled by the brain. Simply put, the brain sends a message to the biceps to contract. If the message does not reach the biceps, then the muscle does not contract. Neuromuscular facilitation is the act of training the brain and the muscle to work as a team.

Muscle memory is fashioned over time through repetition of a given set of fine or gross motor skills. As one reinforces skills through repetition, the neural system learns those movements or skills to the degree that one no longer needs to think about them, but merely to react and perform appropriately. In the context of strength training, muscle memory can also imply that muscle strength can be gained back rapidly (Staron et al., 1991) after one consistently trains for a given period of time, takes a long break from weight training, and then returns to weight training. This occurs because the muscle maintains a "muscle memory" of its previous, trained conditioning.

It is extremely important for instructors to recognize that their class participants are at various stages of muscle memory. Thus, instructors need to offer plenty of options and modifications in particular for challenging or skill related exercises. They should always emphasize mastery of proper resistance training techniques prior to offering more advanced exercise variations.

Primary Movers

In every joint action, there is a muscle that contracts and acts as the primary mover or agonist. To allow this joint action to occur, there is another muscle that acts in opposition to the agonist called the antagonist. There are also stabilizer muscles at work that prevent unwanted movement and allow the agonist and antagonist to perform the movement with full contraction. For example, in a biceps curl performed at shoulder level, the biceps is the agonist, the triceps is the antagonist, and the deltoid acts as the stabilizer of the movement.

Muscle Balancing

Muscle balancing is a foundational concept for resistance training workouts. Think of the body as the center pole of a tent. There are ropes attached to the center pole (muscles) that will pull the tent one way or another depending on which rope is the tightest and strongest. To create a well-stabilized tent, all ropes must be equally strong and stable.

The same is true of the human body. All the muscles of the body work in pairs to create movement. If one part of the pair is stronger than another, a muscular imbalance is created, which leads to improper body alignment and movement mechanics. For example, if the pectoralis (chest) and abdominal muscles are very strong and tight

If working	Be sure to also work
Biceps	Triceps
Deltoids	Latissimus Dorsi
Abdominals	Erector Spinae
Pectorals	Mid-Trapezius/Rhomboids
Iliopsoas	Gluteus Maximus
Abductors	Adductors
Quadriceps	Hamstrings
Gastrocnemius/Soleus	Tibialis Anterior

while the back muscles are very weak and laxed, a postural condition is created called kyphosis or "hump back." To reverse this condition, the pectoralis must be stretched and the back muscles strengthened. These imbalances can also increase the possibility of exercise related injury. In order to prevent muscular imbalance, your class format should include exercises for all of the major muscle groups. You will also need to stretch each major muscle group. Stretches can be integrated in between strength sets (at the completion of a particular muscle group) or at the end of the entire strength routine.

Extra focus can be given to muscles that tend to be weaker or tighter than their opposing group due to life stresses or typical training habits. Muscles that are weaker should be given additional strength or stability exercises while muscles that tend to be tighter should be given extra stretch time. Below is a list of muscles that could use added attention (Yoke, 2006).

Muscles that tend to be weaker than their opposing group and should be given extra strengthening focus are as follows.

- External shoulder rotators
- Rear deltoid
- Mid trapezius and rhomboids
- Lower trapezius
- Abdominals
- Spinal erectors
- Vastus medialis (inner quadriceps group)
- Tibialis anterior

Muscles that tend to be tight and should be given extra stretches are as follows.

- Internal shoulder
- Front deltoid
- Pectorals
- Upper trapezius
- Spinal erectors (can be tight or weak)
- Iliopsoas
- Hamstrings
- Gastrocnemius

Training Intensity

In order to see the results from your strength exercises, it is important to work the targeted muscle group to fatigue, but not to a point of failure. This means the muscle feels tired, but you are able to complete the movement without the loss of proper exercise form and technique. Ideally, the resistance used (e.g., weights, bands, or body weight) is enough to achieve a strong level of fatigue within a reasonable amount of repetitions (e.g., 1–3 sets of 8–16 reps). Once fatigue is reached, it is time to rest prior to performing another set of the same exercise. Rest periods between sets of an exercise can range from a minimum of a few seconds to a few minutes. The greater the fatigue and heavier the resistance, the longer the rest period will need to be between sets. In the group setting, instructors will often alternate between muscle groups using super-sets, tri-sets, and giant sets (a combination of two, three, or more different exercises done back to back without a rest period) to avoid long rest periods and keep the flow of the workout going.

An additional technique often used in group classes to expedite the onset of muscle fatigue is a mid-range isometric hold or short-range pulse. These holds and small pulsing actions are typically added after the final set of full range repe-

Example loads	
Biceps Curl	
For Muscle Strength	
REPS	WT
1 set of 4-8	50 lb
For Muscle Endurance	
REPS	WT
2-4 sets of 8–16	5 lb

titions, in particular, when the resistance available does not sufficiently fatigue the muscle in the recommended rep ranges.

Monitoring Training Intensity

It is the instructor's responsibility to monitor the group throughout the class and help participants select the proper resistance in a non-intimidating way. It will also be important to teach participants to monitor their own form and level of fatigue. Some participants may have trouble initially gauging their resistance training intensity. Fatigue levels can be measured using the Borg RPE scale. A suggested range is 12–13 (on the 6–20/15-point scale) initially, then 15–16 near the end of the set for submaximal training, and up to 19–20 for high-intensity training (Faigenbaum, Pollock, et al., 1999). Refer to Chapter 20, "Monitoring Exercise Intensity" for more information.

Muscle Soreness

Muscle soreness, which occurs during the workout, is known as acute muscle soreness. Stretching the muscle or switching to a different exercise can often relieve this soreness. Another type of muscle soreness is called delayed onset of muscle soreness (DOMS). This usually happens 1 to 2 days after a workout. There is still controversy over what causes this condition and how it can be relieved. Some theories state that there is an actual tearing and inflammation of the muscle during the workout, and that warming up properly and stretching the muscle after training along with using lighter loads will help to alleviate this soreness.

Injury Prevention

Safety and form are of major concern in any resistance training program. Therefore, all exercises should be performed in a slow, controlled manner. Fast, explosive movements can place excessive stress on the muscles, joint structures, and connective tissues. One common cause of injury in a resistance training class is movement that is executed too rapidly (e.g., trying to keep up with the beat of the music) and/or with incorrect body alignment. Movement speeds of 2–4 seconds on the lifting phase (concentric action), a pause at the most contracted position, and 2–4 seconds on the lowering phase (eccentric action) help to maintain good execution.

The most common types of injuries that occur in resistance classes are inflammation problems caused by overuse or "over- reps." Excessive squats and lunges often used in combination work may cause some knee problems. Other commonly over-stressed joints include the shoulder, wrist, and spine. It will be important to keep overhead movement in a range that does not aggravate the shoulder and decrease the stress on areas like the wrist, neck, and low back by maintaining proper alignment during exercise execution. Less common injuries include muscle strains or ligament sprains.

A complete warm-up along with proper body alignment and the use of appropriate resistance are the most important factors in injury prevention. Training participants how to facilitate effective neuromuscular response also aids in decreasing injury.

If injury does occur, recommend they use the RICE method—rest, ice, compression, and elevation—for immediate relief. If pain persists after the provision of such first-aid, advise your participant to seek the advice of a physician.

Breathing Through Resistance

Breathing also plays an important safety role in resistance training. It is advisable to exhale on the exertion (lifting phase) and inhale on the lowering phase. Holding the breath will create muscle fatigue at a faster rate and may illicit the Valsalva maneuver. This is a condition causing the glottis to close and the abdominal muscles to contract, forming an unequal pressure in the chest cavity, reduced blood flow to the heart, and insufficient oxygen to the brain. Dizziness and temporary loss of consciousness may occur. Blood pressure will also increase which may be a concern for participants with a history of coronary artery disease.

The Value of Rest

Rest and repair are necessary for muscle growth and recuperation. Generally, 48 hours is sufficient for this process to occur. Two to 3 non-consecutive days of resistance training (e.g., Monday, Wednesday, and Friday) is an adequate schedule for the average person. If working with heavier resistance, a rest period of 30–90 seconds between exercises is sufficient for immediate muscle recovery.

Types of Equipment

The equipment you choose for the muscle-sculpting segment of class can vary from day to day because the choices are always increasing. Hand-held weights, tubing, weighted poles, balls, balance boards, and benches are just a few of the products on the market. Adding different types of resistive equipment to your routines will enhance training effects as well as reduce the incidence of plateaus and boredom. Remember to instruct your students as to the appropriate use of any new piece of equipment introduced.

Constant vs. Variable Resistance

Constant resistance is a form of dynamic resistance where the resistance directed against the target muscle or muscle group does not vary through the range of motion. Constant resistance training uses free weights, such as dumbbells, barbells, medicine balls, or even your own body weight. Gravity and position play a major role in the effectiveness of this type of resistance. The main disadvantage of constant resistance is the inability to train effectively against gravity through a full range of motion for certain exercises.

Variable resistance exercise is designed to achieve maximum muscular involvement and is usually carried out through the use of specialized machines. When using variable resistance machines, the applied force changes throughout the range of motion due to the special arrangement of pulleys or cams. With variable resistance machines, the resistance design attempts to match the particular muscle's strength curve, allowing for a fuller range of effective training. True variable resistance is hard to duplicate in a group exercise class. The closest thing to variable resistance that is used in a group class would be elastic tubing and bands. Unlike a fixed weight, elastic resistance is variable because the resistance continues to increase as the device is progressively stretched, compressed, bent, or twisted. With tubing, the load or the intensity of the exercise can also be varied by changing the anchor angle as well as the foot or grip positioning. For example, when holding a tube you can vary your grip allowing for less or more working tube length; the less the length, the greater the resistance. Also, by its nature a tube or band becomes less elastic at the end range of its extensibility, making it much harder to pull. This fact works well with muscle groups where the strength curve matches the end range of an exercise motion. Examples include the anterior deltoid during a front raise and the quadriceps during knee extension. In these exercises, the muscle produces the most force at the end range of motion. However, flexors of the elbow (biceps) are relatively weak close to full extension and close to full flexion, and so a band or tubing does not match the capabilities of these muscles. Unfortunately, when the resistance produced by the band is greatest, a large component of the resistance puts stress on the elbow joint, rather than on the contracting muscles. Be aware when using tubing where you feel the exercise. Ideally, you should feel the fatigue in the targeted muscle group(s). If the stress is joint related, ease up on the tension by selecting a lighter resistance, limiting the range of motion or shifting the anchor point.

Action Steps for Designing a Resistance Tubing Class

Tubing Tips

1. Prior to using, check all tubing for holes or tears.
2. Avoid pulling the tubing toward the face.
3. Select appropriate resistance to maintain proper form and alignment.
4. Avoid gripping the handles too tightly as to not elevate blood pressure.
5. Maintain wrist alignment so the hand is in line with the forearm.
6. Maintain continuous tension in the tubing so that movement can be controlled.
7. Maintain a smooth and controlled pace on the lifting and lowering phase.

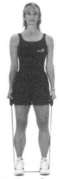

Fig. 28-1. Two-foot Position on Tube

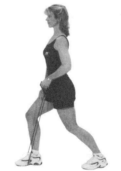

Fig. 28-2. One-foot Position on Tube

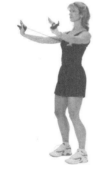

Fig. 28-3. Chest Press (Pectoralis Major, Anterior Deltoid, Triceps)

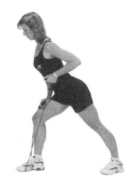

Fig. 28-4. One-arm Row (Latissimus Dorsi, Posterior Deltoid, Biceps)

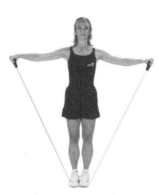

Fig. 28-5. Lateral Raise (Deltoid Group)

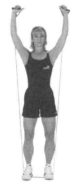

Fig. 28-6. Overhead Press (Deltoid Group, Trapezius, Triceps)

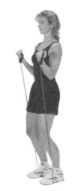

Fig. 28-7. Biceps Curl (Biceps, Brachial Radialis and Brachialis)

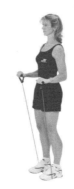

Fig. 28-8. Reverse Curls (Biceps, Brachial Radialis and Brachialis)

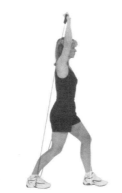

Fig. 28-9. Overhead Triceps Press (Triceps)

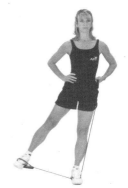

Fig. 28-10. Hip Abduction (Hip Abductors)

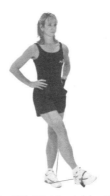

Fig. 28-11. Hip Adduction (Hip Adductors)

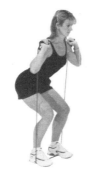

Fig. 28-12. Squat (Gluteals, Quadriceps, Hip Flexor, and Hamstrings

Music

The music you choose for your resistance training class or the muscle strengthening segment of a mixed format class can help motivate your students to work hard and stay engaged in the movement. A strong, driving beat between 120 and 130 beats per minute (bpm) will keep the energy high while allowing instructors to execute the movement with proper form and full range of motion. Participants may find it pleasing to move with the beat and complete the sets and reps with the musical phrase. This is not a must, but does add a level of polish to a body sculpting class. Thus, for example, a 4 beat lift (approximately 2 seconds) with a 4 beat hold (approximately 2 seconds) followed by an 8 beat lowering phase (approximately 4 seconds), would work perfectly with music created for exercise purposes. A verbal count down usually takes 2 beats of music (e.g., hold one and two and three and four) unless you are doing small-range pulsing type move, which can move on the beat. In order to have your sets match the phrasing of the music, it is best to perform 8 or 16 repetition sets.

Example lift count (music 120–130 bpm):
    Single Rep:
    Up for two—4 beats
    Hold for two—4 beats
    Down in four—8 beats
    Total = 8 seconds/counts in 16 beats of music
    Repeat 8 times = 64 seconds/128 beats of music (4 phrases of 32 beats)

This is just one example of many ways you can work with the beat of your music.

Keep in mind that working with the beat takes practice and a higher level of musicality on the part of the instructor. Music linked classes are not for every class or instructor. There are certain classes and exercises that are better taught without adherence to the music. A circuit format where everyone may be doing different exercises at the same time is one such example. Another example would be a class where there is a wide variance in participant abilities. Those participants with heavier weights may not be able to move at the same tempo as the ones who have selected lighter resistance. In these cases, it will be the responsibility of the instructor to direct and remind participants to always work at their own pace and avoid moving at a speed that reduces their ability to maintain good form and alignment. So, whether you prefer moving with the beat or simply having the music in the background, be sure to keep your primary attention and focus on the needs of your class participants.

Effective Cueing

Effective cueing can be tricky in the group environment due to the wide variety of participant goals and abilities. It is a good idea to start with the least challenging version of an exercise then progress appropriately for your group. Once an advanced exercise is introduced the instructor should re-visit the easier version or modification for those who are not ready to advance. It is even trickier to control what the participants think they should be doing. This is where you must utilize your greatest communication skills. You need to find ways of encouraging those who should advance without discouraging those who should not. A phrase such as, "if you are sensing fatigue you are working at the perfect level; if not try adding this variation" may help to encourage all class participants. Watch out for cues that are not inclusive, negative, or overly aggressive, like "come on, you can do it, no pain no gain" or "go for the burn." Keep in mind that the group wants to follow what the instructor is doing, so be sure to demonstrate a variety of options to make everyone feel comfortable.

Exercise Sequencing

Strength training sequences can include the following.
- Moving from one primary muscle group to the next, while performing 1–3 sets of 4–16 reps (traditional weight room format).
- Moving from a single set of one exercise directly into a second, third, or more and then repeating the entire series over again (super-, tri-, or giant sets).
- Moving through a series of exercise patterns including arm combinations, leg combinations, or arm and leg combinations (more choreographed format).
  - arm combinations—2 or more arm movements or movement variations (e.g.,, a biceps curl into an overhead press)
  - leg combinations—2 or more leg movements or movement variations (e.g., a front lunge followed by a side squat)
  - arm and leg combinations – 1 arm and 1 leg movement (e.g., a squat followed by an overhead press) or an arm and leg movement performed simultaneously (e.g., performing a squat while you do a biceps curl)

When designing your class you may choose to keep things simple and stick with a single sequence style or get creative with a variety of sequences and exercise variations. There are many ways to vary a base exercise. These variables of change include:

1. equipment type (e.g., tubes, weights, balls)
2. contraction type—(e.g., isometric, concentric, eccentric)
3. speed of movement (i.e., varying the beats used per contraction phase)
4. range of movement (e.g., full, partial, pulse)
5. lever usage (e.g., long, short)
6. angle or plane of joint action (e.g., front, side, diagonal, supinated, pronated)
7. body positioning (e.g., standing, kneeling, seated, supine, prone)
8. traveling (i.e., movement in space front, side, and back)

Example 1:

An arm and leg combination sequence that uses angle and traveling variations might look like this:

*   4 biceps curls in front of the body with alternating step front lunges (Fig. 28-13)
*   4 biceps curls on the side of the body with alternating step side squats (Fig. 28-14)
*   4 biceps hammerhead curls with palms facing in, hands in front with calf raises (Fig. 28-15)
*   4 biceps preacher curls with raised arms to front, with alternating step back lunges (Fig. 28-16)

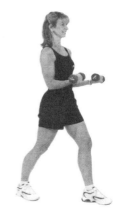 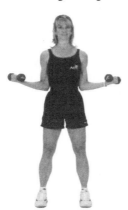 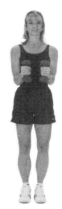 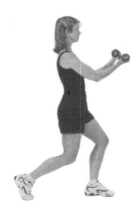

Fig. 28-13.   **Fig. 28-14.**   **Fig. 28-15.**   **Fig. 2-16.**

You would repeat this sequence of four parts for 2–3 sets (a set is completed once all four parts have been executed).

At this point, the biceps should be fatigued. It will be time to move on to another muscle group.

Example 2:

An arm sequence that uses speed and range of movement as variations might look like this:

*   8 full range overhead triceps extension performed with focus on the concentric phase using 8 beats of music on the extension, 4 beats on the hold and 4 beats on the return to start position

Combine movements using several variables of change:
1. equipment type
2. contraction type
3. speed of movement
4. range of movement
5. lever
6. angle or plane
7. body positioning
8. traveling

- 8 full range overhead triceps extension with focus on the eccentric phase using 4 beats of music on the extension, 4 beats on the hold and 8 beats on the return to start position
- 16 pulses, 2 beats per pulse, at mid range of the movement

To superset this exercise you could go immediately into a similar exercise sequence for another upper body muscle group (e.g., biceps curls) or lower body muscle group (e.g., squats).

Selecting the Exercise Order

When designing your overall class format, you will want to consider the order in which you will perform each exercise. There are many options depending on your class goals, the equipment available, and the focus of the workout. In general, any well thought-out and balanced format will work. Shifting the format on a regular basis will keep the class interesting as well as help to prevent training plateaus. Some format suggestions include the following.

- Work the large muscle groups first. For example, perform exercises for the back and chest before isolating the shoulders or arms. Likewise you would isolate the larger hip and buttocks muscles prior to the legs.
- Group exercises according to body position (e.g., standing versus supine). With the exception of a circuit format, classes will flow more smoothly if you complete most or at least a group of exercises from one position before moving on to another.
- Perform challenging core exercises before less or non-core challenging exercises. An example would be to perform a high demand core stability exercise like a bilateral bent-over row prior to a less challenge core exercise such as a seated row with tubing.
- Alternating pull with push exercises. An example would be to do a bent-over lat row (pull exercise) followed by a push-up or chest press (push exercise).
- Alternating upper with lower body exercises. Below is an example of an alternating upper body lower/body format.

Example: Alternating upper/lower body format order

16 reps – overhead press (for trapezius and deltoids)
16 reps – squats (for gluteals, quadriceps, and hamstrings)
16 reps – bent-over rows (for mid-trapezius and latissimus dorsi)
16 reps – lunges (gluteals, quadriceps, and hamstrings)
16 reps- biceps curls (for biceps)
16 reps – calf raises (gastrocniemius)
16 reps – supine bridge for (hamstrings and gluteals)
16 reps – push-ups (for pectoralis major and triceps)
16 reps – ab curls (for rectus abdominus)
16 reps – prone back extension (for spinal erectors)
Repeat sequence for 2–3 sets.

Example Body Sculpting Class Breakdown

A general total body sculpting class might include the following format.

- Warm-up (5–10 minutes). Include a balanced combination of dynamic and prepatory stretching along with rehearsal movement patterns that will mimic the actions to be performed later with resistance.

- Upper Body (10 minutes). Work larger muscle groups followed by smaller groups (latissimus dorsi , trapezius, pectoralis major followed by deltoids, biceps, and triceps).
- Lower Body (10 minutes). Include exercises for the gluteals, hamstrings, quadriceps, tibialis anterior, and calves.
- Upper and Lower Body Work (10–20 minutes). Reach the peak in intensity with combination movements (upper and lower body exercise done simultaneously) or strength sequences (super-sets, tri-sets, and giant sets) utilizing both the upper and lower body in specific muscular fatigue sequences. When performing these combinations, you will need to lower the resistance to accommodate the weaker muscle groups being challenged.
- Floor work (10 minutes). Include upper body exercises (push-ups, chest flyes, and bench presses) as well as core work (abdominal curls, planks, and spinal extension exercises). This section can also include lower body exercises, such as bridge hip lifts and side lying leg work, if time allows.
- Cool-down Stretch (5–10 minutes). Provide a final static stretch with attention given to all muscle groups worked.

Avoiding Plateaus

Throughout the course of any group strength class, it will be important for an instructor to recommend that participants apply the principles of progressive overload. Encourage them to increase their resistance (appropriately), offer more reps or sets of the existing exercises, and/or vary and add new exercises on a regular basis. These progressions should be offered every few workouts for your regular participants. After the initial months of resistance training, when adequate strength levels have been attained, participants may still feel as though they are hitting a training plateau. At this time, it will be important to continue to create new challenges to the musculoskeletal system. This can be accomplished in many ways. You can vary the exercise equipment and/or format design of the workouts. Try using tubing if you were only using free weighs or visa versa. For groups that you see multiple times a week, you can rotate muscle focus. For example, have a heavy upper body focus day followed by a heavy lower body day. Another option could be to shift from a traditional body sculpt format to a cardio/sculpt circuit. As your group progresses, you may also want to offer a greater challenge by incorporating core stability and balance skills. Have them try performing a standing exercise like a biceps curl on one foot or work on a less stable surface like a balance board. By making constant shifts in your class options and routines, your participants will see continual growth and development in muscular strength and endurance, and most importantly, will avoid burnout and overuse injuries.

Summary

Group exercise classes that train the body for muscular endurance and strength activities should be included in a total fitness program. The most important focus of the program is teaching participants where the muscle is, how to properly contract the muscle, and perform the exercise with correct alignment and movement mechanics. It will be important for instructors to apply the same principles used in weight room training (e.g., progressive overload, muscle balancing, injury prevention, and exercise sequencing) while taking into consideration some of the limitations and challenges presented in a group situation (e.g., availability of proper resistance, use of music, monitoring, and cueing). With all these factors in place, we should be able to develop group exercise resistance training classes with a focus on body sculpting and muscle strengthening that yield effective and measurable results.

References

1. Aerobics and Fitness Association of America. (2010). Standards and guidelines for weighted workouts. In AFAA's *exercise standards & guidelines reference manual*. Sherman Oaks, CA: Aerobics and Fitness Association of America.

2. American College of Sports Medicine (2006). The recommended quantity and quality of exercise for developing and maintaining cardiorespiratory and muscular fitness and flexibility in healthy adults. *Medicine & Science in Sports & Exercise*, 30, 975–991.

3. American College of Sports Medicine. (2010). *Guidelines for exercise testing and prescription* (8th ed.). Baltimore, MD: Lippincott Williams & Wilkins.

4. Andersen, J.L., Schjerling, P., & Saltin, B. (2000). Muscle, genes and athletic performance. *Scientific American*, 9, 49.

5. Baechle, T.R., & Grove, B.R. (1998). *Weight training: Steps to success* (2nd ed.). Champaign, IL: Human Kinetics.

6. Dorgo, S., King, G.A., & Rice, C.A. (2009). The effects of manual resistance training on improving muscular strength and endurance. *Journal of Strength & Conditioning Research*, 23(1), 293–303.

7. Luttgens, K., & Hamilton, N. (1997). Kinesiology: Scientific basis of human motion (9th ed.). Boston, MA: McGraw-Hill.

8. McArdle, W.D., Katch, F.I., & Katch, V.L. (1996). *Exercise physiology: Energy, nutrition and human performance* (4th ed.). Baltimore, MD: Williams & Wilkins.

9. Pollock, M., Franklin, B., Baldy, G., et al. (2000). Resistance exercise in individuals with and without cardiovascular disease: Benefits, rationale, safety, and prescription. An advisory from the Committee on Exercise, Rehabilitation, and Prevention, Council on Clinical Cardiology, and American Heart Association. *Circulation*, 101, 828–833.

10. Staron, R.S., Leonardi, M.J., Karapondo, D.L., Malicky, E.S., Falkel, J.E., Hagerman, F.C., & Hikida, R.S. (1991). Strength and skeletal muscle adaptations in heavy-resistance-trained women after detraining and retraining. *Journal of Applied Physiology*, 70 (2), 631–640.

11. Thomas, M., Müller, T., & Busse, M.W. (2005). Quantification of tension in Thera-Band and Cando tubing at different strains and starting lengths. *Journal of Sports Medicine and Physical Fitness*, 45(2), 188–98, June.

12. Westcott, W.L. (1990). *Strength fitness: Physiological principles and training techniques* (3rd ed.). Dubuque, IA: William C. Brown.

13. Williams, M., Haskell, W., Ades, P., et al. (2007). Resistance exercise in individuals with and without cardiovascular disease: A scientific statement from the American Heart Association Council on Nutrition, Physical Activity, and Metabolism. *Circulation*, 116, 572–584.

14. Wilmore, J.H. (1986). *Sensible fitness* (2nd ed.). Champaign, IL: Leisure Press.

15. Winnett, R.A., & Carpinelli, R.N. (2001). Potential health-related benefits of resistance training. *Preventive Medicine*, 33, 503–513.

16. Yoke, M. (2006). AFAA's *personal fitness training: theory & practice* (Laura A. Gladwin, Ed.). Sherman Oaks, CA: Aerobics and Fitness Association of America.

29

Mat Science:
An Integration of Basic Conditioning, Dance, Pilates, and Yoga Activities

Linda Shelton, MS and
Laura A. Gladwin, MS

Focus

Mat Science (I and II) brings to the group fitness instructor a unique integration of a variety of movements derived from the classic disciplines and philosophies of dance, Pilates, and yoga along with basic conditioning exercises to reflect the latest fusion trends within the industry. It is based on a progressive exercise series that can accommodate most, if not all, fitness levels to improve strength and endurance, joint mobility, flexibility, balance, and coordination while focusing on breathing and mindful movements.

Philosophy

The philosophy behind Mat Science is to embrace the original disciplines on which almost every floor exercise used in group fitness today is based on, and update the version back to its roots for a contemporary group training experience both on the floor and standing. It encompasses the Eastern philosophy of yoga, the holistic approach of centering and conditioning from Pilates, and the application of current exercise science and biomechanics to lend for a safe, effective, mind/body-oriented, and more meaningful exercise experience.

Relationship Between Historical Disciplines and Fitness-Based Classes		
YOGA	**PILATES**	**FITNESS**
1. SIMILARITIES		
Exercises		
Many exercises specific only to yoga and Pilates, without calling them yoga conditioning, are now an accepted and common part of a fitness class repertoire of moves and have adopted classical names (e.g., plank, side-plank, roll-up).		Most exercises currently used in fitness (particularly for stretching and flexibility training) are primarily yoga poses.
Benefits		
Increase muscular strength, endurance, tone, flexibility		
Progression		
Include multi-levels of variations, adaptable to all		
Movement Structure		
There is form and structure to each posture; instructors can self-personalize the class.		
2. DIFFERENCES		
Focus		
The quality of movement in yoga and Pilates focus on breath and form, which produce a meditative state, a mindset that is brought about through repetitive rhythmic movement and a constant, focused flow of activity.		Focus, mindset, and meditative flow are absent.
The connection between movement, body and breath as one unit is emphasized.		Separatism and isolation of the body and mind.
Emphasis is on the process.		Emphasis is on the end-product or goal.
Emphasis is on mindfulness and being present with each movement; awareness if the mind has wandered.		Emphasis on finishing; wandering goes unnoticed.

YOGA	PILATES	FITNESS
Competition		
Compare self with self	Compare self with self	Compare self with others
Breath		
Emphasizes nostril breathing, initiated by filling the lungs and expanding the ribs with a deep diaphragmatic breath	Emphasizes a deep diaphragmatic inhale, followed by a forced exhalation through the mouth	Exhale with the most difficult (resistive) part of the movement
Movement Quality		
Both static and movement postures	No static exercises, only flow from one position to the next	Both static and full range of motion are used along with pulsing. For strengthening, the emphasis is on the concentric phase of movement with control of tension during eccentric phase.
Exercise Names		
Postures are commonly named after an animal (e.g., cobra, cat, scorpion, eagle) based on characteristics that the two share.	Exercise names are based on the description of what the movement is (roll-ups).	Exercise names are based on description of what the movement is (directional), and/or what muscle(s) are working (biceps curls), or what position exercise is performed in (side-lying leg lift).
Language (below are some examples of different words that mean the same thing)		
"Engage" your muscles. "Spiral" your shoulders open.	"Engage" your muscles. "Let your shoulders fall away from your ears."	"Contract" your muscles. "Pull your shoulders back."
Yoga and Pilates tend to be more descriptive: "feel your shoulder blades sliding down your back" or "feel a lifting…or feel a broadening."		Fitness is more directive: "squeeze your shoulder blades together" or "relax your shoulders."
3. OVERLAP (between historical disciplines and fitness-based classes)		
Many exercises are **common** between disciplines but **called something different**		
curl-ups	roll-ups	ab crunches
Many exercises are common between disciplines, **named the same** but are **performed differently**		
Cat: emphasis with the breath is to move past neutral in both directions, both arching and rounding the spine		*Cat*: emphasis is to move from rounding to table-top neutral
The **same exercise** is common between disciplines but **performed for different reasons**		
Downward facing dog: emphasis is to stretch hamstrings and open shoulders		*Mountain Climbers*: used to stretch calves in a static position and actively used to strengthen calves and increase muscle endurance
The **same exercise**, common between disciplines, may be **called something different**, yet is performed for the **same reasons and with similar form**		
Side lean in potted palm purpose: to elongate the torso laterally, stretch side and back muscles		Side bend in Indian cross sit purpose: to elongate the torso laterally, stretch side and back muscles
4. SUMMARY: RELATIONSHIP BETWEEN HISTORICAL DISCIPLINES/FITNESS		

Though the physical and mental approach is different, all disciplines maintain the philosophy that:
- movement improves the quality of life.
- body and mind are somehow connected.
- strengthening core muscles is essential to function.
- being fit improves one's mental state and how one feels about self.
- being fit contributes to life function.

Principles of Mat Science

Balance

Balance is achieved when all the body's muscles work synergistically without exerted or strained effort, breathing is tempered and even, and the mind is clear and free of extraneous thought. Within the Mat Science class format, "balance" is when the body, mind, and breath are connected in movement.

Extension

The principle of extension refers to the ability of the muscle to elongate out and away from the joint, creating freedom of unrestricted joint mobility as well as "activating" muscles to full length.

Alignment

The principle of alignment is to achieve proper form by setting posture before movement. This can make the difference in whether the execution of the exercise is performed correctly. Alignment improves the ability of the body to respond efficiently, improves balance, increases mental focus, and stimulates the ability to relax in any exercise and breathe.

Range of Motion

The principle of range of motion states that every exercise has a minimum and maximum boundary, or limitation, which determines personal range of motion. Using breath as a guide, awareness of the body's feedback, sensations, and signals determine when it's time to exceed beyond a certain point of tension, when to pull back tension, and when to maintain a certain range of motion.

Progression

For continued improvements in fitness, an exercise program should provide gradual increases or progressions in frequency, intensity, duration, and/or type of exercise. In Mat Science, progression refers to exercise selection. Every posture (position) consists of a series of exercises that layers the amount of challenge of intensity and difficulty as well as progressively builds on each other so an individual can continue to develop and reap the benefits that this discipline dictates. Recommended progressions will vary depending on age, physical limitations and participant's fitness level.

Flow

The principle of flow refers to the ability to transition smoothly from one posture to the next, using the breath to assist the process. Sequentially, movements that are held and those that move with the breath can be combined.

The Breath

The principle of breath acknowledges the breath as an integral part of every movement. Breathing should be deep, slow, and rhythmical. It is important for one to acquire an ability to regulate the length and duration of the inhalation, exhalation, and the retention of air within the lungs or pauses between breaths as dictated by each particular move or pose.

Class Format Guidelines

A typical Mat Science class is a blend of yoga postures, Pilates exercises, as well as any exercise from a more traditional fitness floor or dance class (like floor/barre work). A class may vary from 30–90 minutes, and the exercise selection is dependent on the instructor's knowledge within the various exercise techniques. For example, a class may be more yoga-based than dance-based or more Pilates-based than yoga-based.

The class format follows AFAA's *Basic Exercise Standards and Guidelines* (BESGs). However, the body of the class will vary depending on length of class, participant fitness levels, and instructor exercise selection. Therefore, AFAA recommends the following.

1. Always begin a Mat Science class with an initial warm-up and breathing.
2. Include a progressive series of exercises that build heat; increase both strength and flexibility in the body of the workout.
3. Always finish a Mat Science class with a final cool-down period to relax and restore.
4. If teaching more than one Mat Science class during the week, vary activities, progression, and intensity levels at each session.
5. Select different objectives or purposes for your class format (e.g., today we'll concentrate a little more on back strengthening, or today let's explore minimal and maximal boundaries during our forward bends).
6. Move fluidly and mindfully with each exercise; speed is not an option.
7. Use the principles of Mat Science to fine-tune your movements.
8. Develop appropriate levels of intensity of progressions for each movement used.
9. Modify movements for participants who need special attention.

Summary

Mat Science can provide a fun alternative to basic floor work by incorporating a variety of exercise techniques from basic conditioning exercises, dance, Pilates, and yoga to enhance fitness and well-being. To provide safe execution of these exercises, it is important to follow the training principles of Mat Science in conjunction with AFAA's *Basic Exercise Standards and Guidelines*. (Refer to Chapter 17.)

Sample Class Format

Warm-Up

Time: 10–15 minutes

Purpose:

- This initial warm-up is to introduce the breath so that body, mind, and breath can be linked for the entire workout.

What to include:

- Some form of breathing activity as part of your warm-up, alone or with a movement.
  Examples: Supine Breathing, Half Sun Breaths, Moving Twist with a Sun Breath
- Movements should include limbering and fluid motion as preparation for more challenging exercises to come (just as with current BESG for traditional fitness).
  Examples: Potted Palm Series, Cat, Cat with Downward Facing Dog in Vinyasa (flow)
- These movements should not be too challenging but bring students into mindfulness of their own bodies and how they're moving.

What to avoid:
- Positions in the first 10 minutes that require more ROM and deep openings of the joints (e.g., hips, shoulders, spine). Save these activities for when the body is more prepared (at least 10 minutes, depending on how much heat and preparation you have done in the initial warm-up).
    Examples: Bound Angular, Sitting Angular, Straight Leg Forward Bend, Back Bending

Body of Workout (based on class goals)

The following types of activities are recommended as part of a complete Mat Science class. Depending on the focus of the class that day (e.g., strength, alignment, back bending, etc.), more of one group of movements may be included than others. For a well-rounded class, however, include activities from each category.

Time: about 40 minutes total for this entire section (time will vary for each type of activity listed).

Heat-Building Movements
- Purpose: Increase core temperature and muscle core temperature.
- Mild heat builders can be utilized as part of the warm-up; more dynamic heat builders are best introduced following initial warm-up.
    Examples: Mild heat builders: Cat, Bridge/Moving Bridge, Bali Seal, Moving Low Lunge
    Dynamic Heat Builders: Cat to Downward Facing Dog, Hundred, Roll-ups
- Dynamic heat builders can also combine two or more movements together in a flow series to increase heat.
    Examples: Plank to Chatarunga to Downward Facing Dog to Cobra, Push-up to Plank Pose (3–6 times).
- Some heat building exercises also increase strength at the same time so include these last as a transition into strength
    Examples: Plank Pose with variations (with alternate leg raises, with a push-up)
- Avoid sacrificing form and stabilization for movement

Strength-Building Movements
- Purpose: To increase dynamic and functional strength of upper, core and lower extremities as both primary movers and stabilizers
- Include these moves at least 20 minutes into class when the body is fully warm and prepared
- Use transition moves, counter-moves (move of opposition to balance muscles worked) or resting poses between series of poses as necessary to relax, refocus or realign
    Examples: Child's Pose after Plank series; Bridge after an abdominal strengthening series; Forward Bend after back bending series
- Upper body strengtheners:
    Examples: Push-ups, Chatarungas slow and completed with hover, Swimming, Downward Facing Dog (held with the breath), Planks and Side Planks

- Torso strengtheners:
  - *Examples:* Scale, Single Leg Stretch, Crisscross, Planks, Back Bends, Knee Drops
- Lower body strengtheners:
  - *Examples:* Low Lunge, Leg Circles (done slowly with active legs), Kneeling Side Kicks, Side-lying Side Kicks

Back Bends

- Purpose: considered energizing movements to increase range of motion, flexibility and strength of the spine, as well as to open up front of the body
- Back bends should be included later in class, when the body is thoroughly warm and prepared; if the body has cooled down, rebuild heat first or begin with a moving back bend series before holding in any position
- These exercises should be performed progressively and slowly. Back bending can be mild (e.g., Low Lunge) or more challenging (e.g., Locust).
  - *Examples:* progression—opposite arm and leg to Sphinx to Cobra
- Back bending can be static, increasing ROM gently
- Back bending can be performed as a flow series with breath
  - *Examples:* Cobra: inhale in 4 counts and lift; exhale and lower in 4 counts. Then repeat 3–6 times; Moving Locust
- Back bending can be performed in a flow series with a forward bend
  - *Example:* in Low Lunge—bring arms forward, bend chest to knee, return to Low Lunge, arms extended above head
- Balance back bending with a counter move of forward bending (active or restoration) for release
  - *Examples:* Staff Pose Forward Bend (active), Child's Pose (restoration)

Forward Bends

- Purpose: lengthen back muscles, increase hamstrings flexibility and for relaxation and calming the mind by using the breath
- Create heat in the body before doing forward bends
- Avoid being overly aggressive; ease into forward bends slowly. Choose progressive exercises for both back and hamstrings
  - *Examples:* Potted Palm Forward Bend to Staff Pose Forward Bend or to Sitting Angular Forward Bend
- Balance forward bends with back bends

Twisting

- Purpose: Torso rotation is an important function of the spine; including rotation (twisting motions) improves spine range of motion, back flexibility and is good way to get the breath deeper in the abdomen and into the thoracic and lower spine, and out of the chest and shoulders
- Twisting can be static or performed with flow and the breath
  - *Examples:* in Potted Palm Twist, then with Sun Breaths
- Twisting for Mat Science is performed sitting or lying supine and can also be used as a cool-down or restorative movement
  - *Examples:* Bent Knee Twist, Long Lying Stretch
- For balance, always twist equally in both directions as part of the movement sequence

Joint Openers

- Purpose: to increase joint range of motion (particularly shoulders and hips) and increase flexibility of muscles that have the tendency to be tight (hamstrings); these stretches are considered "deep" openers
     Examples: Bull Seat Prep, 1/2 Staff Pose Twist, Sitting Angular Leg Extension, Long Lying Stretch
- Include these exercises during the last half of class when you're warm and fluid; the body uses heat created to stretch without straining.
- Use the principle of range of motion to establish minimal and maximal boundaries; ease into each position, carefully and slowly.
- Use the breath to move deeper into position; be cautious of any joint pain

Transition (Resting) Movements

- Purpose: To relax from exertion after a challenging series (example: Plank/Downward Facing Dog Vinyasa, Scale Progression) or movement (joint openers); to reconnect to focus and the breath; and to transition smoothly and easily to another movement.
- Do use these poses when you need to take a break
     Examples: Child's Pose, Extended Seal, supine knees to chest

Cool-Down

Time: 5 to 10 minutes

Purpose: to use the breath to slow down and relax, release from any deep joint openers, twisting, or strength movements.

Choose movements that are more restorative in nature.
     Examples: Bent Knee Twists, Long Lying Stretch, Side-lying Shoulder Circles

What to avoid:

- Building heat
- Moves that are too active or strenuous
- Ending a class in a backbend

Sample Exercises Provided are examples of exercises appropriate for the warm-up, body of the workout, and cool-down segments of a Mat Science class (by number, not order of suggested progression).

Warm-Up

Half Sun Breaths

Roots: Yoga

Benefits: Increases circulation; promotes proper breathing technique, warms up upper torso

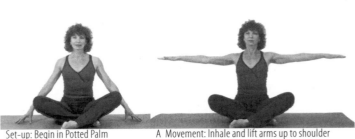 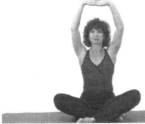

Set-up: Begin in Potted Palm

A Movement: Inhale and lift arms up to shoulder height; exhale and turn palms down.

B Inhale and lift arms up overhead, intertwining fingers, exhale—turn palms up to ceiling, arms remain straight, inhale here, exhale bring arms back down by your sides on the floor.

Cues: Make sure to call the breath. Keep shoulders relaxed. Keep breath smooth and even.

Breathing: Full complete breathing or Ujjayi

Number of reps: 3–4

Variation: Simplified version: inhale, lifts arms above head, palms touch (or arms parallel), exhale, return hands to the floor.

Side Lean

Roots: Yoga

Benefits: Increases circulation; promotes proper breathing technique; warms up upper torso, particularly the lats, sides of torso and shoulders

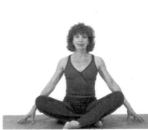 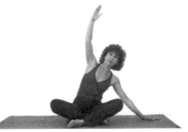 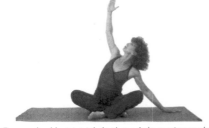

Set-up: Begin in Potted Palm

A Movement: Walk fingertips of one hand out to the side, let hand relax on the floor, scoop other arm up and overhead; continue to stretch laterally.

B To open shoulder joint, inhale, then exhale, moving arm behind you. Look up at your hand. Return to Potted Palm, set position, then repeat other side.

Cues: Initiate the deeper movement by opening at the shoulder, not just pulling arm. Keep equal length on both sides of torso; don't collapse into the stretch. Keep shoulders down and relaxed. Feel length in the back by drawing shoulder blades down and back.

Breathing: Full complete breathing or Ujjayi

Number of breaths: 2–4 held on each side, or a movement series of 3–4 reps.

Moving Cat Seal

Roots: Yoga

Benefits: Synchronizes movement with breath, warms up upper torso, hips and thighs; use also as Mild Heat Builder

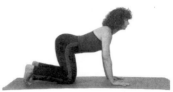 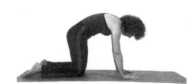 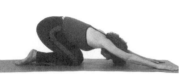

A Set-up: Kneel on all fours; knees are positioned under hips and arms under shoulders. Spread your fingers, fingers pointing forward, palms flat on the floor, elbows not locked. Contract abdominals so head, neck and spine are aligned in one straight line. Curl toes underneath.

B Movement: The beginning of this move is the same as CAT. Inhale, simultaneously tip your sitz bones up and draw your shoulder blades and shoulders back and down away from your ears. Look up without hyperextending neck (see A photo).

C Exhale, tuck chin and pull belly in toward spine as you round spine and drop the tops of your feet onto the floor so you can sit back on your heels, with arms extended overhead, hands on the floor; this is called Extended Cat Seal.

Cues: Keep the roundness in spine as you sit back on heels. It's not necessary to get your seat back onto your heels if you're tight.

Breathing: Full complete breathing or Ujjayi

Number of reps: 4–6

Body of Workout

The Hundred

Roots: Pilates

Benefits: Dynamic Heat-Builder; increases circulation with synchronized movement and breaths. Strengthens abdominals and scapular muscles

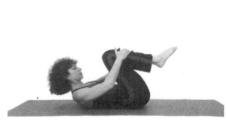 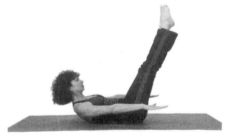

A Set-up: Lying supine, bring knees to chest and grasp legs below your knees. Bring navel to spine, lifting head, neck and shoulders off the floor; tuck chin down and in toward chest. Keep shoulder blades on the mat, and continue to press navel to spine to keep back in contact with mat.

B Movement: Maintain abdominal brace and extend legs in air anywhere from a 90- to 45-degree angle. Extend arms parallel to your torso, palms down; keep arms stiff through fingertips. Maintain this position, inhale for 5 counts, then exhale for 5 counts, pumping arms in short quick movements downward quickly on every count. Repeat for l00 counts.

Cues: Only arms and shoulders are moving. If necessary, build up to 100, stopping when abdominal brace or scapular stabilization is lost.

Breathing: Complete inhalation/forced exhalation

Number of reps: 10 cycles of 10 inhales and exhales, equaling 100

Variation: If necessary, keep knees bent to learn the movement.

Low Lunge

Roots: Yoga

Benefits: Mild Heat-Builder; stretches hip flexors and quadriceps; mild back bend when arms are lifted; strengthens abductors and adductors as hip and knee stabilizers as balance is challenged; becomes a dynamic heat builder and lower body strengthener when combined in flowing movement series

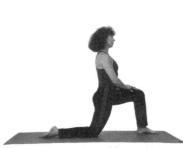 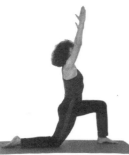

A Set-up: From a kneeling position or all fours position, step forward with one foot, keeping front knee aligned directly over ankle; place hands on front thigh. Contract abdominals to bring spine to a neutral position. Drop shoulder blades down and back, creating space between ears and shoulders, with breastbone lifted.

B Movement: Press forward through front hip to increase stretch on hip flexor, without taking knee past toes. To increase heat of static posture, sweep arms up and out to your sides until arms are extended overhead and parallel to each other. Lengthen arms through fingertips. Hold for recommended breaths. Do as a Flying Lunge or Vinyasa Forward Bends in lunge position for more heat. (see Variations)

Cues: As arms sweep upward, keep shoulders down and away from ears. Press hips forward without leaning forward.

Breathing: 3–5 breaths held or a movement series of 4–6 reps for each variation below

Number of breaths: 3–5 breaths held or a movement series of 4–6 reps for each variation below.

Variation: Lunge in movement (1) keeping hands on thigh, inhale and straighten front knee in 4 counts, bend back to starting position in 4 counts; (2) Flying Lunge: maintain a lunge position, only moving your arms: with arms hanging by your sides, inhale, then exhale, sweeping arms overhead, inhale, lower arms to your sides; (3) Vinyasa Forward Bend 1: maintain a lunge position, intertwine forearms behind the small of your back: inhale, forward folding by bending from the hips to bring chest toward knees, keep back long, not rounded, exhale lifting torso back to starting position; (4) Vinyasa Forward Bend 2: same as (3) except from the forward fold, arms lift overhead, palms to touch or parallel instead of returning behind back.

Double Leg Stretch

Roots: Pilates

Benefits: Strengthens abdominal muscles as stabilizers; synchronizes breath with movement to improve coordination and control

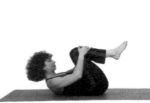 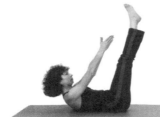 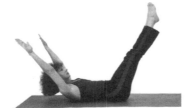

A Set-up: Begin supine with both knees bent in toward chest. Head, neck and shoulder blades lifted off the floor. Abdominals braced and toes gently pointed. Place hands just below knees on lower legs

A Movement—Version 1: Inhale, simultaneously straighten arms and legs without moving torso or changing hip angle, keeping legs together (B): maintain torso and leg position, and circle arms out, around and overhead, back to same extended position (C). Inhale, reach up toward legs with arms, exhale to start position (A).

C Movement—Version 2: Inhale, extend legs and lift arms up and overhead until even with your ears (C): exhale and sweep arms down by your sides and back to start position as you bend your knees in toward chest at same time (A).

Cues: Continue to pull navel to spine as arms and legs straighten and fold. Keep shoulder blades lifted off the mat; stabilize upper torso position by drawing shoulder blades down and back toward spine. Keep legs and arms active, chin toward chest.

Breathing: Complete inhalation/forced exhalation

Number of breaths: 6–10

Knee Drops

Roots: Pilates

Benefits: Develops pelvic stability; strengthens abdominals; strengthen hip lateral flexors and rotators as stabilizers. Use also as a Mild Heat Builder and Warm-Up (Version 1)

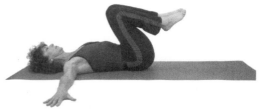 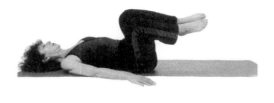

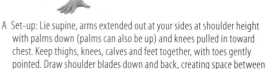

A Set-up: Lie supine, arms extended out at your sides at shoulder height with palms down (palms can also be up) and knees pulled in toward chest. Keep thighs, knees, calves and feet together, with toes gently pointed. Draw shoulder blades down and back, creating space between shoulders and ears; keep shoulders on floor for entire movement

B Movement: Maintain this position, lower knees toward the floor; keep knees aligned and together. Only lower as far as you can keeping pelvis stable, shoulders on the floor and maintain ability to use abdominals to lift legs back up. Bring knees back to center, using your abdominals. Repeat for recommended reps.

Cues: Two breathing patterns: (1) inhale, then exhale as you lower legs. Inhale, then exhale lifting legs back up or (2) inhale, lowering legs, exhale back up to center

Breathing: Complete inhalation/forced exhalation

Number of reps: 10 (1 rep equals a drop to both sides)

Chatarunga

Roots: Yoga

Benefits: Dynamic Heat-Builder; strengthens upper torso and arms; develops core and scapular stabilization; use also as Upper Body Strengthener

Set-up: Begin in Plank Pose or modified on your knees

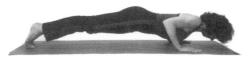 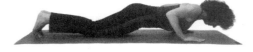

A Movement: Inhale, then exhale, lowering entire body as one unit to the floor. Keep elbows close to body.

B If you lack upper body strength, place knees on floor and perform the same exercise (B). Hover just above the floor, then push back up to starting position, or lower all the way to the floor to combine with another movement.

Cues: Stabilize the torso, maintaining one straight line by contracting your abdominals, keep navel pulled in toward spine. Look at a point right in front of you to avoid dropping head and collapsing chest. Keep chest open. Draw shoulders back and down, avoid forward rounding.

Breathing: Full complete breathing or Ujjayi

Number of reps: 1–6 depending what it is combined with

Roll-Ups

Roots: Pilates

Benefits: Warms up the entire spine; mild hamstring stretch; works the abdominals as stabilizers; use also as a Dynamic Heat Builder and Core Strengthener

Set-up: Lie supine on the floor, legs and feet relaxed and together. Extend arms in the air above shoulders, activated, with fingers pointing toward ceiling. Let shoulder blades drop down your back, creating space between ears and shoulders. Tuck chin.

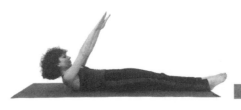 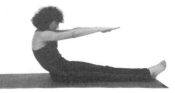 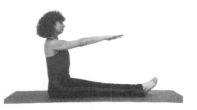

A. Movement: Inhale, then exhale and using your abdominals (keep legs and hip flexors relaxed throughout) by bringing navel to spine, begin to roll upwards.

B Lead with your breastbone and arms and continue to reach forward. Keep the roundness in your spine and chin tucked.

C Extend the spine as you come to a full seated position. Inhale and roll down the same way you rolled up.

Cues: Continue to keep length in the torso, even in roundness as you lift out and away from hips. Balance opposition of back and ab muscles working together to stabilize the movement.

Breathing: Complete inhalation/forced exhalation

Number of reps: 4–6

Variation: Roll part way up and stop, until stronger, at the "sticky point" of exercise when hip flexors want to take over. Use a basket hold (cross arms, place hands on opposite shoulders) to train neck muscles until stronger.

Plank Hip Extension

Roots: Yoga and Pilates

Benefits: Strengthens legs; improves scapular, core and pelvic stability; strengthens upper torso; use also as a Dynamic Heat-Builder and Upper Body and Core Strengthener

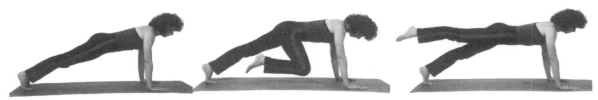

Set-up: Begin in Plank Pose

B Movement: Maintain Plank Pose, inhale and draw one knee in toward chest without changing torso or pelvis position, toes gently pointed.

C Exhale, slowly straighten leg behind you keeping leg at hip height and spine in a neutral position. Inhale, draw knee back toward chest. Complete reps and switch legs.

Cues: Stabilize the torso, maintaining one straight line by contracting your abdominals, keep navel pulled in toward spine. Look at a point right in front of you to avoid dropping head and collapsing chest. Keep chest open. Draw shoulders back and down, avoid forward rounding.

Breathing: Full complete breathing or Ujjayi or complete inhalation/forced exhalation

Number of reps: 8–12 on each leg

One-legged Bridge

Roots: Pilates

Benefits: Strengthens legs, hips and buttocks; improves core and pelvic stability. Use also as a Core Strengthener.

Set-up: Lie supine, knees bent and feet flat on the floor, hip-width apart; relax arms by sides with palms facing down. Cross one ankle over opposite thigh. Draw shoulder blades down and away from ears.

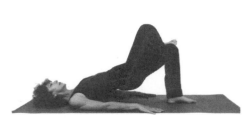 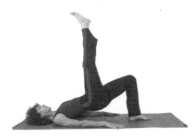

A Movement: Maintain this position and inhale, then exhale as you begin to lift tailbone off floor. Continue to pull navel in toward spine as you lift a neutral spine off the floor to the point where shoulder blades are still in contact with the floor. Contract buttocks as you reach the top of the lift. In the final position, you'll feel a stretch in the hip flexor and rectus femorus of the stabilizing leg.

B Inhale, then exhale, navel to spine as you slowly lower as if to lay vertebrae down in straight line on the floor, starting with upper back to tailbone. To make this same exercise more challenging, extend one leg straight up in the air in line with hips

Cues: Don't arch back as you lift; keep spine neutral. Keep head, neck and shoulders relaxed. The pelvis should be stable in both lifting and lowering motions.

Breathing: Ujjayi or complete inhalation/forced exhalation

Number of reps: 4–6 of each or either movement

Variations: Hold the One-Legged Bridge statically for 3–4 breaths in the lifted position

Superman Series

Roots: Yoga and Pilates

Benefits: Increases range of motion, flexibility and strength of spine; improves core and pelvic stability; opens front of torso; strengthens buttocks and legs

Set-up: Lie prone with arms outstretched palms down; place forehead and tops of feet on the floor. Drop shoulders back and away from ears. Pull abdominals inward, dropping tailbone down toward the floor. Contract buttocks and thighs pressing hips and pubis to the mat (A).

A B

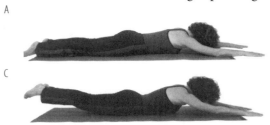 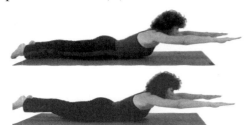

C D

Movement: Do one or all of the following variations: (1) Inhale and lift head, arms, and chest off the floor; keep head aligned with spine, then lower yourself back to the floor (B). (2) Keeping upper torso motionless and arms on the mat, lift legs off floor, only as high as you can without undue tension in spine (C). (3) Balancing on pubic bone, lift both upper torso and legs off the floor, reaching in opposite directions with extremities to create length in spine (D).

Cues: Keep arms and legs active. Do this move in progression slowly to build strength and not overwork lower back. Tune-in to fine points of each part of this movement, always creating length out of the lower back.

Breathing: Ujjayi or complete inhalation/forced exhalation

Number of breaths: 1–2 held or a movement series of 4–8 reps.

Swimming

Roots: Pilates

Benefits: Strengthens back muscles, upper torso, buttocks and legs; improves core and pelvic stability; opens front of torso; use also as an Upper Body Strengthener.

Set-up: Same as set-up for position Superman A, legs and ankles together.

Cues: Keep arms and legs active; keep reaching extremities in opposition for more length. Keep shoulders back and down from ears, with neck long. Do this move half time as an Opposite Arm and Leg Lift to learn the movement.

Breathing: Complete inhalation/forced exhalation

Number of reps: 4–5 count breath inhale and 4–5 count breath exhale

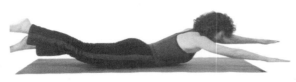

Movement: Lift head, left arm and right leg off the floor, as high as you can and switch. Alternate arms and legs in short, quick, yet long swimming motions, keeping the movements controlled and even.

Bent Knee Forward Bend

Roots: Yoga

Benefits: Stretches back muscles

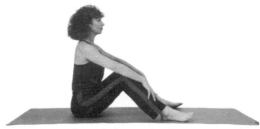

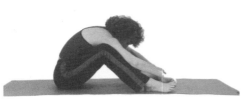

A Set-up: Sit with knees bent and feet on the floor. Reach under your seat and pull the fleshy part of your buttocks out and away from your tailbone so you can feel both sitz bones on floor. Place hands on lower legs, arms straight but relaxed. Lift torso up and off of hip bones, creating length in the spine. Let shoulders fall away from ears to create space between shoulders and ears.

B Movement: Inhale, then exhale as you lean forward from hips toward feet. As chest comes in contact with thighs, grasp inside of feet, rounding spine. Continue to use the breath to exhale deeper into forward bend.

Cues: Begin to round spine when maximum hip flexion in this position is reached. Use feet hold as an anchor to reach deeper in pose. Keep head aligned with spine and no tension in neck.

Breathing: Full complete breathing or Ujjayi

Number of breaths: 4–8 held or a movement flow of 4–6 reps.

Seated Bent Knee Twist

Roots: Yoga

Benefits: Improves spine mobility and relaxation; stretches sides of torso

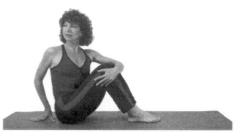 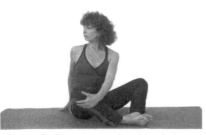

Set-up: Sit with knees bent as close to chest as possible and sit upright without leaning backward, feet flat on floor and together. Place both hands behind buttocks, press hips forward and up onto sitz bones to lengthen torso up off hips. Keeping legs and ankles together, grasp the outside of one knee and gently inhale, then exhale to twist toward that side, letting shoulder and head follow the movement. Use the breath to rotate further into the pose.
Movement: Static posture; hold for recommended breaths.

Variation: Do this same twist in Bound Angular Pose to deepen hip opening and groin stretch at the same time.

Cues: Stay lifted evenly on both sides of torso without collapsing into the movement. Don't lean backwards onto buttocks to increase the rotation. Don't pull yourself around; use the breath to increase the twist.

Breathing: Full complete breathing or Ujjayi

Number of breaths: 4–6

Cool-Down

Child's Pose

Roots: Yoga and Pilates
Cues: Use the breath to deepen and relax.
Benefits: Resting pose; stretches back, neck and thighs. Use also as a Cool-Down static pose.
Cues: Use the breath to deepen and relax.
Breathing: Full complete breathing or Ujjayi
Number of reps: 4–6

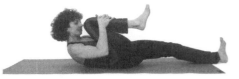

A. Set-up: Kneel with legs and ankles together, then sit back onto your heels (if flexible enough) touching buttocks; tops of feet are on mat. Torso is resting on knees, forehead on the floor, and arms by your sides, palms up.
B Movement: This is a static pose; stay here and rest for recommended breaths.

Single Knee to Chest Stretch

Roots: Yoga

Benefits: Cool-down stretch for hip flexors, buttocks, upper and lower back.

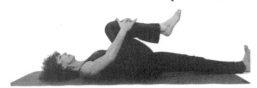 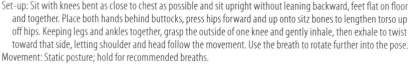

A Set-up: Lie supine with both knees bent in toward chest. Clasp hand around one lower leg just below the knee, then slowly slide other leg straight, toes flexed. Hold knee in toward chest and pelvic tilt, lengthening out through heel of extended leg. Hold here for a few breaths before continuing.

B Movement: From the set-up position, lift head and shoulders off mat, trying to touch nose to knee. Hold here.

Cues: Keep shoulders down and away from ears as you lift upper torso; stay relaxed. Keep lengthening straight leg, pressing out through heel to increase stretch on hip flexors as you pelvic tilt.

Breathing: Full complete breathing or Ujjayi

Number of breaths: 4–6

References

1. Ansari, M., & Lark, L. (1998). *Yoga for beginners.* New York, NY: Harper Collins.

2. Calais-Germain, B. (1993). *Anatomy of movement.* Seattle, WA: Eastland Press.

3. Davis, C. (2009). *Contemporary theories in rehabilitation: Evidence for efficacy in therapy, prevention, and wellness.* Thorofare, NJ: Slack Incorporated.

4. Finger, A., & Bingham, A. (2000). *Introduction to yoga.* New York, NY: Three Rivers Press.

5. Friedman, P., & Eisen, G. (1980). *The Pilates method of physical and mental conditioning.* New York, NY: Doubleday & Co.

6. Gallagher, S.P., & Kryzanowska, R. (1999). *The Pilates method of body conditioning.* Philadelphia, PA: Trans-Atlantic Publications.

7. Luttgens, K., & Hamilton, N. (1997). *Kinesiology: Scientific basis of human motion* (9th ed.). Boston, MA: McGraw-Hill.

8. McGinnis, P.M. (2005). *Biomechanics of sport and exercise.* Champaign, IL: Human Kinetics.

9. Robinson, L., & Thomson, G. (1998). *Body control: Using techniques by Joseph H. Pilates.* Philadelphia, PA: BainBridge Books.

10. Schiffman, E. (1996). *Yoga, the spirit and practice of moving into stillness.* New York, NY: First Pocket Books.

11. Windsor, M., & Laska, M. (1999). *The Pilates powerhouse.* Cambridge, MA: Perseus Books.

12. Yogananda, P. (1993). *Autobiography of a yogi.* Self Realization Fellowship.

30 *Sports Conditioning*

Jill Boyer-Holland and
Sandy Greger, MEd, ATC

Focus

Before participating in any sport, it is important to become involved in a conditioning program. Preseason conditioning will improve performance, increase skill, and help to prevent the injuries most common to that sport. Accidents occur frequently when muscles tire and reflexes slow. Strong muscles do not tire as quickly, so we can spend more time playing and less time recovering.

Learn the Physical Requirements of the Sport

Although there are similarities between all conditioning programs, each sport is unique unto itself, as is its training program. These differences must be recognized and defined. As a fitness professional, you must learn the physiological requirements of each sport. If you are unfamiliar with a sport, watch the game or event carefully to see what muscles are involved and how movements are utilized during actual performance. This will give you valuable clues as to what exercises to select for training.

In any conditioning program, certain factors need to be addressed. They are strength, flexibility, and endurance.

Strength is the maximum amount of force that a muscle is able to exert in a single contraction. By selecting strengthening exercises specific to the chosen sport, you can greatly enhance muscular efficiency and reduce the possibility of injury.

Flexibility is the maximum range of motion available at a joint. Increased flexibility decreases risk of injury to joints and muscles by increasing available range of motion. It helps to improve the quality of performance by reducing muscle tension, which allows for freer, more fluid movements. It is important to note that different sports have different flexibility requirements.

The term "endurance" pertains to both the muscular system and the cardiorespiratory system. Muscular endurance is the ability of a muscle to contract repeatedly over a long period of time. The cardiorespiratory system is the pathway our body uses to get oxygen and other nutrients out to the working muscles. The more efficiently the heart can pump blood, nutrients, and oxygen to the muscle, the greater the cardiorespiratory endurance of the body. Maintaining 64–94% of maximum heart rate (or RPE 5–8) for a period of 20–60 minutes will help to achieve this goal. However, many sports require a high anaerobic capacity as well. This refers to the body's ability to function for a short period of time in a state of oxygen deficit at a high intensity. For these sports, some form of interval training should be considered. The higher the intensity, the shorter the duration of the activity should be. Work intervals must be followed by periods of active recovery to reestablish steady state (normal breathing) before being repeated.

In addition to improving the fitness-related components mentioned above, sports require skill. The skill-related components of fitness are:
- **Agility**—the ability to change body position quickly and efficiently
- **Balance**—the ability to keep the body in equilibrium
- **Coordination**—the integration of the muscular and nervous system to create harmonious movement

- **Power**—the ability to produce maximum force in the shortest time
- **Reaction time**—the time it takes to initiate a response
- **Speed**—the ability to propel the body rapidly from one place to another

Since each component stresses the body in a slightly different manner, specific exercises need to be developed in order to improve the performance and skill requirements of each individual sport.

Alpine Skiing Preconditioning Program

As an example in designing a sport-specific training program, we will look at the demands that downhill (Alpine) skiing puts on one's body and develop a program to meet these special needs.

Alpine skiing is technically difficult and potentially very dangerous. Being in shape for skiing can make these difficulties easier to overcome and help reduce the risk of injury. Gone are the days of skiing your way into shape. "Hitting the slopes" will be far more enjoyable if done figuratively, not literally.

Skiing is a sport that demands tremendous muscle strength and endurance, good flexibility, and a well-developed aerobic and anaerobic capacity. Balance, agility, coordination, and reaction time, as well as muscular power, are also prime factors that must be taken into consideration when developing a training program for this physically demanding sport.

By examining the energy demands of skiing, one can quickly see that it is important to train both the aerobic and anaerobic energy systems. The Alpine skier must be a long distance runner as well as a sprinter. One method of training both systems is Fartlek training or Swedish speed play. In this form of interval training, constant pace periods (submaximal) are interspersed with shorter periods of increased speed (maximal). Movement is continuous, thus placing an anaerobic stress within the context of aerobic training.

To design a sports conditioning program, you must:

1. **Assess the physical demands**. Alpine skiing demands the development of power, strength, and endurance of the legs, thighs, buttocks, hips, abdominals, and lower back. One way of achieving this goal is through circuit training, which emphasizes strength training within an aerobic format by moving rapidly from one exercise to the next using low resistance and high repetition, achieving not only muscle hypertrophy, but a significant increase in aerobic capacity as well.

2. **Match the appropriate exercises**. The ability to sustain isometric contractions of the thigh, calf, buttocks, abdominal, and back muscles to maintain position and control while skiing are necessary, but intermittent bursts of power and dynamic contraction are also required to carve turns. Exercises that stress these muscles isometrically as well as isotonically should be considered along with some form of plyometric training, which will help to develop greater muscular power.

3. **Look for the specific challenge**s. In Alpine skiing, we are constantly subjecting our bodies to quick changes of direction and variations in terrain, and then recovering lost balance. Sometimes, we are successful in overcoming these challenges; sometimes, we are not. If we do not meet the challenge, we may find ourselves hurdling through the air, landing in the infamous "face plant." Since constant terrain changes require great agility, drills can be developed to improve the ability to change position quickly. Training on a Bosu®, core board, or wobble board, for example will dynamically and statically improve balance and hopefully keep us

upright. But if the worst happens and we take a tumble, we increase our chances of surviving these falls without injury if we have good flexibility. When our muscles are tight, the range of motion available at the joint is limited, predisposing us to injury. It is important to keep in mind that flexibility is joint- and direction-specific, and will differ with each individual. One's flexibility is determined by lifestyle, past athletic history, and genetics. For Alpine skiing, an overall flexibility program is recommended. A weekly yoga class can improve overall flexibility and help to reduce the risk of injury.

4. **Determine the total components**. Having examined the physical requirements of our sport, we have determined that the following components need to be addressed.
   a) Aerobic and anaerobic energy systems
   b) Muscular strength, power, and endurance, primarily for the lower legs, thighs, hips, back, abdominals, and buttocks
   c) Core stability
   d) Balance
   e) Agility
   f) Coordination
   g) Flexibility for the total body

The class outlined below has been designed specifically to meet these needs.

Tuned to Ski Circuit

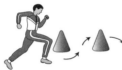

Slalom Running. Develops the ability to shift the body's weight rapidly while moving forward. Fine-tunes turning ability. Proper foot landing is heel, ball, toe.

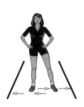

Lateral Slides. Develops the ability to rapidly shift the body's weight laterally. Fine-tunes turning ability.

Air Squats. Conditions the legs to act as shock absorbers over uneven terrain, e.g., moguls, etc. Avoid hyperextension of the knees.

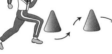

Wall Sits with Heel Raise. Strengthens the quadriceps, hip flexors and calf muscles. Sitting position is held for the one-minute time limit. Heels are raised and lowered in time with music. Never drop the buttocks below the level of the hips.

Step-ups. Strengthens the hip and knee flexors. Enhances climbing ability. Step can be 8-12 inches high depending on participant ability. Angle of step should never exceed 90 degrees from the hip.

Rope Jumping. Stabilizes the forearm and conditions the wrists for poling. Promotes independent leg action, calf, quad and hip extensor strength and endurance.

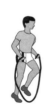

Pole Hopping. Promotes independent leg action and lateral hip movement.

Step-Tap   Step-Tap

Push-ups. Strengthens upper body, abdominals and back muscles. Hips should be slightly piked to avoid low-back strain.

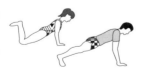

Standing Lunges. Strengthens knee musculature. Weight should be centered in the heel of the front foot during lunge. Do not allow knee to extend beyond the tip of the toes.

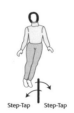

Box Jumping. Plyometric training helps develop muscular contraction and extension of the legs, as well as power and quickness. Box may be 8–10 inches depending on participant ability.

Summary

In conclusion, our world as a whole is becoming more competitive as evidenced by the aggressive approach many of us take to our chosen leisure time activities. George Sheehan, world-renowned physician and runner, once said, "Every individual is an athlete whose event is getting through a 16-hour day." Getting through the rigors of a normal work day and having enough energy and strength left over to play our favorite sports is a goal everyone can work toward. Achieving and then maintaining physical fitness, we enable ourselves to play longer, harder, and ultimately better in any sport we choose.

References

1. Aerobics and Fitness Association of America. (2007). *Kickboxing a manual for instructors.* Sherman Oaks, CA: Aerobics and Fitness Association of America.

2. American College of Sports Medicine. (2010). *ACSM's guidelines for exercise testing and prescription* (8th ed.). Baltimore, MD: Lippincott Williams & Wilkins.

3. American College of Sports Medicine. (2010). *ACSM's resource manual for guidelines for exercise testing and prescription* (6th ed.). Baltimore, MD: Lippincott Williams & Wilkins.

4. Buxbaum, R., & Micheli, L.J. (1979). *Sports for life: Fitness training, nutrition and injury prevention.* Boston, MA: Beacon Press.

5. Noble, B.J. (1986). *Physiology of exercise and sport.* St. Louis, MO: Times Mirror/Mosby College.

6. Pearl, B., & Moran, G. (1986). *Getting stronger: Weight training for men and women.* Bolinas, CA: Shelter.

7. Sheehan, G. (1988). Lecture delivered at The Academy of Osteopathic Sports Medicine Clinical Conference. Palms Springs, CA. 10 Mar.

8. Southmayd, W., & Hoffman, M. (1981). *Sports health: The complete book of athletic injury.* New York, NY: Perigee.

9. Wilmore, J.H., Costill, D.L., & Kenney, W.L. (2008). *Physiology of sport and exercise* (4th ed.). Champaign, IL: Human Kinetics.

31

Step Training

Patti Mantia, EdD and
Laura A. Gladwin, MS

Focus

Since its origin in the late 1980s, step training has continued to be a popular form of high-intensity, low-impact aerobic exercise, and has advanced to new and exciting levels. Although relatively new to the group exercise class setting, bench stepping has been used for decades in athletic training, physical therapy, and as a tool for submaximal testing to assess cardiovascular fitness. As fitness instructors continue to develop step training classes that are interesting and challenging for their participants, they must be aware of, and incorporate, the current safety guidelines.

Step Training Recommendations

Detailed discussions on step training research, choreography, injury prevention, and teaching techniques are found in AFAA's *Step Training: A Manual for Instructors.*

As is true with any form of cardiorespiratory training, programming recommendations for step training should be carefully considered. When beginning such a program, class participants should be advised to begin with a moderate program and to gradually progress the program as they become accustomed to this type of exercise. Table 31-1 outlines step training recommendations.

Table 31-1. Level	Recommended Step Height	Suggested Stepping Duration
Level 1		
Someone who has not participated in a regular exercise program	4 inches	10–20 minutes
Level 2		
A regular exerciser who is new to step training	4 to 6 inches	10–20 minutes
Level 3		
A regular stepper	4 to 8 inches	minimum of 20–30 minutes, no more than 60 minutes
Level 4		
A highly skilled and regular stepper	4 to 10 inches	20–60 minutes

Class Format

The following are the components of a step class.

Pre-class Instructions

Duration: 2–3 minutes
Purpose: To familiarize participants with step training technique and guidelines.

Warm-up

Tempo: 120–134 bpm
Duration: 8–12 minutes
Purpose: To increase core temperature as well as prepare the muscles and joints for movements that will follow. This can be

accomplished by combining movement rehearsal, limbering, as well as light preparatory stretches. A proper warm-up should prepare the body for vigorous exercise and may reduce the risk of injury.

Cardiorespiratory Training

Tempo: 118–128 beats per minute (bpm); 128–135 bpm for advanced, highly-skilled participants since form, technique, and safety can be compromised at fast tempos, especially for novice steppers

Duration: 20–60 minutes

Purpose: To improve the heart, circulatory, and pulmonary systems. This can be accomplished by utilizing a variety of training methods that target cardiorespiratory endurance. (For more information on the various types of training methods, see Chapter 17, "Basic Exercise Standards and Guidelines.")

Muscular Strength and Endurance Training

Tempo: 120–130 bpm

Duration: 15–20 minutes

Purpose: Important component to overall health. Benefits include an improved ability to perform everyday activities, increased muscle mass, increased metabolism, stronger bones, decreased risk of injury, improved posture and symmetry, and improved athletic performance.

Flexibility and Final Class

Tempo: Under 100 bpm

Duration: 5–10 minutes (or time to complete a minimum of 1 set for each muscle group)

Purpose: Flexibility training improves joint mobility and increases range of motion in order to decrease the risk of potential injury and enhance physical performance. The final class segment is designed to promote mind-body awareness and facilitate the relaxation response, a state in which the heart rate and blood pressure are decreased, muscles are relaxed, and physiological stress is reduced. It is an optimal time for participant education. It also provides a sense of completion.

To minimize risk of injury and maximize conditioning benefits of stepping, teach the following body alignment and stepping technique guidelines to step class participants. Continually monitor participants' form, and coach as necessary (Refer to figures 31-1, 31-2, and 31-3).

Body Alignment

- Shoulders back and relaxed
- Chest lifted and body erect
- Abdominal muscles contracted to support torso
- Neutral spine
- Knees relaxed, not locked
- Avoid hyperextension of joints
- Avoid twisting (torque) in the joints

Stepping Technique

- Use a full body lean; do not bend at the waist or hips
- Knee flexion should not exceed 90° when weight-bearing.
- Watch the platform periodically.
- Focus on the feet first. Add arm movements when proficient with the footwork.
- Step to the center of the step; don't let your feet hang off the edge.
- Stay close to the step platform as you step down.*
- Don't step down with your back to the platform.
- Step lightly; avoid pounding your feet on the step.
- Allow your whole foot to contact the floor, and step (except during propulsion/power movements, lunges, and repeaters).
- Use proper lifting techniques. Bend at the knees instead of the back when lifting the step. Carry the step close to the body.

Note: A general guideline of one shoe length is recommended as an appropriate distance when stepping down away from the step. However, as lever length and foot sizes vary, this guideline may not be appropriate for everyone. Individual stride length can be determined in the following manner. Starting with feet together, step forward with the right leg to the point where you feel the gluteals on the left leg engage. This distance will mark the appropriate stride length for an experienced stepper with adequate leg strength and flexibility. The novice should step down with the shorter stride until dynamic strength and mobility are developed.

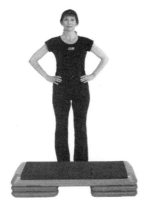

Fig. 31-1.
Body alignment

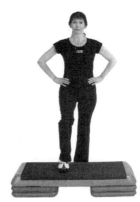

Fig. 31-2.
Stepping technique

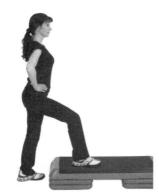

Fig. 31-3.
Proper step posture

Variables that Affect Intensity

As in any form of aerobic activity, the exercise session should begin with a moderate intensity and increase gradually. The participant should remain within the training range for the designated period of time and decrease gradually to the pre-exercise level. Creating the bell-shaped intensity curve will allow the participant to adapt both physiologically and biomechanically to the exercise. The instructor should inform the students of methods to adapt intensity to an appropriate level.

A number of variables were found to affect exercise intensity during step training. The most significant increases occurred with two key variables: (a) step height, and (b) choreography.

Step Height as a Variable to Modify Exercise Intensity

Intensity and step height appear to be linear in relationship. Thus, an increase in step height will produce an increased energy cost. Participants are encouraged to select a step height that will allow an appropriate training stimulus without compromising form and technique.

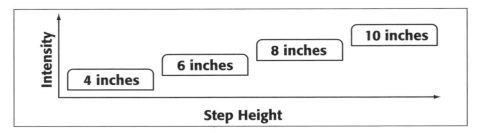

Choreography as a Variable to Modify Exercise Intensity

Movement patterns may be designed to manipulate the intensity of a step class. Factors, such as lever length, elevation of levers, range of motion, speed of movement (e.g., propulsions or power movements), and traveling, will dictate the intensity of the step skill or combination of skills. Smaller movements, such as the basic step and V-step, are generally low-intensity movements that may be used in the building and decreasing phases of the bell curve design. Movements, such as lunges and traveling knee lifts, are higher in intensity and should be interspersed throughout the workout (rather than placed all together) to avoid overworking the class participants. A summary of step movement skills and the measure of intensity for each is provided in Table 31-2.

Step Movement	VO$_2$ (ml/kg/min)	METs
Basic Step	26.2	7.5
Across-the-top	26.6	7.6
Alternating Knee-lift	28.7	8.2
Repeater Knee-lift	32.0	9.1
Alternating Lunge	32.7	9.3
Turn-step with Lunge	35.0	10.1

Table 31.2. Effect of Varying Step Patterns on Exercise Intensity (Caralco et al., 1991)

Effect of Power vs. Traditional Step Aerobics

When step skills are performed quickly, the intensity of the movement is increased. Propulsion movements and power skills demonstrate a higher intensity than when they are performed in a traditional step aerobics manner. A summary of traditional and power step movement patterns and the measure of intensity for each is provided in Table 31-3.

Step Height	Heart Rates		VO$_2$ (ml/kg/min)		METs	
	Traditional	Power	Traditional	Power	Traditional	Power
4 inches	138 bpm	158 bpm	26.5	34.5	7.6	9.9
6 inches	144 bpm	163 bpm	29.0	37.0	8.3	10.6
8 inches	155 bpm	170 bpm	32.4	38.7	9.3	11.1

Table 31-3. Effect of Power vs. Traditional Step Movements (Greenlaw et al., 1995)

As mentioned earlier, choreographic variables, such as lever length, range of motion, elevation, traveling, arm movements, and the inclusion of power movements, will affect intensity. Some fitness instructors also add light hand-held weights into this equation. Research studies done on "stepping with light weights" have shown very small or no increase in VO_2 utilization. Thus, the benefit and appropriateness of adding hand-held weights during step activity has been questioned in the industry. As with any advanced training technique, we must evaluate whether the benefits outweigh the potential risk for increased injury or overuse. Therefore, in those situations where instructors have chosen to add light weights to their step activity, AFAA recommends using a lower music bpm (e.g., 118–124 bpm) and limiting the upper body patterns to a pace that can be controlled in both the concentric and eccentric movements (i.e., typically one arm movement per two steps). Additionally, instructors should reserve the use of weights for the more advanced, highly-skilled participant.

The Effect of Music Tempo on Exercise Intensity

Although increases in step tempo provide an additional energy cost during exercise, the increase is minimal when compared to other variables examined. Be aware that safety may be compromised at faster tempos, as proper form and technique are more difficult to achieve. Evaluate the risk/benefit ratio of increased music tempo and select a music tempo that allows class participants to execute the movements in proper form.

Guidelines currently recommend a stepping cadence of 118–128 bpm to provide sufficient physiological stimulus and allow participants to maintain proper form and body alignment. This guideline is appropriate for the general population in the group exercise setting. The skilled and highly conditioned stepper may be able to maintain form and technique at slightly faster tempos— up to 128–135 bpm. Continually monitor the class. Be aware of participants' form and adjust tempo accordingly.

Biomechanical Considerations

As with any mode of exercise, injury potential in step aerobics is a significant consideration. Minimal research has been performed thus far to examine the immediate and long-term biomechanical effects of step training. Information available to date, however, suggests that step training is a safe mode of aerobic exercise.

Biomechanical Effects on the Feet

Francis et al., of San Diego University, examined the biomechanical forces applied during step training.[1] With the use of a sensitive scale known as a force plate, the initial study compared vertical impact, friction forces, and time to peak force during three different modes of training: (a) walking, (b) running, and (c) step training. The work of Francis suggests that the biomechanical forces of step training are similar to those of walking.

As the first foot down off of the step receives the greatest impact force, a single lead leg should not be maintained for longer than a 1-minute duration. As the novice stepper may experience muscular fatigue quickly, it may be necessary to change the lead leg more frequently when working with this population. As lunges and propulsion movements exhibit greater impact forces and are high-intensity movements, they should be limited in duration (i.e., approximately 1 minute) and interspersed throughout the workout. Movements of this nature should be reserved for individuals with higher skill and fitness levels.

Biomechanical forces discussed in this study were collected at a stepping rate of 120 bpm. As the protective mechanisms within the foot engage at approximately 1/20th of a second after forces are applied, step tempo is a significant consideration. A moderately paced movement will allow the protective mechanisms to engage before peak forces are applied. In contrast, a faster stepping rate will increase the force and decrease the protective mechanism efficiency. Additionally, a moderately paced movement will allow the entire foot to be placed on the floor and provide a greater surface area to absorb the impact forces. There is one exception—only the ball of the foot should be placed on the floor during lunging movements to avoid placing a rapid stretch on the Achilles tendon.

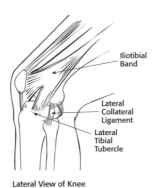

Iliotibial
Band

Lateral
Collateral
Ligament

Lateral
Tibial
Tubercle

Lateral View of Knee

Fig. 31-4.
Anatomy of the Knee

Biomechanical Effects on the Knees

The knee is a structurally complicated hinge joint (Fig. 31-4). The stability of the knee depends primarily on the integrity of the supporting ligaments and musculature. The knee becomes particularly vulnerable as the degree of weight-bearing knee flexion increases.

Flexion beyond 90° provides excessive force (as much as eight times the body weight) to the knee, creating an unnecessary risk of injury. Range of motion at the knee should be limited, therefore, to no more than a 90° angle when weight bearing (Fig. 31-5).

When the knee is supporting the body weight, the foot becomes locked to the floor. Pivoting at this point causes twisting of the support leg and undue stress to the knee. Pivoting movements should only be performed when the leg is non-weight bearing or "unloaded." Participants with prior knee pain or injury should obtain a physician's approval and should stop step training immediately if pain or discomfort is experienced.

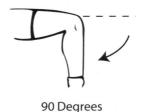

90 Degrees

Fig. 31-5.
Flexion of Knee Joint

Summary

Step training continues to be a form of aerobic activity that is enjoyed by group exercise participants. Instructors have a responsibility to lead participants through a workout that is both physiologically and biomechanically sound. The guidelines provided here and in AFAA's Step Training: A Manual for Instructors reflect current industry guidelines that are based on scientific research performed to date.

References

1. American College of Sports Medicine. (2010). *ACSM's guidelines for exercise testing and prescription* (8th ed.). Baltimore, MD: Lippincott Williams & Wilkins.

2. Arthur C., Guyton, M.D., & Hall, J.E. (2000). *Textbook of medical physiology* (10th ed.). Philadelphia, PA: W.B. Saunders Co.

3. Caralco et al. (1991). The metabolic cost of six common movement patterns of bench step aerobic dance. *Medicine & Science in Sports & Exercise*, 23(4), Abstract #2140.

4. Clapp, J.F., & Little, K.D. (1994). The physiological response of instructors and participants to three aerobic regimens. *Medicine & Science in Sports & Exercise*, 26(8), 1041–1046.

5. Dawson, J., Juszczak, E., Thorogood, M., Foster, C., Marks, S.A., Dood, C., & Fitzpatrick, R. (2003). Distant past exercise in women: Measures may be reliable, but are they valid? *Medicine & Science in Sports & Exercise*, 35(5), 862–866.

6. Engels, H.J., Currie, J.S., Lueck, C.C., & Wirth, J.C. (2002). Bench-step training with and without extremity loading: Effects on muscular fitness, body composition profile, and psychological affect. *Journal of Sports Medicine and Physical Fitness*, 42(1), 71–78.

7. Francis, P. et al. (1994). *Introduction to step Reebok*. San Diego, CA: San Diego University.

8. Greenlaw, K. et al. (1995). The energy cost of traditional versus power bench step exercise at heights of 4, 6, and 8 inches. *Medicine & Science in Sports & Exercise*, 27(5), Abstract #1343.

9. Grier, T.D., Lloyd, L.K., Walker, J.L., & Murray, T.D. (2002). Metabolic cost of aerobic dance bench stepping at varying cadences and bench heights. *Journal of Strength and Conditioning Research*, 16(2), 242–249.

10. Kravitz, L. et al. (1995). Effects of step training with and without hand weights on physiological and lipid profiles of women. *Medicine & Science in Sports & Exercise*, 27(5), Abstract #1012.

11. Kravitz, L., Cisar, C.J., Christensen, C.L., & Setterlund, S.S. (1993). The physiological effects of step training with and without handweights. *Journal of Sports Medicine and Physical Fitness*, 33(4), 348–358.

12. Wang, M.Y., Flanagan, S., Song, J.E., Greendale, G.A., & Salem, G.J. (2003). Lower-extremity biomechanics during forward and lateral stepping activities in older adults. *Clinical Biomechanics*, 18(3), 214–221.

Part 7

Mind/Body Considerations

Holistic Fitness: An Overview

Yoga: Eastern vs. Western Philosophy

32 Holistic Fitness: An Overview

Meg Jordan, PhD, RN

Focus

The holistic fitness movement arose out of a desire to bring increased awareness of mind-body-spirit unity to the exercising public. The goal of teaching exercise in a holistic manner is to broaden the pursuit of a conditioned body to include a more comprehensive commitment to health—physically, mentally, emotionally, spiritually, and communally. Classes taught with this emphasis have the potential for creating a sort of group resonance and heightened sense of connection among participants. For many, holistic fitness has lowered the barriers and excuses to consistent exercise. The more you can address the whole person who is exercising in your class, the greater his or her appreciation and commitment to overall health and vitality.

Holistic Philosophy

The term holism was coined by South African author Jan Smuts to describe the unifying whole of organic life, and it has since extended to include both the material and nonmaterial aspects of the universe.(1) Holism is a complex philosophy that asserts that the whole of something is appreciably larger than the sum of its parts, and that parts are misperceived by us to be discrete entities. However, life forms are so interconnected and interdependent, they are in reality an "undivided wholeness" and have the potential to influence each other even when forcefully divided.

Holistic philosophy has informed the fields of ecology, biology, integrative medicine, psychology, and the social sciences. As a concept representing non-duality (seamless wholeness), holism is an integral part of the wisdom traditions, and a dynamic vision and practice first articulated by Hindu, Buddhist, and Chinese philosophy and several indigenous cosmologies.(2)

By the early 20th century, general systems theorists advanced conventional Western worldviews by mapping out the interconnectedness of natural structures both within the social sciences (e.g., family, community, subculture, culture, earth, solar system) and within the biological sciences (e.g., subatomic waves/particles, atoms, molecules, organelles, cells, tissues, organs, systems).(3)

In the last century, quantum theory was developed by physicists, changing the underlying notions of reality, as well as opening up new fields of scientific paradoxes and mysteries. Now when we say that divided parts of a whole continue to influence each other, we have amazing laboratory experiments to back it up. Paired atoms, when separated, continue to respond as if undergoing the same stimulus. The quantum world is indeed filled with examples of holism that inspire us with metaphors for experiencing oneness.(4)

Holistic Health and Medicine

Professionally, holistic fitness is an offshoot of holistic health and medicine. The American Holistic Medical Association and the Holistic Nurses Association pioneered the first awakenings to weave holistic care into clinical practice.(5) Holistic practitioners help patients balance their emotional and physical state through healthy lifestyles that include a change in attitude combined with the proper diet, exercise, stress management, healthy relationships, and a sense of meaning, purpose, and belonging.

> **Cross-Disciplined**
> Holistic fitness is an enjoyable mix of ideas and techniques from several motor-sensory explorations such as yoga, tai chi, aikido, dance, authentic movement, and bodywork.

Conventional medicine doctor Ralph Snyderman, MD, Chancellor Emeritus of Duke University, said, "It is essential for conventional medicine to recognize the needs of patients who are crying out for more comprehensive and holistic approaches than are currently being provided to them by their physicians. Integrating the best of scientific medicine with CAM (complementary and alternative medicine) strategies is termed 'integrative medicine' and is, in my view, a more effective as well as a compassionate approach to healthcare."(6)

Holistic medical practitioners at the Health Medicine Institute, a nonprofit educational, clinical, and research association, teach a four-faceted approach: (a) a commitment to person-centered care, (b) prevention versus treatment, (c) personal responsibility, and (d) integrative collaboration among complementary fields.

Holistic fitness instructors can borrow from this model and apply lessons in their classes. They can reinforce the importance of daily physical activity as one of the best preventive "medicines" known, and they can encourage participants to accept personal responsibility for their health, while helping build cultural support through networking with local nutritionists, employee wellness programs, civic groups, farmers markets, health fairs, community parks and recreation departments, regional hospitals, clinics, and schools. Holistic health requires the entire village.

Entry into Fitness World

Holistic fitness was not part of the initial launch of the fitness movement. It crept in later quietly and through a side door, so to speak. The early days of the fitness movement in the U.S. were underscored by the publication of cardiologist Ken Cooper's groundbreaking book in 1969, Aerobics, which launched a generation of runners gathering their aerobic points. This was soon followed by a wave of aerobic dance instruction heralded by Jacki Sorensen and Judi Shepherd Misset.(7) Shortly afterwards, AFAA held its first certification workshop and the fitness instruction profession rapidly grew to a worldwide phenomenon.

Conventional exercisers in the decades of the '70s and '80s were fueled with such enthusiasm that people often powered through tightness, pain, and stress in their efforts to grow stronger, faster, and leaner. As a result, bodies broke down almost as often as they became conditioned; complaints of overuse injuries, such as shin splints, stress reactions, and plantar fasciitis, grew more common. AFAA reported on several new exercise injury studies in the 1980s.(8,9,10) Within a year, new guidelines suggested less repetition, slower beats per minute, and a "grounding" of high-impact classes, especially for beginners.

As an emerging movement form, holistic fitness classes draw from a variety of existing disciplines such as authentic dance, somatic education, Eastern energy traditions, and mind/body research in the medical field. Holistic fitness also flowed out of the larger cultural issues that were addressed by new inroads into positive psychology and the human potential movement, along with advocacy work in promoting healthy body image among exercise enthusiasts and professionals.(11)

With the gentler, safer workouts emerging, there was a corresponding wider net thrown, enticing more people to the fitness movement—not just the young and hardy. At the same time, another social force fueled this more conscious attention to the whole body, and that was the graying of the population. People not only needed more attention paid to reducing their risks for chronic disease, they wanted to build cardiorespiratory endurance, musculoskeletal strength, flexibility, and balance. And, they needed to de-stress from their tough workday, to find relief from an overcrowded schedule, and replace tension with relaxation.

As holistic classes flourished, AFAA introduced more continuing education programs that encouraged instructors to avoid exercising in a "disembodied" way, such as counting repetitions in a mindless way. The new holistic emphasis meant being mindfully present to the way our bodies move through space and learning to enjoy the process of attaining a relaxed mind, fit body, and freer spirit. Embracing holistic fitness requires that you reach toward the interior spaces that help you become a more authentic being.

Becoming a Holistic Fitness Instructor

There are many resources for you to adopt holistic teaching skills and movement styles. First, your own mindset might need an adjustment. Be prepared to learn in multiple ways: (a) intuitively (with your right brain), (b) academically (with your left brain), (c) kinesthetically (by going through the motions), and (d) through sensory means (sight, sound, smell, taste, touch). Enhance your auditory holistic skills by listening to different kinds of music, drumming, and chanting.

You might also adopt a daily routine of stress management through the following.

- Meditation
- Guided Imagery
- Visualization
- Positive self-talk learned through audio programs and books
- Yoga
- Relaxation methods
- Breathwork sessions

Consider seeking out workshops in the following techniques. Then pick and choose from what you learn, adding to your personal "toolkit." Holistic fitness is ultimately creative, allowing you to absorb information from various innovators in the human potential field, and adapting the information with your own personal style.

- Feldenkrais Method
- Alexander Technique
- Somatic Education
- Continuum
- Rosen Bodywork
- Rolfing
- Massage Therapy
- Laban Movement Analysis
- Eastern Energy Systems: Tai Chi and Qigong
- Martial Arts: Tae Kwon Do, Aikido

Components of a Holistic Fitness Class

The class itself can take any number of forms, for example, yoga, stretch, body contouring, mat work, even aerobics. Applying holistic principles is what transforms the class instruction, atmosphere, receptivity, and engagement.

Present Awareness: You want to make sure to avoid rushing into class last minute. Set the mood properly, allow people to get present, shake off the stress of getting to class, and make several attempts to acknowledge their commitment to show up with eye contact, smiles, and gestures. Holistic classes have a sweet ritual feeling to them—intentional opening and closures. Then focus on present-time awareness. Learn to be here now, and keep redirecting your energy and attention to the present real-time focus.

Breathwork: Teaching proper breathing is essential to holistic fitness and overall wellness. Breathing rhythmically and taking note to not hold one's breath is taught in all AFAA workshops. In holistic fitness classes, instructors can use the breath as a meditative mantra or focusing device to help participants notice their exertion and make adaptations. San Shin Kai is a meditative-breathing exercise at the start of martial arts classes that helps unify mind, body, and spirit, according to Carol and Mitchell Krucoff in Healing Moves.(12)

Caring: Holistic fitness classes set a new benchmark for caring and compassionate, welcoming instruction. They create a "sacred space" of inner calm, and eliminate the intimidation factors so many participants unfortunately feel when they are newcomers in health clubs. Put out a warm, emotional welcome mat.

Cueing: Well-timed cueing is important in all group exercise. The cueing in holistic fitness classes is non-intrusive and pleasant. It is laced with rich imagery, allowing the participants to generate an integrated experience. It is smooth and seamless.

Grounding: Holistic instructors pay special attention to how they work with their centers of gravity and shift body weight. Learn to move from your center, also known as tan-tien in Eastern energy traditions. Pacing your movements with your breath, and speeding up and slowing down as needed to safely execute the movements will help you stay attuned to body-mind-spirit alignment.

Music: Music is an important motivating feature in all classes, and even more so in holistic fitness classes. From the provocative to the evocative, holistic music is usually free of lyrics, dance-oriented, primal, ethnic, New Age, atmospheric, and elemental. Check out the resources at the end of the chapter.

Variety: To awaken a holistic sense of the body in all its capacities, you will want to include a variety of movements: (a) large, (b) small, (c) fluid, (d) staccato, (e) sharp, (f) graceful, (g) spring-loaded, (h) relaxed, (i) sweeping, (j) syncopated, (k) dynamic, and (l) still. You certainly don't need to perform all of them in each class, but the oppositional tension that is generated with different types of movement can be a powerful tool for building confidence, endurance, strength, and flexibility. In addition, variety of movement styles creates opportunities for more flexibility in the neuromuscular response.

Visualization: Ask participants to be mindfully present to the way their bodies move through space. Teach them to look for the way a naturally spontaneous flow will arise.

Contributors to Holistic Fitness

Becoming a holistic fitness instructor is more of a lifelong journey than a one-time accomplishment. As you learn to think about abandoning stale, customary, or rote ways of exercising, you will challenge yourself to find creative, all-encompassing movement styles and approaches. To do that, you'll need solid mentorship. Take time to explore the following recognized fields of knowledge and expertise that comprise holistic fitness.

Peak Performance

Another contributing body of knowledge behind holistic fitness is the research supporting peak performances and flow states. Internationally recognized researcher Mihaly Csikszentmihalyi (suggested pronunciation: 'chick-sent-me-high-ee'), authored *Flow: The Psychology of Optimal Experience* when he was chairman of the Psychology Department at the University of Chicago. His life's work has been the study of states in which individuals are fully absorbed in an activity. That deep immersion allows them to have feelings of great satisfaction, in which the ego and typical moment-to-moment strategizing falls away. Time seems to be suspended. Csikszentmihalyi explains that athletes who have experienced flow states describe moments in which every action, movement, and thought follows smoothly from one sequence to another. Flow states occur in a variety of experiences from conducting a symphony orchestra to preparing a Thanksgiving meal. The one constant requires that the whole being is involved and all previously learned skills are tapped into effortlessly. Participating regularly in holistic fitness can certainly open a doorway for inviting more flow states into your life.

Positive Psychology

Traditionally, much of the psychotherapeutic profession has focused on defining pathology and treating it for successful management of anxiety, depression, or neurosis. A new branch of therapy—known as positive psychology—attempts to help people concentrate on what is right about their lives.

Ecological Balance

As fitness instructors grow in appreciation of how health is both a personal and cultural creation, they naturally gravitate to a commitment between personal and planetary health. Become an advocate for clean air, water, and safe environments—they go hand in hand with holistic fitness. Becoming engaged with holistic health challenges and possible solutions within your own communities is a first step toward creating sustainable ecosystems on every level (e.g., personal, communal, and planetary). Several health clubs are leading a green initiative, reducing their energy costs, using more natural light, bringing in plants, and starting recycling programs.

Spill-Over Effect

Some research reports a "spill-over effect" when people exercise; they address other aspects of their lifestyle—diet, stress management, relationships, career goals—and start to clean up those areas as well.(13)When you live a more holistic lifestyle, you have more physical and mental energy to tackle neglected areas. Increasing one's commitment to a holistic development process can be accomplished by mapping out short- and long-term goals. Chapter 2, "Wellness, The Big Picture," helps you evaluate many dimensions of a healthy lifestyle.

The Flow

Developed by martial arts master Victor Blome, the Flow provides participants with a biofeedback gauge in the form of a water-filled polyurethane sleeve that looks like a condom sized for a blue whale! As a motion awareness system, the Flow allows you to coordinate movements with rhythmic breathing until the flow of water becomes less unsteady and choppy, and actually starts to glide around you as your coordination and balance become freer and less rigid. Flow instructor Nancy Gillette, MS, an AFAA Advisory Board member, says that the Flow enables you to have a cardiovascular challenge, upper body-workout, moderate lower-body workout, while enjoying a liberating, moving experience.

NIA

Debbie and Carlos Rosas, founders of Nia, are pioneers within the holistic fitness movement, who have always championed our rights to strive for wellness in mind, body, and spirit. Their training techniques incorporate a variety of movement styles including martial arts (e.g., Tae Kown Do and Aikido), dance forms (e.g., jazz and modern dance), yoga, somatics, and conscious breathwork. They offered this advice in an earlier edition of Fitness: Theory & Practice:

"Because 'holistic fitness' is feeling-based, it can be very emotional for participants as they connect to various psychophysical parts of themselves. Often, these parts arise unexpectedly. Personalities, such as the child within, the adolescent, the adult, the warrior, the nurturer, the leader, the follower, and so forth, may surface. For many, this can be the first time they experience a new self, their own emotions and their power to act and make decisions based on what they feel and think. Go slowly and remain compassionate and loving throughout your process." Read about their training programs at www.nianow.com.

Somatic Education

One of the major contributions to healing the classic mind/body split in the Western psyche is somatic education, a collection of sensory motor theories from leading thinkers in the field. Somatic education introduces participants to approaches such as authentic movement, focusing, the Lomi School, continuum, body/mind centering, process-oriented psychology, Gestalt therapy, sensory awareness, Hakomi, Rolfing, Feldenkrais work, and the various branches of Reichian psychotherapy. It interweaves these understandings with psychodynamic, Jungian, and other traditional perspectives.

Professor Don Hanlon Johnson has extended the early work of Thomas Hanna, the founder of somatic theory, with his graduate program in somatic psychotherapy at the California Institute of Integral Studies and publication of his book The Body in Psychotherapy: Inquiries in Somatic Psychology. Somatic approaches, such as authentic movement, allow raw emotions to shift and transform out inner and outer selves. The body-mind is seen as a repository for every memory, emotion, and lived experience, and as such, effective movement instructors are essentially body-oriented therapists.

Not all Kumbaya

There has been a disconcerting criticism in the holistic fitness field, with one side aligned with exercise physiologists who value a more conventional form of exercise that is standardized, tested, and highly qualified to be disseminated to the masses. They have expressed concern that some holistic fitness classes are riddled with uncredentialed instructors who offer touchy-feely nonsense, a haphazard collection of unfounded claims. Sure, there may be some, but the fitness field is eclectic, diverse, and most of the time, well self-regulated by the industry itself. Ineffective or unsafe classes usually come under scrutiny and are quickly dropped by conscientious fitness directors.

While AFAA's stance has always been a strong voice for the safest, most effective forms of exercise, backed by science, AFAA certified instructors and personal fitness trainers also understand that physical activity is to be promoted, and that at a certain point, barriers need to be decreased to attract the non-exerciser. Often innovation occurs at the margin, at places that take initial creative risks, and later those innovations are shaped to conform to respected, evidence-based limits. For over 25 years, the industry has watched the growth of holistic fitness move from a marginalized entry to a respected mainstream offering. It's considered an advantage to cue class participants in the language of many yoga teachers, with rich imagery visualizations and relaxing music. Every class benefits when the instructor embodies a holistic health commitment, and encourages his or her participants to strive for personal and environmental well-being. Experiment with the techniques mentioned above and add a mind-body-spirit dimension to your classes. You're sure to win many converts to holistic fitness.

Resources

Music

Just as music drives and motivates class participants in any group exercise, it is a critical component of holistic fitness classes. However, the selection must be carefully crafted to help participants maintain a state of psychological well-being and physical freedom. There are mind/body music selections offered by many of the fitness industry vendors as well as downloadable online availability.

- **New Age**
  Now We Are Free – Hans Zimmer from "Gladiator"
- **Tribal**
  New Age – Sleepy Sun
  Dawn of a New Age – Dreamcatcher (album)
  Gabrielle Roth
  Gino d'auri
- **Jazz/Dance**
  Artful Balance
- **High Energy**
  Mickey Hart
  Bobby McFerrin
- **Mellow**
  Enigma
  The Mission soundtrack
- **Cool-down/Stretching**
  Meditation – Best of New Age
- **Visualization**
  Beyond Ordinary Nursing
  Academy of Guided Imagery

Summary

Holistic fitness is the conscious application of holistic health principles within group exercise classes, personal training, or any physical activity sessions. It is concerned with the health and well-being of the whole person—mind, body, spirit, and environment in dynamic balance and interdependence. It emphasizes and seeks to enhance the inherent healing ability of each individual and empowers people through teaching principles and skills that enable them to take greater responsibility for their personal development, healing, and health maintenance. Holistic fitness can enrich your life and keep the pleasure principle firmly within the fit life.

Reference Notes

1. Smuts, J.C. (1999). *Holism and evolution.* (first published 1926) reprinted in Sierra Sunrise Press.

2. Schlitz, M., Amorok, T., & Vieten, C. (2007). *Living deeply: The art & science of transformation in everyday life.* Oakland, CA: New Harbinger Publications. p. viii.

3. von Bertalanffy, Ludwig. (1968). *General system theory: Foundations development, applications.* (Allen Lane, Ed.). New York: George Braziller.

4. Kim, L. (2008). *Healing the rift: Bridging the gap between science and spirituality.* New York: Carriage House Press. p. 65.

5.   Dossey, B., Keegan, L., & Guzzetta, C.E. (Eds.) (2000). *Holistic nursing, a handbook for practice* (3rd ed.). Gaithersburg, MD: Aspen Publishers. p. 9.

6.   Snyderman, R. (2009). *The ACP Evidence-based guide to complementary & alternative medicine.* (Bradley Jacobs and Katherine Gundling, Eds.). Philadelphia, PA: American College of Physicians Press. p. xiv.

7.   Jordan, P. (1999). *The fitness instinct.* Rodale Reach.

8.   Francis L.I., Francis P.R., & Welshens-Smith, K. (1985). Aerobic dance injuries: A survey of instructors. *The Physician and Sportsmedicine,*13(2):105-111.

9.   Garrick J.G., Gillien, D.M., & Whiteside, P. (1986). The epidemiology of aerobic dance injuries. *American Journal of Sports Medicine,* 14(1):67-72.

10.   Falsetti, H.L., & Proudit, S. (1985). Injury rate rport for instructors. *Aero Fit J,* 3(5):33-36.

11.   Tucker, L.A., & Mortell, R. (1993). Comparison of the effects of walking and weight training programs on body image in middle-aged women: An experimental study. *American Journal of Health Promotion,* Sep-Oct, 8(n1):34-42.

12.   Krucoff, C., & Krucoff, M. (2008). *Healing moves.* Monterey, CA: Healthy Learning. p. 174.

13.   O'Donnell, M. (2002). *Health promotion in the workplace* (3rd ed.). Albany, NY: Thomson Learning.

14.   Sha, Z.G. (2008). *Soul mind body medicine: A complete soul healing system for optimum health and vitality.* Novato, CA: New World Library.

Additional Reading

1.   Baldwin, C. (1994). *Calling the circle: The first and future culture.* Newberg, OR: Swan Raven & Co.

2.   Berry, T. (1988). *The dream of the earth.* San Francisco, CA: Sierra Club Books.

3.   Brigham, D.D. (1991). The use of imagery in multimodal psychoneuroimmunology program for cancer and other chronic disease. In R. Kunzendorf (Ed.), *Mental Imagery.* New York: Plenum Press.

4.   Dossey, L. (1999). *Reinventing medicine: Beyond mind-body to a new era of healing.*

5.   Loo, M., & Maguire, J. (1991). *East-west healing: Integrating Chinese and western medicines for optimal health.* New York: Wiley.

6.   Macy, J. (1991). *World as lover; World as self.* Berkeley, CA: Parallax Press.

7.   Rossman, Martin. (1990). *Healing yourself: A Step by step program for better health through imagery.* Mill Valley, CA: Insight Publishing.

33 Yoga—Eastern vs. Western Philosophy

Richard Michael Odom

Focus

Never before in history have so many of the world's great healing traditions been so accessible. Their teachers, texts, and techniques afford the opportunity to better understand our own fitness theories and practices in the light of so many other "ways of knowing."

Yoga is just such a light. Despite its comprehensiveness (most of its techniques go far beyond the scope of this text), its antiquity (yoga is at least 3,000 years old), and its cultural ties (to India, China, and Tibet), yoga achieves a level of integration that enables us to bridge aesthetics, performance, and healing—in equilibrium.

The West Differentiates— the East Integrates

"The power of landscape to restore and strengthen, to mind a spirit in turmoil rests primarily in one thing: A receptivity to the medicine it has to offer."
- Richard Strozzi-Heckler

The East keeps us honest. Western Civilization's propensity to fast forward ourselves into the future or to reclaim our past, as the only worthwhile quest, leaves the present as a casualty of oversight. "Anywhere but here, anything but this, and anytime but now" ignores, denies, and dismisses today.

Traditions like yoga anchor us in the present moment. They remind us that to deny the present is to forfeit your freedom to change. Hollywood dubbed it the eternal Groundhog Day. The East calls it karma. We may know it as being "stuck." Our Western culture has wonderful tools to manifest, to convert, and to "make things happen." But without the context of now, you build a house without a foundation.

Contrast this integration with the West's mastery of differentiation addressing fitness. As the West tends to compartmentalize everything, it divides fitness into individual components (e.g., strength, endurance, etc.). Add our appetite for speed and change, apply a generous portion of modern technology, and it is possible to create some amazing results in human performance and aesthetics— quickly. Not surprisingly, all of this results in our preoccupation with the musculoskeletal system.

Yoga, on the other hand, with its emphasis on integration, works particularly well with the aspects of the body that unify (the nervous system), coordinate (the endocrine system), and control (the breath). The potential dialogue between two diverse ways of knowing, East and West, is both exciting and possible.

Mind/Body Dialogue

To affect unity, coordination, and control of the human body, yoga relies on a prolific form of proprioceptive exercise. It is actually a body/mind dialogue that is based on the implicit axiom that if the mind can influence the body (psychosomatics), then the converse is true. In yoga, there is a shift of consciousness from the outside to the inside, from the cerebral cortex and all its analyses to some of the older regions of the brain, to the nervous system, and to the body's innate ability to take care of itself. Thus, the body influences the mind (somatopsychics).

To these ends, yoga created postures or "asanas" which are the equivalent of a gymnastic exercise—but without the movement. Or at least it appears that way to the casual observer. Consider the posture as a "study in stillness" (like a diver, poised at the diving platform, mentally rehearsing the dive, then clearing the mind and body of all superfluous tension). There is no movement of the bones, but all of the soft tissues, fluids, and breath are in symphony. It is the cultivation of the homeostatic ability (the ability to integrate tension successfully) that is the hallmark of the asana.

The posture (asana) is a proprioceptive exercise with endless variations (even though the most popular "classic" postures number less than 40). Any number of asanas can inform the central nervous system of where each part of the body is in space, how it relates to every other part, and the condition each part is in—today. Postures are used to create a continuous flow of proprioceptive sensation that, brought into awareness, enables the student to discern between the troubled workings of the mind and the authentic needs of the body. Knowledge is power and asana provides it.

The energy and the safety of each posture relates to yoga's use of the static and the proximity to, and use of, the ground. This makes yoga appropriate on some level for almost every person.

Asanas (Postures)—Positions and Orientations

Asanas or postures can be classified into four positions and five orientations. The four positions are related to the spine (which yoga places much emphasis on because of the spine's relationship to the nervous system, and is yoga's greatest asset and its greatest liability): (a) forward bends (Figure 33-1), (b) backward bends (Figure 33-2), (c) side bends (Figure 33-3), and (d) twists (Figure 33-4). The five orientations are (a) supine (Figure 33-5), (b) prone (Figure 33-6), (c) kneeling (or sitting) (Figure 33-7), (d) standing (Figure 33-8), and (e) inverted (Figure 33-9). The combination of these with symmetry and asymmetry of the limbs make up the various postures.

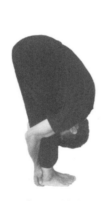

Figure 33-1

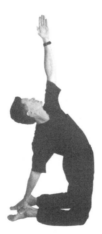

Figure 33-2

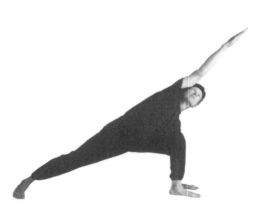

Figure 33-3

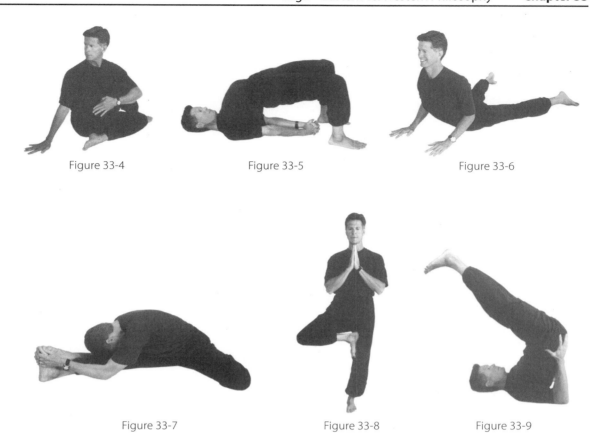

Figure 33-4   Figure 33-5   Figure 33-6

Figure 33-7   Figure 33-8   Figure 33-9

Pranayama is breath control or movement of **prana**, or the life force. With very little precedence in the West (although that may change with the emergence of energetic medicine), it is best to keep it simple. The essence of yoga is simplicity. The breath is our link to that simplicity. To strip each body movement down to its lowest common denominator is the goal of each asana. The softening and deepening of each breath steadies the mind, comforts the body, and is the goal of each breath.

Fitness is a Two-Sided Coin

When you apply posture and breath to your fitness regimen, you will create a whole new vocabulary. Fitness is a two-sided coin. On one side it is a form of controlled injury. Various forms of applied force (intervention) are the basis of this. The most popular, of course, is progressive overload. The other side of the coin is the healing reflex. If walking is one of the most basic forms of overload, then a "good night's sleep" is the body's answer to inducing the healing reflex. (In fact, the replication of certain characteristics of a night's sleep is an important goal of yoga.)

It is not that yoga has taken a separate path from the principle of overload (actually, overload is the primary concern of popular "power" yoga classes); it is just representative of many Eastern healing disciplines not to differentiate, but to produce both effects (overload and healing) as one and the same.

Consider the following: from a yoga perspective, strength becomes not so much a function of bulk (which it certainly is), but a function of flexibility. Endurance has less to do with capacity and more to do with conservation or effortlessness. With yoga, balance has as much to do with "staying in balance" as it does with "catching one's balance." And flexibility is less a concern of creating it as it is to understand and undermine why we keep losing it in the first place. Yoga will add a fresh perspective and test every barometer, cue, and notion of fitness.

Simply put, yoga is a method—a way of attainment. The word "yoga," derived from the Sanskrit word for yoke, means union. To some this could mean to join one's hands to one's feet (to touch one's toes). To another, it suggests to unite with the Divine. And still another might envision the fusion of the physical, mental, and spiritual parts of the self through the practice of yoga. All are part of the yoga experience.

The Four "Ways" of Yoga

Yoga is actually represented as four "ways." The way of harmony, or **Raja Yoga** (of which hatha is one), is the physical component. The way of unity is known as **Jnana Yoga** (the intellectual approach to yoga). **Bhakti Yoga** is the way of devotion (the religious orientation). **Karma Yoga** is the journey of works (the path of cause and effect). They each fit different yoga practitioner's temperaments and form much of the comprehensiveness of yoga.

Styles of Yoga

There are a variety of styles for teaching yoga that center around the efforts and practice of several Indians that came to the West over the past 50 years. **Iyengar** teachers are the "engineers" of yoga, paying attention to precision and alignment. They will usually give you a good foundation. **Bikram** teachers take "heat and repetition" to a whole new dimension, giving you a way to measure progress. **Satchadinanda** teachers attempt to "integrate" the various components of yoga practice—asana, chant, breathing, relaxation, meditation—giving you a feeling of completion. **Ashtanga** teachers put "overload" back into the definition of yoga (this style will remind you of plyometrics). There is also the "therapeutic" value of **T.K.V. Desikachar** trained teachers, the "spontaneity" of some **Kripalu** teachers, and a wonderful sense of "belonging" in the **Sivanada** classes, to name just a few.

Yoga Education in Baby Steps

How do you learn to teach yoga? Do you take a weekend certification program or a home study course? Not completely, first and foremost, yoga is about practice over time, not merely discussion or observance. Consider whether you want to be a yoga instructor or whether you want to simply integrate the philosophy and postures into your present work. Either way, approach yoga in baby steps—a very Eastern approach to learning anything. Practice a little bit, and then a little bit more, allowing for continuity over time—tortoise mind, hare brain.

There are three things you must keep in mind when attempting to integrate an Eastern method like yoga into your lifestyle: (a) comprehensiveness (the Indians have a method for everything and most go far beyond the scope of this text), (b) antiquity (yoga is at least 5,000 years old and although some things are timeless, some things like language and context do age), and (c) cultural ties (e.g., the Sanskrit, incense, and hip flexibility of India, Tibet, and China). Keeping these in mind, study all that you wish or have time to achieve. However, keep the actual work (your practice) task specific. To identify the task, look to the people you wish to serve (including yourself). What are the present demands being made on their (and your) lives, and what are their (and your) symptoms? The symptoms include exhaustion, stiffness, pain, and distraction while the demands relate to personal attention, time, and energy. Choose wisely from Eastern techniques so as not to replicate the demands. Also, choose techniques that help to alleviate and better manage the symptoms. The many ways of yoga are fascinating and sometimes helpful. However, to be "yogic" is to use discretion.

Incorporating Yoga into Fitness Classes

How can an instructor slowly begin to incorporate yoga into a regular fitness class? First, begin to raise participants' awareness of breath. The quality and the depth of the breathing pattern will indicate the quality of attention to the current activity. Succession of breath usually is a red light that the participant is ignoring pain, and experiencing fear or anxiety. A second element of yoga that can be incorporated is the quality of stillness. The end of class cool-down segment is an excellent place to practice the art of letting go. Learning how to ground the body is fundamental, so place participants' supines on the floor in their most relaxed positions. Learn what stillness feels like; begin to create a muscle memory of it. The third step is to integrate actual yoga exercises that you have practiced over time into a class (even between or before strength exercises). As you will learn with practice, each yoga exercise has sequential variations.

Rules of Engagement – The Use of Postures

"Traditions have great power precisely because they present us with possibilities and guides that can support invention…"
 - Charles Moore, Gerald Allen, Doylyn Lyndon

Physiological Effects of Yoga

1. Improves proprioception
2. Makes muscles more pliable
3. Facilitates joint lubrication and hydration
4. Reduces perception of effort
5. Allows you to access your health status before you hurt yourself
6. Releases stress through preparation rather than exhaustion
7. Replicates play—slow, deliberate, and conscious cross-training

Psychological Effects of Yoga

1. Freedom from time
2. Inherent attraction—makes you feel good
3. A more positive outlook on life
4. More "connection" to others (empathy)
5. Self-acceptance
6. Improved listening skills
7. The power of moments

The following is a listing of a few yoga principles regarding:

1. **Intensity**—The stress level that you apply to each posture has value in proportion to the understanding or enlightenment that it yields. The critical moment is when "understanding" is sacrificed in order to "withstand" stress. One becomes desensitized, and the intensity becomes more important than the understanding of "what is in there."
2. **Form**—Most of us (especially instructors) suppose there is a "right way" of doing a posture. From another perspective, there is a wrong way (tissue damage). Every other way is an act of intelligence by the body that helped one through a difficult moment sometime in the past. It is for the participant (not the instructor) to determine that it is no longer "helpful." Intelligence should rule, not protocol. Sometimes it might not look as pretty, but "form" should be the opportunity to "inform," not to merely display.
3. **Progression**—The actual physical progression of the postures looks just like the human journey from the womb to the vertical adult. The measurement of progress is a little more tricky. Progress is much more subtle in yoga. The degree of difficulty is less important than execution with grace, mental clarity, serenity, and evenness of breath.
4. **Intervals**—There is a luxury to properly spacing two asanas. It feels good and is therapeutic. However, so many of us are sleep deprived that in the interval, we're gone. Therefore, please keep it brief.
5. **Order**—You can begin standing up or lying on the floor; there are benefits to both. Some prefer to unload the spine, to get into the horizontal plane, and to enter into an alternate state of awareness (receptive) as soon as possible. Muscle memory and subconscious mind training blossom in this environment.

6. **Duration**—Brevity maximizes attention. This is true for both posture and class length. Greater duration has some health benefit. Time priorities should figure in here.

7. **Content**—Specificity can be beneficial, but some prefer variety to induce a fireworks display of proprioception.

Summary

There is much to learn about the integration of Western and Eastern philosophies and practices. Yoga is one form of activity that brings comprehensiveness, antiquity, and culture together to achieve a level of integration that enables us to bridge aesthetics, performance, and healing—in equilibrium.

Recommended Reading and References

1. Criswell, E. (1989). *How yoga works…an introduction to somatic yoga.* Novato, CA: Freeperson Press.

2. Desikachar, T.K.V. (1999). *The heart of yoga.* Rochester, VT: Inner Traditions International.

3. Devereux, G. (2000). *15-minute yoga.* Hammersmith, London: HarperCollins.

4. Kogler, A. (1995). *Yoga for every athlete.* St. Paul, MN: Lewellyn Worldwide.

5. Lidell, L. (1983). *The Sivananda companion to yoga.* New York, NY: Simon and Schuster.

6. Mehta, S., Mehta, M., & Mehta, S. (1990). *Yoga: the Iyengar way.* New York, NY: Alfred A. Knopf.

7. Mishra, R.S. (1987). *Fundamentals of yoga.* New York, NY: Julian Press.

8. Roundtree, S. (2008). T*he athlete's guide to yoga: An integrated approach to strength, flexibility, and focus.* Boulder, CO: VeloPress.

9. Scaravelli, V. (1991). *Awakening the spine: The stress-free new yoga that works with the body to restore health, vitality, and energy* (2nd ed.). New York, NY: HarperOne.

Other Resources

1. Grilley, P. (2004). *Anatomy for yoga.* (DVD format); Pranamaya, found at http://www.amazon.com

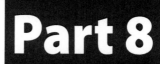

Part 8

Special Populations

Adaptive Exercise for the Physically Challenged

Exercise and Chronic Disease

Exercise Programming for the Large-Sized Participant

Healthy Backs—Fit for a Lifetime

Older Adult Fitness

Pregnancy: Fitness Programming within a Continuum of Care

Youth Fitness

34 Adaptive Exercise for the Physically Challenged

Kathy Normansell, MS
Nancy Gillette, MA

Focus

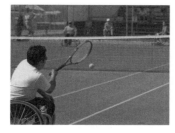

Not all persons can readily join and receive benefits from a traditional group exercise class. The recognition of groups with unique needs has increased the offerings of "specialty classes" for seniors, persons who are overweight, pregnant women, and those with cardiac problems. However, the specific needs of those with physical disabilities have not been fully addressed by any of these classes. Some of these (e.g., cerebral palsy and spinal chord injuries) are complex conditions that make exercise response quite unique, and limited research is available to guide fitness programming for them. Therefore, the purpose of this chapter is to outline some of the physiological implications and related concerns associated with activity for those who are in need of special attention, including those with specific disabilities, and provide helpful instruction and safety tips. This is a clientele with complex and unique conditions requiring instructors with advanced training and certification, who should work in conjunction with physical therapists to provide effective, safe, and enjoyable maintenance exercise programs for participants who have successfully completed a therapeutic exercise program. Activity for such persons should also be rendered only in conjunction with a health care provider's prior approval and after consultation. Services must be rendered with the explicit understanding that the non-medically licensed fitness professional is providing service only to improve levels of fitness and physical well-being of clients—not for medical treatment, as that would be outside the fitness instructor's professional scope of practice.

Physiological Responses to Exercise

Without a basic understanding of how disabilities can affect physiological responses to exercise, the fitness instructor has no way of judging whether the aerobic needs of the disabled participant are being met. While both acute and chronic physiological responses to exercise can be predicted for able-bodied men and women, such responses cannot necessarily be generalized for the disabled person. Depending upon the extent and the type of disability, the degree of physiological response possible will vary from the able-bodied norms.

The rationale for an aerobic workout is to exercise the body hard enough to create a demand for a targeted amount of oxygen to be consumed (VO_2), thus positively stressing the cardiovascular system. It is the role of the cardiovascular system to deliver oxygenated blood to the working muscles and remove the waste products of the energy metabolism from these muscles. With the able-bodied population, the limiting factor during aerobic workouts usually involves the efficiency of the cardiovascular system. In simple terms, conditioning (training) strengthens the heart muscle, allowing it to pump more blood per stroke, and improves the efficiency of the skeletal muscles in extracting and utilizing the oxygen.

During exercise, arterial circulation redistributes blood and oxygen from inactive organs to active muscles to support aerobic metabolism. If the oxygen demands exceed the ability of the heart to supply oxygenated blood, then the aerobic metabolism will be limited, resulting in fatigue and diminished work capacity. Thus, any condition or disability that affects the control of the heart rate

(HR), blood pressure, or myocardial contractibility can reduce the cardiac output response and the overall ability to perform aerobic exercise.

In some cases of spinal cord injury (SCI) above the sixth thoracic vertebra, the autonomic nervous system (ANS) may be damaged to the extent that the HR cannot be stimulated above 100–110 bpm, obviously impairing the ability to distribute large quantities of oxygenated blood in a timely manner. Additionally, lack of sympathetic nervous control affects the maintenance of blood pressure through improper regulation of vasodilation and vasoconstriction. With any lower body paralysis, the skeletal venous pump is absent, resulting in venous pooling and edema which further limits the circulating blood volume.

The amount of oxygen utilized during exercise, and ultimately the degree of stress to the cardiovascular system, is determined by the amount of muscle activity. The more muscle mass working, the higher the demand for oxygen, the more "aerobic" is the activity. If a person is limited in the amount of functioning muscle available, then a large oxygen demand cannot be created and the cardiovascular system will not be fully stressed. Such conditions that limit functional muscle mass include full or partial paralysis, such as with spinal cord injury, spina bifida, polio or cerebral vascular injury (CVA), muscle denervation as with multiple sclerosis (MS), atrophy as with muscular dystrophy (MD), muscle spasticity, common with head injury (HI), CVA or cerebral palsy (CP), or amputation. In these cases, both the acute and chronic responses to an exercise session would be limited.

If a reduced muscle mass is attempting to do the work of what is normally conducted by a larger muscle mass, then the energy cost of the relatively high work load on the remaining musculature may actually result in an anaerobic, rather than an aerobic, response. Because of the relatively smaller muscle mass involved, the physiological responses to maximal exercise are less for upper body work than for whole body or even lower body work. While the maximal, aerobic potential from exercise may be limited, research has shown that even spinal cord injured quadriplegics can benefit with increases in their cardiac output from an upper body training program.

Assuming that enough muscle mass can be utilized to create an aerobic demand and that there is no damage to the ANS, then long-term physiological responses/improvements will be dependent upon adherence to training principles. When a progressive disability is involved, long-term improvements in fitness level may not be seen. To date, no definitive research has indicated that exercise participation either increases or decreases the speed or severity of the rate of progression.

> *While exercise may not directly affect the progressive nature of the disability, it may help the person cope with the progression.*

If an individual is slowly losing muscle functioning due to MD, exercise should help to prevent added loss caused by deconditioning. It is important to remember, however, that a temporary worsening of the condition may occur in cases such as MS and MD if the muscle is worked to total fatigue. Thus, resistance work should be submaximal and not to fatigue. With rest, a complete return to the participant's pre-exercise condition should occur. In almost all cases, health care providers and medical associations have supported the participation in regular exercise programs for persons with progressive physical disabilities.

FITT Principles

To achieve a training effect from exercise participation, the FITT (Frequency, Intensity, Time, and Type of activity) principle is generally recommended. For apparently healthy adults, the American College of Sports Medicine (ACSM,

2010) recommends an exercise frequency of 3–5 days a week, but takes it a step further regarding heart rate. The recommended maximun exercise heart rate (HRmax) range for persons who are:

- sendentary/extremely deconditioned is 57–67%.
- minimally active is 64–74%.
- periodic exercisers is 74–84%.
- regular/habitual participants is 65–80%.

(For more detailed information, refer to *ACSM's Exercise Management for Persons with Chronic Diseases and Disabilities* which accompanies AFAA's self-study course on this subject matter.)

While the frequency of exercise should not be affected by most disabilities, the recommended intensity levels will be changed with many. Typically, the target heart rate (THR) for exercise is determined using a percentage of the maximal heart rate, estimated by the formula of "220 - age." Because the upper body is not capable of working to the same maximal levels as the lower body, ACSM recommends using the adapted formula of 200 minus your age to determine the HR_{max} for upper body work rather than the traditional formula.

The HR may not always be a reliable guide to use to set target heart rates for participants with some disabilities. The use of the THR during group exercise classes is based on the linear relationship between HR and VO_2 established during lower and full body work. With upper body work, when the arms are raised above shoulder level for prolonged periods, the HR may be inflated relative to VO_2 due to the increased stress on the heart, which is not coincident with an increased oxygen demand. Thus, the use of the rating of perceived exertion (RPE) may be more accurate than the HR in most seated group exercise classes. Professionals should consider using the RPE Borg scale in Chapter 20, "Monitoring Exercise Intensity."

The RPE is recommended for use with persons with a spinal injury above the sixth thoracic vertebra, for persons who have limited tactile sensation, persons with attention deficits, and for persons with coordination difficulties that cause them problems in finding their pulse. The use of the RPE should be carefully explained before it can be utilized effectively. With patience and practice, persons who are developmentally and intellectually disabled can also successfully use the RPE scale.

Regardless of whether the HR or RPE is used, persons with MS and MD should be encouraged to work at the lower end of their target zone. If they begin exercising at too high an intensity, fatigue may develop early and preempt the remainder of the workout. At other times, they may not realize that they have overexerted until several hours later when total exhaustion occurs causing a temporary worsening of their condition. With rest, a complete return to the participant's pre-exercise condition should occur; therefore, an added rest period may be required for them on days of exercise.

The time and duration of aerobic exercise is recommended to be 20–30 continuous minutes or an accumulation of several 10-minute bouts for the sedentary participant. The ACSM recommends beginning a new exercise program for sedentary, deconditioned adults using discontinuous intervals of "hard" to "easy" exercise bouts. Since the sedentary, disabled person will likely be even more deconditioned than the sedentary, able-bodied person, an exercise program should be started conservatively. Over time, the length of the "hard" phase should be increased while the length of the "easy/recovery" phase is reduced until a continuous period can be achieved. When muscle paralysis or weakening, or a progressive disability is involved, a continuous period may never be achievable and intervals may always be the best option. Further discussion on intervals will be addressed later in the section on movement adaptations. Keep in mind, that it is highly recommended that fitness instructors refer certain participants with conditions they are unfamiliar with or untrained to address to other professionals (e.g., clinical exercise physiologists).

Associated Concerns

Other associated concerns may accompany some disabilities. The prevention of most of these problems is the responsibility of the participant. However, an instructor should be aware of the potential for such occurrences. Exercising in high heat and humidity can be dangerous for anyone, especially persons with injury to the ANS, which might occur with a spinal cord injury or MS. Such individuals may have a reduced ability to sweat. The production of sweat and its evaporation is one of the ways the body rids itself of excess heat to maintain the core body temperature.

Another source of heat dissipation is the radiation that occurs as vasodilation and blood flow diversion bring the heat to the body surface. With ANS damage, both of these sources of heat reduction may be absent or reduced, thereby increasing the risk of heat exhaustion or heat stroke. Overheating may also increase the fatigue level for persons with MS and limit their endurance and ability to work hard. Conversely, working out in cold environments can tighten arthritic muscles or the spastic muscles of someone with cerebral palsy, making fluid movement even more difficult.

Persons with impaired circulation need to be cautious of creating skin irritations that can take a prolonged time to heal. If impaired sensation is involved, the individual may be unaware that an abrasion has developed until a large sore appears. Persons with amputations can develop irritations from sweat increasing friction against the prosthesis. If severe enough, such sores can prevent the ability to wear the prosthesis until healing occurs.

Pressure sores from prolonged sitting are serious problems for wheelchair users who should relieve the pressure with frequent chair "push-ups." A full bladder may increase the heart rate and/or blood pressure of someone with a spinal cord injury. Emptying the bladder or catheter bag before exercising may also help prevent a bladder accident. Should such an accident occur, the fitness instructor should try to minimize any embarrassment to the participant and call as little attention as possible to any necessary clean up.

Seizure disorders may be an associated condition with many disabilities. While medication controls the majority of seizures, the fitness instructor should be aware of any class members who have a history of seizures. Seizures are not medical emergencies and do not require medical attention unless they continue for prolonged periods (10–15 minutes) or seem to be following one after another. Long-term exercise tends to reduce seizure activity. Seizures during exercise itself are rare, but post-exercise seizures are fairly common. Multiple seizures may also occur. Following a grand mal seizure, an individual will likely be tired and need rest. Therefore, the fitness instructor should discourage the person from leaving the facility immediately and alone. It is not uncommon during a grand mal seizure for an individual to lose control of the bowel and bladder. The most important intervention during a seizure consists of protecting the individual from injury without restraining him or her. Remove any objects nearby that could cause injury. Help protect the head from banging on the floor, but again, do not restrain. The fitness instructor can also play an important role in helping relieve any embarrassment that a seizure may cause.

Pre-Class Instruction

The more a fitness instructor knows about his/her participants prior to the start of a class, the better prepared the instructor can be to help meet the participants' needs. While it is time consuming, a pre-class interview with a new participant is very beneficial.

Do not assume that a physical disability causes a person to be unhealthy or at unusual cardiovascular risk. Many disabilities are stable, non-progressive, and cause no more inherent risks than occur with an able-bodied person. Follow the guidelines established by AFAA to determine when a physician's clearance is needed. Increased legal liability should not be an undue concern provided fitness instructors work in consultation with the participant's health care provider, are properly trained, and follow established guidelines.

A medical history/health risk screening should be required of all new fitness class participants. A few extra questions may elicit helpful background information which need medical clearance prior to the start of a program or special programming. Questions might address whether any special assistance is needed in class or in the locker room, whether or not the individual can transfer in and out of his/her wheelchair independently, and/or whether the individual is currently under a therapist's treatment. The usage of medication should be noted and any possible effects related to exercise, overexertion, or heat should be determined. Fitness instructors should refer certain participants with conditions they are unfamiliar with or untrained to address to other professionals (e.g., clinical exercise physiologists).

A pre-class interview is a good time to check the degree of balance and stability of the person while standing or sitting. Although the participant may be active in other sports activities, the group exercise class may involve many new movements. A seat or chest belt may provide an added measure of security, provided the material has some give and is not constrictive. Immobilization of a wheelchair may or may not be desirable depending upon personal preference. Certainly, the power switch to an electric chair should be shut off before exercise is begun.

Many movements in a group exercise class can be easily adapted—almost automatically—to fit someone who is exercising while sitting down, while other movements will need special adaptation. At the pre-class interview, alternative moves can be explored. Any movement in which the majority of the power/aerobic demand is being created by the lower body will need adjustment for someone exercising while seated.

> ### Balance
>
> *Even though an individual may walk unassisted or even with the use of canes, he or she may not have enough balance to perform cardio movements to tempo while standing. Many ambulatory persons who have had a stroke, head injury, or who have CP may not be able to control their balance while attempting to perform the cardio routines. Thus, sitting for at least part of the class may provide better stability, allow freer movement, and contribute to a more aerobic workout.*

Movement Adaptations

Traveling moves. Effective in a traditional cardio class, traveling moves are difficult to perform for those who are seated. On a level surface, a wheelchair is very efficient—even several pushes would not likely be very aerobic for most wheelchair users. Additionally, most classes incorporate traveling moves in sets of four to eight counts. Such short-duration travels consist of only one or two pushes on the wheelchair before braking to reverse the movement direction. Such stop and start moves will be anaerobic at best. During traveling moves, the seated participant will need to find an upper body alternative. Similarly, many low-impact classes utilize power moves that involve flexion/extension of the knees and hips to work the body up and down against gravity. It is not recommended that someone seated attempt to mimic this type of move by raising up and down with the trunk—a move that would undoubtedly compromise the back.

Intervals. The use of intervals is an important part of most adapted routines. Because the upper body musculature is relatively small, even when unaffected by disability, overuse of the muscles can easily result in fatigue. If a disability is involved, over fatiguing the muscles could result in an inability to complete the workout and obtain the cardiovascular benefits. This is especially a risk in individuals with muscle weakness and muscle paralysis. Interval usage of the muscles will help reduce the fatigue risk. The important point is to avoid prolonged repetition using the same muscle group. Repeated moves with the arms raised overhead should be followed by moves in which the arms are kept low, allowing the deltoid muscles to relax. Intervals of repeated biceps curls could be followed by triceps work (opposing muscle group). Large movement patterns should be followed by smaller patterns, fast moves by slower.

Balance and coordination. A different problem occurs with ambulatory and non-ambulatory persons with balance and coordination problems, such as found with CP, HI, and CVA. Transitioning from one movement pattern to the next can be quite difficult. Often, persons with balance/coordination problems will lag a few counts behind the rest of the class due to their difficulty in coordinating all the components of the movement. If the movement pattern is changed too quickly (e.g., every 8 counts), the reaction delay and slowness in coordinating the new movement may make it very difficult for the person to keep up. Thus, prolonged repetition is more appropriate. Persons with balance/coordination problems may also have trouble with any intricate foot patterns, dance moves, or multi-part combinations. Simplicity of movement patterns is the key to a successful workout.

Warm-up and cool-down. During the warm-up when lower body limbering or static stretching is being conducted, seated individuals who will not be doing any leg work may substitute arm/shoulder limbering and stretches. Many classes incorporate floor work near the end of class before the final cool-down. If a person does not have any voluntary movement in the lower body, he or she may want to leave class when the floor work begins. If this occurs, the fitness instructor has a responsibility to explain to the participant the importance of a full cool-down and encourage him/her to conduct some stretching out of the wheelchair once at home. Most wheelchair users have chronic tightness from prolonged sitting and are vulnerable to contractures of the hip and knee flexors. Additionally, many paraplegics and some quadriplegics do have some active abdominal muscles and should be encouraged to do as much of a curl-up as possible, even if the shoulders can just barely be lifted off the floor.

Most wheelchair users can benefit from some floor work, but many need some assistance in **transferring in or out of their chairs.** Proper technique must be followed in assisting in a transfer to prevent injury to the disabled participant or to the person conducting the transfer. Body mechanics in a good lift include using the leg muscles (not the back), keeping a wide base of support, keeping a firm grasp on the individual, and keeping the weight close to the body. For safety of the individual being assisted with the transfer, care should be taken not to scrape the body against the wheelchair or drop the person on the floor. Transfers should be done on soft (matted) surfaces.

The disabled individual should give the directions and feel comfortable with the transfer. There are several different ways transfers can be conducted, utilizing partial to total assistance. Before attempting to give assistance in a transfer,

---

Use of Wheelchair

Not all persons who exercise seated do so because of paralysis. Weakness, lack of coordination, or amputation may cause some persons to use a wheelchair. In these cases, the seated exerciser should be encouraged to incorporate leg movements, or, when possible, to increase the aerobic demand. Such leg moves could include marching, small kicks, toe taps, step-outs, and knee lifts. Those who do not have functioning leg movement should be encouraged to use trunk movement when possible to increase the aerobic demand. Gentle side-to-side or forward and back rocking can be done.

proper training and practice is important. Consultation with a physical therapist or other health care provider for instruction in how to safely perform a transfer may be necessary.

Within a traditional fitness class, much concern is given to **proper postural alignment** in order to prevent undue stress and injury. Malalignment is a symptom of some disabilities, thus postural deviations may be seen and need to be accepted. It is not the role of the fitness instructor to try to correct such deviations, rather the instructor should help the participant achieve as effective and safe a workout as possible. For example, a person with a quadriplegic SCI may need to lean back in the chair for stability due to lack of trunk and abdominal muscles. Toe walking due to excessive tightness in the Achilles tendon and internal rotation of the legs due to tightness in the hip adductors are common with CP. Therefore, many people with CP will not be able to stand in "proper alignment" during class. A fitness instructor is not a therapist and should not attempt therapeutic intervention, since it is outside their scope of practice. On the other hand, the instructor must be aware of contraindicated movements that could have adverse results. When in doubt fitness instructors should refer participants to more advanced trained professionals or seek consultation.

Administrative Concerns

Several issues that are not directly related to the fitness instructor's abilities can affect the success of an integrated program. Such issues include facility accessibility, advertising/promotion, and the type of class taught. Accessibility is discussed in the next chapter. Legal advice concerning service requirements dictated by the Americans with Disabilities Act and similar state laws should be obtained by each programmer.

Advertising and promotion. Spreading the word that a program is open to persons with physical disabilities can be an arduous task. Many may feel intimidated to attend a club that is perceived to be a place for "perfect bodies" only. Others may not wish to attend if they think it is going to be a "special" segregated class. Probably the best marketing approach to take is a varied one. Use as many different media sources as possible. If one or two disabled persons are already interested in the class, arrange to have them involved in a photo with the fitness instructor. A resource for participant referrals includes local physical, occupational, or recreational therapists and any local affiliate of Disabled Sports USA or the Veterans Administration. If there is a rehab center nearby, offer to conduct several free sample classes for the patients who are nearing discharge. Some facilities have had success in recruiting by holding demo classes in area malls. As with any new program, word of mouth will probably be one of the best advertisers.

Type of class. If a class limited to those with special conditions is to be considered and is going to be offered, careful thought must be given to the time and day it is scheduled. Most facilities' "down time" is also the time that is most inconvenient for working adults.

Once the participant is ready, the type of class he/she enters will affect successful integration. For obvious reasons, step classes will probably be the hardest to adapt for persons who are lower body mobility impaired. Similarly, a class that utilizes a predominance of traveling moves will put the disabled member at a disadvantage when it comes to achieving a good workout. Classes consisting of movements that stay in one spot and offer variety in arm and leg moves are more easily adapted for disabled participants. A circuit class may be the best alternative, with a few of the stations modified specifically for the disabled members. Such stations could include arm cycling (with a bicycle secured to the top of a table and the pedals turned by hand) or a rower machine (with the seat stabilized).

If a large number of participants are disabled, a team teaching approach may be beneficial, fun, and initially easier than teaching solo. While the main instructor is teaching class as usual, the co-instructor can make modifications for the disabled participants where necessary. Team teaching can allow for a much more individualized approach, as well as increase motivation and excitement in the class. The ideal technique would be to utilize a properly trained disabled person as a co-instructor if such a trained person is available. To promote the feeling that all participants are equal members of the class, the lead may be changed at times (e.g., have the main instructor teach seated, with the co-instructor providing alternatives for those standing). Over time, as the participants learn to make adaptations on their own, the co-instructor may be phased out.

Instructor Attitude

A fitness instructor can make or break any class. An instructor can make a workout fun, during which participants are motivated and challenged, or make it an hour of pure sweat and strain. Likewise, an instructor's attitude can determine whether a person who is disabled participates successfully in a fitness class. Disabled persons are not "special" or amazingly brave just because they carry on in life with a disability. Persons with disabilities are not always friendly, just as those who are able-bodied are not always friendly. The instructor needs to be relaxed and comfortable and treat a person with a disability as he or she treats any other participant.

The bottom line is that a person is a person first, the disability is secondary. A specific comment does need to be made regarding persons with communication problems. If a fitness instructor does not understand an individual's speech, then he or she should say so. Pretending to understand is condescending, and will not be appreciated by the individual.

Summary

It would be difficult in this chapter to describe all the specific concerns and adaptation suggestions for various disabilities. The fitness instructor is encouraged to learn as much as he or she can about the disability, think through the implications, and most importantly, seek additional training. Providing adapted classes can be rewarding for both the instructor and the participant. Proper training can help ensure that it is also safe and effective. Check out the resources that follow for updated information from experts on these medical conditions.

References

1.   American College of Sports Medicine. (2009). *ACSM's exercise management for persons with chronic diseases and disabilities* (3rd ed.). Champagne, IL: Human Kinetics.

2.   American College of Sports Medicine. (2010). *ACSM's guidelines for exercise testing and prescription* (8th ed.). Baltimore, MD: Lippincott Williams & Wilkins.

3.   Franklin, B. (1985). Exercise testing, training and arm ergometry. *Sports Medicine, 2*, 100–119.

4. Glaser, R., Sawka, M., & Laubach, L. (1972). Metabolic and cardiopulmonary responses to wheelchair and bicycle ergometry. *Journal of Applied Physiology*, 46 (6), 1066–1070.

5. Gordon, N.F. (1993). *Diabetes: Your complete exercise guide.* The Cooper Clinic and Research Institute Fitness Series. Champaign, IL: Human Kinetics.

6. Korn, M.J. (1999). Selected neuromuscular disorders. In D. Cotton (Ed.), *Clinical exercise specialist.* San Diego, CA: American Council on Exercise.

7. Lasko, P.M., & Knopf, K.G. (1988). *Adapted exercises for the disabled adult.* Dubuque, IA: Eddie Bowers Publishing.

8. Lepore, G., Gayle, G.W., & Stevens, S.F. (2007). *Adapted fitness instruction: A manual for group exercise leaders.* Champaign, IL: Human Kinetics.

9. Miller, P. (Ed.) (1995). *Fitness programming and physical disability.* Champaign, IL: Human Kinetics.

10. Paciorek, M., & Jones, J. (1994). *Adapted exercise for the disabled adult.* Dubuque, IA: Eddie Bowers Publishing.

11. Pimental, N. et al. (1984). Physiological responses to prolonged upper-body exercise. *Medicine & Science in Sports & Exercise*, 16(4), 360–365.

12. Sawka, M.N. (1986). Physiology of upper body exercises. *Exercise and Sports Sciences Review*, 14, 175–210.

13. Shephard, R.J. (1990). *Fitness in special populations.* Champaign, IL: Human Kinetics.

14. Winnick, J. (2005). *Adapted physical education and sport* (4th ed.). Champaign, IL: Human Kinetics.

15. Zwiren, L.D., Huberman, G., & Bar-or, O. Cardiopulmonary functions of sedentary and highly active paraplegics. *Medicine & Science in Sports & Exercise*, 5, 63.

Web-Based Resources

Arthritis Foundation, www.arthritis.org

Amputee Coalition of America, www.amputee-coalition.org

Spina Bifida, Spina Bifida Association of America, www.spaa.org

Poliomyelitis, Post-Polio Health International, www.post-polio.org

Spinal Cord Injuries, National Spinal Cord Injury Association, www.spinalcord.org

Cerebral Vascular Injury, www.stroke.org, American Stroke Association, www.strokeassociation.org

Multiple Sclerosis, National Multiple Sclerosis Society, www.nmss.org

Muscular Dystrophy, Muscular Dystrophy Association, www.mda.org

Cerebral Palsy, United Cerebral Palsy, www.ucp.org

Wheelchair Users, Disabled Sports USA, www.dsusa.org, www.wheelchair-sportsandrecreation.com

Seizure Disorders, Epilepsy Foundation, www.epilepsyfoundation.org

Scott O. Roberts, PhD,
Mary Yoke, MA, and
Deanna Lowe, MA

35

Exercise and Chronic Disease

Focus

An abundance of scientific literature has overwhelmingly confirmed the health-related benefits of exercise for apparently healthy populations. And likewise, individuals with a diagnosed chronic disease or disability benefit as much if not more from regular physical activity as do apparently healthy individuals. As a result, these individuals as determined and directed by their physician often choose health club settings to carry out their exercise program. As a fitness instructor, it is imperative to develop a basic understanding of certain chronic diseases and disabilities, and the effects that exercise has on them. Understanding the precautions that exist with those individuals with a chronic disease will help to provide safe and effective exercise instruction. Although an in-depth discussion of the specific diseases is warranted, it is beyond the scope of this manual. The following discussion is to provide a brief overview of some of the major chronic diseases fitness instructors might encounter in a fitness facility. For further information and a comprehensive discussion, please refer to the reference list at the end of this chapter. Fitness instructors should keep in mind that their role is to improve participant well-being through the design and implementation of exercise services—not to treat or alleviate adverse health conditions or disease.

Asthma

General Guidelines

- Review the medical history questionnaires before the first exercise session.
- Follow the American College of Sports Medicine's (ACSM) guidelines for risk factor stratification and the recommendations for seeking a medical clearance.
- Know the emergency procedures of your facility.
- Use the Borg RPE scale and be able to teach participants how to use it.
- Don't pretend to know everything; ask questions. If you don't feel comfortable working with certain individuals, explain why, and have them obtain specific exercise recommendations from their doctors, or refer them to a medically supervised program or to a clinical exercise physiologist.
- Remember the team approach–physician, participant or patient, and instructor all work together to make the exercise training safer and more effective.

Asthma is a common respiratory problem affecting more than 20 million Americans, including 9 million children under the age of 18 (American Lung Association, 2005). It is a reactive airway disease caused by constriction of the smooth muscle around the airways, swelling of the mucosal cells, and increased secretion of mucus. Persons diagnosed with asthma experience defining characteristics, including coughing, wheezing, and dyspnea (shortness of breath). Extrinsic or intrinsic factors cause asthma. Extrinsic factors are external irritants, such as pollen, cigarette smoke, and air pollution, whereas intrinsic asthma is the result of internal factors, such as a bacterial respiratory tract infection attacking the body. A large percentage of the population experiences exercise-induced asthma (EIA, also known as exercise-induced bronchospasm) which is a moderate obstruction of the airway that is not life threatening. Although asthma is not a contraindication to exercise, those who have been diagnosed with asthma should first consult with a physician, then follow specific guidelines for their exercise program.

Exercise Guidelines for Asthma

1. Prior to beginning the exercise program, the participant should consult with his/her physician and, in accordance with that consultation, develop a medication and treatment plan to prevent EIA attacks.
2. A bronchodilating inhaler should be available at all times during the exercise session. It should be used at the onset of symptoms.
3. Exercise intensity should start low then gradually increase as the participant's body adapts to physical activity.
4. Avoid exercising outdoors in extreme cold or when pollen levels are high.
5. A humid exercise environment is best. Many people with asthma find that water exercise is especially well-tolerated.

6. Use of an inhaler prior to exercise often reduces the likelihood of experiencing an EIA attack.

7. Breathing through the nose or with pursed lips may reduce or dissipate symptoms during exercise.

8. An extended warm-up and cool-down should be practiced.

Heart Disease

Heart disease affects one out of every two people in the United States. It is the leading cause of death in the U.S. and in most of the developed world, and the number of cases continues to increase despite repeated warnings reported by scientific research. Atherosclerosis, narrowing of the coronary arteries, is the primary contributing factor for the development of the disease. This narrowing causes reduced blood flow to the heart, producing angina (chest pain), and ultimately myocardial infarction or heart attack. Atherosclerosis of the cerebral blood vessels can lead to a stroke, or death of brain tissue. The risk of stroke is greatly increased with people with hypertension (high blood pressure). Cardiorespiratory fitness has been found to significantly influence risk of death, and offers strong support that both regular physical activity and high levels of fitness protect against atherosclerotic heart disease. As a result, sedentary lifestyle, or physical inactivity, has been labeled a primary risk factor for heart disease. Other risk factors are (a) age, (b) family history, (c) hypertension, (d) high cholesterol, (e) cigarette smoking, (f) prediabetes, and (g) obesity.

Exercise Guidelines for Heart Disease

1. Participants should be screened for heart disease risk factors prior to beginning an exercise program. Participants who are male and 45 years of age or older, or who are female and 55 years of age or older, or who report two or more major atherosclerotic cardiovascular disease (CVD) risk factors are considered to be at moderate risk for heart disease. Participants with known cardiac, pulmonary, or metabolic disease and/or symptoms suggestive of heart disease are considered to be at high risk for heart disease and complications. The ACSM recommends that both moderate- and high-risk participants obtain a release from a physician before starting an exercise program.

3. Guidelines prescribed by the physician for a participant with heart disease, pulmonary disease, or metabolic disease should be strictly followed.

4. A record of current medications and their effects on exercise should be developed and reviewed with a participant in conjunction with his/her health care provider before initiating the exercise program.

5. Comply with the target heart rate range and RPE guidelines for each participant, recommended by his or her physician.

6. The participant should be instructed to alert the fitness instructor should any signs or symptoms develop before, during, or after exercise.

7. Do not exceed your level of expertise. It may be more prudent to refer high-risk participants to a medically supervised program or to a clinical exercise physiologist.

8. Exercise intensity should start low then gradually increase as the participant's body adapts to physical activity. High-intensity exercise is not recommended without specific permission from the participant's physician.

Arthritis

Two of the most common forms of arthritis are osteoarthritis (degenerative joint disease) and rheumatoid arthritis. Osteoarthritis affects nearly every adult over 70 years of age, and rheumatoid arthritis affects about 3% of women and 1% of men in the U.S. population. A degenerative process, osteoarthritis is the wearing away of cartilage between two bones, allowing bony contact to occur, whereas rheumatoid arthritis is caused by inflammation of the membrane surrounding joints. This inflammation is often associated with pain and swelling in one or more joints. Exercise is generally recommended by health care providers for those with arthritis to improve muscular strength and endurance around the affected joints, increase joint range of motion and flexibility, decrease pain and stiffness, improve motor coordination, and improve total body fitness. During a severe arthritic bout, vigorous exercise should be avoided as it can exacerbate flare-ups. However, gentle stretching is usually well tolerated and may help relieve pain.

Exercise Guidelines for Arthritis

1. Exercise classes, such as low-impact cardio, stationary indoor cycling, and water exercise, should be encouraged. These classes should avoid quick, ballistic movements that can be painful for the arthritic participant.
2. Frequent, low-intensity exercise sessions should be performed.
3. Decrease intensity and duration of exercise during severe bouts of pain or inflammation.
4. Stretch daily, if possible. Gently move every joint every day, enhancing mobility of both muscles and joints.
5. Isometric exercises may be preferable, especially for joints that are chronically painful.
6. An extended warm-up and cool-down period is advised to help minimize pain.
7. Monitor all changes in medication and fluctuations in pain levels with the disease, and have the participant consult with his or her appropriate medical professional.
8. Be aware of the 2 hour pain rule: if pain persists 2 or more hours after an exercise session, reduce the intensity or duration in future sessions.
9. Obesity and overweight are risk factors for osteoarthritis. Help the participant with appropriate weight loss and weight management strategies, if necessary.

Diabetes Mellitus

The two most common forms of diabetes mellitus include (a) insulin dependent diabetes mellitus (IDDM), or type 1, and (b) non-insulin dependent diabetes mellitus (NIDDM), or type 2. Both types of diabetes are characterized by high blood glucose levels, also known as hyperglycemia. Approximately 7% (21 million) of the American population has diabetes mellitus, and the numbers continue to increase (National Diabetes Fact Sheet, 2005). IDDM, commonly known as juvenile-onset diabetes, occurs when the body does not produce insulin. As a result, daily injections of insulin must be taken to regulate glucose levels in the body. Approximately 10% of people with diabetes are diagnosed with type 1 diabetes. Type 2 diabetes is the most common form, affecting about 90–95% of those with diabetes. Largely due to obesity and physical inactivity, persons with type 2 diabetes cannot efficiently use the insulin they produce. Type 2 diabetes usually requires nutrition therapy and occasionally pharmacological therapy. However, current research suggests that type 2 diabetes can be prevented, and even alleviated, through proper nutrition and regular participation in an exercise program. While the provision of service to prevent or treat such conditions by non-licensed personnel is prohibited by law, fitness professionals can assist in improving the well-being of people with diabetes. It is important to note that individuals with diabetes require special attention in exercise programming due to special needs. As a fitness instructor, adherence to these guidelines will provide safe and effective exercise for the participant with diabetes.

Exercise Guidelines for Individuals with Diabetes

Frequency: 3–7 days per week

Intensity: 50–80% HRR or RPE of 12–16 on the 6–20/15-point scale

Duration: 20–60 minutes per day continuous or accumulated in bouts of at least 10 minutes to total 150 minutes per week of moderate physical activity

Type: Activities that use large muscle groups in a rhythmic and continuous fashion

Resistance training should be encouraged, following the general guidelines for apparently healthy individuals, as long as the participant is free from any contraindications (e.g., signs/symptoms of cardiovascular disease, retinopathy, and recent laser treatments).

Frequency: 2–3 days per week

Intensity: Low resistance; gradual progression; 2–3 sets of 8–12 repetitions (at 60–80% 1-RM)

Time: 20-60 minutes (or time to complete 8–10 multi-joint exercises; sessions may vary based on training protocol)

Type: Free weights, weight machines, elastic tubing

Special Precautions for Persons with Diabetes

1. Blood glucose should be monitored frequently when beginning an exercise program.
2. It is recommended that insulin be injected into a muscle that is not active during exercise (e.g., the abdomen) in those individuals requiring daily insulin injections.
3. Exercise should be avoided during periods of peak insulin activity.
4. Participants should be encouraged to always carry a carbohydrate snack to alleviate hypoglycemia should it occur.
5. Exercise sessions should be scheduled the same time of day for those with type 1 diabetes.
6. Encourage participants to consume a carbohydrate snack prior to, and possibly during, exercise to reduce the occurrence of hypoglycemia.
7. Increase carbohydrate intake or decrease insulin dose (as directed by physician) before exercise.
8. Work with the participant's physician, carefully following all recommendations.
9. Keep the emergency response number and plan handy.
10. Know the symptoms of hypoglycemia, including: excessive fatigue, nausea, lightheadedness, dizziness, profuse perspiration, spots in front of eyes, confusion, shakiness, headaches, sudden rapid heart rate, and even seizures. If any of these occur, call 911 immediately.

11. Encourage participants to check feet often; wear polyester or blend socks along with silica gel or air midsoles to help prevent foot ulcers. Participants should contact their physician immediately should foot ulcers occur.

Hypertension

Hypertension, or high blood pressure, is a disease affecting approximately 65 million individuals in the U.S. It is defined as having a resting systolic blood pressure (SBP) greater than or equal to 140 mmHg and/or a resting diastolic blood pressure (DBP) greater than or equal to 90 mmHg. Hypertension occurs more frequently in African American individuals, and it is a major risk factor for cardiovascular disease and stroke. Hypertension places undue stress on the heart, increasing left ventricular wall thickness, and reducing diastolic filling. Recent research reports that regular physical activity can decrease blood pressure.

Exercise Guidelines for Hypertension
1. Emphasize cardio exercise, such as walking, jogging, cycling, or swimming, in order to help reduce high blood pressure. Individuals exhibiting elevated blood pressure should exercise at lower intensities (40–70% of HRR).
2. Exercise should be performed on most days of the week in 30–60-minute sessions.
3. High-intensity activities and isometric activities should be avoided.
4. For resistance training, repetitions should be high and weight should remain low. Avoid resistance training to the point of failure, even if the weights are light.
5. Avoid the Valsalva maneuver, as it increases vascular pressure.
6. Utilize RPE as certain hypertensive medications alter heart rate during exercise.
7. Avoid positions in which the feet are higher than the head.
8. Teach relaxation and stress management techniques.

For additional information see Chapter 13 on Risk Appraisal and Medical Considerations of Exercise

Summary

Exercise therapy for individuals with chronic disease is accepted and practiced by clinicians in many diverse health care settings. More than likely, fitness instructors will encounter individuals who have been diagnosed with a disease that requires special considerations and guidelines regarding exercise. It is to such instructors' advantage to continue learning about special populations. For more information on certification programs and workshops in this field, instructors should contact the American College of Sports Medicine.

References

1. American College of Sports Medicine. (2009). *ACSM's exercise management for persons with chronic diseases and disabilities* (2nd ed.). Champaign, IL: Human Kinetics.
2. American College of Sports Medicine. (2010). *ACSM's guidelines for exercise testing and prescription* (8th ed.). Baltimore, MD: Lippincott Williams & Wilkins.
3. America College of Sports Medicine. (2010). *ACSM's reference manual for guidelines for exercise testing and prescription* (6th ed.). Baltimore, MD: Lippincott Williams & Wilkins.

4. American Lung Association. (2005). Epidemiology and statistics unit, research and program services. *Trends in asthma morbidity and mortality.* Retrieved April 4, 2009, from http://www.lungusa.org/atf/cf/% 7B7A8D42C2-FCCA-4604-8ADE-7F5D5E762256%7D/ASTHMA1.PDF

5. Centers for Disease Control and Prevention. (2005). National diabetes fact sheet: General information and national estimates on diabetes in the United States. Retrieved April 4, 2009, from http://www.cdc.gov/ diabetes/pubs/pdf/ndfs_2005.pdf

6. Ehrman, J.K., Gordon, P.M., Visich, P.S., & Keteyian, S.J. (2003). *Clinical exercise physiology.* Champaign, IL: Human Kinetics.

7. Howley, E.T., & Franks, B.D. (2003). *Health fitness instructor's handbook* (4th ed.). Champaign, IL: Human Kinetics.

8. Ram, F.S., Robinson, S.M., & Black, P.N. (2000). Effects of physical training in asthma: A systematic review. *British Journal of Sports Medicine*, 34(3), 162–167 (June).

9. Ram, F.S., Robinson, S.M., & Black, P.N. (2000). Physical training for asthma. Cochran Database Syst Rev. DC001116 Journal Code: DJ9; 2.

Web Sites

American Diabetes Association: http://www.diabetes.org
American Lung Association: http://www.lungusa.org
American Heart Association: http://www.aha.org

36 Exercise Programming for the Large-Sized Participant

Gail Johnston and
Mary Yoke, MA

Focus

The primary goal of any exercise program should be to improve or maintain the wellness of the individual who is exercising. Many instructors have lacked the knowledge and confidence to provide safe and effective fitness programs for the large-sized exerciser. Coupled with the embarrassment and anxiety many large-sized participants feel when they begin exercising, the number of programs suited for this special population's needs has been rather small. However, new approaches and programming alternatives are being developed all the time as we expand movement options for this group.

Addressing the needs of this population is a matter of growing urgency, as the number of adults classified as overweight and obese is rapidly increasing. Currently, more than 66% of adults are overweight and 32% of adults are obese (Ogden et al, 2006). Obesity is a condition characterized by excess body fat and is associated with an increased incidence of high blood pressure, high cholesterol, diabetes, degenerative arthritis, many cancers, reduced life expectancy, and early death. It increases the likelihood of hernias, hemorrhoids, gallbladder disease, varicose veins, and makes breathing more difficult. Excess weight can make everyday activities problematic. Obese people are hospitalized more frequently than are people of average weight, and they have more surgical complications. The direct and indirect costs of obesity are estimated to be more than $117 billion annually. It is imperative that fitness professionals learn to work with this population and help to increase the health and fitness of large-sized exercisers everywhere.

Destroying the Myths

Because of the pervasive fat bias that exists in this country, it is important to dispel some myths at the start.

Fat people are all out of shape. While obesity and lower fitness levels often go hand in hand, it is possible to be "fat and fit" or heavy and healthy. Several studies have shown that regular exercise of 60–90 minutes per week in overweight people lowers the risk of death more than for individuals who are normal weight but inactive. It is important to note, though, that being fit or active doesn't completely eliminate the risks of being obese.

Fat people are all uncoordinated. The size of the body is not the determinant of grace, coordination, or physical ability. While each person brings his or her own physical limitations to activities, physical ability is also enhanced by repetition and practice.

Thinness is the goal of exercise. As long as this myth continues, there will be an enormous number of people who will not be able to succeed at exercise. Finding pleasure in movement is the process, and the process of integrating pleasurable exercise into a healthy lifestyle is the ultimate goal. Instead of emphasizing thinness, it is more appropriate to promote feeling strong, fit, and empowered.

Guiding Your Clients and Class Participants Towards Success

As a fitness professional, your job is to support your client through his or her process of changing from an inactive lifestyle to an active one. This requires a variety of attitudes and skills.

A non-judgmental attitude sets up a psychologically safe environment. Only harm can come from evaluating an individual's worth according to his or her size, lifestyle, speech, appearance, color, ethnicity, or gender. Lectures, criticism, and reprimands have no place in this process of positive change. Work on dropping judgment and blame; practice self-acceptance and acceptance of others. Show respect, sensitivity, compassion, and patience with every participant. Attending an exercise class can be a stressful experience for the large person who is new to exercise. Try, by listening and reassuring, to alleviate as much stress as possible. Provide support and encouragement.

Address your own fat bias. If you have a bias against overweight or obese individuals, it will get in the way of successful communication with your clients and participants. Be aware of your language: watch how you talk about your own body, or your own fears about being fat, your desire to make everyone thin, and/or the jokes you tell.

Effective listening skills help to facilitate the change process because your clients feel as if they're being heard. Active listening takes practice because it requires total concentration. It places a greater importance on hearing what other people say than on what you feel you need to say to them. Allow yourself to drop all expectations and projections of what you might say next; simply relax and be completely present for your clients. This skill helps your clients develop a bond with you based on the assurance that your listening is proof that they are worthy human beings.

Support your clients as they move toward their goals. Don't project your own goals onto your clients. Let them determine the exercise intensity that is comfortable for them, especially at first. Give them time to decide which exercises give them pleasure and to determine their own level of satisfaction with their performances. Allow them to feel successful for just being there with you.

Role modeling healthy lifestyle practices shows your clients that the lifestyle they are struggling to achieve is possible. It also gives you an opportunity to practice what you preach. In your life, do you give as much attention to your spiritual and emotional health as you do to your physical health? Are you forgiving of yourself when you aren't perfect? Do you totally accept and appreciate your body as it is? Are you patient with yourself when you're learning something new?

An ongoing hunger for knowledge helps you avoid fads, educate your clients, and maintain a full array of options for problem-solving.

Wear appropriate attire when leading large-size participants. This generally means covering yourself with a large, loose T-shirt. Studies show that very obese participants are not motivated by thin, lean instructors; in fact, they often find being around a perky, hard-body instructor demotivating and more likely to increase their sense of hopelessness.

Participant Screening

A current health assessment and health risk appraisal is essential for all clients. Please refer to Chapter 17, "Basic Exercise Standards and Guidelines," regarding pre-class procedures and medical clearance. The guidelines are appropriate for large individuals. Anyone with a pre-existing medical condition, family history, or other risk factors should be screened by his or her physician prior to beginning an exercise program.

The primary responsibility for the individual's overall health management should lie with the individual and his or her physician. Requiring physician approval may be one of the first barriers to fitness for your large participants. Many large people are reluctant to approach their physicians for an exercise recommendation for fear that the medical approval will be wrapped in prejudicial language, such as "Of course you should exercise. You'll lose that weight and look a lot better." To help your participants past this barrier, maintain a list of names of physicians who are "fat-friendly" to whom you can refer.

Fitness testing (e.g., body composition, step tests, muscular strength, flexibility, and endurance tests) is commonly offered prior to beginning an exercise program as a motivational tool for the participants. Some participants, however, will push beyond their current fitness levels in order to "pass" the tests. Also, it may not be inspiring for a client to learn that his or her body fat is over 30%. Therefore, it is recommended to either perform waist circumference or BMI as a baseline measurement. Because fitness testing may be demotivating for some and uncomfortable for others, it should be administered only on an individual basis as your participants request it. In most instances, however, group exercise instructors may not be trained in or have the opportunity to administer fitness assessments.

Frequency of Exercise

Cardiorespiratory Training. Three times a week at first is recommended, even if the duration is only 10–15 minutes each time. *Too much, too soon is the major cause of drop-out and/or injury.* Slow, gradual progression is the key to success. When a participant is comfortable with 3 times per week, then he or she can increase the frequency to 4–5 times per week, keeping the intensity relatively low. Eventually, he or she can be encouraged to walk at a low intensity every day, although more vigorous exercise should be limited to no more than 5 times per week.

Resistance Training. To enhance muscular strength and physical function, incorporating resistance training into group fitness classes is recommended. Refer to Chapter 17, "Basic Exercise Standards and Guidelines."

Monitoring Intensity

Fatty deposits in the area of the wrist and neck make pulse monitoring the least effective method of evaluating exercise intensity. Additionally, heart rate monitor chest straps may be too small and/or inaccurate due to fat mass. The preferred method for intensity monitoring is the Borg Rating of Perceived Exertion (RPE) Scale. On the 0 to 10 scale, the recommended level is 3–4 (moderate to somewhat hard); on the 6 to 20 scale, the recommended level is 12–14 (light to somewhat hard). Remember that overly deconditioned people may become anxious and stressed when they feel their heart rate beating rapidly and they may have difficulty pacing themselves. It is best to help them avoid over exercising and overexertion. See Chapter 20, "Monitoring Exercise Intensity," for more on RPE.

Exercise Duration

It is well known that a longer duration is better for general weight loss, since more work is being performed and more calories are being burned. However, very large participants will be unable to exercise for long durations at first. It is very likely that some exercisers will only be able to sustain 5 minutes or so of cardiorespiratory conditioning. This is to be expected, and every effort to move should be applauded and encouraged. Eventually, the 5 minutes can increase to 10, then 15, 20, and so on. The ACSM recommends as much as 50–60 minutes per day on most days of the week for weight loss. It is also recommended that at least 2,000 kcals be expended through exercise each week for long-term weight control.

In the early stages of training, exercises that are easily accomplished are preferable to those that offer a challenge. Feelings of inadequacy are then avoided and the participant's confidence can grow. Deconditioned exercisers may also prefer exercises that are repetitive over a period of time so they can notice improvements in coordination, strength, flexibility, and confidence immediately.

It's important to note that a number of studies have shown that physical activity and exercise are essential for sustaining significant weight loss and in preventing weight regain. An important message for deconditioned large-sized exercisers is that any amount of physical activity is better than nothing. Start slowly and conservatively, and follow the principles of progression.

Five Questions for the Large-Sized Participant

There are no specific exercises that can or should be done by larger people. The key to appropriate fitness programming is to learn how to modify exercises for each individual based on the answers to the following five questions for that individual.

- What is the most effective position in which to work this muscle group considering the weight distribution?
- Is the spine protected?
- What is the leverage to be considered?
- What is a reasonable speed of movement?
- What is a reasonable range of motion?

Additional Exercise Considerations

Don't limit the movement options. Without your assistance, your clients are successfully navigating a wide range of daily activities that includes standing, sitting, bending, lifting, climbing stairs, and getting in and out of cars. Your role is to expand on these movements. Avoid putting your participants in a chair unless nonweight-bearing exercise is recommended.

Four elements of a safe and effective exercise class should be integrated in the following order.

- Safety first, because pain and injuries are some of the most common reasons for dropping out of an exercise program.
- Motivation next, to help the participant focus on the social and pleasurable aspects of movement.
- Alignment is next because most new participants feel as if they've done something wrong when their alignment is pointed out and corrected.
- Education is last, not because it is unimportant, but because education does not usually motivate new participants to stay with their programs. When participants are ready for education, they usually start asking questions.

Include movements that open the body, such as stretches for the pectoralis major and anterior deltoid muscle groups. Because of the fat bias in our society, it is common for the posture of larger individuals to be closed, as if they are trying to hide their bodies.

Consider the speed of the movement. Moving too quickly may cause an exerciser to use momentum to keep up. Backed by substantial body mass, a movement executed too quickly could lead to injury.

High-impact exercise is generally contraindicated. A compression of three times body weight on the lower leg could lead to injury over time.

Exercises that teach kinesthetic awareness are helpful for individuals who are out of touch with their bodies. For example, place a hand on the working muscle to feel for the contraction.

Balancing exercises help clients find their center of gravity to assist with grace and confidence in movement. These exercises should be done with the option of a ballet barre, wall, or other support.

Adapt exercises to allow body mass to move for greater range of motion. For example, when an individual with greater abdominal body mass is performing spinal flexion in a seated position, one or both legs should be in a straddle position so range of motion is not limited by the abdomen contacting the thighs.

For certain large people, the supine position is recommended only for limited periods of time. Compression of internal organs from large torso body mass may inhibit breathing if the position is held for long periods of time. Note that some large-sized participants will feel very exposed and uncomfortable on the floor, and may have difficulty getting up and down. Sequence your class to minimize floor-to-standing transitions.

Last, but certainly not least, don't forget the fun factor. The actions of stretching and contracting are not necessarily fun for someone who has been inactive for a long time. You can add fun to your class through music, movement, instruction, versatility, personality, and a little craziness.

Nutrition and Weight Management

According to the American Dietetic Association, "successful weight management to improve overall health for adults requires a lifelong commitment to healthful lifestyle behaviors emphasizing sustainable and enjoyable eating practices and daily physical activity." Fitness professionals can assist their participants by providing credible resources related to healthful nutrition. One of those resources is www.MyPyramid.gov. Your participants will be able to locate a personalized plan to assist them in weight loss management. For more information on nutrition refer to Chapter 8, "General Nutritional Needs."

Summary

Movement options for the large-sized exerciser are constantly expanding as our knowledge of this special population increases. A comprehensive exercise program can meet the needs of the large-sized participant by providing safe and effective fitness activities.

References

1. American College of Sports Medicine. (2001). Position stand. Appropriate intervention strategies for weight loss and prevention of weight regain for adults. *Medicine & Science in Sports & Exercise*, 33, 2145–56.

2. American College of Sports Medicine. (2010). *ACSM's guidelines for exercise testing and prescription* (8th ed.). Baltimore, MD: Lippincott Williams & Wilkins.

3. American Dietetic Association. (2009). Position of the American dietetic association: Weight management. *Journal of the American Dietetic Association*, 109(2), 330–346.

4. Andersen, R., & Franckowiak, S. (1999). "Obesity." In ACE's *clinical exercise specialist manual.* San Diego, CA: American Council on Exercise.

5. Brownell, K.D. (1995). "Exercise in the treatment of obesity." In K.D. Brownell and C.G. Fairburn (Eds.), *Eating disorders and obesity: A comprehensive handbook* (pp. 473–478). New York, NY: The Guilford Press.

6. Ogden, C.L., Carroll, M.D., Curting, L.R., McDowell, M.A., Tabak, C.J., & Flegal, K.M. (2006). Prevalence of overweight and obesity in the United States, 1999-2004. *Journal of the American Medical Association,* 295, 1549–55.

7. U.S. Department of Agriculture & U.S. Department of Health and Human Services. (2005.). *Dietary guidelines for Americans.* Retrieved April 11, 2009, from www.healthierus.gov/dietaryguidelines

37 Healthy Backs— Fit for a Lifetime

Dorette Nysewander, EdD

Focus

Chapter 7, "The Musculoskeletal System: Structure, Function, and Exercise Application," provided an overview of a healthy spine with deviations associated with abnormal curvatures. A critical link to a successful work/life balance is a healthy, fit back. So if 4 out of every 5 people experience back pain in a lifetime, what does it take to stay healthy (Medical News Today, 2009)? Identified in this chapter are five considerations for being kind to your spine as well as promoting spine health to your class participants: (a) lifestyles, (b) daily activities, (c) ergonomics, (d) recreational sports, and (e) fitness levels, concluding with a series of recommended back exercises.

Lifestyles

Standing erect and walking on two legs presents some unique challenges, as the pressure on the lower spine is equal to more than half an individual's total body weight. While back health affects individuals of all ages, let's look at what can aggravate the back and recommendations for improvements.

- *Obesity or being overweight* pulls the body forward exaggerating the back's natural curves causing the muscles trying to correct the imbalance to strain.
- *Inactivity or sedentary* increases the pressure on spinal discs by about 40% more than standing. The sling muscles (e.g., psoas, iliacus, rectus femoris) become tight, thus when standing, the body is pulled forward and off balance.
- *Smoking* tends to lead to the development of spinal degeneration at an earlier age.
- *Stress* can increase tension of tight muscles or cause spasms, thus adding to the physical problem occurring or increasing the perception of the discomfort.
- *Improper posture* takes the spine out of neutral causing stress to bones and muscles.

Many of these lifestyles can dramatically change the health of the back. If an individual has no pre-existing health issues, then moderate changes in nutrition, increased daily and physical activity, with attendance in a smoking cessation class can minimize aggravations and prevent health degradation.

To ease stress to the back, massage or myofascial release techniques are recommended. Both of these techniques increase blood and oxygen supply to the muscles with a gentle sliding pressure to stretch the tissues. Tennis balls and foam rollers are effective tools to use.

From this point forward, it is important to incorporate the use of the fourth question of the AFAA 5 Questions™. Question 4 asks, "Can you maintain proper form and alignment for the duration of the exercise?" Using this evaluation method can potentially provide the greatest back health benefit whether during exercise or performing daily activities.

Imagine your shoulders and hips or torso as a box, with the spine running down the center. Stand tall, with relaxed shoulders and think in terms of your box with scapular and pelvic stability. Scapular stability is defined as the isometric contraction of the rhomboids and serratus muscles engaged simultaneously so that the shoulder girdle becomes stabilized. Pelvic stability is the neutral point between anterior (arching of the low back) and posterior (flattening or tucking the tailbone). To maintain this pelvic tilt, perform an isometric contraction of the abdominals and erector spinae muscles simultaneously.

To apply this concept, stand facing a barre attached to the wall. Hold onto the barre at shoulder level. Pull back with your shoulders as if to pull the barre off the wall. Your shoulder blades will engage. Now, pretend to hold a newspaper underneath your arm. Squeeze it tightly as if not to drop it. Put these two movements together (pull back and squeeze) to stabilize your shoulder girdle. Hold this position, while you shift your focus to your pelvis. From your neutral pelvic point, pull upwards with your abdominals and lengthen slightly with erector spinae as your tailbone points downward. Use an isometric contraction with these muscles to maintain pelvic stability without flattening out the natural curve of your lumbar spine.

It is with scapular and pelvic stability along with maintaining the four natural curves of the spine that an individual needs to ensure proper form, alignment, and stabilization of their torso regardless of exercise movements or activities of daily living. So what does it mean to have perfect posture?

Daily activities. Perfect posture is a system to minimize wear and tear on the body, and maintain a healthy spine. To achieve this, keep the feet shoulder or hip distance apart to broaden the base of support, knees bent, abdominals tight, spine neutral, rib cage lifted, shoulders back and down, and your head upright. From the side, you should be able to draw a straight line from your ankle, up through the knee, hip, rib cage, shoulder, and ear.

To ensure back health during daily activities, remember the following.

- *Backpacks*—were designed for convenience and should not contain items that are greater than 10% of your body weight. If your posture changes, the backpack is too heavy (Moore et al., 2007).
- *Cars*—purchase cars that have an ergonomically correct back support. Be aware that sitting in bucket seats place the knees higher than the hips, putting more pressure in the low back.
- *Chores*—while dusting, vacuuming, or cleaning use proper body positions during these activities; brace the abdominals, maintain a neutral spine, and use your legs.
- *High heels*—when wearing high heels contract your abdominals as the pitch of the head will place your spine in a forward pelvic tilt. Wearing a ¾ inch heel increases pressure on the back by 22% more than being barefoot.
- *Laundry*—before lifting a laundry basket make sure to keep it close to your body as you lift; If living in a two-story house or larger use a laundry shoot.
- *Position changes*—move from a side-lying position to your knees, place one foot forward, from the kneeling position and push up to stand; reverse to get back down to the floor.
- *Purses*—women who hold a heavy purse or carry it over one shoulder, strain back muscles on the opposite side of the body which pulls the spine out of alignment. Be sure to include only important items and change sides often.
- *Sleep*—in a supine position, place a pillow under the knees and use a cervical pillow for the neck; in a side-lying position place pillow between

the knees, under the waist and the neck. Make sure you sleep on a good orthopedic or TempurPedic® mattress.

- *Wallets*—men who place a wallet in their back pocket will experience a shift in the hips while sitting. Minimize this stress by using a money clip or placing your wallet in a front coat pocket.
- *Yard work*—be sure to hold equipment in a position that supports the body; take frequents breaks and stop when fatigued.

Ergonomic

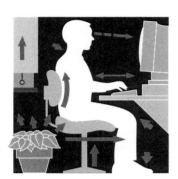

Ergonomics. Ergonomics looks at fitting the job to the person verses the person to the job. Occupations in which individuals are sedentary or physically exerting can pose risks to back health. The key to minimizing these risks is awareness.

To understand better how to design your workstation within ergonomically correct principles, review the following points and make changes accordingly.

Chair—as you sit, adjust arm pads to a level position. Feet should rest firmly on the floor. The back of the chair should adjust to maintain the natural curves of the spine. Adjust the lumbar pad to support the low back.

Copyholder—place at the same level and distance as the monitor, and within a visual to keep your head in neutral.

Footrest—feet should be flat on the footrest to maintain the knees at a 90° angle.

Lighting—to prevent glare use a monitor screen.

Monitor—place the monitor directly in front of the keyboard. The level of the screen should adjust and be at eye level. You should maintain a neutral position of the head and be able to see the entire screen. The distance from you to the monitor is 18–24 inches, or approximately your arm's length.

Mouse—operate without stretching your arms or putting the body into awkward positions. If necessary, use a palm/wrist pad for support.

Telephone—use a headset to eliminate awkward positions of the head and neck.

Printer—receive documents without placing the body in a compromising position.

Work surface—at your workstation, check to make sure your arms are not repeatedly moving above shoulder height, and that elbows are at a 90° angle. Additionally, your work surface should move to accommodate proper posture. If you stand, the desk surface should rise; conversely, if you sit, it should lower. Every tool that you need to be able to perform your job should be in arms reach. Allow between 7 to 10 inches of thigh clearance between your seat and the bottom or your desk. When standing, be sure to change your weight often by placing your foot up on a step.

As you work throughout the day, remember to move often. Walk around for a few moments every hour and practice a few stretches (e.g., reach arms overhead or side to side; push back into your chair and round your upper body down over your knees; stand up and place your hands to your lower back and lift the top of your head to the ceiling while arching slightly backwards).

Lifting Techniques

Described below are steps to think about before performing a lift. Whether a load is heavy or light think through the following.

- Test the load you are about to lift; then plan the lift.
- Ask for help if necessary, or use a piece of equipment to help with the lift.

- Stand close to the object and make sure you have a firm stance.
- Stabilize your torso, bend your knees, and squat to grasp the object.
- Keep the load close to your body; lift with your legs to a standing position.
- Slowly lower the object and bend your knees when setting the object down.

Driving Techniques

Think about your posture, seat design, and vibration to maintain back health. Remember to position the seat to where your legs are not reaching for the pedals, avoid the use of bucket seats, make sure your seat has the appropriate ergonomic padding, and take frequent breaks.

By practicing these ergonomic principles and staying in shape you will be able to work free of stress or strain to the body.

Recreational Sports

In order to progress in a sport, muscles should be trained to respond to the activity. Participation in sports is a great way to raise levels of endorphins, improve sleep, reduce stress, and improve mental outlook. In addition, it is a great way to reconnect with the neighbors, friends, or families. To manage the care of the back, you should remember four factors: (a) change (allowing the body to adapt to a sport over time); (b) alignment (practicing proper posture); (c) twisting (training muscles in rotation); and (d) speed of progression (gradually increasing activity, if there has been a lapse in training) (Guten, 2005). Start with a warm-up, approximately 5–10 minutes to increase blood flow and core temperature, as well as gradually increasing heart rate and blood pressure. Finish with a 5–10 minute cool-down to gradually decrease intensity followed by an additional period of stretching for flexibility. As with any activity, you will need to pace yourself on how long they participate and remember to stop at any signs of discomfort (AFAA, 2010).

Fitness Levels

The best exercises are those in which you enjoy doing. To achieve physical fitness, you should include cardiorespiratory, muscle strength/endurance, and flexibility exercises into a program design. The design should include frequency, intensity, and duration of these components. Refer to Chapter 17, "Basic Exercise Standards and Guidelines," for training recommendations at a glance. Exercises should be appropriate to your skill level.

Exercise activities that provide many health benefits with reduced stress to the back include low- impact group exercise classes, cycling, walking, cross-country skiing, yoga, Pilates, and swimming. Often eliminated from fitness programming is the training of balance. Slips, trips, and falls can cause injuries or musculature tears when balance is lost. Try performing some of these exercises for 30 seconds (Tinetti, 1986). A plus (+) is given for each exercise you can perform for 30 seconds; a minus (-) is given if you needed support either with hands or feet during the 30 seconds. Rate yourself as follows: Low Risk – 30 seconds; Moderate Risk – 15 to 25 seconds; High Risk – < 15 seconds or did not attempt. Exercises include the following.

- Tandem stance (one foot in front of the other)—eyes open; eyes closed
- Rise on toes—eyes open; eyes closed
- Seated sway to one side hold/repeat—eyes open; eyes closed

- Standing sway to one side/repeat—eyes open; eyes closed
- Sway forward hold/ back hold—eyes open; eyes closed
- One-legged stance—shift weight—eyes open; eyes closed
- Kick to the side—eyes open; eyes closed

Commonly, tight muscles are associated with discomfort in the upper, middle, and lower back. In the neck and upper (or thoracic area), if you have overly tight pectorals and anterior deltoids, this would indicate that the shoulder retractors (trapezius III and rhomboids) muscles are weak. For the middle to lower back, if you have overly tight erector spinae, iliopsoas (hip flexors), and hamstrings, the rectus abdominis and oblique muscles are weak. The design of a healthy back program should focus on muscle symmetry.

Recommended Back Exercises

Provided in the table below are progressions of back strengthening and stretching exercises per body position. Before beginning these exercises, whether it is the instructor or class participants, a self-administered health history for any back problem or pain should be performed. Many people have a history of low-back pain and this bears careful assessment before decisions should be made about contraindications to specific exercises (including those meant to promote healthy backs), the need for medical referral and review, or modifications of certain exercises in a participant's program. Anyone exhibiting a history of back problems and/or pain should be cleared by their physician prior to beginning the exercises listed below. For those who have received physician clearance, perform these in a neutral spine and practice scapular and pelvic stability. Choose one body position daily, and spend about 10 minutes moving through the levels and finish with flexibility stretches. With all strengthening exercises, perform 3 sets of 10; with all stretches, perform one to four times holding for 15–60 seconds.

Body Position	Type of Exercise	Level I	Level II	Level III	Level IV
Supine (face up)	Strengthen	ATL heel slides	ATL heel slides w/ alternating arms	ATL Toe taps	ATL toe taps with ATL arms
	Strengthen	Bridge	Bridge ATL marches	Bridge ATL arms w/marches	Bridge ATL arms w/leg extensions
	Stretch	Supine spinal stretch	Supine spinal stretch	Supine spinal stretch	Supine spinal stretch
	Strengthen	Partial curl-up Arms reach to knees	Partial curl-up Arms across chest	Partial curl-up Arms behind head	Partial curl-up Arms reaching behind head
	Strengthen	Partial curl-up w/spinal rotation	Partial curl-up w/spinal rotation; ATL knees	Partial curl-up w/spinal rotation; ATL leg extensions	Partial curl-up w/spinal rotation; w/ knees bent up over hips
	Stretch	Supine spinal stretch	Supine spinal stretch	Supine spinal stretch	Supine spinal stretch
Prone (face down)	Strengthen	ATL leg extension	ATL arm extension	ATL arm/leg extensions	ATL arm/leg extensions W/1-lb wt
	Strengthen	Modified cobra Hold 10 seconds	Modified cobra Hold 20 seconds	Modified cobra Lift hands up	Modified cobra Arms extension
Quadruped	Strengthen	Single arm extension	Single leg/toe slide	Alt arm, w/leg/ toe slide	Alt arm, w/leg extensions
	Stretch	Cat stretch	Cat stretch	Cat stretch	Cat stretch
	Stretch	Kneeling reach Or child's pose	Kneeling reach Or child's pose	Kneeling reach Or child's pose	Kneeling reach Or child's pose
Seated	Strengthen	Hip hinge seated	Hip hinge lift off seat	Hip hinge lift off seat w/ALT arm extension	Hip hinge lift off seat w/both arms extending
Seated (on ball)	Strengthen	Hip hinge seated I	Hip hinge lift off seated	Hip hinge lift off seat w/ALT arm extending	Hip hinge lift off seat w/both arms extending
	Stretch	Lateral torso & hip flexor stretches	Lateral torso & hip flexor stretches	Lateral torso & hip flexor stretches	Lateral torso & hip flexor stretches
Standing	Strengthen	Wall squats 45°	Wall squats 90°	Wall squats w/ ball 45°	Wall squats w/ball 90°
	Stretch	Lateral torso & hip flexor stretches	Lateral torso & hip flexor stretches	Lateral torso & hip flexor stretches	Lateral torso & hip flexor stretches

Key—*Alt (alternate) *w (with) *lb (pound) *wt (weights)

NOTE: Some of these exercises can be viewed in Chapter 17, "Basic Exercise Standards and Guidelines."

Sample Exercises

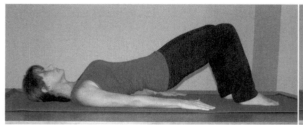

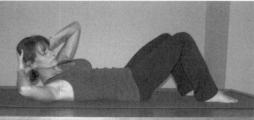

Supine. Bridge (level I)

Supine. Partial curl-up with spinal rotation(level I)

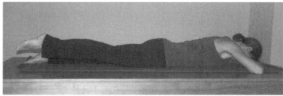

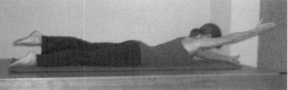

Prone. Alternating leg extension (level I)

Prone. Alternating leg and arm extension (level III)

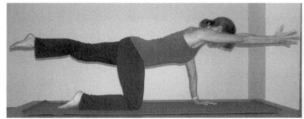

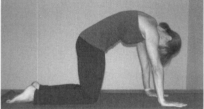

Quadruped. Alternating arm and leg extension (level IV)

Quadruped. Cat stretch

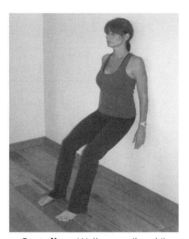

Standing. Wall squat (level I)

Summary

To maintain the health of your spine as well as promote spine health to your participants, remember to consider the five areas of back health: (a) lifestyles, (b) daily activities, (c) ergonomics, (d) sport activities, and (e) fitness levels. Practice performing scapular and pelvic stability, and incorporate balance training in your fitness workouts. If getting to the gym is difficult, take 10 minutes to go through recommended progression of back exercises, as this will provide support during activities of daily living.

References

1. Aerobics and Fitness Association of America. (2010). Basic exercise standards and guidelines. In L.A. Gladwin (Ed.), *Fitness: Theory & practice.* Sherman Oaks, CA: Aerobics and Fitness Association of America..

2. American College of Sports Medicine. (2010). *ACSM's resource manual for guidelines for exercise testing and prescription* (6th ed.). Baltimore, MD: Lippincott Williams & Wilkins.

3. Guten, G. (2005.). *Injuries in outdoor recreation.* Guildford, CT: Globe Pequot Press.

4. McKenzie, R. (1997). *Treat your own back.* New Zealand: Spinal Publications.

5. Medical News Today. (2009). *The myths of back pain: 80% of adults experience back pain in a lifetime.* Retrieved April 16, 2009, from http://www.medicalnewstoday.com/articles/134732.php

6. MedlinePlus. (2009). *Ergonomics.* Retrieved April 11, 2009, from http://dohs.ors.od.nih.gov/ergo_computers.htm

7. Moore, M., White, G., & Moore, D. (2007). Association of relative backpack weight with reported pain, pain sites, medical utilization, and lost school time in children and adolescents. *The Journal of School Health,* 77(5), 232–239.

8. Occupational Health and Safety Administration. (2008). *Ergonomic solutions: Computer workstations e-tool checklist.* Retrieved April 12, 2009, from http://www.osha.gov/SLTC/etools/computerworkstations/checklist.html

9. Tinetti, M.E. (1986). Performance-oriented assessment of mobility problems in elderly patients. *Journal of the American Geriatrics Society,* 34,119–126.

38 *Older Adult Fitness*

Laura A. Gladwin, MS

Focus

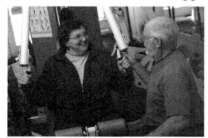

It is well documented that physical activity is essential for healthy aging, yet the older adult population (65 years of age and older) is among the least active (CDC, 2002; Nelson et al., 2007; USDHHS, 2008). This makes for a great opportunity for fitness professionals to expand their horizons and consider a career in working with older adults. Over the years, more resources have become available to assist fitness instructors in understanding the group dynamics, exercise programming, communication, and motivational techniques to improve exercise adherence (Rikli & Jones, 2001; Rose, 2003; Jones & Rose, 2005; AFAA, 2008). This chapter provides a brief overview of recommendations for pre-exercise screening and exercise programming for older adults, and compliments AFAA's Longevity Training for Seniors (2008) instructor workshop.

Pre-Exercise Screening

As in any age group, health and fitness levels vary from individual to individual, especially in the widely diverse older adult population. Physical abilities can range from the deconditioned frail to the highly active and elite athlete. This population also presents itself to chronic diseases (e.g., cardiovascular disease, hypertension, diabetes, cancer) and the use of medications that can affect exercise intensity. Therefore, AFAA recommends that participants initially receive consent from their doctors, approving them for exercise participation. Unfortunately, for some, this could be a barrier. Therefore, steps should be taken to identify any potential health risks or limitations to exercise testing and performance by implementing a self-administered questionnaire. For participants 65–69 years of age, the Physical Activity Readiness Questionnaire (Canada, 2002) would be appropriate. For those over 70 years of age, a more specific health history and activity questionnaire which focuses on lifestyle, chronic illnesses, medications, functional activities, physical exercise, and perception of falling (to name a few) would be more appropriate (Rogers, 2005). Those found to be in need of medical clearance based on questionnaire results should be referred to their physician for clearance prior to further participation.

To assist group exercise instructors in class format and design, AFAA recommends the use of the Senior Fitness Test (Rikli & Jones, 2001) which assesses both physical and functional performance. The test is fairly simple and can be administered in a group setting providing for a "meaningful and motivating" experience. Results will help to ensure inclusion of appropriate exercises to improve not only cardiorespiratory endurance, muscle strength and endurance, and flexibility, but also the activities we perform on a daily basis, such as ambulation, sitting and standing, stair climbing, reaching, and dressing, to provide enhanced well-being and quality of life.

Exercise Programming

Due to the varying fitness levels among older adults, the FITT recommendations for cardiorespiratory, resistance, and flexibility training have been expanded (refer to Table 38.1). A need for the inclusion of skill-related components, such as balance, agility, coordination, power, reaction time, and speed, has also been under discussion as an integral part of program design. Based on research, skill-related components have resulted in improved performance in daily activities and quality of life (Rikli & Jones, 1999; Spirduso et al., 2005; Baker et al., 2007; Katula et al., 2008).

In general, all older adults should participant in some form of physical activity because research supports some is better than none. In addition, those who participate in any amount of physical activity gain some health benefits. The following table represents a summation of the recommendations developed by the American College of Sports Medicine (ACSM), the American Heart Association (AHA), and the U.S. Department of Health and Human Services (USDHHS) for older adults.

Table 38.1 AFAA At-a-Glance: F.I.T.T. Summary Chart for Aging Adults

Cardiovascular Training

Health and Disease Prevention Recommendations

5–7 days per week; accumulation of 30 minutes of moderate-intensity activity

Fitness Improvement Recommendations

F: 3–5 days per week of continuous training (5 days for moderate; 3 days for vigorous; or 3–5 days of a combination of moderate to vigorous intensity)

I: Based on RPE 0–10: 5–6 for moderate; 7–8 for vigorous

T: 20–60 minutes: 30 min up to 60 min for moderate activity; 20–30 min for vigorous; or start with 10-minute bouts resulting in 2 ½ – 5 hrs/wk

T: Non-, low-, and light-impact

Strength Training

F: 2–3 days per week

I: To the point of mild fatigue typically in 10–15 reps

T: 20–45 minutes or time to complete 1–3 sets of one exercise for each major muscle group

T: Progressive static and dynamic forms of resistance training

---

Flexibility Training

F: Minimum of 2–3 days per week (preferably every day)

I: Edge of discomfort, holding each static stretch for 10–60 seconds

T: 10–20 minutes or time to complete 1–3 sets of one stretch for each major muscle group

T: Static and dynamic (slow movement) forms of stretching

Balance Training

F: 2–3 days per week (preferably every day)

I: To a level that challenges one's balance without continued loss of form and alignment

T: 5–10 minutes or time to complete 1–3 sets of 8–10 balance exercises

T: Static and dynamic exercises

(Adapted from ACSM & AHA, 2007, Physical Activity and Public Health in Older Adults: Recommendation from the American College of Sports Medicine and the American Heart Association; USDHHS, 2008, Physical Activity Guidelines for Americans; ACSM, 2010. *ACSM's Guidelines for Exercise Testing and Prescription*, 8th ed.)

Cardiorespiratory Conditioning

As we age there tends to be a decrease in cardiorespiratory function due to a decrease in maximum heart rate, decrease in stroke volume and cardiac output, and a decrease in VO_{2max}. Therefore, it is important for group exercise instructors to be abreast of the latest guidelines to ensure safety in older adult cardiorespiratory programming.

For the average, healthy, mature adult (over 50 years of age), recommendations for the sedentary/less active participant is to begin cardiorespiratory (aerobic) training at a low to moderate intensity (40–59% of HRR or 64–84% HR_{max}). However, due to this population having higher incidences of medication usage and chronic illness, the Rating of Perceived Exertion (RPE) is the preferred method for monitoring exercise intensity in both group and individual settings (ACSM, 2010). An RPE of 5–6 that "noticeably" increases heart rate and breathing is the current guideline for moderate intensity (Nelson et al, 2007). Sessions should be conducted at least three to five times per week for a minimum of 30 minutes or a minimum week's total of 2 hours and 30 minutes (ACSM, 1998; USDHHS, 2008; ACSM, 2010). Individuals who are sedentary and/or deconditioned should start at lower intensity levels. For those at a higher fitness level, intensity may range from 60–85% HRR and 85–94% HR_{max} or 7–8 RPE (with higher increases in HR and breathing) which constitute vigorous exercise intensity. If exercise intensity is being monitored using heart rate, a heart rate monitor can prove to be a very useful tool.

A more frequent, longer duration activity (up to 60 minutes), at a low to moderate intensity, will produce positive physiological changes within an aging body with less injury occurring. Activity-related injuries may occur more frequently among older adults due to poor flexibility, osteoporosis, or other musculoskeletal disorders (ACSM, 1998). Therefore, exercises that utilize the large muscle groups over an extended period of time, such as walking, swimming, stationary cycling, low-impact aerobic dance, tai chi, qigong, and seated-chair aerobics, are recommended along with an adequate warm-up and cool-down period.

Muscular Strength and Endurance

With normal aging, a general reduction in muscle mass occurs, frequently referred to as sarcopenia. The loss of muscle mass is thought to be due to atrophy from disuse resulting in a decrease in the number of muscle fibers and in the diameter of the remaining fibers. The loss of muscle fiber has been reported to be as high as 30% between 30 and 80 years of age (Abrass, 1990). The good news is that it is never too late to gain strength through exercise. In a landmark study that changed the minds of many practitioners, Maria Fiatarone (1990) studied 10 men and women, all 90 years of age, relative to their strength development potential. After completing an 8-week, high-intensity weight-training program (focusing on the quadriceps), results showed a 174% strength gain in the trained leg of the subjects. The lower extremity strength gain ranged from 61–374%, demonstrating a three- to four-fold increase in strength overall (Fiatarone et al, 1990).

Resistance training utilizing concentric and eccentric exercises are preferred over isometric exercises since isometric exercises have a tendency to elevate blood pressure leaving the older adult at possible risk. However, individuals suffering from musculoskeletal disorders, such as arthritis and osteoporosis, may be an exception (AGS, 2001; Swezey, 2000). Concentric and eccentric

Recommendations for strength training in the healthy senior participant are as follows. A progressive training format, at a frequency of two to three times per week, a minimum of one set per muscle group of 10–15 repetitions per set, at moderate to slow speed, exercising 8–10 different muscle groups with an intensity based on RPE between 5–6 (moderate) and 7–8 (vigorous).

strengthening of muscle groups at inflamed joints can aggravate tenderness and pain. In this instance, employment of slow stretching and very conservative isometric exercises helps to prevent muscle atrophy (Minor & Kay, 1997).

Progressive resistance training using multiple sets and repetitions with workloads of 60– 80% RM (repetition maximum) can be safely performed by healthy sedentary adults, as well as frail older adult populations with multiple chronic diseases, when performed under proper supervision (Charlotte et al., 1991; Hyatt, 1996; Kohrt et al., 2004; Coe & Fiatarone Singh, 2010). A variety of equipment may be used depending on the individual's fitness level and equipment availability. Equipment may range from weight training machines, handheld weights, elastic bands, weighted bars and balls to the natural resistance of water and one's own body against gravity such as in Pilates and yoga.

Strengthening exercises that incorporate multi-joint exercises, involving more than one muscle group, are recommended to enhance functional activities in older adults. For example, working the muscles in the lower extremities (e.g., lunges and squats) helps improve balance, strength, and endurance, which are needed for sitting, standing, walking, and climbing. Include exercises for the upper body (e.g., push-ups, rows, and the overhead press) to aid in reaching, lifting, and carrying objects. In addition, include exercises for the muscles in the hands and fingers (e.g., gripping a tennis ball, pressing fingers into a soft rubber ball, or extending them against an elastic band). These muscles are needed to open doors; change light bulbs; prepare meals; button, zip, and snap clothes; and more.

Balance, Flexibility, and Postural Stability

Balance, a physical performance variable, is typically found to decrease with age and is thought to be an important factor relative to the prevention of falls (Tinetti et al., 1994; Kannu, et al., 2005). In the United States, one out of every three adults 65 years of age or older fall each year. Exercise, and even simple activity, has been found to significantly reduce the loss of balance in seniors, particularly older women. It is extremely valuable, therefore, for the fitness professional to discuss proper body mechanics as they relate to balance as well as to develop exercises that specifically focus on improving balance (Rose, 2005). Activities, such as progressive resistance training, walking, dancing, Pilates, tai chi, yoga, stability ball exercises, core-strengthening, and flexibility training, have shown to improve balance in older adults (Jarnlo, 1991; Judge et al., 1993; Wolf et al., 1996; Rose, 2003; Orr et al., 2008).

Flexibility is another area of concern. Flexibility tends to be lost due to connective tissue stiffening and a decrease in mobility with age. With sedentary aging, muscles tend to shorten and contract, and connective tissues tend to weaken, leading to joint stiffness, limited range of motion, and general changes in posture, balance, and gait (Denner & Edwards, 1992; Buckwalter et al., 1993; Holland et al., 2002).

Stretching exercises performed may regularly help maintain, improve, and prevent declines in flexibility and range of motion, which, in turn, help prevent muscular imbalances that may lead to injurious falls. Slow range of motion exercises (dynamic stretching), Proprioceptive neuromuscular facilitation (PNF), and static stretching are the most commonly used methods. However, static stretching and slow (dynamic) movements are recommended (ACSM, 2010).

Exercise Adherence

Exercise adherence for the older adult participant is necessary to ensure positive physical results. Factors that influence exercise adherence include changes in fitness and health status of the participant, increased feelings of competence and personal growth (self-efficacy), commitment, and goal-setting (Martin & Sinden, 2001). Exercise programs specifically designed for the older adult, that are enjoyable, offer tasks that are fairly easy to accomplish, accessible, lend social support, and have little to no cost associated with participation may create a positive effect on exercise adherence as well. The group dynamics of an older adult fitness class can play a vital role in the success of your program. An environment where older adults reach out to one another through fostering, mentoring, socializing, and camaraderie can create a wonderful bonding situation with the desire for continued participation. Instructors who provide a caring and warm environment, as well as demonstrate a sense of humor tend to improve exercise adherence. In addition, those who provide positive reinforcement, easy-to-follow choreography directives, compliments, praise, and encouragement will keep their participants coming back for more

However, there are exceptions within the young at heart, active, and fit seniors who are more apt to attend fitness classes designed for the younger adult crowd in their 20s, 30s, 40s, and 50s (e.g., step aerobics, spinning, Pilates, low-/high-impact aerobics, muscle conditioning, and advanced yoga). They do not consider themselves "old." They are healthy, active individuals. Recommending they attend older adult fitness classes (supposedly designed for their aging needs) may actually be interpreted as an insult instead of a positive gesture on the instructor's part. Keep in mind that a very active senior participant in his or her 70s can demonstrate the fitness level of a moderately-fit 30-year-old (Butler et al., 1998). The older adult fitness class may be more appropriately named and reserved for the sedentary, less-fit mature adult with physical ability and limitations, not age, as the prerequisite. The more active, young at hearts actually may feel more comfortable in a less structured environment as well as exercising in the privacy and comfort of their own home.

Physiological adaptations come about more slowly in older adults, so implementation of an exercise program should start gradually and then progress at a slower rate than would be implemented for younger adults. Participants should be encouraged to work at their own pace and stay within their "comfort zone." Gradually building into an exercise program and providing exercises that participants can successfully perform empowers your participants. If your participants become empowered, you will find they will continue a life-long commitment to physical activity.

> ### Enjoyable and Pain-Free
>
> *Always remind participants that they are welcome to stop whenever discomfort arises or they feel tired and fatigued. Gradually build intensity and develop enjoyable, but realistic challenges in order to maintain interest.*

Class Format

The class format will vary depending on the dynamics of the group, the exercise environment, and the goals of the program. No matter how the class is organized, always begin with a warm-up and end with a cool-down, final stretch, and relaxation segment.

Sequencing

Transition from a standing position to the floor is not always easily accomplished in the less fit older adult. Therefore, it may be preferable in some cases to do the complete class in either a standing or seated position, or a combination of both to avoid the strain of lifting and lowering the body off the floor. If floor work is to be included, place it at the end of class to allow adequate time to recover and return to a standing position.

Types of Activity

There is an array of physical activities to choose from that support cardiorespiratory conditioning in a group exercise setting. From group walking programs, line dancing, circuit training, step, and water fitness, to tai chi, qi qong, and more.

Good program design incorporates both aerobic and anaerobic weight-bearing exercises for bone health, particularly to enhance bone density in older adult participants. Group settings include weighted bars, balls, hand-held weights, elastic tubing, and bands for improving muscle strength and endurance. Weights and bands should only be introduced when the participant has reached a fitness level that will enable him or her to add the extra force and/or when correct alignment and execution can be maintained throughout a full range of motion. More information is available in AFAA's *Standards and Guidelines for Senior Fitness.*

Balance and flexibility exercises should be a standard part of any group exercise class.

Balance (neuromuscular training) is an important factor relative to the prevention of falls, which is a major concern among older adults. Therefore, include progressive resistance training and progressive balance exercises that address the multisensory systems (vision, somatosensory, and vestibular). Instructors should also take into consideration the four dimensions of balance (voluntary postural control, anticipatory postural control, reactive postural control, and sensory organization) during the exercise selection process. A series of exercises referred to as "narrowing the base of support" provides for progressive balance training and includes the following.

1. Standing with feet hip width apart with eyes:
   a. open; hands on a barre or back of a chair for support
   b. open; no support
   c. closed; with support
   d. closed; no support
2. Standing with feet together with eyes:
   a. open; hands on a barre or back of a chair for support
   b. open; no support
   c. closed; with support
   d. closed; no support
3. Semi-tandem stance with eyes open (feet are touching with toe of one foot at the instep of the other foot) with no support
4. Full tandem or toe-to-heel (where one foot is touching the heal of the foot in front) with no support
5. One-legged stand with no support
6. Toe stand on two feet and progress to one-legged toe stand with no support

NOTE: The most important thing for instructors to maintain when implementing balance activities is a safe environment utilizing appropriate exercise selection and proper spotting techniques.

Other balance training modalities may include (a) directional changes, (b) stepping, (c) stability ball activities, and (d) tai chi. Progressing the difficulty of standing balance activities would be to perform various tasks on an unstable surface (e.g., cushioned mat, balance disc, half foam roller, or BOSU® ball for advanced participants). Dr. Debra Rose, one of the world's experts in balance and mobility training, has made available to fitness professionals her knowledge and techniques in her book titled, *Fall proof! A Comprehensive Balance and Mobility Training Program.*

Flexibility can be achieved by selecting a variety of statically held stretches, slow (dynamic) movements, or PNF exercises that address all areas of the body from head-to-toe. The ACSM recommends a 6-second contraction followed by a 10- to 30-second assisted stretch when performing PNF exercises. (Refer to Table 38.1 for frequency, intensity, and duration.)

Program Design Guidelines Beyond FITT

It has been discussed that it is important to follow the FITT principles of training to achieve health and fitness benefits. However, there are some other variables to consider as well to ensure a safe and enjoyable exercise experience for your older adult participants. They include, but are not limited to, the following.

1. Make sure participants know how to monitor their workloads at a comfortable pace throughout the class.

2. New exercisers often have difficulty pacing their fitness program. Be alert for signs of overexertion.

3. Monitor intensity every 4 to 5 minutes during cardiorespiratory conditioning.

4. Slow and controlled movements working through a full range of motion are recommended when performing resistance activities. During the cardio workout, keep movements simple and easy to follow while enabling participants to maintain good posture and alignment. Keys to successful choreography include the following.
   - Arm and leg elevation should directly correlate with the range of motion, flexibility, and fitness level of the individual.
   - Arm and leg elevation should be varied to control heart rate and reduce the stress on the joints.
   - Combination moves requiring coordination of both arms and legs should be entered into slowly, starting with either the arms or the legs, and then adding the other.
   - Utilize only a few moves when building a combination.
   - Use lateral movements with caution (e.g., grapevines), and simplify movement patterns whenever possible (e.g., modified grapevines).
   - Repeat directions and movement patterns often, and use verbal and nonverbal cues.

5. Avoid forward spinal flexion movements if known spinal osteoporosis is present.

6. Dizziness may occur if a participant closes his or her eyes, lowers his or her head below the heart, performs twisting motion of the neck and head, or rises off the floor or from a chair too quickly.

7. Participants with prosthetics (e.g., hip or knee replacement) need to follow their doctor's exercise recommendations pertaining to joint action and range of motion.

8. If incorporating stepping exercises utilizing equipment, such as the bench, with older adults:
   - get physician's clearance—step choreography can be hard on hips, knees, and feet.
   - refer to AFAA's Step Training and Basic Exercise Standards and Guidelines.
   - keep music beats per minute (bpm) low (118–124 bpm).

- use just the floor (no step platform) or no more than a 4-inch platform for novice participants.
- choreography should be simple and easy to follow.
- provide a longer warm-up and cool-down period.

Summary

As researchers continue to look at the process of aging, we see that everyone ages differently. In addition, the human body, no matter what age, can respond to and receive positive effects of training through regular exercise. With America growing older, physical activity can play a major role in maintaining health and independence among the older adult population. As a fitness professional, you can make a major contribution towards the quality of life in seniors by providing a warm, supportive, and motivating environment that delivers safe and effective functional exercise programs.

Sample Workout for Active Seniors
Janie Clark, MA

Warm up for approximately 10 minutes with:
1. Rhythmic limbering movements (such as shoulder shrugs, hip shifts, and arm circles)
2. Gentle activity designed to increase circulation (such as walking in place and easy-does-it arm swings)
3. Conservatively executed stretches (including mild stretches for the back, the hamstrings, and the calves)

Aerobics for approximately 20 minutes. Develop creative patterns by combining the steps shown below (as well as other low-impact movements).

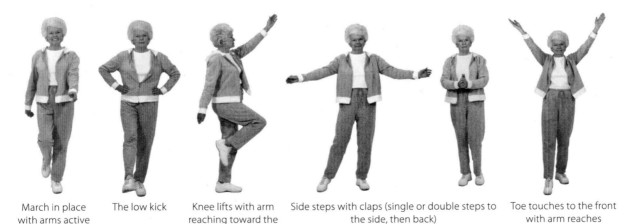

| March in place with arms active | The low kick | Knee lifts with arm reaching toward the front | Side steps with claps (single or double steps to the side, then back) | Toe touches to the front with arm reaches overhead |

Note: Observe a post-aerobic cool-down period for 5 to 10 minutes using non-strenuous movements similar to those performed during the warm-up. Gradually decrease the intensity level with light activity that engages the lower body along with gentle stretches.

Strengthening exercises for approximately 15 minutes. The following senior-specific modality considerations apply:

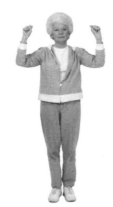 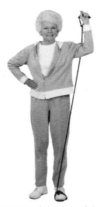 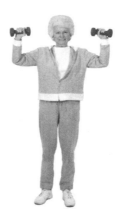

Initially, senior should practice exercises without the use of resistive devices.

As strength and confidence increase, easy tension bands may be introduced.

Upon further conditioning, light hand weights may be employed.

Note: Seniors with shoulder issues may not be able to achieve full range of motion in the overhead press movement. Modifications should be made to accommodate them (e.g., non-weighted or reduced range of motion).

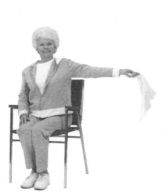 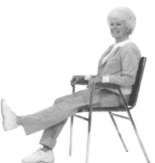 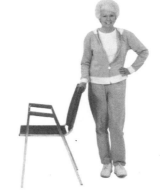

Additional accessories (such as dowels, neckties, scarves, towels and foam-type balls) may be used.

A viable alternative may be to combine seated, chair activity with standing exercise.

Standing knee extension exercise for lower body strengthening

Note: Floor work is appropriate when well tolerated. When getting up and down for floor work is difficult, chair routines may be developed.. Modifications should be made to accommodate them (e.g., non-weighted or reduced range of motion).

Below is a sample list of well-known, standard strengthening exercises appropriate for most older adults:
1. Open and Close Hands
2. Biceps Curl
3. Triceps Extension
4. Upright Row
5. Single-arm Bent-over Row (with spinal support supplied by placing the opposite hand and knee on a weight bench)
6. Standing Push-up with Hands against Wall (pushing away from a wall is easier on delicate wrists than the traditional floor push-up)
7. Modified Bent-knee Sit-up (include forward curls as well as curls toward both sides)

8. Reverse Curl
9. Hamstring and Gluteus Contraction
10. Knee Flexion
11. Knee Extension
12. Leg Lift Engaging the Outer Thigh (abduction)
13. Leg Lift Engaging the Inner Thigh (adduction)
14. Calf Lift (raise onto toes)
15. Shin Strengthener (With heel on floor, energetically tap toe to floor at a steady pace.)

Enjoy a **cool-down stretch** for 5 to 10 minutes. Below is a sample stretch routine suitable for almost all older adults. With reference to well-conditioned seniors, the chair stretches shown here may be modified for safe execution on the floor or in a standing position:

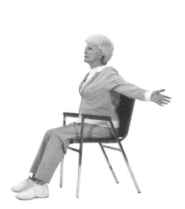 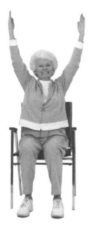 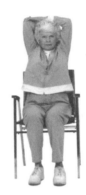

The backward reach–chest stretch   The upward reach– torso stretc   The gentle pull–shoulder girdle stretch

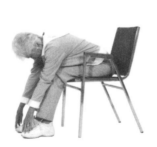 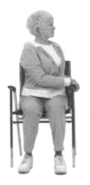 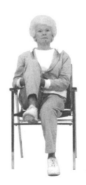

The forward stretch with continuous hand contact for spinal support
Note: Some seniors with spinal issues may not be advised to flex forward at the spine.

The turn–torso stretch   The leg hug–hip stretch

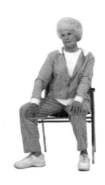
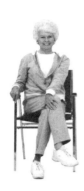
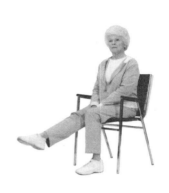
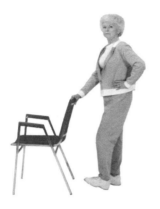

The leg-out inner thigh stretch   The leg-over outer thigh stretch   The point–shin stretch   The flex–calf stretch

References

1. Abrass, I.B. (1990). The biology and physiology of aging. *Western Journal of Medicine*, 153, 641–645.

2. Aerobics and Fitness Association of America. (2002). Standards and guidelines for senior fitness part 1: "Healthy sedentary older adults." In *AFAA's exercise standards & guidelines reference manual* (4th ed.). Sherman Oaks, CA: Aerobics and Fitness Association of America.

3. American College of Sports Medicine. (1998). Position statement on the recommended quantity and quality of exercise for developing and maintaining cardiorespiratory and muscular fitness, and flexibility in healthy adults. *Medicine & Science in Sports & Exercise*, 22(2), 265–274.

4. American College of Sports Medicine. (2001). Exercise recommendations for flexibility and range of motion. In *ACSM's resource manual for guideline for exercise testing and prescription* (4th ed.). (pp. 468). New York: Lippincott Williams & Wilkins.

5. American College of Sports Medicine (2006). *ACSM's guidelines for exercise testing and prescription* (7th ed.). Baltimore, MD: Lippincott Williams & Wilkins.

6. American College of Sports Medicine. (2010). *ACSM's resource manual for guidelines for exercise testing and prescription* (6th ed.). Baltimore, MD: Lippincott Williams & Wilkins.

7. American Geriatrics Society. (2001). Exercise prescription for older adults with osteoarthritis pain: Consensus practice recommendations. A supplement to the AGS clinical practice guidelines on the management of chronic pain in older adults. *Journal of American Geriatric Society*, 49(6), 808–23.

8. Armbruster, B., & Gladwin, L.A. (2001). More than fitness for older adults: A whole-istic approach to wellness. *ACSM's Health & Fitness Journal*, 5(2), 6–12.

9. Baker, M.K., Atlantis, E., & Fiatarone Singh, M.A. (2007). Multi-modal exercise programs for older adults. *Age Ageing*, 36(4), 375–381.

10. Beckett, L.A., Brock, D.B., Lemke, J.H., Mendes de Leon, C.F., Guralnik, J.M., et al. (1998). Analysis of change in self-reported physical function among older persons in four population studies. *American Journal of Epidemiology*, 143, 766–778.

11. Brown, M., & Rose, D.J. (2005). Flexibility training. In C.J Jones & D.J. Rose (Eds.), *Physical activity instruction of older adults* (pp. 155–174). Champaign, IL: Human Kinetics.

12. Bucksch, J. (2005). Physical activity of moderate intensity in leisure time and the risk of all cause mortality. *British Journal in Sports Medicine*, 39(9), 632–638.

13. Buckwalter, J.A., Woo, S.L., Goldberg, V.M., Hadley, E.C., Booth, F., Oegema, T.R., et al. (1993). Soft tissue aging and musculoskeletal function. *Journal of Bone and Joint Surgery*, 75, 1533–1548.

14. Buckwalter, J.A. (1997). Decreased mobility in the elderly: The exercise antidote. *The Physician and Sportsmedicine*, 25(9), 44–52.

15. Butler, R.N., Davis, R., Lewis, C.B., & et al. (1998). Physical fitness: Benefits of physical fitness for the older patient. *Geriatrics*, 53, 46–62.

16. Centers for Disease Control and Prevention. (2002). *Promoting active lifestyles among older adults*. Handout (quoting BRFSS 2000 unpublished data). Available at CDC on the World Wide Web: http://www.cdc.gov/nccdphp/dnpa/physical/pdf/lifestyles.pdf

17. Charlotte, S.L. et al. (1991). *Muscle hypertrophy response to resistance training in older women*. Palo Alto, CA: American Physiological Society.

18. Denner, R., & Edwards, D. (1992). Life is movement: Exercise for the older adult. *Activities, Adaptation and Aging*, 17, 15–25.

19. Estabrooks, P.A., & Carran, A.V. (2001). Predicting scheduling self-efficacy in older adult exercise: The role of task cohesion. *Journal of Aging and Physical Activity*, 8, 41–50.

20. Fiatarone, M.A., Marks, E.C., Ryan, N.D., et al. (1990). High intensity strength training in nonagenarians: effects on skeletal muscle. *Journal of American Medical Association*, 262(22), 3029–3034.

21. Fiatarone Singh, M.A. (2002). Exercise comes of age: Rationale and recommendations for a geriatric exercise prescription. *Journal of Gerontology Series A: Biological Sciences and Medical Sciences*, 57, (A), M262–282.

22. Gladwin, L.A. (1996). Stretching: A valuable component of functional mobility training in the elderly. In J. Clark (Ed.), *Exercise programming for older adults*. Binghamton, NY: The Haworth Press, Inc.

23. Holland, G.J., Tanaka, K., Shigematsu, R., & Nakagaichi, M. (2002). Flexibility and physical function of older adults: A review. *Journal of Aging and Physical Activity*, 10, 169-206.

24. Hyatt, G. (1996). Strength training for the aging adult. In Clark, J. (Ed.), *Exercise programming for older adults*. Binghamton, NY: The Haworth Press, Inc.

25. Jarnlo, G.B. (1991). Hip fracture patients: background and function. *Scandinavian Journal of Rehabilitative Medicine*, 24 (Suppl.), 1–31.

26. Judge, J.O. et al. (1993). Balance improvements in older women: effects of exercise training. *Physical Therapy*, 73, 254–265.

27. Kannus, P., Sievanen, H., Palvanen, M., et al. (2005). Prevention of falls and consequent injuries in elderly people. *Lancet*, 366(9500), 1885–1893.

28. Katula, J.A., Rejeski, W.J., & Marsh, A.P. (2008). Enhancing quality of life in older adults: A comparison of muscular strength and power training. *Health and Quality of Life Outcomes*, 13(6), 45.

29. Kohrt, W.M., Bloomfield, S.A., Little, K.D., Nelson, M.E., & Yingling, V.R. (2004). ACSM's position stand on physical activity and bone health. *Medicine & Science in Sports & Exercise*, 36(11), 1985–1996.

30. Martin, K.A., & Sinden, A.R. (2001). Who will stay and who will go? A review of older adults' adherence to randomized controlled trials of exercise. *Journal of Aging and Physical Activity*, 9, 91–114.

31. Minor, M.A., & Kay, D.R. (1997). "Arthritis." In *ACSM's exercise management for persons with chronic diseases and disabilities* (1st ed.). Champaign, IL: Human Kinetics.

32. Monane, M., Matthias, D.M., Nagle, B.A., & Kelly, M.A. (1998). Improving prescribing patterns for the elderly through an online drug utilization review intervention. *Journal of the American Medical Association*, 280, 1249–1252.

33. Nelson, M.E., Rejeski, W.J., Blair, S.N., Duncan, P.W., Judge, J.O., King, A.C., Macera, C.A., & Castaneda-Sceppa, C. (2007). Physical Activity and Public Health in Older Adults: Recommendation from the American College of Sports Medicine and the American Heart Association. *Medicine & Science in Exercise & Sports*, 39(8), 1435–1445.

34. Rikli, R.E., & Jones, C.J. (1999). Development and validation of a functional fitness test for community-residing older adults. *Journal of Aging and Physical Activity*, 7, 129–161.

35. Rikli, R.E., & Jones, C.J. (2001). *Senior fitness test*. Champaign, IL: Human Kinetics.

36. Rogers, M. (2005). Preexercise and health. In C.J. Jones & D.J. Rose (Eds.), *Physical activity instruction of older adults*. Champaign, IL: Human Kinetics.

37. Rose, D.J. (2003). *Fall proof! A comprehensive balance and mobility training program*. Champaign, IL: Human Kinetics.

38. Spirduso, W., Francis, K., & MacRae, P. (2005). *Physical dimensions of aging* (2nd ed.). Champaign, IL: Human Kinetics.

39. Swezey, R.L. (2000). Osteoporosis: Diagnosis, pharmacological, and rehabilitation therapies. *Critical Reviews in Physical and Rehabilitation Medicine*, 12, 229–269.

40. Tinetti, M.E., Baker, D.I., McAvay, G., Claus, E.B., Garrett, P., Gottschalk, M., Koch, M.L., Trainor, K., & Horwitz, R.L. (1994). A multifactorial intervention to reduce the risk of falling among elderly people living in the community. *The New England Journal of Medicine*, 331, 821–827.

41. von Stengel, S., Kemmler, W., Kalender, W.A., Engelke, K., & Lauber, D. (2007). Differential effects of strength versus power training on bone mineral density in postmenopausal women: A 2-year longitudinal study. *British Journal in Sports Medicine*, 41(10), 649–55.

42. Ward, A., Taylor, P., & Rippe, J. (1991). How to tailor an exercise program. *The Physician and Sportsmedicine*, 19(9), 64–74.

43. Wolf, S.L. et al. (1996). Reducing frailty and falls in older persons: an investigation of tai chi and computerized balance training—Atlanta FICSIT Group: Frailty and Injuries—cooperative studies of intervention techniques. *Journal of American Geriatrics Society*, 44, 489–497.

44. U.S. Department of Health and Human Services. (2008). *2008 physical activity guidelines for Americans*. Washington, DC: Office of Disease Prevention and Health Promotion (U0036)/www.health.gov/paguidelines.

References for Janie Clark's Sample Workout

1. Aerobics and Fitness Association of America. (1994). Standards and guidelines for senior fitness. In AFAA's *Reference manual* (5th ed.). Sherman Oaks, CA: Aerobics and Fitness Association of America.

2. Aerobics and Fitness Association of America. (2007). Standards and guidelines for senior fitness. In AFAA's *Longevity training for seniors workshop outline*. Sherman Oaks, CA: Aerobics and Fitness Association of America.

3. Clark, J. (1992). *Full life fitness: A complete exercise program for mature adults*. Champaign, IL: Human Kinetics.

4. Clark, J. (2008). *Quality-of-life fitness* (2nd ed.). New Smyrna Beach, FL: American Senior Fitness Association.

Recommended Reading

1. American College of Sports Medicine. (2009). *ACSM's exercise management for persons with chronic diseases and disabilities* (3rd ed.). Champaign, IL: Human Kinetics.

2. Baechle, T.R., & Westcott, W.L. (2010). *Fitness professional's guide to strength training older adults* (2nd ed.). Champaign, IL: Human Kinetics.

3. Brill, P.A. (2004). *Functional fitness for older adults*. Champaign, IL: Human Kinetics.

4. Clark, W.R. (2002). *A means to an end: The biological basis of aging and death*. New York: Oxford University Press.

5. Coe, D.P., & Fiatarone Singh, M.A. (2010). In *ACSM's resource manual for exercise testing and prescription* (pp. 682–687). Baltimore, MD: Lippincott Williams & Wilkins.

6. Jones, C.J., & Rose, D.J. (Eds.). (2005). *Physical activity instruction of older adults*. Champaign, IL: Human Kinetics.

7. Rose, D.J. (2003). *Fall proof! A comprehensive balance and mobility training program*. Champaign, IL: Human Kinetics.

8. Spirduso, W., Francis, K., & MacRae, P. (2005). *Physical dimensions of aging* (2nd ed.). Champaign, IL: Human Kinetics.

39 Pregnancy: Fitness Programming within a Continuum of Care

Dorette Nysewander, EdD
and
Michael T. Phelan, MD

Focus

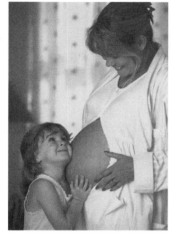

In this chapter, discussions will include health and exercise topics for the child-bearing year. Perinatal clients ask fitness professionals many questions during this time, so it is important to provide appropriate guidance within the industry's scope of practice and know when to refer a client back to their physician. Fitness professionals working within this special population need specialized training and education beyond a basic certification. This comprehensive overview focuses on the planning for pregnancy, nutritional guidelines, special exercise considerations, fitness programming, and postpartum recovery.

Introduction. Obstetricians provide perinatal care to thousands of women. In doing so, these professionals stress that while being a natural process, pregnancy is much like an athletic event. The better prepared you are mentally and physically, the easier and more tolerable the process will be.

Pregnancy can be a wonderful and joyous experience. A woman's attitude is important in how she perceives the experience to be. Taking a proactive approach to fitness, nutrition, and self-care will make each pregnancy easier, safer, and more enjoyable.

The ideal results within this childbearing year and beyond is to have a pregnancy to term without unnecessary interventions, a healthy baby, and a supportive environment that addresses the physical and emotional needs of both the mother and infant. Fitness professionals can compliment medicine by assisting clients with program specific guidelines and support.

Planning For Pregnancy

Women who are thinking about becoming pregnant should plan early and consult with their physician. All aspects of a woman's well-being should be addressed. Topics during this visit can include, however are not limited to, diet and exercise, nutritional supplements, avoidance of certain medications and/or substance abuse, immunizations, and genetic counseling.

There are many healthy babies born annually. Subject to a physician's advice and counsel, some recommendations for a planned pregnancy that prove to be most beneficial for clients include the following.

1. Get into shape prior to pregnancy. Pregnancy is the hardest work a woman's body will go through. Becoming physically fit will keep a client's energy levels high.(1)

2. Take folic acid or folate (400 micrograms) at least 4 weeks prior to conception and continue this throughout the pregnancy. Folic acid has been shown to reduce the risk of birth defects in a baby's spinal cord and skull by 70%.(2)

3. Supplement a strict vegetarian diet with necessary vitamins and minerals, for example, B_{12}. Without the intake of eggs or dairy products, there is a greater risk of neural tube defects (a class of birth defects affecting the brain and spinal cord.)(3)

4. Manage conditions of diabetes, high blood pressure, or other circulatory problems. It becomes increasingly more difficult to try to begin to manage these conditions during pregnancy.(4)

5. Avoid certain medications or over-the-counter therapies. From conception to about the 8th week of gestation, the baby is vulnerable to teratogens (drugs or viruses that can cause malformity). For a reference list see Table 39-1.(5)

6. Change lifestyle to eliminate tobacco, alcohol, and/or illicit drug use. Research has associated these behaviors with miscarriage, premature and low birth weight, and birth defects.(6,7)

7. Obtain titers to ensure vaccinations are up-to-date, that is, rubella (German measles) and chickenpox. Having no immunity to these diseases can cause complications during pregnancy.(8)

8. Inquire about genetic counseling; regardless of a client's health status there might be certain health problems that run throughout the families (e.g., cystic fibrosis and sickle cell anemia).(9)

Table 39-1. Teratogenic Agents

Alcohol	fetal alcohol syndrome
Aminoglycosides	deafness
Aminopterin	Intrauterine growth retardation, CNS defect, cleftlip/palate
Antineoplastics	
Birth control pills	VACTERL syndrome (Vertebral, Anal, Cardiac, Tracheoesophageal, Renal and Limb malformations)
Carbamazepine	fingernail hypoplasia, craniofacial defects
Cigarettes	IUGR, low birth weight, prematurity
Cocaine	cerebral infarcts, mental retardation
Diazepam(Valium)	cleft lip/palate
Diethylstilbestrol (DES)	clear cell vaginal cancer, adenosis, cervical incompetence
Iodine	goiter, cretinism
Isotretinoin (Accutane)	CNS, craniofacial, ear, and cardiovascular defects
Lithium	cardiac(Ebstein's) abnormalities
Phenytoin	craniofacial and limb defects
Progesterone	masculinzation of feminine fetus
Radiation	IUGR, CNS and face defects, leukemia
Tetracycline (antibiotic)	teeth discoloration
Thalidomide	phocomelia
Trimethadione	craniofacial and cardiovascular defects, mental retardation
Valproic acid	spinabifida, hypospadias
Warfarin	IUGR, stillbirth, craniofacial, and CNS defects

Since some women may be uncomfortable with consulting a physician to discuss a planned pregnancy, they can receive health information via e-mail every other week for 3 months in preparation for pregnancy, by going to www.ihealthrecord.org. While this is no substitute for medical care, the Center for Disease Control and Prevention (CDC) and other medical societies have developed e-mail-based education programs that are offered through this Interactive Health Record(10).

Nutritional Guidelines

Good health demands an approach to eating nutritionally that begins with pre-pregnancy, includes breast feeding, and extends to old age. Nutrition seems most appealing if taken in small, frequent meals, as this helps to stabilize blood sugar. The table below provides macronutrient levels for healthy women, pregnant women, and lactating mothers. Caloric intake will need to be adjusted based on the weight of the woman, her activity levels, and her physician's specific recommendations. Fitness professionals can assist in helping to educate their clients about these guidelines without stepping into a licensed professional's areas of practice. Another source to help with developing a customized nutritional regimen is www.mypyramid.gov, plan for moms Web site.

Table 39-2.					
Nutrient	**Healthy Women**	**Pregnant Women**	**Lactating Mothers**	**Function**	**Food Source**
Calories	1800–2000	2100–2500	2400–2800	Energy, growth, ↑metabolic requirements	Protein, fat, carbohydrates
Protein	46 g	76–100 g	66–80 g	Builds and repairs tissue, forms antibodies, placenta, amniotic fluid, ↑blood volume	Lean meat, cheese, eggs, beans
Carbohydrates	45–65% of total daily calories	45–65% of total daily calories	45–65% of total daily calories	Primary source of energy, ensures protein is used efficiently, metabolizes more quickly in pregnancy	Fruits, vegetables, whole grain breads, cereals with high fiber
Water/Fluids	6–8 c	8–10 c	10–12 c	Fluid for BV, AF, transports nutrients, aids in digestion, core temp	Water, juice, milk
Folic Acid/ Folate	400–800 mg . 4mg	400–800 mg .4mg	600 mg . 6mg	Red blood cells, aids in DNA, RNA, amino acid synthesis	Leafy green vegetables, melons, wheat germ
Vitamin D	.005 mg 200 IU	.01 mg 400IU	.01 mg 400IU	Absorb calcium, strengthen bones/teeth	Fortified milk, butter, exposure to sun
Calcium	800 mg	1200 mg	1200 mg	Builds bones and teeth, blood clotting, nerve transmission	Milk, cheese, spinach, collards, whole grains
Iron	30–60 mg	30–60 mg	30–60 mg	hemoglobin oxygen delivery, growth	Liver, dried beans, fruits
Potassium	1875–5600 mg	1875–5600 mg	1875–5600 mg	Muscle contractions, electrolyte balance, releases energy	Fruits, dried peas, beans, bran
Sodium	1100–3300 mg	1100–3300 mg	1100–3300 mg	Regulates balance of water, acids, bases	Salt, MSG, soups, fish, snacks

Recommended servings for pregnancy include: whole grains, pasta, fortified cereals-six-nine (6–9), vegetables-four (4), fruits-two-four (2–4), milk and dairy-three (3), meat and beans, fish, eggs or nuts-three-four (3–4); fats oils and sweets [eat sparingly]. Also include a daily intake of between 20–30 grams of fiber.

Other nutrition considerations include the following.

Caffeine—leads to dehydration, as it's a natural diuretic; limit consumption or avoid all together.

Food cravings—during pregnancy there is a desire for specific foods in large quantities and while not harmful, consumption should be integrated with healthy eating.

Lactose intolerance—some women will have sensitivities to milk, substitute with lactose intolerant products or spinach, salmon, fortified juices, and sardines rich in calcium.

Listeriosis—is an illness caused by bacteria. To prevent listeriosis during pregnancy, wash all fresh fruits and vegetables prior to eating, avoid unpasteurized milk or soft cheeses, raw or undercooked meat, poultry, shellfish, and prepared meats (e.g., hot dogs or deli meats).

Mercury—it is best to stay with canned tuna, and farm-raised fish or smaller ocean fish to avoid consumption of mercury. Swordfish, king mackerel, orange roughy, halibut, and shark all have high levels resulting in harm to the baby's brain or nervous system.

Organic nutrition—"organic" is a labeling term that denotes products are produced under the authorization of the Organic Foods Production Act; methods are used to reduce pollution from air, soil, and water, while optimizing health and productivity of independent communities of plants, animals, and people. This is a healthier option for mother and baby.

Phyenylketonuria (PKU)—is a genetic disorder and pregnant women with this condition are unable to metabolize phenylalanine properly. Recommendations are to limit intake of all foods that contain this amino acid including meat, fish, dairy, eggs, and especially products containing artificial sweeteners (e.g., diet sodas, sugar-free chewing gum).

Pica—refers to strong urges to eat non-food items such as clay, ice, laundry starch, or cornstarch. Pica can be harmful to a pregnancy, as it affects intake of nutrients and can lead to constipation and anemia.

Plastic bottles—substitute with glass whenever possible; if using plastic the #2 Hope (high-density polyethylene) is the safest choice; look for the recycle triangle stamped on the bottom.

Supplementation—when food is not enough additional nutrients may be recommended or prescribed.

Vegetarians—need to ensure that they are getting enough of the right kind of protein in addition to taking the following supplements—iron, B_{12}, and Vitamin D.

Breastfeeding benefits for baby and mother. Nutrition for the baby is just as important as nutrition for the mother. Breastfeeding can be beneficial by providing a ready-to-eat, easily digested, and immune-boosting source of food. Additionally, moms benefit from more efficient involution of the uterus, allowing faster recovery to their postpartum body. Studies have also shown breastfeeding lowers the incidence of breast and ovarian cancer. Alternatively, there are many formulas on the market, each specific to the infant's nutritional demands.[11,12,13,14,15,16,17]

Special Exercise Considerations

Advocates of exercise. The American College of Obstetricians and Gynecologists (ACOG) and the U.S. Department of Health and Human Services advocate exercise for women experiencing a healthy pregnancy.[23] Women who experience absolute and relative contraindications during pregnancy are to work directly with their physicians who in turn provide the appropriate guidance and care. For a list of the conditions, see Table 39-2.[28] All pregnant women should be given written permission to exercise, and sedentary pregnant women should not begin an exercise program in the first or third trimesters.

The following special exercise considerations have been provided for pregnant women in their second and third trimesters of a **healthy** pregnancy.

Women who are inactive should start slow when starting to exercise. ACOG recommends (a) to begin with as little as 5 minutes of exercise a day and add 5 minutes each week until a woman can stay active for 30 minutes a day; (b) get at least 150 minutes of moderate-intensity aerobic activity a week or try 30 minutes of aerobic exercise on most, if not all, days; (c) habitually engage in vigorous-intensity aerobic activity or for those who are highly active continue physical activity during pregnancy, provided that they remain healthy and discuss with their physicians how and when activity should be adjusted over time.[18,19,20]

Cardiovascular changes. During pregnancy blood volume will increase from 30–50%. This places increased demands on the cardiovascular system. Some changes include increased heart rate and increased cardiac output. Specifically, heart rate goes up by 10–15 beats per minute (bpm), whereas cardiac output can increase up to 50%. In addition, pulmonary reserve is decreased because respi-

Absolute Contraindications to Exercise during Pregnancy
- Hemodynamically significant heart disease
- Restrictive lung disease
- Incompetent cervix
- Multiple gestations at risk for premature labor
- Persistent second or third trimester bleeding
- Placenta previa after 26 weeks of gestation
- Premature labor during the current pregnancy
- Ruptured membranes
- Pregnancy-induced hypertension [PIH]/Pre-eclampsia

Relative Contraindications to Exercise during Pregnancy
- Severe anemia
- Unevaluated maternal cardiac dysrhythmia
- Chronic bronchitis
- Poorly controlled type 1 diabetes
- Extreme morbid obesity
- Extreme underweight (BMI < 12)
- History of extremely sedentary lifestyle
- Intrauterine growth restriction in current pregnancy
- Poorly controlled hypertension
- Orthopedic limitations
- Poorly controlled seizure disorder
- Poorly controlled hyperthyroidism
- Heavy smoker

ratory rates are elevated at rest. These additional demands on the pregnant body should be considered during any physical activity.(21)

ACOG recommends that pregnant women exercise at a moderate intensity of 12–14 "somewhat hard" using the Borg rating of perceived exertion (RPE) 6–20 scale. So, if pregnant women are able to talk normally while exercising, the heart rate is at an acceptable level. Because of these changes, it is recommended to avoid prolonged standing or crossing of the legs.(22,23)

Studies show that women who voluntarily continue weight-bearing exercise during pregnancy maintain their long-term fitness to exercise over time at a higher level, gain less weight (3.4 vs. 9.9 kg), deposit less fat (2.2 vs. 6.7 kg), and have increased fitness levels than those who stop.(24)

Hormonal and anatomical changes. During pregnancy there is an increased secretion of various hormones to include relaxin, estrogen, progesterone, and elastin. Elastin and relaxin causes connective tissues and joints to soften, thus increasing the risk for potential injuries. Some changes women will experience include an expanding rib cage, pelvic instability, and an increased shoe size.(21)

With the enlarging weight of the uterus and breast, special attention should be paid to strengthening and stretching exercises to minimize stress to the spine. This includes exercises to stretch the chest and strengthen the upper back (trapezius, rhomboids) while maintaining strong abdominals and gluteal muscles to help prevent added strain to the low back. To help minimize stress during pregnancy, women should maintain a neutral pelvic position by performing an isometric contraction of the abdominals and erector spinae muscles simultaneously. Stretching these muscles often, wearing supportive shoes, and elevating the legs during rest will provide additional comfort.

Pelvic floor muscles. These puboccygeal muscles are located in the perineum floor, attached to the pubic bone in front and coccyx in back, providing a base of support for the pelvic organs (e.g., uterus, bladder, and bowel), as well as forces incurred by straining, coughing, and more. In addition, they provide sphincter control (i.e., a ring like muscle that normally maintains constriction of a body passage or that relaxes as required by normal physiological functioning) for perineal openings (e.g., urethra, vagina, and rectum).

Maintaining the health of these muscles is essential for pregnancy and a lifetime, as women will have increased tonicity and support for their pelvic organs. Encourage 50 to 100 repetitions of kegel exercises throughout the day. These can be performed in any position, and are best identified as those muscles that contract to stop the flow of urine. Clients should contract these muscles and return to a neutral pelvic floor between repetitions.(25)

Syndromes

Supine hypotensive syndrome occurs because of the expanding uterus and added weight compressing the vena cava (vein) carrying blood back to the heart. As women lie supine after 20 weeks of gestation, many begin to feel uncomfortable, faint, or nauseous. Therefore, exercising in this position should be avoided. Should women experience this, they need to roll to one side until the condition improves.(26)

Carpal tunnel syndrome is a condition resulting from pressure on the median nerve where it passes into the hand via a gap under a ligament at the front of the wrist. This is typically caused by edema in the wrists and women experience tingling and/or numbness in their hands. It may be uncomfortable for pregnant women to put any pressure or rely on support from their hands. Therefore, weight-bearing exercises using the hands will need to be modified.(12)

Round ligament syndrome refers to pain or discomfort caused by stretching of the round ligaments on the sides of the uterus from a fetal growth spurt. Bringing the legs up toward the abdomen often relieves this discomfort.(26)

Leg cramps. During pregnancy up to 30% of women can experience a sharp, painful cramp or "charley horse" in the calf, foot, or both—especially at night. Causes for these cramps include dehydration, electrolyte imbalance, metabolic, vascular, and neurologic disorders. Stretching the legs before going to bed can help relieve cramps. Other recommendations are to drink plenty of water, wear supportive stockings, and rest when tired. To increase blood flow, clients should lie on their left side and flex their feet gently to improve circulation. When exercising, have clients keep feet flexed and encourage them to minimize the amount of time sitting with their legs crossed.(27)

Diastasis recti. The rectus abdominis covers the front surface of the abdomen stretching from the crest of pubis to the xiphoid process. Holding these two muscles together is a fibrous tissue called the linea alba. As the uterus enlarges, the muscles will stretch to a point, however, to prevent the muscles from over stretching the linea alba splits. This is not painful to the mother: however, as women exercise they notice a change in this area of their abdomen and will have questions.

As the head, neck, and shoulders lift up, the abdominal muscles tense and a gap will be apparent. By placing a hand on the abdomen below the navel with the fingers pointing towards the feet, a gap can be felt. If the gap is one finger or less, this is considered normal. However, if the gap is two fingers wide oblique work should be omitted, and if the gap is three fingers or more eliminate curl-ups and head raises. Performing pelvic tilts and bracing the abdominals will help to support the transverse abdominis (i.e., muscle that wraps around the torso from front to back and from the ribs to the pelvis) and stretch the low back without any further tearing. Muscles typically return to a pre-pregnant state during the postpartum period.(28,29, 30)

Hydration and heat. Pregnant women should take time to drink before, during, and after exercise. It is important to stay hydrated. With weight gain, women increase in mass producing a rise in core temperature. While this would be a concern during exercise, pregnancy actually produces partial acclimation which causes sweating to occur sooner and lowers the core temperature. Women should avoid saunas, steam rooms, and whirlpools. Core temperature should not exceed 38° C or 101° F, whether experiencing a fever or not. The most vulnerable time during development is from the 23 to 28 days of gestation, when the neural tube is forming.(31)

Fitness Programming

When a pregnant woman has been cleared for exercise, an appropriate fitness program should be designed so that it includes the special considerations mentioned above, any guidelines the physician has given, and a client's goals.

It is recommended that a client new to exercise begin her exercise program after the first 12 weeks of gestation. About 15% of recognized pregnancies will end in a miscarriage with more than 80% of miscarriages occurring within the first 3 months of pregnancy (first trimester) depending on maternal age and parity. Miscarriage has been associated with chromosomal defects in about a half or two thirds of cases.(32,33) While there is no conclusive evidence to support the notion that exercise causes miscarriage, the loss of a baby can be a traumatic experience, and as such, this recommendation is given to fitness professionals. For current clients that become pregnant, it too will be necessary for them to consult with and receive clearance from their physician on the appropriate intensity and duration of a program. Whether a new or current exerciser, walking and kegels are low-intensity exercises that can be performed at any time.

Fitness professionals should consider a few thoughts prior to working with pregnant clients. These include the following.

1. Pregnancy is not a time where tremendous fitness adaptations will occur. Thus, the goal should be to have a client experience a renewed energy from exercise and avoid exhaustion.
2. What is 9 months, compared to a lifetime? Sometimes this will be a question that you pose to a client that still continues to exercise at the same rate prior to pregnancy.
3. Watch for warning signs of overexertion should a client be exercising to strenuously (e.g., pain, dizziness or feeling faint, increased shortness of breath, rapid heartbeat, chest pain, uterine contractions, or difficulty walking). Should a client experience overexertion, you should stop exercise immediately and provide the appropriate care.
4. With each exercise modality it will be important to monitor the client and provide modifications to her exercise program as she progresses.
5. Uncertain or adverse reactions to an exercise program should be referred back to the client's physician before continuing with a program.

Provided below are popular fitness modalities with recommended exercise suggestions for pregnant women to exercise safely. With some of these exercise modes, high-risk moves have been listed with suggested modifications. For movements of daily living as well as exercise, transitioning from one position to the next will assist in blood flow and comfort. From a standing position, kneel to one knee, lower the other knee and sit to the side, walk down to a side-lying or quadraped position, and reverse the movement to stand.

Group Exercise Formats

Aqua. For participation in water classes, pregnant women experience a center of gravity change and significant reduction of pressure to the low back. Other benefits include buoyancy, blood pressure stabilization, and—through movement—the alleviation of swelling. Water pressure against the body in motion creates a hydrostatic effect, causing body fluids to move effortlessly upward and a massage effect to reduce swelling.

Participants should perform movements with proper posture, hydrate often, and have a snack available. Encourage clients to wear water shoes during exercise as well as into the locker room to avoid slipping; progress slowly when exiting the pool, transition to gravity as gradually as possible. Recommended depth of the water is between the sternum (70% of body weight lifted) and navel (50% of body weight lifted); water temperature should be 83–86° F (28–30° C) and avoid temperatures that exceed 90° F (32° C).(34)

High Risk	High-impact movements (e.g., hopping, jumping); quick or sudden changes of body movements due to the greater surface area and antagonist water inertia; avoid twisting movements; limit or avoid long lever moves (e.g., hip extension)
Modifications	Low-impact movements—no hops or jumps; controlled ranges of motion; use buoyancy devices on the extremities; perform exercise movement with short levers (e.g., leg curl)

Dance-exercise classes. There are multiple variations of dance-exercise classes being taught from high-/low-impact aerobics to rhythmic jazz, ballroom, ballet, Latin, and so many more. Progression and speed of movement should be appropriate for the pregnant exerciser. Modifications can and should include tempo, choreography, change of direction, and the elimination of jumping or hopping.

Indoor cycling. Many women enjoy this modality as it provides support to the joints. Recommendations include a proper set-up of the cycle with handlebars raised at least one notch higher than the norm. This will decrease the possibilities of discomfort from the knees being too close to the abdomen. Participants are encouraged to wear a pregnancy support belt, perform endurance and recovery rides, and change the intensity as often as needed.(35)

Pilates. This method incorporates certain principles of movement that allow women the opportunity to bring balance into their pregnancy: (a) physically, (b) emotionally, and (c) physiologically. Some physical benefits include increased strength and flexibility with better coordination; emotionally women feel more in control and at peace; physiologically women experience improvements in biometric measures. Pilates uses both mat and equipment methods. It will be important to modify supine movements after 20 weeks gestation. Suggested exercises include seated breathing, bridge, seated roll-up/roll-down, spine stretch, saw, side-lying leg lift, spine twist, side-lying leg circle, and cat.(36,37)

Step. For participation in step aerobics, the height of a client's platform should be no greater than 6 inches, reducing to 4 during the last trimester. At any time a client cannot see her feet, participation should be continued by performing movements on the floor without the step. The music speed should be of a tempo in which full range of motion can be demonstrated, that is, 118–122 bpm. Movements that require tremendous pelvic stability or pressure to the perineum floor should be avoided.(38)

High Risk	Propulsions, straddle downs, repeaters, abduction/adduction leg work, jumps to or off the step, pivots, squats, fast footwork with tempo changes
Modifications	Basic step, V-step, turn step, over-the-top, touches, heels, curls, kicks (traveling or in place), L-step, slowed low-impact movements on and off the step

Yoga. This practice of over 5,000 years emphasizes the "union of the mind and body," something pregnant women can recall during labor and delivery. Benefits include increased fitness levels, flexibility and tonicity of the pelvic floor, increased circulation, and control of the breath during exertion and relaxation. Clients should maintain proper body alignment and avoid any exercise that is uncomfortable. Movements should be performed slowly and with control.(39,40)

High Risk	Down dog, plank, side plank, hover, back bends, inverted poses, revolving twists, jumps, or headstands
Modifications	The mountain; spine prep; warrior I, II, and III; reverse warrior; modified triangle pose; modified extended angle; runners lunge; tree; finger-to-big-toe; child's pose; modified camel; seated spine twist; staff; half fish; stretches for the upper body, torso, and leg muscles

Weight or resistance training. With pregnant women, the recommendation is to use equipment which provides the most support to the body. Weight machines keep the body in proper alignment while isolating the primary muscle group for endurance conditioning. As clients workout on machines, fitness professionals should ensure that no joints hyperextend, by using foot pedals to bring forward the arms of equipment. This will alleviate any risk of potential injury due to the laxity of connective tissue.

Other options are to use hand weights or resistance tubes. If there is allergic reaction to latex, use tubing with nylon handles. Light weights of 1–3 pounds and the strength of a resistance tube should be used appropriately for the various muscle groups. Caution is given to wrapping tubing around the hands as this will increase blood pressure. Ankle weighted boots or wraps should only be used to strengthen the legs during a workout. Make sure clients are exhaling on their effort as they perform lifts. The recommendation is to perform higher repetitions with lighter weight, that is, 12–15 per set.(21)

High Risk	No supine weight work after 20 weeks of gestation. Free weights, deep squats; machines to avoid prone leg curl, supine leg press, abduction/adduction, abdominal/oblique, chest fly without range limiter, 10° chest, any machine that is tight or cumbersome around the midsection of the body or those without range limiters
Modifications	Incline leg press, leg extension, seated leg curl, chest press/fly with range limiters, low- and high-seated row, overhead press, lat pull down, back extension, smith press, biceps, triceps

Flexibility and relaxation techniques. Stretching at the end of a workout should be for at least 10 minutes in duration. Repeat stretches two to four times per muscle group and hold for 15–30 seconds. Ideally, it is best to stretch daily. Relaxation techniques can include meditation, guided imagery, and massage. Incorporate these techniques as appropriate.(21)

Other fitness activities. Participation in golf and tennis are activities many pregnant women continue as long as they are comfortable. Running can be modified to include longer duration walking programs. Cardiovascular activities that provide non-impact or low-impact options include swimming and the use of a stationary cycle, elliptical, or treadmill. For clients that need a connection to other pregnant women and newborns, there are community fitness programs (e.g., Baby Boot Camp, StrollerFit, YMCA You and Me Baby).

Activities that are too strenuous or create an unstable platform for the pregnant exerciser should be avoided. Some of these include kickboxing, horseback riding, water or snow skiing, core board, trampoline, and skating (ice or roller).

Postpartum recovery. A physician's medical clearance is important for returning to exercise after child birth. For most women this is 4–8 weeks postpartum depending upon the birth process. However, kegel exercises can be performed shortly after delivery to assist in rehabilitating pelvic floor muscles and increasing blood flow to the area. Hormonal changes continue, so ensure that joints and connective tissues are protected from injury. It will be important to focus on muscle symmetry and posture to strengthen weak muscles and stretch those that are tight. New moms will want to focus on their core, especially the abdomen. For women wanting to increase their tone or those that might have experienced diastasis recti, they might benefit from the well-researched Tupler Technique. Cardiovascular exercise should start slow and gradually progress once the client's energy level increases. Stretching and relaxation techniques will help with muscle tension and common discomforts. Along with exercise, rest, proper nutrition, and adjusting to parenthood are all factors to be considered.

Summary

The miracle of life and delivering a healthy baby begins with a physician's involvement and support in the planning for pregnancy, nutritional guidelines, special exercise considerations, fitness programming, and postpartum recovery. A fitness professional can assist women by helping to develop/carry out safe and effective fitness programs before, during, and after pregnancy. This can help to improve a women's mood, self-esteem, and adjustments to physical changes. Fitness professionals should be sure to provide a continuum of care by referring to a client's physician when appropriate or other professionals as questions arise beyond the industry's scope of practice.

Reference Notes

1. Barclay, L. (2009). *Few women follow healthy lifestyle guidelines before pregnancy.* Retrieved June 24, 2009, fromhttp://www.medscape.com/viewarticle/588266

2. American College of Physicians. (2009). *Folic acid for the prevention of neural tube defects: U.S. preventive services task force recommendation.* Retrieved June 22, 2009, from http://www.annals.org/cgi/reprint/ 150/9/I-50.pdf

3. The National Institutes of Health. (2009). *Low levels of vitamin B12 may increase risk for neural tube defects.* Retrieved June 22, 2009, from http://www.nih.gov/news/health/mar2009/nichd-02.htm

4. National Diabetes Information Clearinghouse. (2008). *For women with diabetes: Your guide to pregnancy.* Retrieved June 24, 2009, from http://www.diabetes.niddk.nih.gov/dm/pubs/pregnancy/

5. Brochert, A. (2007). *Crush step 2: The ultimate USMLE step 2 review* (3rd ed.). Mosby Inc. pp. 194.

6. American College of Obstetricians and Gynecologists. (2009). *Tobacco, alcohol, drugs, and pregnancy.* Committee on Patient Education. Retrieved June 22, 2009, from http://www.acog.org/publications/patient_education/bp170.cfm

7. National Institution on Alcohol Abuse and Alcoholism. (2006). *Drinking and your pregnancy.* Retrieved June 25, 2009, from http://pubs.niaaa.nih.gov/publications/DrinkingPregnancy_HTML/pregnancy.htm

8. American College of Obstetricians and Gynecologists. (2009). *Routine tests during pregnancy.*

9. Kids Health from Nemours. (2007). *Genetic counseling.* Retrieved June 29, 2009, from http://kidshealth.org/parent/system/medical/genetic_counseling.html#

10. Center for Disease Control and Prevention. (2009). *Pregnancy-Planning Education Program.* Retrieved June 23, 2009, from http://www.cdc.gov/ncbddd/pregnancy/

11. American College of Obstetricians and Gynecologists. (2008). *Nutrition during pregnancy.* Retrieved June 22, 2009, from http://www.acog.org/publications/patient_education/bp001.cfm

12. Simkin, P., Whalley, J., Keppler, A., Durham, J., & Bolding, A. (2008). *Pregnancy, childbirth and the newborn: The complete guide.* New York: Meadowbrook Press.

13. March of Dimes. (2002). *Baby basics: You month-by-month guide to a healthy pregnancy.* The What to Expect Foundation: New York.

14. Dolan, D., & Zissu, A. (2006). *The complete organic pregnancy.* HarperCollins: New York.

15. American Academy of Family Physicians. (2004). *Pregnancy: Things to think about before you're pregnant.* Retrieved June 29, 2009, from http://familydoctor.org/online/famdocen/home/women/pregnancy/basics/076.html

16. U.S. Department of Agriculture. (n.d.). Retrieved June 22, 2009, from http://www.mypyramid.gov/mypyramidmoms/pyramidmoms_plan.aspx

17. Barclay, L. (2009). *Folic Acid–Containing Supplements May Reduce the Risk for Neural Tube Defects.* Retrieved June 22, 2009, from http://www.medscape.com/viewarticle/702651

18. U.S. Department of Health and Human Services. (2008). *Physical activity guidelines for Americans summary: Key guidelines for women during pregnancy and the postpartum period.* Retrieved June 29, 2009, from http://www.health.gov/paguidelines/guidelines/summary.aspx

19. Medlineplus. (2008). *Should I exercise during my pregnancy.* Retrieved June 29, 2009, from http://www.nlm.nih.gov/medlineplus/magazine/issues/winter08/articles/winter08pg26.html

20. American College of Obstetricians and Gynecologists. (2003). *Exercise during pregnancy.* Retrieved June 29, 2009, from http://www.acog.org/publications/patient_education/bp119.cfm

21. Lewis, B., Avery, M., Jennings, E., Sherwood, N., Martinson, B., & Crain, L. (2008). The effect of exercise during pregnancy on maternal outcomes: Practical implications for practice. *American Journal of Lifestyle Medicine.* Retrieved June 29, 2009, from http://www.medscape.com/viewarticle/580466

22. Weissgerber, T., & Wolfe, L. (2006). Physiological adaptation in early human pregnancy: adaptation to balance maternal-fetal demands. *Applied Physiology, Nutrition, and Metabolism.* 31:1–11.

23. American College of Sports Medicine. (2010). *ACSM's resource manual for guidelines for exercise testing and prescription* (8th ed.). Baltimore, MD: Lippincott Williams & Wilkins.

24. Clapp, J. (2008). *American Journal of Obstetrics and Gynecology.* Long-term outcome after exercising throughout pregnancy: fitness and cardiovascular risk. 199(5). Mosby, Inc.

25. American College of Obstetricians and Gynecologists. (2007). *You and your baby: Prenatal care.* Retrieved June 24, 2009, from http://www.acog.org/publications/patient_education/ab005.cfm

26. Aerobics and Fitness Association of America. (2008). *Perinatal Fitness.* Sherman Oaks, CA: Aerobics and Fitness Association of America.

27. Hensley, J. (2009). Leg cramps and restless legs syndrome during pregnancy. *Journal of Midwifery & Women's Health,* Vol(54), Issue 3, pp. 211–218.

28. American College of Obstetricians and Gynecologists. (2002). Exercise during pregnancy and the postpartum period. Washington, D.C.: *ACOG Committee Opinion,* 99, 171–173.

29. Marx, J. (2006). *Rosen's emergency medicine: Concepts and clinical practice* (6th ed.). St. Louis, MO: Mosby.

30. Tupler, J., & Gould, J. (2004). *Lose your mummy tummy.* Da Capo Press.

31. Aerobics and Fitness Association of America. (2007). *Personal fitness training: Theory & Practice.* Sherman Oaks, CA: Aerobics and Fitness Association of America.

32. WebMD Medical Reference provided in collaboration with the Cleveland Clinic. (2005). *Pregnancy: Miscarriage.* Retrieved June 23, 2009, from http://www.webmd.com/infertility-and-reproduction/guide/pregnancy-miscarriage

33. Aleman, A., Althabe, F., Belizán, J.M., & Bergel, E. (Last assessed 2007). Bed rest during pregnancy for preventing miscarriage. *Cochrane Database of Systematic Reviews 2005*, Issue 2. Art. No.: CD003576. DOI: 10.1002/14651858.CD003576.pub2.

34. Aerobics and Fitness Association of America. (2008). *Aqua fitness outline.* Sherman Oaks, CA: Aerobics and Fitness Association of America.

35. Aerobics and Fitness Association of America. (2005). *Indoor cycling outline.* Sherman Oaks, CA: Aerobics and Fitness Association of America.

36. Segal. N., Hein, J., & Basford, J. (2004). The effects of Pilates training on flexibility and body composition; an observational study. *Archives of physical medicine and rehabilitation*, 85(12), 1977–1981.

37. Aerobics and Fitness Association of America. (2006). *Practical pilates outline.* Sherman Oaks, CA: Aerobics and Fitness Association of America.

38. Aerobics and Fitness Association of America. (2008). *Step training outline.* Sherman Oaks, CA: Aerobics and Fitness Association of America.

39. Aerobics and Fitness Association of America. (2006). *Practical yoga: Instructor training.* Sherman Oaks, CA: Aerobics and Fitness Association of America.

40. Miller, O. (2003). *The prenatal yoga deck: Poses and mediations.* San Francisco, CA: Chronicle Book.

40 *Youth Fitness*

Scott O. Roberts, PhD
and Deanna Lowe, MA

Focus

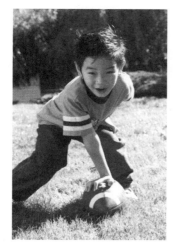

Over a third of children today are overweight, and another third are at risk for becoming overweight. Physical inactivity is now recognized as one of the leading causes of childhood obesity, diabetes, and elevated chronic disease risk in children. In 2003–2004, 33.6% of children and adolescents in the United States were classified as overweight or obese. Those at risk of chronic health conditions, or diagnosed as obese, are often found to have elevated blood pressure, blood lipids, plasma insulin, unhealthy diets, and sedentary lifestyles. These conditions at youth tend to carry over into adulthood. Recent research has found that most children (those under 13 years of age) participate in adequate amounts of physical activity. However, the downward trend of inactivity tends to be within adolescents (children 13–18 years of age) who are falling short in meeting sufficient amounts of physical activity to achieve health benefits.

Children and adolescents are more apt to exercise if adults, teachers, and other role models (especially parents) encourage children to participate in healthy and active lifestyles. Fitness should be a learning experience that encourages good habits, positive attitudes, and fun. This chapter provides fitness instructors with important information regarding pediatric exercise science and program implementation. For more detailed information, refer to AFAA's *Standards and Guidelines for Youth Fitness.*

Cardiorespiratory Training

Significant evidence suggests that children and adolescents can increase their aerobic capacity by following a regular exercise program. Increased capacity results from enhanced oxygen transport and enhanced metabolic capacities. Measurement of maximal oxygen uptake (VO_{2max}) in children provides an accurate analysis of aerobic power in children.

Research conducted by Payne and Morrow found that a typical child can improve VO_{2max} by 2.07 ml/kg/min from aerobic training. Clinicians agree that a certain amount of cardiovascular training is beneficial to children as reinforced in the American College of Sports Medicine's 1988 opinion statement on the quality and quantity of exercise required to maintain adequate fitness levels in children. Since then both ACSM and the U.S. Department of Health and Human Services (USDHHS) have continued to establish youth fitness guidelines for fitness professionals.

The amount of exercise required for optimal functional capacity and health at various ages has not been precisely defined. Until more definitive evidence is available, current recommendations (USDHHS, 2008; ACSM, 2010) are that children and adolescents:

- Participate in 60 minutes (1 hour) or more of physical activity 3–4 days per week or daily. The majority of the 60 minutes should comprise of moderate- to vigorous-intensity (or 30 minutes of each) to total an accumulation of 60 minutes.
- Moderate intensity refers to activity that "noticeably" increases breathing, sweating, and heart rate while vigorous intensity is that which "substantially" increases breathing, sweating, and heart rate.

Benefits

- Improved cardiorespiratory and muscular fitness
- Improved bone health
- Reduced symptoms of anxiety, depression, and tension
- Improved self-image and self-confidence
- Reduced risk for developing chronic health conditions

- Children and adolescents who are obese may not be able to achieve these recommendations. Therefore, gradually progress the frequency and duration in order to address each individual's fitness level.
- Children should be encouraged to participate in sustained activities that use large muscle groups (e.g., swimming, jogging, aerobic dance) and that are age-appropriate. Emphasize active play and intermittent bouts of activity rather than sustained exercise for younger children.
- Other activities, such as recreational sports and fun activities that develop components of health and performance (speed, power, flexibility, muscular endurance, agility, and coordination), should also be incorporated.
- Heart rate monitoring may be optional due to low cardiac risk in non-obese children and adolescents; RPE is preferable and helps children to monitor themselves. The OMNI scale for children may act as an alternative method to monitoring exercise intensity.

Resistance Training

Over the years, scientific research concerning resistance training in children (6–17 years of age) has focused on safety issues and injury prevention for children and adolescents who participate in resistance training. In the past decade, research has been conducted on the benefits of resistance training in children and has found that increases in neuromuscular adaptations occur in children compared to hypertrophic adaptations in adolescents when participating in structured and supervised resistance training programs.

Children and adolescents should be encouraged to participate in regular resistance training that involves repetitive movements against an opposing force. It is important to note that children and adolescents can develop strength through a variety of activities including (a) participation in sports, (b) weight training, (c) calisthenics, (d) manual resistance exercises, and (e) simply playing. According to ACSM (2010), resistance training for children and adolescents is similar to adults (refer to Chapter 17, "Basic Exercise Standards and Guidelines"), and recommends performing a minimum of 8–15 repetitions in good form to a point of moderate fatigue.

General Definitions and Guidelines

Resistance training utilizing weights is recommended in children who display emotional maturity and the ability to follow directions. It is important that a trained adult supervise children who participate in resistance training programs at all times. An adequate warm-up should be performed followed by a sufficient cool-down that includes flexibility exercises. The ACSM recommends that children avoid power lifting and bodybuilding until developmental maturity is reached.

- **Resistance Training Movements**—Those performed against an opposing force should be encouraged in children who participate in regular physical activity. Resistance training utilizes various forms such as calisthenics, tubing, and weighted balls. Exercises should be performed in a slow, controlled manner to maximize muscular strength and endurance.
- **Free Weight Training**—When children have demonstrated a level of maturity (around 10–12 years of age) they may perform exercises involving free weights if correct form and technique are employed. Light weights (1–2 lb) are recommended at the onset of training.

- **Weight Training Machines**—If children are developmentally able (usually around 10–12 years of age) they should be allowed to use weight training machines. However, most machines are designed for the adult body, and children cannot properly perform the exercise intended. If this is the case, children should not use the weight training machines.
- **Manual Resistance Training**—Children may perform these activities with the help of a partner if they are mature enough to safely follow directions. One child performs the exercise while the other child offers resistance. Example: Hip Abduction—one child lies on the ground while the other child applies resistance to the leg being raised (abducted).
- **Isometric Training** —Appropriate for children if they adhere to proper breathing techniques. Isometric training is described as sustained muscular contraction with no change in muscular length.

Special Considerations

Children who have been previously diagnosed with a medical disease, disability, or musculoskeletal condition should have a physician's clearance prior to beginning an exercise program. Other considerations, provided by the National Strength and Conditioning Association (NSCA) and American Alliance of Health Physical Education Recreation and Dance (AAPHERD), are outlined below.

- Equipment and activity should be varied and appropriate to the age, size, and strength of a child and/or adolescent, as well as to his or her maturity level.
- Training should be comprehensive to increase motor skills and fitness level.
- Only when good form has been achieved should the resistance/weight be increased. If a prepubescent (i.e., of age preceding puberty) child cannot perform a minimum of 8 reps in good form, the resistance is too heavy and should be reduced.
- Focus should be on participation and proper technique versus the amount of resistance.

Children's thermoregulatory response to exercise should be monitored more closely as children do not have the ability to dissipate heat as efficiently as adults do. Therefore, exercise should not be performed in extreme environmental conditions, such as high temperature and humidity.

Proper hydration should be encouraged before, during, and after exercise. Past research has shown that children will inadvertently dehydrate themselves because they do not understand the body's need for hydration during exercise.

A weight that allows less than 8 repetitions should never be used. Heavy weights can be extremely dangerous to the growth plate and joint structures of prepubescent children.

Exercises should not be performed to the point of momentary muscular fatigue.

Special Populations

Keeping in mind that children with special conditions are in need of medical evaluation prior to commencing an exercise program, the general guidelines below may be of assistance to professionals working with these populations. Treatment of disease and other health conditions, however, needs to be provided by health care providers.

- **Asthma**—Children who experience exercise-induced asthma (EIA) should be encouraged to participate in exercise programs. Evidence shows that regular exercise can improve their overall fitness level and decrease the incidence of EIA attacks. (See Exercise Guidelines for Asthma in Chapter 34, "Exercise and Chronic Disease.")
- **Diabetes**—Children with diabetes should perform regular exercise to expend energy, reduce body fat, and improve metabolic control over their diabetes.
- **Obesity**—Excess adipose tissue is associated with increased health risks and disease. Children involved in exercise programs not only shed excess fat, but also decrease blood cholesterol levels, decrease blood pressure, and increase self-worth and self-esteem.

Summary

Children who adhere to an exercise program learn lifestyle habits that decrease risk for disease and increase the likelihood of physical activity throughout life. Children receive a training effect from exercise when exercise is performed properly and safely. Although physiologic changes have been observed in children, the primary focus of children who exercise should be to achieve health-related goals. As fitness instructors, conservative strategies should be employed when designing aerobic and strength training programs for children emphasizing safety and adult supervision.

References

1. American Academy of Pediatrics. (2001). Strength training for children and adolescents. *Pediatrics*, 107, 1470–1472.
2. American Academy of Pediatrics. (2006). Active healthy living: Prevention of childhood obesity through increased physical activity. *Pediatrics*, 117(5), 1834–1841.
3. American College of Sports Medicine. (1988). Opinion statement on physical fitness in children and youth. *Medicine & Science in Sports & Exercise*, 20, 422–423.
4. American College of Sports Medicine. (2006). *ACSM's guidelines for exercise testing and prescription* (7th ed.). Baltimore, MD: Lippincott Williams & Wilkins.
5. American College of Sports Medicine. (2010). *ACSM's guidelines for exercise testing and prescription* (8th ed.). Baltimore, MD: Lippincott Williams & Wilkins.
6. Bar-Or, O. (1989). Trainability of the prepubescent child. *The Physician and Sportsmedicine*, 5, 64–82.
7. Gilliam, T.B. (1977). Prevalence of coronary heart disease risk factors in active children 7-to-12-years of age. *Medicine & Science in Sports & Exercise*, 9, 21–25.
8. Gortmaker, S.L. (1987). "Increasing Pediatric Obesity in the United States." *ADJC*, 141, 535–540.
9. Healthy People 2010 mid-course review on physical activity and fitness. Retrieved August 28, 2008, from http://www.healthypeople.gov
10. Kraemer, W.J., Fry, A.C., Frykman, P.N., Conroy, B., & Hoffman, J. (1989). Resistance training and youth. *Pediatric Exercise Science*, 1, 336–350.
11. National Strength and Conditioning Association. (1985). The NSCA's position paper on pre-pubescent strength training. *National Strength and Conditioning Association Journal*, 7, 27–29.

12. Payne, V.G., & Morrow, J.R. (1993). Exercise and VO_{2max} in children: A meta-analysis. *Research Quarterly for Exercise and Sport*, 64, 305–313.

13. President's Council of Physical Fitness and Sports. (2004). Physical activity for children: Current patterns and guidelines. *Research Digest*, 5(2).

14. Robertson, R.J., Goss, F.L., Andreacci, J.L., Dube, J.J., Kowallis, R.A., Rutkowski, J.J., Snee, B.M., Crawford, K., Aaron, D.J., & Metz, K.F. (2005). Validation of the children's OMNI RPE Scale for stepping exercise. *Medicine & Science in Sports & Exercise*. Retrieved May 4, 2009, from http://www.faqs.org/abstracts/Sports-and-fitness/Validation-of-the-childrens-OMNI-RPE-Scale-for-stepping-exercise.html

15. Roberts, S.O. (1997). Exercise prescription recommendations for children. *American College of Sports Medicine Certified News*, 7, 1–5.

16. Roberts, S.O., Ciapponi, T., & Lytle, R. (2008). *Strength training for children & adolescents*. Reston, VA: National Association of Sport and Physical Education.

17. Rowland, T.W. (1985). Aerobic responses to endurance training in prepubescent children: a critical analysis. *Medicine & Science in Sports & Exercise*, 17, 493–497.

18. Tolfrey, K., Campbell, I.G., & Batterham, A.M. (1998). Exercise training induced alterations in prepubertal children's lipid-lipoprotein profile. *Medicine & Science in Sports & Exercise*, 30, 1684–1692.

19. U.S. Department of Health and Human Services. (2008). 2008 physical activity guidelines for Americans. Washington, DC: Office of Disease Prevention and Health Promotion (U0036)/ www.health.gov/paguidelines.

Recommended Reading

1. Faigenbaum, A.D., & Westcott, W.L. (2009). *Youth strength training*. Champaign, IL: Human Kinetics.

Part 9

Essentials of Exercise

Program Management Basics

Marketing and Promoting Your Business

Advancing Your Fitness Career

Substitute Teaching

Law and Exercise

41 Program Management Basics

Kathy Stevens, MA

Focus

This chapter will give an overview of the basic information and skills necessary to make the leap from group exercise instructor to group exercise program manager/director.

Assessing the Role and Responsibilities

As a group exercise program manager/director you may find yourself responsible for class scheduling; hiring and firing; training; making and enforcing policy; marketing; financial aspects such as payroll, bill paying, and budgeting; facility design; equipment selection; and a myriad of other general maintenance or office duties. Even if you hire others to do some of these jobs, you may still be responsible for overseeing each area. The larger the facility or chain of facilities you are working for, the more likely there will be centralized policies and procedures for you to follow as the director of the group exercise program. This means that many of the policies and materials we will discuss in this chapter may already be set in place for you to follow.

It is extremely important to make a realistic assessment of your individual skills before embarking into management. This will enable you to devote your energies and talents to those jobs you are good at and enjoy. Teaching every day of the week is a far cry from directing a program. While the teaching experience helps, when you manage a program, you may find that you no longer have time to teach. You're too busy observing new instructors, making schedule changes, balancing the budget, dealing with customer complaints, or organizing the fitness room. The experience you have as an instructor will enable you to be good in that one area of operation, but you'll need to either become well versed in the other areas or hire and manage others who are.

Be sure to understand the overall mission statement and goals of the business you will be working for. The mission statement of the business must be compatible with your own personal goals and standards. If your personal goals and standards are different from those of the business, you'll find your job is suddenly at odds with what's important to you. Being in harmony with the long-term goals of a business means quality job performance, an enjoyable work environment, and great personal satisfaction.

Planning

Planning is done before, during, and after a business operation has begun. Planning and follow-through are critical to the long-term success of any business. Planning meetings should include key personnel, management, and business owners. The group exercise department will be an integral part of any fitness facility plan. The following is a list of areas that need to be considered.
- Business Plan: mission statement, short-term goals, and long-term goals
- Operational Plan: specific to each department
- Financial Plan: fiscal goals and P & L (profit and loss) statements
- Marketing Plan: in-house and community advertising

The **business plan** develops out of the mission statement and business goals. A "mission statement" helps chart the course of a business. A mission statement is a short paragraph or sentence that describes what the business is all about, including the vision of what the business will become. Mission statements are important because every decision made, every policy created, everything done in the business, must contribute to the vision of the mission statement. Out of the mission statement evolves the short- and long-term goals of the business. This is where yearly, monthly, weekly, and even daily goals are specified. The more specific, measurable, and realistic these goals are, the easier it will be for the group exercise manager to do his/her job. It will be important for you as the program manager to be aware and stay in alignment with these goals, as well as the overall vision of the business. Employee and employer satisfaction will often be determined by this congruency. Many a program manager has been misguided by working on personal goals that are not of importance to the business owner(s). The manager ends up feeling unappreciated for the work effort he or she has put forth, while the owners feel that they are not getting the job done that they are paying for. Thus, it will be important for a program manager and owner(s) to stay in alignment and have a way of measuring the status of the program goals in relation to the overall business plan.

This is where an **operational plan** for the group exercise department comes in. The operational plan will cover what needs to be done for this area of the facility to run efficiently and effectively. Within this plan will be details such as hiring, training, and scheduling instructors; developing and updating the schedule; and designing and maintaining the exercise room/s and related equipment. We will discuss these areas in further detail later in the chapter.

The **financial plan** may include (a) establishing appropriate pay rates for the instructors, (b) processing pay roll, (c) budgeting for equipment, and (d) execution of club marketing strategies. In any business, income is the bottom line. Regardless of the quality of instruction or the high-tech equipment, if the business doesn't make enough money, it simply can't stay in business. Although the program director is not personally responsible for the cost of running the group exercise program, he/she needs to understand and respect the effect that this area has on a facility's overall profit and loss statement (P & L).

The **marketing plan** crosses over all of the other plans. A strong marketing plan can help deliver the vision of the business plan, propel the operational plan, and impact the financial plan. As the group exercise director, you will want to help with both the in-house and community marketing strategies. In-house strategies may include member incentives such as participation-based contests and guest recruitment rewards. It will also include the proper posting and marketing of the existing schedule to ensure class attendance. Community marketing can be accomplished through print ads that communicate the benefits or specialties of the group exercise program. It can also include community outreach by the director or other appropriate staff members. Community speaking engagements, local cable TV segments, races, and sporting events are all great ways and places to get the message out about your excellent program while establishing your staff and facility as industry leaders.

Customer Service

The fitness industry is a service-oriented business, which means you need a keen understanding of just who your customers are, what their needs are, and what you can do to service those needs. All too often managers get so involved in the day-to-day running of a program that they overlook the very reason for the business. Members are the purpose of our business. Stay close to your members; take time to listen to them after class. Work at the front desk; answer the phones; be available when they want to talk to you. Make it easy for members to access program information. This includes, but may not be limited to, class schedules and descriptions, rules of class etiquette, class substitutions or cancellations, membership or class fees, and other services offered like babysitting. An informed member will be less likely to have problems with the policies of your program. Consider every class policy from the viewpoint of a customer. Be consistent in the way you treat the members; from the first visit to the 50th there should not be a change in attitude or service. As the program manager, it will be your responsibility to impart this attitude to your staff members. Remind them that the customer is always right unless it is a matter of member safety. Even in those situations where safety is an issue, it will be important that members are handled in a professional and courteous way. If the service quality and class procedures are not consistent, members will go somewhere else. On the other hand, if service and procedures are regarded and respected, your existing members will be your best form of advertising.

Personnel Management

According to statistics, one of the main reasons people continue to go to a fitness facility is the staff. It's not the expensive equipment or the suspended floor. It's the people servicing the members. The group exercise program has a huge impact on a large portion of the facility membership. This is clearly measured by the high attendance rate and many classes scheduled in most facilities. As a manager, you are the one who ultimately positions and controls the staff that will have these opportunities. It will be your responsibility to make sure your staff is qualified, informed, customer friendly, and satisfied with their work environment.

The following is a list of areas we will cover in this chapter.
- Recruitment and Hiring
- Class Pay Rate, Benefits, and Bonuses
- Expectations
- Training
- Leadership and Communication Skills

Recruitment and Hiring

Recruitment and hiring is a critical component of a group exercise program. As more facilities open up, it becomes harder for a group exercise director to find and recruit qualified instructors. This is probably one of the biggest complaints heard in the industry when it comes to group exercise program management. Therefore, it will be important to cover some strategies for recruitment. In the past, new instructors were often plucked right out of the front row of class participants. Those days are far gone due to the higher standard of expectation and increased demands for professional training and certification. No longer can a person wing it through a class and be hired the next day. So where is a director to go? The first place to start is within the existing staff. Often a staff member will know of another great instructor that is looking to pick up more classes. Next, would be the local in-house workshops and certification programs. Ideally, a facility should host its own in-house programs. This is a great time to recruit and make applications available. Many of the fitness education agencies also have job postings available on their Web sites. And, last but not least, a facility can place an ad in the local papers or on Internet job finding websites.

Once the recruitment process has been successful, you will need to have a hiring process in place. If you hire the right person for each job, half of your responsibility is met. Never underestimate the importance of the hiring process. You should require all instructors to provide a personal resume along with the department application. Your department application should include pertinent personal and professional information such as the applicant's name, address, years instructing, certifications, type of classes preferred, type of classes able to teach or substitute teach, times available, most current pay rate at other facilities, and work references. You will also need to meet with the applicant for an interview and/or class audition. The audition can take place privately between the director and instructor or be completed in a regularly scheduled class by having the applicant team teach or substitute teach. If this is not conducive or convenient, the director may opt to go watch the instructor in a class he or she teaches outside of the facility, or ask the instructor to tape his/her class and provide a DVD or downloadable clip of the class. Find out as much as you can about the person you are considering. Make sure to check references. Ask the references to give you the names of some co-workers of the applicant and call them for additional testimonials. Ask the references to rate the instructor's past performance in each of the following areas: (a) customer satisfaction, (b) skill level, (c) availability, and (d) responsibility. The more you know about the applicant prior to hiring, the better the chances are for proper scheduling and participant satisfaction.

Class pay rates, benefits, and bonuses

If you market your facility as a place where clients can receive high quality instruction, then you must be ready to pay for highly qualified, competent fitness professionals. Be competitive with fitness instructor class pay rates in your area. You don't have to pay the highest, but good pay along with other benefits will keep the top instructors and fitness staff satisfied and committed. If an instructor attracts and keeps customers and is in tune with the philosophy of your program, then he or she is worth a competitive class rate. That appropriate rate will be a matter of area research. It will be your job as a program manager to find out what is a competitive rate for your area. This information is relatively easy to find out by asking the local instructors. In addition to the base class pay rate, your staff will be motivated by **benefits and bonuses** that are both tangible and intangible. Tangible benefits include health insurance; paid vacation time; cash bonuses; free in-house workshops for continuing education; music, shoe, and clothing discounts at local stores; facility memberships for spouse/children; babysitting during class hours; and more. Intangible benefits and bonuses include praise, support, and recognition. The intangible benefits are so simple and inexpensive, yet they are often the most overlooked. Be generous in your praise to employees who are outstanding in the performance of their jobs. If a member tells you something positive about a class, pass it along to the instructor immediately! Positive feedback encourages more of the behavior that prompted the favorable report. Immediate recognition reinforces and supports that behavior. Publicly recognize instructor accomplishments on a staff or facility bulletin board. You will also need to establish a fair and consistent pay raise policy. All too often, the matter of pay raises is more subjective than objective. The squeaky wheel may be the only one getting the grease (or the pay raise). Thus, it may help smooth the decision making process if management and the facility owner(s) have predetermined what constitutes a pay raise.

It is commonly based on continued education/certifications, class recruitment and positive feedback, and longevity and/or exclusivity to the facility. Whatever the case, it is important to your policies in writing and to make sure all instructors are aware of these policies. With that said, it is also important that you as the director adhere to the policy in a non-bias manner. If instructors sense that they are not being treated fairly or equally, it could result in extreme employee dissatisfaction, which may end up being communicated to the class participants.

Expectations

Understanding the rules of any game not only makes the game enjoyable, it also gives it a sense of order. Your group exercise program is no different. Instructors want to know the rules of the game. They want to know exactly what is expected of them. Most of your program expectations should be discussed during the interview and hiring process. It's better to know if an applicant has a problem with the responsibilities and compensation before you hire him or her. Before applicants are assigned specific classes, they should be given a written description of the class format as well as pre- and post-class responsibilities. They should also have a copy of your general staff policies and procedures. These policies and procedures may include, but are not limited to, the following.

- Class Pay Scale and Pay Raise Policy
- Class Coverage/Substitution Procedure
- Certification and Continuing Education Requirements or Recommendations
- Professional Insurance Requirements or Recommendations
- Class Attire and Grooming Recommendations
- Class Sign In or Check In Procedure
- Pre- and Post-Class Responsibilities
- Class Etiquette Policies
- Emergency Response Protocols
- Incident Report Procedure
- Performance Evaluation Procedures

The more detailed your expectation materials, the easier it will be for you to manage your staff properly and the more likely it will be that your staff will do their job right.

In order for your staff to continue to meet your program expectations, you will need to have some form of on-going performance evaluation. This can be done through class observations and evaluations, participant feedback forms, and attendance tracking. Once again, the more detailed and consistent your evaluation, the more sure you can be of program adherence and customer satisfaction. It will be important that you have a policy in place for handling both positive and negative performance evaluations. In most cases, a written notification along with verbal communication is recommended. In the case of a positive evaluation, the communication might include a well-deserved pay increase or posting of recognition. In the case of a negative evaluation, the written and verbal communication should include suggestions for improvement and recommendations for corrective actions, if any. All written evaluations and notifications should be kept in an instructor file for future reference.

Training

Staff training is a must in the competitive fitness industry. More and more smart businesses are offering in-house training programs and continuing education opportunities to their group exercise staff members (e.g., CPR/AED, first-aid, certifications, workshops). Providing opportunities for your certified instructors to receive continuing education credits at a reduced cost without having to travel is a wonderful employee benefit. Many fitness facilities offer a scholarship for one instructor to attend an industry convention at the facility's expense. That instructor then reports back to the group as a whole by conducting a mini-workshop on what he/she learned (e.g., new choreography). It's an opportunity to reward a loyal, productive instructor and encourage all staff members (knowing they may be next to be awarded a scholarship).

An important aspect of your staff training and program management is regular staff communication and meetings. All instructors should be addressed on a monthly, bimonthly, or quarterly basis. This communication can be in the form of newsletters and email blasts, but should culminate in on-site department meetings. The written agenda for the meetings should include department reports, schedule updates, announcements of facility promotions and upcoming trainings, and perhaps even include a social hour that enhances staff spirit. These meetings may include group exercise specific idea and choreography exchanges or more formal interdepartmental staff updates. A written overview should be provided for those instructors that could not attend the meeting. It is also a nice perk to reward those who do attend with a bonus or product.

Leadership/Communication Skills

As a manager, it is imperative that you develop effective leadership and communication skills. Your primary job is to lead and create a desirable working environment. Lead by example—what you do and what you say, how you do it and say it—communicate your ideas, philosophies, expectations, and concerns. Always be willing to follow any direction you might give a staff member.

Clear communication is key—say what you mean and mean what you say. Be straight forward in your policies, and consistent in the way you handle employee issues and directives. Poor communication in the business place leads to confusion and dissolution among your staff members.

Program managers need to be available when a staff member calls or emails you. Respond to emails and return all missed calls within 24 hours. In all dealings with staff (whether one-on-one or in group meetings), managers must be effective listeners. When listening to staff concerns or problems, repeat what you hear to make sure that you understand what they are saying Ask staff members for input and get them involved. Clear communication, exemplary leadership, and open-minded exchanges will lead to an effective and rewarding work environment for everyone.

Selecting Group Exercise Equipment

Group exercise equipment includes all nonpermanent items or props that are necessary to enhance the activities that take place within a group exercise class. Items can include stereo equipment, music, mats, charts, resistance products, cardio props, and aqua aerobic or outdoor training equipment. Consider the following when selecting group exercise equipment.

- Locating manufacturers
- Costs

- Product quality and warranty
- Usage
- Storage
- Overall program enhancement

Specific Equipment

Music Systems—Typically, a fitness setting needs some type of music system. A much-appreciated feature is a speed or pitch control on the tape or CD player. This is available in both fixed and portable units. An audio design company can advise you of necessary amplification and speaker needs based on the dimensions and acoustics of your room. Units that are also compatible to portable units such as downloadable devices (e.g., iPod®) are able to stay abreast of improved technology. Consideration should also be given to a microphone system. Microphone options include corded hand-held, cordless hand-held, cordless headset, or cordless clip-on. The corded microphone is the least expensive and most durable option, yet does not offer the ability to travel around the room or have freedom of arm movement. The cordless microphone is more conducive to the group exercise situation, although is often more sensitive to abuse and expensive than the corded models.

Music—Music may or may not be supplied by the club or organization. In most group exercise situations, music should be professionally mixed so that the songs accommodate the beats per minute of specified classes. Some instructors choose to download or burn their own music. There are various companies that specialize in professionally mixed and downloadable fitness music. They are convenient and cost-effective (ranging from $15 to $50). It is important that one checks with ASCAP and BMI as to the copyright regulations and rules when purchasing or using recorded artists (ASCAP: 1 Lincoln Plaza, New York, NY 10023, (212) 621-6000; http://www.ascap.com/index.html ; BMI: 320 W. 57th St., 3rd Floor, New York, NY, 10019, (212) 586-2000; http://www.bmi.com/).

Mats—Mats are necessary if the exercise surface does not have adequate cushion for floor exercises. Mats are available in a variety of densities and sizes.

Charts—Charts are important as a training tool for class safety and education. They can be purchased laminated in a variety of dimensions. Popular charts are muscle and anatomy guides, target heart rate (also available specific to children and older adults), rate of perceived exertion, and CPR.

Resistance Devices—This category includes all types of free weights (typically in the 1–15 lb range), resistance bands and tubing, weighted bars, balls, and gloves. Resistance devices are an optional type of equipment that can greatly increase the variety of classes offered, as well as allow instructors to continue to challenge students through basic principles of overload (see AFAA's *Basic Exercise Standards and Guidelines* in this text). Storage is a consideration. Some type of shelf, rack, or box—preferably with a locking system—needs to be provided to keep equipment in order.

Cardio and Balance Props—Cardio and balance props, which include all equipment that is used for cardiovascular or balance training, support a growing market that is reflective of the need for variety and cross-training. Cardio props include steps, jump ropes (weighted and non-weighted), slide boards and mini trampolines, springboards, and cycles. This type of equipment provides optional methods of adding variety and intensity to a program. Balance props include core and wobble boards, Bosu® and therapy balls, foam rollers, and soft disks. This list will continue to grow as the industry continues to find new and unique ways to add a new challenge in a group exercise environment. Again, space and storage are major considerations. One must evaluate how many pieces can fit into the workout room and if this number is cost-effective when considering the amount of members it will benefit. Then, storage space must be provided in order to keep equipment in proper condition and out of the way of other activities.

Specialized Equipment—Examples of these types of products are aqua equipment (flotation belts and webbed gloves), kid fitness devices (tumbling mats and running cones), kickboxing and martial arts derived products (wraps, gloves, bags), and cross-training equipment (circuit equipment, medicine balls, weighted vests). Much like the cardio and balance props, this list will continue to grow.

With the growing need for variety and specificity have come many innovative products that may or may not have a use in your program. When considering these products, the cost of each piece needs to be compared to the benefits such items offer. Program managers should work firsthand with the product and evaluate its safety and effectiveness before employing it within the program. In some cases, information about such products and any recalls or injuries associated with certain products should be reviewed by reference to the U.S. Consumer Product Safety Commission. In addition, instructors in some cases will need proper training and product usage guidelines prior to using the equipment in classes. This may be another cost that needs to be considered.

Summary

This overview of program management responsibly and skills is just a start. It is highly recommended for you to further your knowledge and skills through reading, attending management classes, and consulting with other business leaders and asking questions. It is these skills that will enable your group exercise program to run smoothly and stay fiscally fit while you keep your members physically fit!

References

1. American College of Sports Medicine. (2007). *ACSM's health/fitness facility standards and guidelines* (3rd ed.). Champaign, IL: Human Kinetics.
2. Grantham, W.C., Patton, R.W., York, T.D., & Winick, M.L. (1998). *Health fitness management*. Champaign, IL: Human Kinetics.
3. Whyman, W. (2008). *Outdoor site and facility management—tools for creating memorable places*. Champaign, IL: Human Kinetics.

42 *Marketing and Promoting Your Fitness Business*

Lawrence Biscontini, MA

Focus

This chapter outlines key marketing and promotional concepts for instructors, trainers, and business owners. The question often asked by fitness professionals worldwide is, "How can I continue to grow and watch my business succeed with all the competition that pops up daily?" The answer derives first from the creation of a consistently updated quality product, and, second, from obtaining consistent and effective public relations with strategic marketing. Whether one is looking to promote either a single individual or an entire business, the ideas that follow serve as a point of departure for the evolving world of fitness business marketing.

Consistent Positive Publicity

Establishing contacts and relationships with both the media and other people in the wellness profession is critical for networking. In many cases, the differences between the classes and sessions that two individuals or facilities offer in the fitness arena really may be quite negligible. Incorporating the following techniques, however, will help you set yourself apart from the competition by helping you adapt the role of publicist for business marketing. Any publicist first must have a detailed understanding of the attributes that make his or her product unique and superior to any competition. The following sections can assist in securing promotional success for the fitness career.

Self-Promotion

Be sure to keep an objective, positive outlook regarding all business strengths. Use both personal visits and the Internet to get a thorough understanding of what the competition currently offers in terms of both product and pricing. Make a list of your own strengths that the competition does not offer, and contemplate creating additional Unique Selling Points (USPs). Try to be different. Truly, what often separates and distinguishes is not the WHAT (everyone trains a bicep), but the HOW (actual trainer specific, unique approaches). Consider the untapped market of special populations (including youth and elderly) that may benefit in unique, unexplored ways from your business. Without this knowledge, coupled with a plan of action, it is almost impossible to sell your strengths consistently to the media. When you describe your USPs in all printed material, use language uniquely; consider creative, catchy names and unique, colorful descriptions that focus on results. People ultimately want to know what you can do for them in terms of visible, measured outcome on their bodies.

Printed Materials and Press Releases

Develop your own mission statement, vision statement, and business logo to summarize your philosophy towards fitness and wellness. A mission statement summarizes what your business is about today. Your vision statement explains to others the direction in which you plan to be moving tomorrow. A business logo summarizes what you are about, and you can get assistance in creating your own at Web sites like Vistaprint.com. Consider putting both mission and vision statements on business cards with your logo. Web sites such as Vistaprint.com and Shutterfly.com allow you to do this at nominal charges. Create a press release of your personal or company strengths. In addition to your contact information, mission statement, and business logo, list all attributes, education, abilities, equipment, and experience in short, detailed sentences, succinctly answering not only how you will create results, but also the five W's: who, what, when, where, and why. Emphasizing your AFAA certifications on your resume, Web site, and business cards (if you are certified by AFAA state on your business card: "AFAA Certified," since certified professionals may not reproduce the actual AFAA logo on such material) brings international credibility to your business and helps to justify your own pricing system. If you can secure any testimonials from prominent, recognizable figures from your community whom you currently train, seek permission to include a quotation on your press release, as such endorsements add valued credibility to your business.

Note that press releases need to follow specific guidelines—consult the sources listed in the reference section of this chapter for further information. Examine the "bullet points" of your strengths, and keep them readily available on a word-processing program so that updating becomes both continual and effortless. Always keep a data back-up. In the rapidly changing fitness environment today, information must be updated at least every 4 months or else it will sound stale. Wherever you go, keep both your business cards and press releases handy. For ideas on different formats, try consulting Web sites of your favorite personal fitness training and group fitness industry leaders by going directly to their Web pages, like this: www.xyz.com, in which you substitute the full name of the person for the xyz, such as www.jayblahnik.com, for example.

Internet Plan of Action

The Internet offers affordable marketing and networking options to build your business. Having at least one electronic tool in today's market speaks favorably about your company's success. Consider, for example, a simple web page that can serve as an electronic press kit which provides an overview of what you offer, a few action shots, a valid testimonial, and your pricing structure. Costs can add up quickly when building an Internet site, so plan on investigating all alternatives carefully before committing to investment, although most Internet service providers offer the option of a simple web page at no extra charge. Such providers usually offer Internet tutorials explaining how to create a Web site (e.g., homepage, additional page). Again, visit the sites of industry leaders to consider various options for organizing your site.

To promote your services, use both Internet and slower forms of communication (e.g., regular mail, fax, phone). Remember to often consult afaa.com which holds a wealth of valuable fitness information. Other incredibly useful Internet resource options to assist today's professional include: ptonthenet.com, mindbodyonline.com, fitfiend.com, fitizens.com, and onlinehealthclub.com offer total solutions for instructors and personal fitness trainers just getting started in the business.

Contacting the Media

Locate the various media, first in your immediate area and state, and then on a national and international level if appropriate. Given the direct publicity links for all major media networks around the country that are instantly available on the Internet via search engines, forwarding and attaching your personal press releases today means both speedy and effortless work. Some fitness professionals rely completely on electronic media kits that display both text and graphics (e.g., headshots, equipment, services), all readily available in one quick download. Some offer clients the option of paying directly and inexpensively through their Web site by using paypal.com. However you send your finished product advertising your services, use the Internet to obtain names of contact people (including addresses and phone numbers) who can benefit from what you offer.

When searching the Internet for media sources to which you can advertise, remember to incorporate the following into your plan.
- Television
- Radio
- Theater
- Newspapers
- Pertinent magazines
- Internet news sources

When you do make contact, tell specific people in the press about yourself, answering the famous newsworthy questions of "Why you?", "Why this?", and "Why now?" If possible, make direct follow-up calls to the appropriate person at each media contact. Confirm that the information sent was the information received, and volunteer to answer any further questions. Document names of every person with whom you speak, and always be prepared to ask for the name of someone else in that organization that may be better prepared to listen. Remember professional courtesy, and also remember that this is not a time to be shy. A timely letter, email, or fax that summarizes the information included in the initial contact can do wonders, both to show your determination and to keep your product from finding a place on someone's back burner. If the message is critical to your business, attract the attention of the press with an express delivery service or certified priority U.S. mail.

Financial Planning

Set aside a monthly promotional budget to pay for printing, telephone calls, mailing, Internet access, and Web hosting for the above. If you hire someone to do your financial books, be sure to verify his or her fees up front and include these in your budget. Some of these fees may be tax deductible—consult your tax advisor.

Promotional Strategies

Charity Events

By helping others, you also have the opportunity to help yourself. Have your name closely associated with worthwhile charities at least two to four times a year. Offer your services to lead the warm-ups or stretches for major events like AIDS awareness rides, marathon runs for cancer cure efforts, and sport outings during seasonal periods of the year. In addition, you can sponsor activities, appear in speaking engagements (including beyond any facility at which you normally work), and offer your services planning committee meetings associated with charity events. To foster a relationship over time, you may choose to work with just one charity to help build brand recognition and association of your name with that specific charitable organization

In the group fitness setting, consider hosting a special class every month to benefit a chosen charity, and thematically tie in all aspects of the event with that charitable organization. For example, on the last Friday of the month, you could dedicate one particular class to benefit a charity by promoting "warm yoga," in which the entry ticket for each participant in the class is a gently used, "warm" winter coat placed in a large bin that the club would donate to the Salvation Army. Invite the press, the Salvation Army staff, and all members of the facility to the event. Consider putting together similar events with shoes, non-perishable food items, and even cash for worthwhile causes.

Continual Dialogue with Special Events

A. Ask for help: Involve all staff in planning promotional events that will attract the media's interest. Plan ahead, and remember that the more eyes you have involved, the clearer the vision will be for the company's direction.

B. Feedback from the professionals: After forming a relationship with the media, ask for input regarding the impact of your particular press releases. "How can I make this information even more stimulating for the public?" is an excellent question for them.

Piggy-backing

This technique refers to two individuals or companies that come together, forming a symbiotic relationship, with little or no expense to either party. Each may offer a necessary skill without which the other would be rendered less effective, and thus more attention is drawn to the successful pairing.

Personal Fitness Trainer: For example, the personal fitness trainer who uses Swiss balls in fitness programming would do well to pair with a Swiss ball manufacturer as a personal or club sponsor. As a result, both companies would gain from double exposure and profit.

Group Exercise Instructors: For example, instructors can piggy-back with personal fitness trainers by inviting personal fitness trainers and their clients to classes and, in exchange, promoting the personal fitness trainers to all of the members in their classes. Both the personal fitness trainers and instructors get free advertising with little time invested and no expense.

Fitness Facilities

Whole facilities could engage in a mutual promotion program with local supermarkets of choice by agreeing to put discount coupons to the supermarket throughout the fitness facility in exchange for the supermarket allowing the facility's fitness brochures and group exercise schedules to be prominently posted at all check-out counters. Both the supermarket and the facility profit from the high-exposure advertising, and neither company has to invest money other than their printing costs for marketing materials.

Sponsorships and References

Occasionally, some products and services do well when backed by a sponsor. For example, a new facility offering specialized equipment in a particular demographic would do well to approach that equipment company with an inquiry regarding sponsorship, and thus profit from yet another source of publicity. A personal fitness trainer may wish to approach a particular clothing line for sponsorship by first creating a preliminary contact letter. Closely linked with sponsorships are references from celebrities and other high-profile clients, so be sure to approach them to secure permission to name them in your promotional materials. Naming recognized figures on your promotional material can bolster your exposure. Similarly, instructors who integrate specialized equipment into group classes may contact that manufacturer for free promotional materials, posters, music, and other items.

Trade Shows/Conventions/Expos

With your fitness business, you have a commodity. Consider the worthiness of investing in a booth at a large fitness trade show, convention, or expo to market your product as personal fitness trainer/instructor and/or to promote specific products. The exposure and contacts generated may more than return the initial expenditure. You may also consider expanding your career path by applying to present lectures or movement workshops at these conventions.

Foreign Language

If your organization's personnel can speak a language other than English, market this skill. Many fitness facilities in the United States and abroad continuously search for employees who may be multilingual. Stating on promotional materials, "Spanish available," or "All training available in Italian," for example, instantly increases the accessibility of your product and makes you more marketable to those markets. Make sure your Web site also contains keywords in the other pertinent languages so that search engines will call out your site.

Going Green

Today's fitness market follows the global trend of "going green", which is taking into consideration using sustainable resources and demonstrating ethical business practices which incorporate the Three R's: (a) reduce, (b) reuse, and (c) recycle. Consider printing all materials on recycled paper. You could also include a green note in your email signature encouraging readers not to print out every email they receive (e.g., "Please consider the trees of the forest before printing out this and all emails."). As a personal fitness trainer and instructor, everyone notices everything you do, so you may wish to get more ideas for implementing greener practices into your fitness business at thegreenguide.com, voltaicsystems.com, noonsolar.com, and thinkgreen.com. Implementing such steps will help you be able to call yourself a "green instructor/personal fitness trainer" and perhaps be among the first in your facility to initiate such practices, which alone is worthy of press for your business.

Summary

In conclusion, the success of a fitness product depends primarily on its effective marketing. Word of mouth is no small contributing factor to success, and after this, the media and Internet provide the two most significant sources of attention. Telling others about the benefits of a business depends largely on the efficacy of composed press releases, and these should be timely and unique. Setting apart one fitness tool from hundreds like it requires careful thought. In today's fitness market, staying abreast of these merchandising tactics is key.

References

1. Archer, S. (2000). Who wants to be a millionaire? *IDEA Health & Fitness Source*, 32–42, July/August.
2. Atkinson, D. (2001). Personal training: The time crunch. *American Fitness*, 37–39, May/June.
3. Biscontini, L. (2000). Fitness @ your fingertips. *Asiafit*, 32–34, May/June.

4. Biscontini, L. (2008). *Running the show: Outstanding customer service for fitness professionals.* New York: FG2000.

5. Biscontini, L. (2009). *Cream rises: Excellence in private and group fitness education.* New York: FG2000.

6. Cotton, R.T. (Ed.). (1996). *Personal trainer.* San Diego, CA: American Council on Exercise.

7. Gavin, J., & Gauvin, F. (2001). The first industry-wide work satisfaction study of fitness professionals. *IDEA Health & Fitness Source,* 29–37, July/August.

8. Gerard, J. (2001). The psychology of exercise. *ACE Fitness Matters,* 12–13, March/April.

9. Hultin, L. (2000). Creating an attention-grabbing press kit. *IDEA Health and Fitness Source,* 83–86, July/August.

10. Jones, J. (1999). Asses the value of your business. *IDEA Personal Trainer,* 24–35, November/December.

11. Jung, A. (2000). An evaluation of home exercise equipment claims. *ACSM's Health & Fitness Journal,* 4(5), 14–16, 30–31.

12. O'Brien, R. (1977). *Publicity—How to get it.* New York, NY: Harper & Row.

13. Street, R., & Kravitz, L. (2000). The ways of print and broadcast media. *ACSM's Health & Fitness Journal,* 7–11, 30, May/June.

14. Wirth, D. (2001). The Internet can be your tool. *NSCA Bulletin,* 22(4), 7–8.

15. Wright, H. (1990). *How to make 1,000 mistakes in business and still succeed.* IL: Wright Track.

43 *Advancing Your Fitness Career*

Nancy Gillette, MA

Focus

Research questionnaires from the early 1980s showed that the average fitness instructor had a "career span" of 2 ½ years, and that the instructor was generally a woman in her early twenties. As the field of fitness and aerobics matured, the career path for instructors and trainers has widened, and the average career time has lengthened.

Career Choices

Once thought of as a "sideline," or an "avocation" for most, fitness instruction has grown from a part-time, low paying job, to one with possibilities as broad as the minds that have created them over the past 30 years. Credit for these new career choices is due in large part to the aging baby boomers who found that these "part-time" exercise teaching jobs were where their passions lay. As they chose to extend these avocations into careers, to take these second income sources and make them into their primary sources of revenue, some started their own small businesses while others took their accumulated expertise "on-the-road." Many of these new paths came from instructors who, upon reaching 35 or 40 years of age, decided to become behind-the-scenes producers, rather than to remain in the fitness and exercise demonstration spotlight forever. The reevaluation of preferences, strengths, skills, and talents led instructors down a variety of career paths. Some moved into corporate boardrooms, others in front of cameras or behind podiums, rather than in front of exercise class mirrors.

Where to Begin

There are many career paths from which to choose, should an instructor or personal trainer want to diversify or specialize in the professional world of fitness. Some possibilities depend solely on the instructor's inner motivations and goal orientation. The following checklist might help direct an exercise instructor or trainer toward the general path most suited to him or her. Does the instructor/trainer want to:

- be in the spotlight or behind-the-scenes?
- pursue a paid or volunteer position?
- work alone or with a group/association?
- own his/her own business, be in partnership, or work for someone else?
- invest his/her own capital or have others support his/her endeavor financially?
- work locally or travel?
- move and demonstrate exercises himself/herself, remain behind a podium or desk, or work in a laboratory setting?
- make presentations that are entertaining or strictly educational?
- have local, regional, domestic, or international reach?
- connect with clients or exercisers in-person, or through books, magazines, DVD/videos, audio tapes, broadcast, Webcast, or other Internet exposure?

It is advisable to read a variety of books that are career-oriented. For an example, books addressing (a) how to select a career in general; (b) worksheets to determine professional strengths and weaknesses; (c) how to write a resume;

(d) how to successfully conduct oneself in a job interview; (e) dressing for success; (f) how to negotiate salary, perks, benefits, compensation, and retirement package; (g) finding a mentor; (h) how to work as a team member; (i) moving up the corporate ladder; (j) staying motivated; and (k) avoiding job burn out. These resources will be valuable to instructors whether they are in the fitness field short- or long-term, part- or full-time, as a vocation or an avocation. See the recommended reading list that follows.

Broad Options

In the past, there were limited options for an individual who desired to instruct exercise or dispense fitness information to others. Today, a myriad of paths are available, depending upon an individual's desires, other degrees or expertise, ability to travel, monetary goals, and group interactive skills. Once an individual enters a fitness career, usually as an exercise instructor, it is common to begin to specialize in one particular area or direction.

Many instructors may want to become a(n):

- fitness/group exercise coordinator
- director of group exercise classes/fitness for clubs
- health club manager
- health club owner/operator
- fitness coordinator of a chain of clubs
- instructor trainer
- on-the-road workshop/seminar presenter
  - lecture circuit presenter (non-movement orientation)
  - workshop circuit presenter (lecture and movement)
  - certification presenter/specialist (for a certifying body)
  - certification examiner (for a certifying body)
  - leader of local/regional sites
  - on-the-road domestic leader on site
  - international leader on site
- choreographer
- music mixer for cassette tapes, CDs, and iPods
- author of magazine articles
- author of books
- publisher of newsletters or informational brochures
- model for fitness/exercise oriented advertisements
- public service announcer for health and fitness on local cable or network TV, radio, or print media
- part of the production team for exercise DVD/videos as: the script writer, consultant, choreographer, back-up principal, sponsor, fitness product representative, editor, technical director
- star/choreographer of locally released fitness DVD/video
- star/choreographer of internationally released fitness DVD/video
- resource to local business on wellness programs
- on-site coordinator or instructor for corporate fitness programs
- one-on-one personal fitness trainer
- multiple participant or small group exercise leader/trainer
- spokesperson for a product or facility
- representative of a professional organization
- sales representative for a fitness product
- inventor of exercise equipment, devices, or paraphernalia

- fitness Web site designer
- fitness Web site content developer
- Internet consultant for corporations and foundations
- computer programmer for fitness oriented software
- computer programmer for interactive personal training Web sites
- Internet liaison for fitness club chains
- Internet advertising or marketing consultant
- fitness club coordinator of computer membership data collection
- kinesiologist or biomechanist
- exercise physiologist performing laboratory tests or data collection
- coordinator of local charity events, 10K runs, triathlons, walk-a-thons, boot camps, etc.
- exercise/fitness competitor—regional, national, or international athlete
- public relations representative or advertiser for local groups/events
- researcher for academic exercise/fitness studies at local universities and colleges
- volunteer in a research study or data collection activity
- higher education student, teacher's assistant, teacher, instructor, professor, administrator, or dean
- school teacher—high school, middle school, elementary, preschool, or day care in physical education, health, or recreation

Single Ladder to Climb?

If instructors choose to associate themselves with an organization that certifies or holds workshops/seminars, they can climb the ladder of expertise within that organization.

In many career fields, there are clearly defined ladders of success—solitary hierarchies of money, power, and status. For fitness professionals, there is more of a horizontal branching of the tree's ladder—a diversifying or a specializing of focuses less clearly marked.

Within each specialty, for example, exercise DVD/video production, there will be those who create, produce, and star in their own videos using a total individual budget of, let's say, $20,000, or those who are hired as celebrities for $1.5 million up front plus a percentage of the sales revenue, not to mention incredible exposure worldwide. The financial success ladder is clear. Yet, in the fitness "profession," the celebrities are not necessarily the ones who gain respect, status, or credibility. The mentors, power holders, and admired are the fitness educators and professionals with credentials, degrees, and theoretical knowledge to match their success—the "ghost writers" behind the well-known faces. To date, there seems to be a disparity between financial success and "fitness career" success within the inner circle of the exercise field.

Success in the professional fitness world must be measured individually. Since each step requires additional credentials, training, desire, skills, or education, an instructor must be prepared to spend additional time and money to seek out appropriate conferences, workshops, books, individuals to meet, information to know, mentors, and so forth in order to make the next move. With each new path ventured, additional information needs to be learned, assimilated, and dispersed, which in turn creates additional jobs. It is this dynamic change that has kept the fitness industry in its growth phase for more than 30 years.

AFAA Education

Over 250,000 fitness professionals have become certified by AFAA, and have developed careers or part-time work through their association with AFAA. At the basic level, individuals achieve AFAA certification and specialty education, and then go on to any of the career options listed in the previous section. There are a variety of certifications, workshops, self-study programs via hard copy as well as online through e-afaa.com and the Distance Education Center that deliver the education and training necessary for success in the fitness industry. Development of new programs is on-going. Go to www.afaa.com to view latest course offerings.

AFAA CERTIFICATIONS
Primary Group Exercise, KickBoxing, Step, Personal Fitness Trainer, TeleFitness, Military Fitness Specialist Certifications

AFAA SPECIALTY WORKSHOPS
Aqua Fitness; Floor, Core & More for Personal Trainers; Extension; Indoor Cycling; Kickboxing Skills & Choreography; Longevity Training for Seniors; Mat Science I; Mat Science II; Mechanics of Injury Prevention; Midlife Fitness for Women; National Board Review Course for PFTs; Perinatal Fitness; Practical Pilates; Practical Skills & Choreography; Practical Yoga Instructor Training; Resistance Training—the Class Format; Step Skills & Choreography; The Metabolic Connection to Obesity

AFAA SELF-STUDY COURSES
Hard Copy Format: Fitness Gets Personal® Series I & II, Building Client Relationships, ACSM's Health/Fitness Facility Standards & Guidelines, Prenatal Fitness, Stress Management, Eating Disorders, Exercise and Obesity, ACSM Exercise Management for Persons with Chronic Diseases and Disabilities, Nutrition Fundamentals, Aqua Fitness, Step Training, Exercise Science Fundamentals, Senior Fitness, Youth Fitness, Body Composition and Weight Management, OsteoBall® Training for Bone Health, A Taste of...Zumba®, A Taste of...Turbo Kick®, Standards and Guidelines Reference Manual (plus 3 corresponding exams)

DISTANCE EDUCATION CENTER (DEC) and E-AFAA ONLINE COURSES
The DEC: Personal Fitness Trainer Online Preparatory Course, Telexercise® Resistance Training Online Course, Multitraining Live® Web Conferencing
E-AFAA: Multiple Client Training, Music Essentials for Group Exercise, Resistance to the Core, Stress Gets Personal, Yoga Essentials I & II, Emergency Response Preparation, TeleFitness Internet Software Certification, CEU Corners CEU Video Corners

AFAA Opportunities

AFAA EXAMINER NETWORK
AFAA examiners are certified instructors throughout the world who evaluate candidates during AFAA certification practical exams. Examiners are independent contractors who take local assignments on a part-time, fee-for-service basis.

AFAA CONSULTANT NETWORK OF PRESENTERS
The AFAA consultant network of presenters is comprised of AFAA certified instructors with degrees in health- and fitness-related fields, and expertise as educators. The professionals in this network deliver the certification and specialty workshops at the on-site programs and workshops. There is a range of positions within this network that reflect different levels of expertise, experience, education, and accomplishment. All professionals in this network are independent contractors who take local and global assignments on a part-time, fee-for-service basis.

AFAA EDUCATION ADVISORY BOARD

The AFAA Education Advisory Board is a group of degreed, credentialed, and industry expert professionals, who develop, evaluate, update, and oversee the quality and content of all AFAA educational programs. Membership on this board is by invitation only.

AFAA CONTINUING EDUCATION PROVIDERS

AFAA continuing education providers are educators who have received authorization to award AFAA continuing education units (CEUs) for their own fitness workshops and lectures.

AFAA FITNESS PRACTITIONER

An AFAA Fitness Practitioner (AFP) is a degreed professional dedicated to providing a full range of fitness education services that bridge the gap between health care and fitness. The curriculum for this elite level of certification includes a variety of AFAA certifications and special population courses.

PROFESSIONAL AFFILIATE COORDINATORS

A Professional Affiliate Coordinator (PAC) is a part-time AFAA employee (in select states) who brings face-to-face AFAA representation to local instructors, fitness directors, and club owners. PACs visit fitness facilities to set up and promote AFAA workshops, answer questions, demonstrate products, and are available as local AFAA representatives.

PROFESSIONAL INTERNET PORTFOLIO

The Professional Internet Portfolio (PIP) provides fitness professionals (in select states) with the opportunity to conduct business on the Internet, powered by afaa.com. Features of this opportunity include a personalized Web page, inclusion in an online locator service, and the ability to earn referral fees when Web page visitors purchase AFAA products, workshops, and memberships.

EMPLOYMENT AT AFAA HEADQUARTERS

The AFAA headquarters in Sherman Oaks, CA has occasional openings for a variety of jobs, such as event planning, publishing, registration representatives, customer service, data entry, accounting, music and video production, Internet technology, and general office administration.

Summary

As with any specialty, additional training, education, research, networking, practice, time, and energy are important to success. However, the most crucial step when contemplating a career is to evaluate the fitness instructor's strengths, goals, and preferences.

Although a hierarchy does seem to exist among the more visible career selections, and especially among the most lucrative ones in which "celebrity" status comes into play, generally people do what they do because it meets their most basic needs, such as to help, to teach, to be in the spotlight, to have power, to control the purse strings, to lead, to create, to organize, and to communicate.

Whatever motivates a person deep down inside and keeps him or her within the fitness field will lead that individual to the appropriate new career branch. Many instructors find that their greatest joy is in the class setting and remain there long after most people in other careers have retired or moved into "administrative" positions. It's the love of what one does that keeps the newness and vitality in the chosen path, not the newness of the choice itself.

References

1. American College of Sports Medicine. (2007). ACSM's *health/fitness facility standards and guidelines* (3rd ed.). Champaign, IL: Human Kinetics.

2. Association for Worksite Health Promotion. (1992). *Guidelines for employee health promotion programs.* Champaign, IL: Human Kinetics.

3. Bolles, R.N. (2001). *What color is your parachute?* Berkeley, CA: Ten Speed Press.

4. Caple, J. (1993). *Finding the hat that fits: How to turn your heart's desire into your life's work.* Plume Publishers.

5. Dail, H.L. (1989). *The lotus and the pool.* Boston, MA: Shambhala.

6. Fields, J. (2009). *Career renegade: How to make a great living doing what you love.* New York, NY: Broadway Books.

7. Grantham, W. et al. (1998). *Health fitness management.* Champaign, IL: Human Kinetics.

8. Peters, T. (1982). *In search of excellence.* New York, NY: Harper and Row.

9. Plummer, T. (2003). *The business of fitness: Understanding the financial side of owning a fitness business.* Monterey, CA: Healthy Learning Publisher.

10. Pollan, S.M. (1990). *The field guide to starting a business.* New York, NY: Simon and Schuster.

11. Rieger, L. (1999). *Aerobic program coordinator's handbook.* Corvallis, OR: National Intramural Recreational Sports Association.

12. Ruge, K.C. (1998). *Where do I go from here? An inspirational guide to making authentic career and life choices.* Boston, MA: McGraw-Hill.

13. Sol, N., & Gladwin, L. (Eds.). (1996). *An emerging profession: The fitness practitioner.* Sherman Oaks, CA: Aerobics and Fitness Association of America.

14. Stevens, P., & Kennedy, S. (1995). *Beating job burnout: How to turn your work into your passion.* VGM Horizons.

15. Yoke, M. (2001). *A guide to personal fitness training.* Sherman Oaks, CA: Aerobics and Fitness Association of America.

16. Yoke, M. (2006). *AFAA's personal fitness training: Theory & practice.* Sherman Oaks, CA: Aerobics and Fitness Association of America.

17. Zichy, S., & Bidou, A. (2007). *Career match: Connecting who you are with what you'll love to do.* New York, NY: Amacom Publisher.

44 *Substitute Teaching*

Kathy Stevens, MA

Focus

Substitute teaching can be a convenient way to expand one's opportunities and abilities as a fitness instructor. By its very nature it can offer instructors a flexible work schedule, a change of pace, and a chance to develop new teaching skills. On the other hand, it can be an intimidating situation, leading to feelings of apprehension and self-doubt. Thus, this chapter will offer insights and tips to help ensure a positive experience when substitute teaching.

Substitute teaching consists of those occasions for which an instructor covers a class that is not his or hers on a permanent or semi-permanent basis. This can be particularly challenging when an instructor is new to the group and/or the participants are devoted followers of the regular instructor. We will look at four factors that can influence the success of such situations.

1. Having consistent policies in place
2. Evaluating the situation
3. Developing self-confidence
4. Making the right connection

Having Consistent Policies in Place

It is important to have consistent substitution policies in place to smooth the way for both the instructors and class participants. There should be a clearly defined method for choosing and contacting substitutes. Many fitness facilities have instructors cover their own classes. Other facilities have subbing assignments controlled by the group exercise director. Selection should be based on a substitute's capabilities as well as availability. The benefit of having instructors cover their own classes is that they can ask their participants which substitutes they prefer and contact those instructors first. On the other hand, the group exercise director will have a larger pool of instructors to choose from and is typically the best judge of the skills and abilities of the various instructors that might be available.

Once a substitute instructor is assigned, it is then the responsibility of the regular instructor or group exercise director to impart all relevant information about the class to the contracted substitute. This includes, but is not limited to, class type, time, and intensity level. It is important for the substitute to understand the specific needs of the class, and accept the commitment only if he or she feels able to meet those needs. Some facilities utilize pre-designed class formats because it is easier to meet participant expectations when instructors are teaching a consistent format.

The facility should have a method by which it can notify participants of the substitute situation prior to the class. Psychologically, participants adapt better and have less negative reactions to controlled situations. When they are notified prior to an instructor change, they can choose to show up or opt for a different workout. This leaves the participant with a sense of control. The earlier the knowledge is gained, the better the chances of acceptance. Notification can be in the form of announcements by the regular instructor prior to the substitution, but should also be posted at the facility and/or on the Internet. Even in the case of last minute substitutions, efforts should be made to post the change of events.

The facility, the regular instructor, and the substitute should all have a clear and binding understanding/agreement as to whether the substitute will be an independent contractor or an employee. Facility and/or instructor documents such as assumption or risk agreements and/or releases, informed consents, membership agreements, etc. should all cover the substitute and be for his/her benefit as well as the others. Matters of substitute liability insurance coverage or the need for substitutes to secure their own liability insurance coverage, all need to be resolved in advance of service provision by substitutes.

Evaluating the Situation

There are many important elements to consider when evaluating a substitute situation. First, is the basic class information. Substitute instructors will need to know what type of class they will be covering, including the equipment used, start time, finish time, and approximate length of each segment of the class. The more specific and detailed this information, the better.

It is also important to evaluate the physiological and psychological needs of the participants. The substitute instructor should ask a few questions about the participants that frequent the class. What intensity or pattern complexity will they expect? Are there participants with special needs such as senior adults or pregnant women? What type of music do they appreciate? It is also a good idea to find out what teaching characteristics the regular instructor uses to motivate the class. For example, are they humorous, technical, hands-on, or high-energy motivators? Although it would be hard for a substitute to completely change their style of teaching, they may be able to adapt it slightly, if they know what the group is accustomed to. It is ideal if the substitute instructor can observe the class prior to the substitute assignment.

Developing Self-Confidence

In order to develop the self-confidence necessary to be a successful substitute, the instructor must be well prepared. He/she must feel comfortable in their ability to lead a proper and constructive class. This comfort level grows out of having the previously mentioned class information as well as one's overall teaching experience. As in any instructional situation, practice makes perfect. Thus, it will be important for substitute instructors to practice and rehearse their class routines as much as possible prior to an assigned class.

It is also important for substitute instructors to show up with the right attitude and know how to handle potential negative attitudes from the participants. Participants can easily spot an insecure or negative instructor. They will often feed off of these attitudes, which can make the situation worse. If instructors are feeling insecure, they can address it in their opening statement. Let the group know that they are a bit nervous, but excited about teaching for them; convey that they are going to do everything possible to make it a great experience; and mention how glad they are to be helping out the regular instructor. The instructor can also let the group know that he or she would appreciate feedback to help the class go smoothly (e.g., music the right volume, exercises the right intensity, cueing easy to hear and follow). This will give the group a chance to empathize with the instructor's position while also encouraging him/her to make a positive contribution.

On the other hand, the substitute instructor needs to expect and understand possible negative attitudes. Often participants feel disappointed or abandoned if they were not prepared for an instructor change. Their reactions may have little to do with the substitute's abilities. If participants choose this position, it will be important for the instructor to avoid yielding his or her power as the class leader. The instructor needs to recognize the attitude for what it is, pacify the behavior of these participants, and avoid taking it personal. In other words, accept the grumbles with an accommodating attitude and move on. Instructors may also want to find and focus on a friendly face in the crowd or bring a friend that can lend moral support and a positive attitude.

Don't forget the power of humor. This is especially true in a crisis situation. By using a bit of humor you can find a new perspective on a troubled, embarrassing, or discouraging situation. Keeping an upbeat outlook gives you a sense of security in the middle of disturbance. Using humor in the tense first minutes of a substitute class can help the participants take another look at the temporary change that they may be taking too seriously. If you can humor them into accepting the situation and giving you a chance, you will instruct with greater self-confidence, which results in improved instructor performance and participant satisfaction.

Making the Right Connection

All instructor/participant relationships depend on the interaction and ultimate connections made in class. Remember that the first few moments of interaction with others is when their attention spans and powers of retention are the highest. These are the things psychologists tell us that people notice first: a) What they see (in fact, a surprising 55% of the meaning of your message is conveyed by facial expressions and body language); and b) what they hear (38% of which is based on the characteristics of one's voice: rate or tempo, loudness, pitch, articulation, and tone). Instructors should be aware that the last thing people notice, and therefore, the least important for a first impression are the words they are using (the words contribute only 7% of the meaning of your message). It is not that their words are unimportant. Yet, in order for them to be heard, the participants must first like what they see and what they hear. Instructors need to think about their attire and overall appearance, that is, is it appropriate for the group or class they are about to teach? Will he or she make the right impression in those first few seconds of interaction? The tight fitting or midriff-exposing outfit that an instructor might wear for an advanced sculpting or abs class may not be as appropriate for a senior or pregnancy fitness class. Often a group's mind may be made up before you speak. Emerson wrote, "What you are speaks so loudly, I can't hear what you are saying." Therefore, it is easy to see how the first 30 to 60 seconds that you spend with a class may determine the rest of the hour.

Tips to Help Ensure Successful Substitute Teaching

- Lower risk of early death
- Know as much as you can about the class format and participant expectations.
- Get to class early, fully prepared, and ready to greet participants.
- Dress appropriately for the type of class you are teaching.
- Introduce yourself with a short, positive opener.
- Have your class routine well rehearsed.
- Focus on a friendly face.
- Don't take negative attitudes personally.
- Keep your routine simple and easy to cue.
- Make sure you can be clearly seen and heard by all participants.
- Have fun, and let it show.

References

1. Anthony, R., & Ay, R. (1988). *Magic power of super persuasion.* New York, NY: Berkeley Books.

2. Brenot, J. (1985). *Substitute's handbook: a survivor's guide.* Saratoga, CA: R & E Publishers.

3. Hergenhahn, B.R., & Olson, M. (2006). *Introduction to theories of personality* (7th ed.). Englewood Cliffs, NJ: Prentice-Hall.

4. Kennedy-Armbruster, C., & Yoke, M.M. (2009). *Methods of group exercise instruction.* Champaign, IL: Human Kinetics.

45 *Law and Exercise*

David L. Herbert, JD

Focus

The purpose of this chapter is to give fitness professionals, including group exercise instructors, personal fitness trainers, fitness facility managers, and fitness club owners/operators an overview of selected legal issues concerning the exercise industry and profession. The legal status of service providers and their agents/employees/contractors, taxes, insurance, standards of care, negligence, incident reports, releases or so-called waivers of liability, informed consent forms, "legal" music sources, issues dealing with discrimination, and selected employment issues will be addressed. Despite the discussion of all the foregoing within this chapter, what is presented is not meant to be a substitute for individualized legal advice which should be obtained every time the need arises. It should, however, provide a broad overview of selected issues surrounding relevant aspects of the fitness profession.

Legal Status of Service Providers: Corporations, Limited Liability Companies, Partnerships, Sole Proprietorships

There are now four principal types of business entities through which fitness related services may be provided by fitness professionals to consumers. In descending order of legal formality, complexity and cost, these are: corporations, limited liability companies (which for legal and tax purposes can also be a type of partnership), partnerships, and sole proprietorships.

Corporations are distinct legal entities formed by registering/filing articles of incorporation for each such corporation with a state agency which provides authorization to the corporation to form and begin doing business within that state. Corporations are legal entities separate and apart from the individuals who may serve or be employed by such corporations as directors, officers, employees, agents, or contractors. Such corporations are also separate and distinct legal entities from the shareholders who own such corporations through ownership of the capital stock or shares of such entities. A corporation is also a separate taxable entity that must have a tax identification number and file tax returns separate and apart from its owner(s).

Corporations can either be called "C" corporations, and taxed independently of their owners or shareholders, or "S" corporations, which merely report income/loss on an informational basis only. In such circumstances, "S" corporations pass through any income or loss to their shareholders to report on their individual income tax returns.

Limited liability companies are a form of a corporation, but are owned by members rather than shareholders. Such entities operate with very limited liability for their members, and often operate without directors or officers. Such entities may be composed of one or more members, and may also operate if there are two or more individuals as a partnership. Such companies may have a separate tax identification number, but report taxable income on individual tax returns.

Partnerships are composed of two or more individuals/corporations that carry on business and service provision under a particular name and with a separate tax identification number. If a partnership business is carried on in a name different from that of the individuals who are its partners, registration with a state agency of a trade or fictitious name under which business will be carried on may be required. Like "S" corporations, partnerships file informational tax returns only and pass through income/loss to partners to report on their own individual income tax returns but partnerships may also have separate tax identification numbers.

Sole proprietorships are simply businesses carried on by one owner either under a trade/fictitious name or the individual's own name. If a trade or fictitious name is used, registration of the name may also be required as with some fictitious or trade partnership names. Income/loss for income tax purposes is reported on the proprietor's own tax return and usually through the individual's social security number, although a tax identification number may be secured for such businesses.

The services of a lawyer and an accountant should be considered for the formation of any of these operational entities, particularly for corporations, partnerships, and the so-called limited liability hybrid of either. The services that will be necessary in this regard and the costs associated with those services will vary with the operational entity chosen to provide service. The sole proprietorship should be the least costly and the easiest to form and operate. Legal advice, however, may still be necessary, and personal liability concerns are the greatest with sole proprietorships and the least with corporations and limited liability corporations and/or partnerships.

Legal Status of Agents: Employees/ Independent Contractors

Determining the legal status of a fitness professional in reference to his or her employer, or contracting business entity engaged in providing service to consumers, is extremely important when identifying legal liability, insurance needs, and tax responsibilities. To determine if someone is considered an employee or an independent contractor, the Internal Revenue Service (IRS) and the courts frequently look at a variety of factors to make such determinations. In the course of making such classification decisions, the activities of those carrying on business activity will be examined to determine whether or not they are directly monitored or supervised by their principals. Such examinations focus on whether or not the principal exercises enough control over the agent to have the later considered to be an employee of the former.

A relatively new guidance document applicable to such determinations, at least from a federal income tax perspective, has been developed. The guidelines have been published in a revised IRS publication entitled *Publication 15-A, Employer's Supplemental Tax Guide*, 2009 or later edition. Among other things, the publication provides information on the following.

Who Are Employees?
Before you can know how to treat payments that you make to workers for services, you must first know the business relationship that exists between you and the person performing the services. The person performing the services may be:
- an independent contractor;
- a common-law employee;
- a statutory employee; or
- a statutory nonemployee.

This discussion explains these four categories. A later discussion, *Employee or Independent Contractor?* (section 2), points out the differences between an independent contractor and an employee and gives examples from various types of occupations.

If an individual who works for you is not an employee under the common-law rules (see section 2), you generally do not have to withhold federal income tax from that individual's pay. However, in some cases you may be required to withhold under the backup withholding requirements on these payments. See Publication 15 (Circular E) for information on backup withholding.

Independent Contractors

People such as lawyers, contractors, subcontractors, and auctioneers who follow an independent trade, business, or profession in which they offer their services to the public, are generally not employees. However, whether such people are employees or independent contractors depends on the facts in each case. The general rule is that an individual is an independent contractor if you, the person for whom services are performed, have the right to control or direct only the result of the work and not the means and methods of accomplishing the result.

Common-Law Employees

Under common-law rules, anyone who performs services for you is your employee if you have the right to control what will be done and how it will be done. This is so even when you give the employee freedom of action. What matters is that you have the right to control the details of how the services are performed. For a discussion of facts that indicate whether an individual providing services is an independent contractor or employee, see section 2.

If you have an employer-employee relationship, it makes no difference how it is labeled. The substance of the relationship, not the label, governs the worker's status. It does not matter whether the individual is employed full time or part time.

For employment tax purposes, no distinction is made between classes of employees. Superintendents, managers, and other supervisory personnel are all employees. An officer of a corporation is generally an employee. However, an officer who performs no services or only minor services, and neither receives nor is entitled to receive any pay, is not considered an employee. A director of a corporation is not an employee with respect to services performed as a director.

You generally have to withhold and pay income, social security, and Medicare taxes on wages you pay to common-law employees. However, the wages of certain employees may be exempt from one or more of these taxes. See *Employees of Exempt Organizations* (section 3) and *Religious Exemptions* (section 4).

Misclassification of Employees

Consequences of treating an employee as an independent contractor. If you classify an employee as an independent contractor and you have no reasonable basis for doing so, you may be held liable for employment taxes for that worker (the relief provisions, discussed below, will not apply). See section 2 in Publication 15 (Circular E) for more information.

Relief provisions. If you have a reasonable basis for not treating a worker as an employee, you may be relieved from having to pay employment taxes for that worker. To get this relief, you must file all required federal information returns on a basis consistent with your treatment of the worker. You (or your predecessor) must not have treated any worker holding a substantially similar position as an employee for any periods beginning after 1977.

Employee or Independent Contractor?

An employer must generally withhold federal income taxes, withhold and pay social security and Medicare taxes, and pay unemployment tax on wages paid to an employee. An employer does not generally have to withhold or pay any taxes on payments to independent contractors.

Common-law rules. To determine whether an individual is an employee or an independent contractor under the common law, the relationship of the worker and the business must be examined. In any employee-independent contractor determination, all information that provides evidence of the degree of control and the degree of independence must be considered.

Facts that provide evidence of the degree of control and independence fall into three categories: behavioral control, financial control, and the type of relationship of the parties. These facts are discussed below.

Behavioral control. Facts that show whether the business has a right to direct and control how the worker does the task for which the worker is hired include the type and degree of the following.

- Instructions that the business gives to the worker. An employee is generally subject to the business's instructions about when, where, and how to work. All of the following are examples of types of instructions about how to do work.
- When and where to do the work.
- What tools or equipment to use.
- What workers to hire or to assist with the work.
- Where to purchase supplies and services.
- What work must be performed by a specified individual.
- What order to sequence to follow.

The amount of instruction needed varies among different jobs. Even if no instructions are given, sufficient behavioral control may exist if the employer has the right to control how the work results are achieved. A business may lack the knowledge to instruct some highly specialized professionals; in other cases, the task may require little or no instruction. The key consideration is whether the business has retained the right to control the details of a worker's performance or instead has given up that right.

- Training that the business gives to the worker. An employee may be trained to perform services in a particular manner. Independent contractors ordinarily use their own methods.

Financial control. Facts that show whether the business has a right to control the business aspects of the worker's job include the following.

- The extent to which the worker has unreimbursed business expenses. Independent contractors are more likely to have unreimbursed expenses than employees. Fixed ongoing costs that are incurred regardless of whether work is currently being performed are especially important. However, employees may also incur unreimbursed expenses in connection with the services they perform for their business.
- The extent of the worker's investment. An independent contractor often has a significant investment in the facilities he or she uses in performing services for someone else. However, a significant investment is not necessary for independent contractor status.
- The extent to which the worker makes his or her services available to the relevant market. An independent contractor is generally free to seek out business opportunities. Independent contractors often advertise, maintain a visible business location, and are available to work in the relevant market.
- How the business pays the worker. An employee is generally guaranteed a regular wage amount for an hourly, weekly, or other period of time. This

usually indicates that a worker is an employee, even when the wage or salary is supplemented by a commission. An independent contractor is usually paid by a flat fee for the job. However, it is common in some professions, such as law, to pay independent contractors hourly.

- The extent to which the worker can realize a profit or loss. An independent contractor can make a profit or loss.

Type of relationship. Facts that show the parties' type of relationship include the following.

- Written contracts describing the relationship the parties intended to create.
- Whether or not the business provides the worker with employee-type benefits (e.g., insurance, pension plan, vacation pay, sick pay).
- The permanency of the relationship. If you engage a worker with the expectation that the relationship will continue indefinitely, rather than for a specific project or period, this is generally considered evidence that your intent was to create an employer-employee relationship.
- The extent to which services performed by the worker are a key aspect of the regular business of the company. If a worker provides services that are a key aspect of your regular business activity, it is more likely that you will have the right to direct and control his or her activities. For example, if a law firm hires an attorney, it is likely that it will present the attorney's work as its own and would have the right to control or direct that work. This would indicate an employer-employee relationship.

While this new IRS publication may be helpful, the services of an attorney and/or accountant may also be necessary to assist in making determinations regarding whether or not service providers are employees or independent contractors. Despite a probable need to consult with such professionals as to this issue, the following discussion should assist those engaged in making at least tentative determinations regarding this matter.

When is an Instructor an Employee?

If a health and fitness facility collects all membership dues and training fees from consumers and the facility engages an instructor to teach specific classes or sessions at established regular times, with a club manager overseeing the delivery of services and the training of staff, the service provider may well be regarded as an employee of the facility which probably will be deemed to be an employer of such a service provider. Given such a designation, health and fitness facilities will usually be liable for any injuries occurring to consumers that are proximately caused by such professionals in their delivery of services, where those individuals are carrying on activities for the benefit of the employer. This means that the employer would be responsible for paying all legal fees and damage awards should an injured consumer sue a health and fitness facility/employee and prevail upon such a suit where a provider is providing service within the scope of his/her employment. If a facility carries liability insurance, the insurance company would have the obligation to defend the action through attorneys hired by it and pay the necessary legal fees and costs associated with the proceeding, as well as any damage award depending upon the extent and limits of the available insurance coverage and any applicable deductible. Based upon the foregoing, health and fitness facilities should secure adequate liability insurance that covers all of the activities that are carried on within such facilities by those who are deemed to be its employees or agents.

An employer of an employee—as opposed to a principal contracting with an independent contractor—is also responsible for withholding and paying out to the Internal Revenue Service and other governmental entities such as worker's compensation bureaus, applicable taxes, and other withholdings from an employee's pay check. The employer is also required to submit the employee's withholdings, together with the employer's contribution as to same, to the appropriate governmental taxing authorities at established time intervals. Should a health and fitness facility fail to make the necessary withholdings or to remit same to taxing authorities when due, these authorities may well assess interest on past due obligations, certain penalties, and other charges against health and fitness facilities in addition to the required tax payments.

When is an Agent an Independent Contractor and What are the Responsibilities of Such Service Providers?

Fitness professionals who are indeed independent contractors are responsible for determining how, where, and when services will be provided to or for the person with whom they contract. They are also responsible for their own income tax and other governmental tax or payment withholding responsibilities, and for any negligent acts or omissions that occur in their delivery of service to consumers. When health and fitness facilities contract with such service providers, health and fitness facilities should insure that these providers have applicable liability insurance in force to cover contractor acts and omissions and that such coverage also extends protection to those facilities. Contract terms, for example, should provide that such coverage may not be canceled without prior written notice (for example, 30 days) and that facilities will be named as additional insureds, if possible, and indemnified from any defense costs/expenses/awards in connection with suits filed against facilities as well as its independent contractors.

As previously stated, it is often very difficult to determine whether or not service providers are employees or independent contractors. To illustrate a situation where a service provider may indeed be an employee rather than an independent contractor, consider the following example: An aerobics instructor is contacted by a health and fitness facility to provide service to facility customers. All services are set at specific times to be rendered by the provider within the health and fitness facility and pursuant to a detailed schedule of what services shall be provided. The actual delivery of services is carried out during these times by the service provider at the health and fitness facility under the supervision of a fitness director at the facility. There is no written contract in place between the facility and the service provider. The service provider is paid an hourly wage and if no services are provided, no remuneration is given to the instructor. The instructor provides service approximately 25 hours per week and provides no similar services for any other health and fitness facility. Under these circumstances, the service provider is probably an employee and will be treated as an employee for tax and liability purposes.

Notwithstanding the foregoing, consider the following different example: A service provider, who delivers fitness services for a dozen health and fitness facilities and others, contracts in writing with a health and fitness facility to provide service to some of the facility's customers. The services are carried on both at the health and fitness facility and at the contractor's place of business, which is separate and apart from that of the health and fitness facility. The service provider is paid a flat fee for service provision and determines what activities shall be provided to the customers of the health and fitness facility and without supervision by the fitness director of the facility. The service provider has his/her own place of business, stationary, advertising brochures, billing statements, and business cards, and collects/reports his/her income separately from that of the health and fitness facility. The service provider also carries liability insurance, and has agreed by contract with the facility to indemnify the facility for any claims/suites related to injuries and/or other untoward events that occur to customers while the provider delivers services to them at the facility. Under these circumstances, the service provider is probably an independent contractor and the facility should ensure that the service provider has the necessary liability insurance in place to cover his/her activities while carrying out the terms of the contract for the facility.

The foregoing examples (as well as actual determinations as to legal relationships between a health and fitness facility and those who provide service for it) are often complex and dependent upon particular nuances of fact and law. As a consequence, the services of competent legal counsel and accountants should be secured for the purposes of determining such matters. However, as a general rule, when facilities contract with third parties to deliver services on an independent contractor basis, facilities should ensure that a written contract is in place, that no direct supervision is provided as to the activities to be carried on by such an independent contractor, that they are not paid an hourly based wage, that the contractor maintains adequate liability insurance and agrees to indemnify the health and fitness facility as to all activities carried on by the contractor, including any failure to withhold or pay taxes when due. While facilities may still be joined in lawsuits filed by consumers related to the provision of services by an independent contractor based upon legal theories dealing with agency concepts, the foregoing steps should minimize facility exposure in this regard and assist in related determinations for tax and withholding purposes as to who is and who is not an employee.

The Standard of Care Owed by Health and Fitness Facilities

Health and fitness facilities, as well as their officers, agents, and employees, and under some circumstances, even their independent contractors (who might under some circumstances be considered "ostensible" or "apparent" agents), owe a duty to deliver services to consumers in accordance with the so-called "standard of care." Standard of care issues are often determined by reference to established industry benchmarks of expected behavior that have previously been published or established for the delivery of services. Sometimes such statements are minimal standards, below which a facility may not go in their provision of services. Others may be optimal standards that are designed to improve the delivery of services beyond a certain minimal or established threshold level. Care must consequently be taken in the review and application of such standards to determine what are base line statements and whether the facility is obligated to comply with them.

In the health and fitness industry, a variety of standards have been published by, among others, the Aerobics and Fitness Association of America (AFAA), the American College of Sports Medicine (ACSM), the International Health and Racquet Sports Association (IHRSA), the American Council on Exercise (ACE), the National Strength and Conditioning Association (NSCA), and a number of other professional associations and entities including most significantly, the American Heart Association (AHA). In the operation of fitness facilities and the delivery of services in the health and fitness industry, the third and most recent edition of ACSM'S Health/Fitness Facility Standards and Guidelines should be particularly helpful as well as a 1998 scientific statement of the AHA/ACSM published in Circulation. Separate standards and guidelines have been developed by the Medical Fitness Association (MFA) for use in medically based facilities. A relatively new organization, the National Board of Fitness Examiners (NBFE) has developed a set of service delivery expectations in the form of a written and practical examination for personal trainers followed by a "registration" maintained by the NBFE of those who successfully pass the examination process. Such testing has been proposed for use in potential licensing processes for such professionals in at least a few states which have considered the issue. As of 2009, a new effort has emerged for the development of new standards for health and fitness facilities by NSF International.

Despite the development and publication of such statements, the standard of care (and deviations therefrom) is subject to expert witness definition and interpretation in the event of litigation and is something that changes from time-to-time. As a consequence, health and fitness professionals must stay abreast of changes in the industry so that services are delivered in accordance with the developing, evolving, and ever changing standard of care.

While the fitness industry has developed standards and guidelines covering the delivery of fitness services to consumers, the question of the actual duty owed to such consumers is one reserved for determination by judges in the course of their evaluation of particular allegations in individually filed case. At least two court decisions from California have called into question the issue of whether fitness professionals have a duty to screen and properly prescribe/supervise exercise activities for personal trainer clients since these cases determined that the trainer's clients assumed the risks of their activity. One of these decisions has also called into question the duty of a fitness facility to render emergency care to its customers, beyond simply calling 911 for emergency response. While decisions from other states may well indicate that courts in those states may recognize the existence of such duties by fitness professionals to their clients, litigation against fitness professionals, at least in California may not lead to jury determinations on the actual facts of potential cases due to these two decisions. Since judges determine whether or not a particular duty is owed by one person to another, the breach of which might be actionable, determinations about the breach of any such duty as owed by fitness professionals may never reach the determination stage for jury deliberation—at least in California.

Fitness instructors and others in the profession must adhere to the so-called standard of care in their delivery of service. The service to be delivered in accordance with industry expectations in this regard undoubtedly includes screening, recommendation of activities, recordation of activities, record keeping, leadership, supervision, and emergency response concerns. This is true because such professionals, when involved in the rendition of services to consumers, have a duty, once they determine to provide service, to render care in accordance with industry standards. Deficiencies in the provision of care in accordance with the standard required of such professionals which proximately causes harm or damage to consumers, may be actionable not only against the professional, but frequently against his or her employing entity or principal as well.

In the event of litigation, industry standards and guidelines are often cited through expert witness testimony based upon a comparison of particular facts and circumstances that occurred in individual circumstances to such standards which in that sense are used as service delivery expectations. Such witnesses examine the facts, compare those facts to expected methods and modalities of service provision and express an opinion as to whether or not there has been a failure or deficiency to render service in accordance with the standard of care.

Departures from the standard of care or failures to render service in accordance with established duties are deemed to be actionable where they directly, or in a legal sense, "proximately" cause harm to a consumer. Examples of such deficiencies in the health and fitness industry may include those situations where an instructor did not screen or even offer screening to consumers; where an instructor did not recommend appropriate activity; where he/she did not properly supervise or instruct consumers as to their use of exercise equipment or activity; where such instructors did not properly lead consumers in activity; where instructors provided deficient leadership for activity; where fitness professionals failed to "spot" consumers in their use of free weights or similar equipment; where professionals recommended or "prescribed" an exercise regimen that was too rigorous or too dangerous for the consumer; or even where the health and fitness facility or its professionals did not prepare for nor respond properly to an untoward event nor provide proper emergency care to those individuals under their care who needed such service.

In the assessment of whether or not fitness professionals can be held liable to consumers, a variety of damage claims may be considered. These damage claims include medical expenses incurred in the treatment of an injury, pain and suffering, lost wages, temporary and permanent disability, and other items. Under some circumstances, damages may be very significant. In at least one such case against a fitness professional and a facility among others, damages were sought equaling $320 million, although the case was reportedly resolved for less than 10 % of that figure.

If facility or professional conduct is deemed to be wrongful, willful, malicious, intentional, or even criminal, punitive damages may also be awardable against such entities or individuals in addition to compensatory damages. While such an award may be somewhat unusual in most cases against health and fitness facilities, punitive damages have been awarded in fitness related litigation, where for example, a piece of defective exercise equipment was not removed from consumer use which caused later injury, where the facility knew of its dangerous condition, but didn't either repair it or remove it from service. While all similarly situated cases do not always result in such awards, claims for punitive damages can raise the stakes in relevant litigation.

Lawsuits based upon personal injuries must generally be filed in a court of law within a particular period. States define these periods by reference to so-called "statutes of limitation", which define a time frame within which personal injury and wrongful death actions must be filed. These statutes also specify time periods for filing other kinds of actions based upon, for example, an assault and battery that may also occur within a health and fitness facility.

Statutes of limitation for actions such as assault and battery or wrongful death vary from state to state, but are generally for a period of time that is shorter than that which is available for "ordinary" negligence actions. In some states, for example, an assault and battery or wrongful death action must be filed within 1 year of the occurrence of the incident, while in other states an action for personal injury based upon negligence must be filed within 2 years. The services of competent legal professionals practicing in the state where services are provided must be utilized for the purposes of determining the length of applicable statutes of limitation and related questions. Even when there are defined statutes of limitation for specified injuries and actions, facilities should not, for example, blindly destroy consumer records based solely upon statutory time periods that may change or be interpreted via later court decisions to periods beyond an established number of days. For example, statutes of limitation for set periods do not apply to or begin to run for minors until they reach the age of majority; other statutes of limitation do not run or even begin to expire in some states until injury or responsibility (liability) is discovered. As a consequence, records related to service provision should be retained in accordance with advice from legal counsel about the jurisdiction where service is provided and in some cases, ideally, in perpetuity.

Other Litigation Concerns

In the event that a consumer is injured in a health and fitness facility or during the provision of service by a fitness professional, such consumers may institute claim and suit seeking to recover monetary damages for their injuries. In order to recover, such consumers must establish a "cause of action" against the facility and/or the fitness professional. In order to establish such a cause of action four elements must be present. These elements include: (1) proof of a duty owed by a fitness professional or facility to a consumer; (2) a failure of the facility or the fitness professional to perform that duty in accordance with the standard of care; (3) which failure proximately causes actual harm to the consumer; and (4) as a result of the failure to perform the duty the consumer is injured/damaged.

Once a facility/fitness professional undertakes the provision of service to a consumer, (usually pursuant to a contractual document) that provider will have a duty to provide service in accordance with the standard of care. If service is not provided in accordance with that standard, which proximately causes harm and damage to the consumer, then an action may be established, which will be compensable as determined by a judge or jury. The existence of duty is determined by a judge which, if so determined, then leads to a jury determination as to whether any breach of that duty occurred which proximately caused damage, compensation for which, if any is assessed by such a jury. Since lawsuits based upon these elements may be filed long after particular incidents took place, it is an advisable practice for fitness facilities and their personnel to establish a system of incident reporting to memorialize what unusual events take place on any given day and to transcribe statements as to those events that may well be preserved beyond periods that would otherwise be limited by individual memories of events and happenings. Records as to such events, as previously stated, should be preserved indefinitely.

Incident Reports

Incident reports should be utilized by health and fitness facilities and individuals providing service within such facilities or otherwise to make accurate and contemporaneous records of any untoward events that may take place during the provision of service. Such reports may not, under some circumstances, be "discoverable" or in other words disclosed to the other side in the event that litigation is filed related to the incident which is memorialized by the incident reports. However, regardless or whether or not these reports must be disclosed, such reports will be helpful to fitness facilities and will provide an accurate description of what happened in a facility when an incident took place. Such incident reports should be maintained indefinitely or in accordance with the advice provided by attorneys providing service to such facilities based upon their interpretation of applicable statutes of limitation. Similarly, those records that are maintained by facilities as to personnel's interactions with consumers should be maintained either indefinitely or in accordance with the advice provided by their legal counsel based upon these same principles.

Screening Duties and Responsibilities

The expected standard of care established for the provision of service by fitness professionals undoubtedly includes a duty to screen consumers prior to the provision of service. Industry standards from, for example, AFAA, ACSM, AHA and IHRSA, all provide that screening is part of the standard of care that is required for consumers prior to a facility's recommendation or prescription of activity for a consumer and prior to the provision of service.

Par-Q type forms can be utilized for the purposes of obtaining sufficient information to make consumers aware as to whether or not they need to seek medical clearance prior to engaging in activity. While at one time, some within the industry contended that no such screening should be done because it would create a record of medical type information which they contended had to be interpreted by the facility or its personnel (and would therefore perhaps impose additional duties upon them if they did not accurately interpret or utilize that information), it now seems clear that screening is part and parcel of the standard of care established by industry expectations as set forth in written standards and guidelines. Moreover, Par-Q type forms and even some health history question-naires are not designed to empower or require fitness professionals to make medically based or diagnostic decisions as to consumers but rather are utilized either as a self-assessment, informational tool or a screening device, by which consumers are referred to health care providers for clearance decisions when such documents, according to pre-established criteria, demonstrate the need for referral and medical clearance.

Screening devices should provide a written notice to the consumer to complete the forms accurately since the provision of inaccurate information may lead to unnecessary injury and/or other untoward events. If consumers refuse to complete such screening devices, some within the industry contend that only equipment and access to a facility should be provided and that fitness profes-sionals should not prescribe activity or engage in leadership activities with persons that are unwilling to engage in screening processes. Some within the industry also contend, however, that if such screening devices are not completed by consumers, then consumers must execute either an express assumption of risk type document, or preferably, a prospective waiver or release of liability form or be excluded from activity. Exclusion from activity may result in claims related to alleged violations of the Americans with Disabilities Act and facts related to such decisions need to be assessed by individual legal counsel. At least one court decision has touched upon aspects of this issue, however, and indicated that authoritative and objective medical data might well justify some restrictions upon activity or even exclusions from activity where the medical evidence objec-tively indicates the medical/health conditions requiring such decisions.

Prospective Waivers/Releases of Liability

In years gone by, many lawyers and even some within the fitness profession would make the blanket statement that "waivers of liability were not worth the paper that they were written on." Today, however, courts in virtually all states, have issued decisions that may give full legal affect to properly written waivers or releases of liability that are given prospectively by consumers to facilities prior to their engaging in activity.

Even though the rules pertaining to releases may vary significantly from state to state, as a general rule, any competent adult may execute such an agreement provided that at the time the agreement is signed he or she intends to release and give up his or her right to sue a health and fitness facility for any injuries that may occur to these consumers within those facilities. If it is the intent of the facility and the consumer to also give up the consumer's right to successfully institute a suit against a facility for "negligence," waiver documents must clearly so provide if suits based upon negligence are to be effectively precluded.

Since the law varies from state to state as to this and many other legal subjects, since waiver and release documents must be properly written to be effective and since such documents are not recognized in some settings in some states (e.g., New York, Virginia, Montana), the services of a competent lawyer to draft such documents is absolutely imperative. Facilities should not proceed with drafting or utilizing such forms or documents without individualized legal advice. An example of a release form that was "approved" and given legal effect in two separate California cases follows, as does a sample form based upon analysis of the law in Illinois.

"YMCA OF METROPOLITAN LOS ANGELES"
RELEASE AND WAIVER OF LIABILITY AND INDEMNITY AGREEMENT

"IN CONSIDERATION of being permitted to enter the YMCA for any purpose, including, but not limited to observation, use of facilities or equipment or participation in any way, the undersigned; hereby acknowledges, agrees and represents that he or she has or immediately upon entering will, inspect such premises and facilities. It is further warranted that such entry in the YMCA for observation, participation or use of any facilities or equipment constitutes an acknowledgment that such premises and all facilities and equipment thereon have been inspected and that the undersigned finds and accepts same as being safe and reasonably suited for the purposes of such observation or use.

"IN FURTHER CONSIDERATION OF BEING PERMITTED TO ENTER THE YMCA FOR ANY PURPOSE INCLUDING, BUT NOT LIMITED TO OBSERVATION, USE OF FACILITIES OR EQUIPMENT, OR PARTICIPATION IN ANY WAY, THE UNDERSIGNED HEREBY AGREES TO THE FOLLOWING:

"THE UNDERSIGNED HEREBY RELEASES, WAIVES, DISCHARGES AND COVENANTS NOT TO SUE the YMCA; (hereinafter referred to as 'releasees') from all liability to the undersigned; for any loss or damage, and any claim or demands therefor on account of injury to the person or property or resulting in death of the undersigned, whether caused by the negligence of the releasees or otherwise, while the undersigned is in, upon, or about the premises of any facilities or equipment therein.

"[ ] THE UNDERSIGNED HEREBY AGREES TO INDEMNIFY AND SAVE AND HOLD HARMLESS the releasees and each of them from any loss, liability, damage or cost they may incur due to the presence of the undersigned in, upon or about the YMCA premises or in any way observing or using any facilities or equipment of the YMCA whether caused by negligence of the releasees or otherwise.

"[ ] THE UNDERSIGNED HEREBY ASSUMES FULL RESPONSIBILITY FOR AND RISKS OF BODILY INJURY, DEATH OR PROPERTY DAMAGE due to the negligence of releasees or otherwise while in, about or upon the premises of the YMCA and/or while using the premises or any facilities or equipment hereon.

"THE UNDERSIGNED further expressly agrees that the foregoing RELEASE, WAIVER AND INDEMNITY AGREEMENT is intended to be as broad and inclusive as is permitted by the law of the State of California and that if any portion thereof is held invalid, it is agreed that the balance shall, notwithstanding, continue in full legal force and effect.

"THE UNDERSIGNED HAS READ AND VOLUNTARILY SIGNS THE RELEASE AND WAIVER OF LIABILITY AND INDEMNITY AGREEMENT, and further agrees that no oral representations, statements or inducement apart from the foregoing written agreement have been made.

"I HAVE READ THIS RELEASE

"DATE: _____ "   _____
                                              "Signature of Applicant"

This waiver has been upheld in two separate cases from California: <u>Randas v. YMCA of Metropolitan Los Angeles</u>, Cal., 1993; and <u>Los Angeles v. The Superior Court of Los Angeles County</u>, Cal., 1997.

The following represents another form of a release document.

Club Name _____

Address _____

USER'S REPRESENTATIONS, EXPRESS ASSUMPTION OF ALL RISKS AND RELEASE OF LIABILITY AGREEMENT

PURPOSE OF THIS BINDING AGREEMENT:

By reading and signing this document, "You", the undersigned, sometimes also referred to as "User" or "I", will agree to release and hold [Club Name] ("Club" or "We") harmless from, and assume all responsibility for all claims, demands, injuries, damages, actions or causes of action to persons or property, arising out of, or connected with your use of the Club's facilities, premises or services. The agreement and release is for the benefit of the Club, its employees, agents, independent contractors, other users of the Club and all persons on the Club's premises. This agreement includes your release of these persons from responsibility for injury, damage or death to yourself because of those acts or omissions claimed to be related to the ordinary negligence of these persons. This agreement also includes your representations as to important matters which the Club will rely upon.

A. REPRESENTATIONS

The undersigned, You, represent: (a) that you understand that use of the Club premises, facilities, equipment, services and programs includes an inherent risk of injury to persons and property, (b) that you are in good physical condition and have no disabilities, illnesses, or other conditions that could prevent you from exercising and using the Club's equipment/facilities without injuring yourself or impairing your health, and (c) that you have consulted a physician concerning an exercise program that will not risk injury to yourself or impairment of your health. Such risk of injury includes, but is not limited to, injuries arising from or relating to use by you or others of exercise equipment and machines, locker rooms, spa and other wet areas, and other Club facilities; injuries arising from or relating to participation by you or others in supervised or unsupervised activities or programs through the Club; injuries and medical disorders arising from or relating to use of the Club's facilities including heart attacks, sudden cardiac arrests, strokes, heat stress, sprains, strains, broken bones, and torn muscles, tendons, and ligaments, among others, and accidental injuries occurring anywhere in the Club including lobbies, hallways, exercise areas, locker rooms, steam rooms, pool areas, Jacuzzis, saunas, and dressing rooms. Accidental injuries include those caused by you, those caused by other persons, and those of a "slip-and-fall" nature. If you have any special exercise requirements or limitations, you agree to disclose them to the Club before using the Club's facilities and when seeking help in establishing an exercise program, you hereby agree that all exercise and use of the Club's facilities, services, programs, and premises are undertaken by you at your sole risk. As used herein, the terms "include," "including," and words of similar import are descriptive only, and are not limiting in any manner.

You also acknowledge and represent that you realize and appreciate that access to and use of the Club's facilities during non-supervised times increases and enhances certain risks to you. You realize that if you use the Club during non-supervised hours, any emergency response to you in the event of need for same may be impossible or delayed. While we encourage you to use the Club's facility with a partner during non-supervised times, you may choose to do so without a partner, therefore enhancing and increasing the risks to you as to the provision of first aid and emergency response. You realize that a delay in the provision of first aid and/or emergency response may result in greater injury and disability to you and may cause or contribute to your death. Use of the Club with no one else present to supervise or watch your activities is not recommended and would not be allowed unless you agree to assume all risks of injury, whether known or unknown to you.

You do hereby further declare yourself to be physically sound and suffering from no condition, impairment, disease, infirmity or other illness that would prevent your participation or use of equipment or machinery except as hereinafter stated. You do hereby acknowledge that you have been informed of the need for a physician's approval for your participation in an exercise/fitness activity or in the use of exercise equipment and machinery. You also acknowledge that it has been recommended that you have a yearly or more frequent physical examination and consultation with your physician as to physical activity, exercise and use of exercise and training equipment so that you might have his recommendations concerning these fitness activities and equipment use. You acknowledge that you have either had a physical examination and have been given your physician's permission to participate, or that you have decided to participate in activity and use of equipment and machinery without the approval of your physician and do hereby assume all responsibility for your participation and activities, and utilization of equipment and machinery in your activities.

YOU HAVE READ THE FOREGOING, ACKNOWLEDGE THAT YOU UNDERSTAND THE TERMS AND CONDITIONS SET FORTH IN THE PRECEDING PARAGRAPHS AND AGREE TO SAME. Initials: _____

(cont.)

USER'S REPRESENTATIONS, EXPRESS ASSUMPTION OF ALL RISKS AND RELEASE OF LIABILITY AGREEMENT (cont.)

B. EXPRESS ASSUMPTION OF ALL RISKS

You have represented to us and acknowledged that you understand and appreciate all of the risks associated with your participation in various activities at the Club and in the use of equipment/facilities at the Club, including the risks of injury, disability, and death. You have also acknowledged that there are greater, enhanced and even other risks to you if you decide to use the Club's facility during non-supervised times. Knowing and appreciating all of these risks and enhanced risks, you have knowingly and intelligently determined to expressly assume all risks associated with all of your activities and use of equipment/facilities at the Club.

You understand and are aware that strength, flexibility and aerobic exercise, including the use of equipment is a potentially hazardous activity. You also understand that fitness activities involve the risk of injury and even death, and that you are voluntarily participating in these activities and using equipment and machinery with knowledge of the dangers involved. We have also reviewed the risks with you on the date when you signed this Agreement and answered any questions that you may have had. You hereby agree to expressly assume and accept any and all risks of injury or death including those related to your use of or presence at this facility, your use of equipment and your participation in activity, including those risks related to the ordinary negligence of those released by this Agreement and including all claims related to ordinary negligence in the selection, purchase, set up, maintenance, instruction as to use, use and/or supervision of use, if any, associated with all equipment and facilities.

YOU HAVE READ THE FOREGOING, ACKNOWLEDGE THAT YOU UNDERSTAND THE TERMS AND CONDITIONS SET FORTH IN THE PRECEDING PARAGRAPHS AND AGREE TO SAME. Initials: _____

C. AGREEMENT AND RELEASE OF LIABILITY

In consideration of being allowed to participate in the activities and programs of the Club and to use its equipment/facilities, machinery in addition to the payment of any fee or charge, you do hereby waive, release and forever discharge the Club and its directors, officers, agents, employees, representatives, successors and assigns, administrators, executors, and all others from any and all responsibilities or liability from injuries or damages resulting from your participation in any activities or your use of equipment/facilities or machinery in the above-mentioned activities. You do also hereby release all of those mentioned and any others acting upon their behalf from any responsibility or liability for any injury or damage to myself, including those caused by the negligent act or omission of any of those mentioned or others acting on their behalf or in any way arising out of or connected with my participation in any activities of the Club. This provision shall apply to ordinary acts of negligence but shall not apply to gross acts/omissions of negligence, willful or wanton acts/omissions or those of an intentional/criminal nature.

YOU HAVE READ THE FOREGOING, ACKNOWLEDGE THAT YOU UNDERSTAND THE TERMS AND CONDITIONS SET FORTH IN THE PRECEDING PARAGRAPHS AND AGREE TO SAME. Initials: _____

D. LOSS OR THEFT OF PROPERTY

The Club is not responsible for lost or stolen articles. You should keep any valuables with you at all times while using the facilities. Storage space or lockers do not always protect valuables. Consequently, by executing this Agreement and any accompanying documents, you do hereby agree to assume all responsibility for your own property and that of any dependent(s) and to insure that property against risk of loss as you see fit. By the execution hereof, you expressly, on behalf of yourself, and any dependents, do hereby knowingly agree to forego, waive, release and prospectively give up any right to institute any claim or action against the Club relating to lost or stolen property, including property lost or stolen due to the negligent act or omission of the Club. You agree to indemnify and save the Club and all of its personnel harmless from any action, claim, suit or subrogated claim or suit instituted at any time hereafter against the Club related to the theft or loss of your or your dependents' property at the Club. The Club shall be indemnified by you for all costs, expenses, fees, including attorney fees, incurred by the Club or its personnel by reason of any such action.

YOU HAVE READ THE FOREGOING, ACKNOWLEDGE THAT YOU UNDERSTAND THE TERMS AND CONDITIONS SET FORTH IN THE PRECEDING PARAGRAPHS AND AGREE TO SAME. Initials: _____

User shall receive a copy of the foregoing Agreement at the time of its initialing and signing and hereby acknowledges User's receipt of same.

YOU HAVE READ THE FOREGOING, ACKNOWLEDGE THAT YOU UNDERSTAND THE TERMS AND CONDITIONS SET FORTH IN THE PRECEDING PARAGRAPHS AND AGREE TO SAME. Initials: _____

(cont.)

USER'S REPRESENTATIONS, EXPRESS ASSUMPTION OF ALL RISKS AND RELEASE OF LIABILITY AGREEMENT (cont.)

This Agreement shall be interpreted according to the laws of the State of . If any part of this Agreement should ever be determined by a court of final jurisdiction to be invalid, the remaining portions hereof shall be deemed to be valid and enforceable.

YOU HAVE READ THE FOREGOING, ACKNOWLEDGE THAT YOU UNDERSTAND THE TERMS AND CONDI-

TIONS SET FORTH IN THE PRECEDING PARAGRAPHS AND AGREE TO SAME. Initials: _____

ACKNOWLEDGMENT

I have read and received a completed copy of this Agreement and all of its Exhibits, as well as any Rules and Regulations of the Club which are incorporated herein by reference. I agree to be bound by the terms and conditions of the Agreement and the Rules and Regulations of the Club, as same exist or as same may be amended from time to time here-after. This Agreement shall be binding upon me and my spouse, my heirs, my estate, my executors, my administrators and my successors and/or assigns. I realize that this Agreement is designed to prevent me and/or them from filing any personal injury or other lawsuit based upon ordinary negligence, including negligent battery, or even negligent wrongful death, loss of consortium or any other similar lawsuit arising out of any injury to me which I or they may possess hereafter.

The undersigned, on behalf of myself and my heirs, executors, administrators, successors and assigns hereby agree to indemnify the Club and all those hereby released and to hold them absolutely harmless if anyone, including the under-signed, should hereafter file suit against the Club or those released hereby for any matter intended to be released by this Agreement including claims based upon ordinary negligence such as but not limited to personal injury, wrongful death, loss of consortium or other similar actions.

Signature _____ Date: _____

Print Name: _____

Address: _____

Phone Number: (_____) _____

In those states that do not recognize or give legal effect to properly executed releases/waivers of liability, programs may wish to consult with their legal advisor for the preparation of a written or express assumption of risk document. Such a document may assist in preventing or defending against injury/death claims where prospectively executed releases are not recognized. An example of such an assumption of risk form follows:

Club Name _____

Address _____

USER'S REPRESENTATIONS AND EXPRESS ASSUMPTION OF ALL RISKS AND
RELEASE OF LIABILITY AGREEMENT

PURPOSE OF THIS BINDING AGREEMENT:

By reading and signing this document, "You," the undersigned, sometimes also referred to as "User" or "I," will agree to release and hold [Club Name] ("Club" or "We") harmless from, and assume all responsibility for all claims, demands, injuries, damages, actions or causes of action to persons or property, arising out of, or connected with your use of the Club's facilities, premises or services. The agreement and release is for the benefit of the Club, its employees, agents, independent contractors, other users of the Club and all persons on the Club's premises. This agreement includes your assumption of the risks associated with your activities at the Club including those related to injury, damage or death. This agreement also includes your representations as to impor-tant matters upon which the Club will rely upon.

(cont.)

USER'S REPRESENTATIONS AND EXPRESS ASSUMPTION OF ALL RISKS AND RELEASE OF LIABILITY AGREEMENT (cont.)

A. REPRESENTATIONS

The undersigned, You, represent: (a) that you understand that use of the Club premises, facilities, equipment, services and programs includes an inherent risk of injury to persons and property, (b) that you are in good physical condition and have no disabilities, illnesses, or other conditions that could prevent you from exercising and using the Club's equipment/facilities without injuring yourself or impairing your health, and (c) that you have consulted a physician concerning an exercise program that will not risk injury to yourself or impairment of your health. Such risk of injury includes, but is not limited to, injuries arising from or relating to use by you or others of exercise equipment and machines, locker rooms, spa and other wet areas, and other Club facilities; injuries arising from or relating to participation by you or others in supervised or unsupervised activities or programs through the Club; injuries and medical disorders arising from or relating to use of the Club's facilities including heart attacks, sudden cardiac arrests, strokes, heat stress, sprains, strains, broken bones, and torn muscles, tendons, and ligaments, among others, and accidental injuries occurring anywhere in the Club including lobbies, hallways, exercise areas, locker rooms, steam rooms, pool areas, Jacuzzis, saunas, and dressing rooms. Accidental injuries include those caused by you, those caused by other persons, and those of a "slip-and-fall" nature. If you have any special exercise requirements or limitations, you agree to disclose them to the Club before using the Club's facilities and when seeking help in establishing an exercise program, you hereby agree that all exercise and use of the Club's facilities, services, programs, and premises are undertaken by you at your sole risk. As used herein, the terms "include," "including," and words of similar import are descriptive only, and are not limiting in any manner.

You also acknowledge and represent that you realize and appreciate that access to and use of the Club's facilities during non-supervised times increases and enhances certain risks to you. You realize that if you use the Club during non-supervised hours, any emergency response to you in the event of need for same may be impossible or delayed. While we encourage you to use the Club's facility with a partner during non-supervised times, you may choose to do so without a partner, therefore enhancing and increasing the risks to you as to the provision of first aid and emergency response. You realize that a delay in the provision of first aid and/or emergency response may result in greater injury and disability to you and may cause or contribute to your death. Use of the Club with no one else present to supervise or watch your activities is not recommended and would not be allowed unless you agree to assume all risks of injury, whether known or unknown to you.

You do hereby further declare yourself to be physically sound and suffering from no condition, impairment, disease, infirmity or other illness that would prevent your participation or use of equipment or machinery except as hereinafter stated. You do hereby acknowledge that you have been informed of the need for a physician's approval for your participation in an exercise/fitness activity or in the use of exercise equipment and machinery. You also acknowledge that it has been recommended that you have a yearly or more frequent physical examination and consultation with your physician as to physical activity, exercise and use of exercise and training equipment so that you might have his recommendations concerning these fitness activities and equipment use. You acknowledge that you have either had a physical examination and have been given your physician's permission to participate, or that you have decided to participate in activity and use of equipment and machinery without the approval of your physician and do hereby assume all responsibility for your participation and activities, and utilization of equipment and machinery in your activities.

YOU HAVE READ THE FOREGOING, ACKNOWLEDGE THAT YOU UNDERSTAND THE TERMS AND CONDITIONS SET FORTH IN THE PRECEDING PARAGRAPHS AND AGREE TO SAME. Initials:_____

B. EXPRESS ASSUMPTION OF ALL RISKS

You have represented to us and acknowledged that you understand and appreciate all of the risks associated with your participation in various activities at the Club and in the use of equipment/facilities at the Club, including the risks of injury, disability, and death. You have also acknowledged that there are greater, enhanced and even other risks to you if you decide to use the Club's facility during non-supervised times. Knowing and appreciating all of these risks and enhanced risks, you have knowingly and intelligently determined to expressly assume all risks associated with all of your activities and use of equipment/facilities at the Club.

(cont.)

USER'S REPRESENTATIONS AND EXPRESS ASSUMPTION OF ALL RISKS AND RELEASE OF LIABILITY AGREEMENT (cont.)

You understand and are aware that strength, flexibility and aerobic exercise, including the use of equipment is a potentially hazardous activity. You also understand that fitness activities involve the risk of injury and even death, and that you are voluntarily participating in these activities and using equipment and machinery with knowledge of the dangers involved. We have also reviewed the risks with you on the date when you signed this Agreement and answered any questions that you may have had. You hereby agree to expressly assume and accept any and all risks of injury or death including those related to your use of or presence at this facility, your use of equipment and your participation in activity, including those risks related to the ordinary negligence of those released by this Agreement and including all claims related to ordinary negligence in the selection, purchase, set up, maintenance, instruction as to use, use and/or supervision of use, if any, associated with all equipment and facilities.

YOU HAVE READ THE FOREGOING, ACKNOWLEDGE THAT YOU UNDERSTAND THE TERMS AND CONDITIONS SET FORTH IN THE PRECEDING PARAGRAPHS AND AGREE TO SAME. Initials:_____

C. LOSS OR THEFT OF PROPERTY

The Club is not responsible for lost or stolen articles. You should keep any valuables with you at all times while using the facilities. Storage space or lockers do not always protect valuables. Consequently, by executing this Agreement and any accompanying documents, you do hereby agree to assume all responsibility for your own property and that of any dependent(s) and to insure that property against risk of loss as you see fit.

YOU HAVE READ THE FOREGOING, ACKNOWLEDGE THAT YOU UNDERSTAND THE TERMS AND CONDITIONS SET FORTH IN THE PRECEDING PARAGRAPHS AND AGREE TO SAME. Initials:_____

User shall receive a copy of the foregoing Agreement at the time of its initialing and signing and hereby acknowledges User's receipt of same.

YOU HAVE READ THE FOREGOING, ACKNOWLEDGE THAT YOU UNDERSTAND THE TERMS AND CONDITIONS SET FORTH IN THE PRECEDING PARAGRAPHS AND AGREE TO SAME. Initials:_____

This Agreement shall be interpreted according to the laws of the State of. If any part of this Agreement should ever be determined by a court of final jurisdiction to be invalid, the remaining portions hereof shall be deemed to be valid and enforceable.

YOU HAVE READ THE FOREGOING, ACKNOWLEDGE THAT YOU UNDERSTAND THE TERMS AND CONDITIONS SET FORTH IN THE PRECEDING PARAGRAPHS AND AGREE TO SAME. Initials:_____

ACKNOWLEDGMENT

I have read and received a completed copy of this Agreement and all of its Exhibits, as well as any Rules and Regulations of the Club which are incorporated herein by reference. I agree to be bound by the terms and conditions of the Agreement and the Rules and Regulations of the Club, as same exist or as same may be amended from time to time hereafter. This Agreement shall be binding upon me and my spouse, my heirs, my estate, my executors, my administrators and my successors and/or assigns.

Signature _____ Date: _____

Print Name: _____

Address: _____

Phone Number: (_____) _____

Informed Consents

Fitness professionals may believe that waivers of liability and informed consent forms are in essence the same document. This is not the case. Waivers of liability are specific agreements between consumers and facilities/professionals whereby consumers agree not to sue and whereby they prospectively give up their right to successfully sue facilities should they be injured while engaged in activity at those facilities. An informed consent form on the other hand, is a document evidencing the completion of an informed consent process, normally associated with medical or medical type procedures, pursuant to which a consumer gives authorization and consent for a facility to engage in a particular procedure or program with that consumer.

Often times, for example, if fitness testing or similar activities are carried on within a health and fitness facility, informed consent type documents, which disclose the procedure to be performed, the risks and benefits associated with that procedure and other similar information, are provided to consumers for execution by them as part of an informed consent process. If an untoward event results from such a procedure, and an informed consent has been previously obtained, the consumer should not be able to successfully allege that he/she was not informed of the risks associated with the procedure or that he or she did not consent to the procedure. Such forms are also effective in helping to preclude battery actions that might otherwise be filed that are related to those procedures where an actual or constructive touching of the consumer by the fitness professional takes place. On the other hand, if informed consent documents are not obtained as to such procedures, facilities could be responsible for all untoward events that are associated with the provision of service.

Due to their legal complexities, informed consent documents, prospective waivers of liability/releases and assumption of risk type documents should be drafted by competent legal professionals based upon their analysis of state law. An example of an informed consent form for exercise testing of an apparently healthy adult follows:

Informed Consent For Exercise Testing of Apparently Healthy Adults
(without known heart disease)

Name _____

1. Purpose and Explanation of Test

I hereby consent to voluntarily engage in an exercise test to determine my circulatory and respiratory fitness. I also consent to the taking of samples of my exhaled air during exercise to properly measure my oxygen consumption. I also consent, if necessary, to have a small blood sample drawn by needle from my arm for blood chemistry analysis and to the performance of lung function and body fat (skin fold pinch) tests. It is my understanding that the information obtained will help me evaluate future physical activities and sports activities in which I may engage.

Before I undergo the test, I certify to the program that I am in good health and have had a physical examination conducted by a licensed medical physician within the last _____ months. Further, I hereby represent and inform the program that I have accurately completed the pre-test history interview presented to me by the program staff and have provided correct responses to the questions as indicated on the history form or as supplied to the interviewer. It is my understanding that I will be interviewed by a physician or other person prior to my undergoing the test who will in the course of interviewing me determine if there are any reasons which would make it undesirable or unsafe for me to take the test. Consequently, I understand that it is important that I provide complete and accurate responses to the interviewer and recognize that my failure to do so could lead to possible unnecessary injury to myself during the test.

The test which I will undergo will be performed on a motor driven treadmill or bicycle ergometer with the amount of effort gradually increasing. As I understand it, this increase in effort will continue until I feel and verbally report to the operator any symptoms such as fatigue, shortness of breath or chest discomfort which may appear. It is my understanding and I have been clearly advised that it is my right to request that a test be stopped at any point if I feel unusual discomfort or fatigue. I have been advised that I should, immediately upon experiencing any such symptoms or if I so choose, inform the operator that I wish to stop the test at that or any other point. My wishes in this regard shall be absolutely carried out.

(cont.)

Informed Consent For Exercise Testing of Apparently Healthy Adults (without known heart disease) (cont.)

It is further my understanding that prior to beginning the test, I will be connected by electrodes and cables to an electrocardiographic recorder which will enable the program personnel to monitor my cardiac (heart) activity. During the test itself, it is my understanding that a trainer observer will monitor my responses continuously and take frequent readings of blood pressure, the electrocardiogram, and my expressed feelings of effort. I realize that a true determination of my exercise capacity depends on progressing the test to the point of my fatigue.

Once the test has been completed, but before I am released from the test area, I will be given special instructions about showering and recognition of certain symptoms which may appear within the first 24 hours after the test. I agree to follow these instructions and promptly contact the program personnel or medial providers if such symptoms develop.

2. Risks

It is my understanding and I have been informed that there exists the possibility of adverse changes during the actual test. I have been informed that these changes could include abnormal blood pressure, fainting, disorders of heart rhythm, stroke and very rare instances of heart attack or even death. Every effort, I have been told, will be made to minimize these occurrences by preliminary examination and by precautions and observations taken during the test. I have also been informed that emergency equipment and personnel are readily available to deal with these unusual situations should they occur. I understand that there is a risk of injury, heart attack, stroke or even death as a result of my performance of this test, but knowing those risks, it is my desire to proceed to take the test as herein indicated.

3. Benefits to be Expected and Alternatives Available to the Exercise Testing Procedure

The results of this test may or may not benefit me. Potential benefits relate mainly to my personal motives for taking the test, that is, knowing my exercise capacity in relation to the general population, understanding my fitness for certain sports and recreational activities, planning my physical conditioning program or evaluating the effects of my recent physical activity habits. Although my fitness might also be evaluated by alternative means (e.g., a bench step test or an outdoor running test), such tests do not provide as accurate a fitness assessment as the treadmill or bike test nor do those options allow equally effective monitoring of my responses.

4. Confidentiality and Use of Information

I have been informed that the information which is obtained from this exercise test will be treated as privileged and confidential and will consequently not be released or revealed to any person without my express written consent or as required by law. I do, however, agree to the use of any information for research or statistical purposes so long as same does not provide facts which could lead to the identification of my person. Any other information obtained, however, will be used only by the program staff to evaluate my exercise status or needs.

5. Inquiries and Freedom of Consent

I have been given an opportunity to ask questions as to the procedure. Generally these requests which have been noted by the testing staff and their responses are as follows:

_____

_____

I further understand that there are also other remote risks that may be associated with this procedure. Despite the fact that a complete accounting of all remote risks is not entirely possible, I am satisfied with the review of these risks which was provided to me and it is still my desire to proceed with the test.

I acknowledged that I have read this document in its entirety or that it has been read to me if I have been unable to read same.

I consent to the rendition of all services and procedures as explained herein by all program personnel.

Date _____ Patient's Signature: _____

Witness's Signature _____Test Supervisor's Signature _____

Reprinted with permission from Herbert & Herbert, Legal Aspects of Preventive, Rehabilitative and Recreational Exercise Programs, fourth edition (PRC Publishing Inc., Canton, Ohio, 2002). Copyright 2002 PRC Publishing. All other rights reserved.

Legal Music Sources

Copyright laws provide that "the copyright owner has the right to charge a fee for the use of his or her music in public performance." Public performance is defined as "a place open to the public or as any place where a substantial number of persons outside a normal circle of family and its social acquaintances are gathered." Health clubs, studios and even church basements, where some fitness classes may be offered, fall into these categories.

Licensing fees for the use of copyrighted music must be paid to major performing rights organizations, such as ASCAP and BMI. ASCAP and BMI should be contacted prior to playing music in a public place even though, currently, there are usually no late penalties or retroactive fees charged. When one or both of these agencies contacts a facility or a fitness professional as to the use of music for fitness related purposes, fees should be paid according to preestablished charges.

If a professional is planning to get into music tape production and sales, such a professional should investigate his or her legal responsibilities carefully. The copyright owner, the composers, lyricists and publishers of the songs should receive remuneration for their talent. To make sure that the talent that produced the songs receives their just monies, music tape companies and video production businesses are required to pay for each and every song that they use. The music tape companies pay for the right to use the music from the record labels (like Virgin Records) directly. While this can be quite expensive, fines for using unlicensed music run as high as $10,000, and not less than $250, for each song.

Protected Handicaps, Disabilities, and Related Issues

It is important for health and fitness facilities to understand that there exists in virtually all of the states and on a federal level, certain statutory enactments, such as the Americans With Disabilities Act, which protect individuals with defined disabilities from discrimination in the provision of accommodations and services. Many disabled individuals (those who are afflicted with conditions adversely impacting a major life activity) are protected by these statutes and regulations. Access to and participation in life activities is protected by such laws. These individuals generally include those who are infected with HIV/AIDS.

In order to comply with other legal requirements, health and fitness facilities must establish a uniform policy to protect consumers and employees from blood borne pathogens that may exist within health and fitness facilities. Such rules and regulations have been established to avoid discrimination against those who are afflicted or infected with such a disease while protecting others from infection. So long as the requirements of the blood borne pathogen rule are complied with, health and fitness facilities will adhere to the requirements of law and provide service to all consumers without discriminating against those with protected disabilities (the rule provides for the application of universal precautions when handling blood, bodily fluids or other materials that may contain such substances, e.g., the use of rubber gloves when cleaning up blood spills). Any effort to segregate or discriminate against those with protected disabilities should be subject to careful consideration. Legal counsel should be consulted prior to any such effort inasmuch as discrimination based upon such a classification in the health/fitness industry clearly appears to be unwarranted and in fact prohibited.

Emergency Response Planning

In the late 1980s–1990s and into the present decade, a number of actions have been instituted against health and fitness facilitates related to failures to provide appropriate and proper emergency response care. Since it appears that health and fitness facilities have a clear duty to recognize injuries and other untoward events (such as heart attacks) which may take place within facilities, and to timely respond to such events, they are charged with the duty to plan ahead of time to react to such foreseeable events. Therefore, facilities must comply with their duties and responsibilities by engaging in emergency response planning in advance of their provision of service to consumers.

Standards from a wide variety of organizations, including AFAA, AHA, and ACSM, provide that emergency response planning is part of the standard of care owed to consumers regardless of a least one California court decision seemingly indicating otherwise. As a consequence, facilities must develop written emergency response plans and rehearse those plans so that appropriate emergency response may be provided to stricken consumers. Such planning will require access to an emergency communication system (911) and the presence of staff members trained in and prepared to carry out first aid and CPR. Failures to engage in such planning and to actually provide service when necessary can result in rather large damage awards as was exemplified by a 1996 jury verdict in favor of the plaintiff in excess of $5 million in a case from Arizona, Spiegler v. State of Arizona, related to a facilities failure to deliver appropriate emergency response after a young lady collapsed while exercising at the facility.

At present, the standard of care for health and fitness facilities is moving toward requiring the presence and use of automated external defibrillators (AEDs) in health and fitness facilities to respond to incidents of need. Several states such as, New Jersey, have adopted statutes mandating the presence of such devices in health and fitness facilities. Even in the absence of such statutes, alleged failures to have and/or use such devices have resulted in a variety of claims and suits to date. More litigation in this area can be expected in the future.

Summary

There are a wide variety of legal concerns facing health and fitness facilities and professionals who provide services to consumers. While the services of knowledgeable and competent legal counsel and other professionals are often necessary to assist facilities and personnel in meeting their expected standard of care, facility owners and operators as fitness professionals must engage in a program of self-education as well. Such a program must assist professionals to first learn and then comply with the expected standards of care as which will pertain to their activities as such standards evolve, while realizing the potential legal concerns that may arise in the course of their provision of service.

References

1. American College of Sports Medicine. (2007). *ACSM's health/fitness facility standards and guidelines* (3rd ed.). Champaign, IL: Human Kinetics Publishers.
2. American Heart Association/American College of Sports Medicine. (1998). Recommendations for cardiovascular screening, staffing and emergency policies at health/fitness facilities. *Circulation*, 97, 2283–2293.
3. Cotten, D., & Cotten, M. (1997). *Legal aspects of waivers in sport, recreation, and fitness activities.* Canton, OH: PRC Publishing.
4. *The Exercise Standard and Malpractice Reporter.* (Newsletter). Canton, OH: PRC Publishing.

5. Herbert, D.L., & Herbert, W.G. (2002). *Legal aspects of preventive, rehabilitative, and recreational exercise programs* (4th ed.). Canton, OH: PRC Publishing.

Part 10

Appendices

Instructor Evaluation

AFAA's Nutritional Supplement Policy

Glossary of Terms

Appendix A

Instructor Evaluation Form

Lawrence Biscontini, MA

Instructor Name _____ Date _____

Location _____

Class Name/Type _____

Evaluator _____

Class Statistics

Instructor Arrival Time _____

Class Scheduled Start Time _____ Instructor Started Class Time _____

Class Scheduled End Time _____ Instructor Ended Class Time _____

Class Introduction

Class Introduction and Instructions (Was the purpose of the experience explained?) _____

_____

_____

"Intensity" explained?   ❏ YES ❏ NO   "Modifications" explained?   ❏ YES ❏ NO

"Special populations" addressed? ❏ YES ❏ NO   "Legal" music sources?   ❏ YES ❏ NO

Pertinent announcements made?   ❏ YES ❏ NO   Class maintained appropriate cohesiveness? ❏ YES ❏ NO

Number of Participants _____ Counted at _____(time)

Beats Per Minute of Music (if applicable) _____ Counted at _____(time)
(Guidelines: Step 118–126, Low Impact 130–145, High/Low Impact 140–155)

Instructor Qualifications & Presentation

Instructor Certification(s) _____ Exp. _____

CPR Certifying Body _____ Exp. _____

Instructor Apparel (uniform, professional, etc.) _____

_____

Evaluation Summary

Additional Comments/Evaluator Summary _____

_____

_____

_____

_____

_____

_____

_____

Follow-up _____

_____

_____

By What Date _____

I have read, understand, and acknowledge the above evaluation. The Evaluator has reviewed all major sections of this evaluation with me.

Evaluator Initials _____ Instructor Initials _____

Please enter a number for each box below.
1 = **Needs Improvement/Unacceptable**   2 = **Acceptable**   2+ = **Proficient**   3 = **Exemplary**   N.O. = **Not Observed**

	Warm-up	Class Body	Cool-down	Totals	Comments
Movement General attention to **Safety** (no high-risk movements)					
Balanced Muscle Groups selected					
Range of Motion safely and progressively manipulated					
Intensity safely and progressively manipulated					
Choreography and/or Complexity safely and progressively manipulated					
Movement Transitions smooth and within guidelines					
Instructor **Form** (posture, alignment, range of motion, precision, and strength) Stretching (as appropriate)					
Class Design/Class Flow					
Music **Music Volume and Tempo**					
Instructor Musicality (awareness of phrasing, movement on downbeat, counting, mic., minimal playlist manipulation)					
Communication					
Instructor Cueing (Overall Score) verbal/directional/preview					
Use of Voice (enunciation, diction, quality)					
Instructor as Leader (enthusiasm, role model with guidelines, fair treatment of all)					
Instructor as Educator (precise terminology, referrals as appropriate)					
Instructor as Personal Coach (modifications, personalizes class, eye contact)					
Appropriate Timing for and closure to each section					
			Total		

Scoring

51–70 Instructor Needs Improvement   102–136 Above Average Instructor
70–102 Average Instructor   136–153 Superior to Exemplary Instructor

Do more of this (suggestions for creating a true experience):

_____

_____

_____

_____

_____

Do less of this:

_____

_____

_____

_____

_____

Keep this:

_____

_____

_____

_____

_____

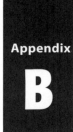

Appendix

B

AFAA's Nutritional Supplement Policy

Policy Statement on the Sale, Provision, or Recommendation of Nutritional Supplements by AFAA Certified Fitness Professionals to Clients

Copyright © 1999, 2006, 2007, 2009 by AFAA, Sherman Oaks, California

As part of its mission, the Aerobics and Fitness Association of America (AFAA) is committed to assisting AFAA certified fitness professionals in their provision of exceptional fitness-related services to clients. To assist in this process, AFAA gathers and publishes information on a wide variety of topics to inform such professionals and help them to provide the best possible services to their clients.

In 1999, AFAA originally developed this Policy Statement regarding the recommendation, provision, and/or sale of nutritional supplements to consumers. In 2006, 2007, and 2009, AFAA determined to review and update the statement. As with its first work on this subject, this revised Policy Statement is intended to assist fitness professionals in determining how they might, in the exercise of independent professional judgment, provide relevant services or products to their clients. However, this statement is not intended to limit the recommendation or sale of nutritional supplement products by knowledgeable entities which use computerized programs or algorithms to recommend the use of nutritional products to individual clients, nor to limit the provision of relevant service by those who are qualified by reason of education, training, licensure, or other form of regulation to provide nutritional supplement advice or dietary advice. By reason of the development and publication of this Policy Statement, neither the authors nor AFAA shall be deemed to be engaged in the practice of any form of health care or law; nor do they assume any duty toward clients of fitness professionals or fitness professionals themselves who consider the materials within this Policy Statement for adaptation to their professional practices. Fitness professionals considering these issues should consult with their individual medical and legal advisors for guidance.

As a starting point, fitness professionals must acknowledge that some manufacturers of nutritional supplements as well as others often encourage health and fitness facilities and fitness professionals to sell a wide range of nutritional products to their employees and customers. Many facilities and professionals have undertaken to do so for a variety of reasons. However, AFAA believes that the recommendation, sale, or provision of such products must be based upon a number of factors.

The sale of nutritional supplements in the United States involves literally thousands of products sold to most adult Americans through a variety of retail and service establishments as well as over the Internet. The range of nutritional supplement products is extremely diverse. As reported by the United States Government Accountability Office (US GAO), the greatest growth in supplement sales in the United States was in weight loss products. As of 2007, according to the NUTRITIONAL BUSINESS JOURNAL, the industry has been reported to be nearly $24 billion in sales in the United States and perhaps as large as $228 billion worldwide. Growth in the industry is expected to continue at least through

2011 due to increasing interest in personal health and wellness, the aging of the population, and perhaps consumer efforts at weight loss.

Nutritional supplements include vitamins, minerals, herbs, and even hormones. There are 13 vitamins, 15 minerals, and untold numbers of herbal and other similar products available for sale in this market. While vitamins and minerals may be the most studied, and perhaps the best understood of all nutritional supplements, controversy continues to surround all such products.

As a general rule, but subject to ever developing research findings which may indicate otherwise, vitamin and mineral supplements are not harmful unless taken in excessive doses, in which case, actual damage can result. Several herb products, such as aspirin, have proven medicinal properties, while many other herbs and even hormones can be clearly harmful, or are not yet well understood. Moreover, some nutritional products can be harmful when ingested along with other such products, prescriptions, over-the-counter medications, or even foods or beverages. Those with certain health conditions should not ingest some nutritional products. In addition, those who ingest certain nutritional products may have increased surgical and anesthesia-related risks. Consequently, it is necessary to obtain health care provider advice, approval, and monitoring of product use.

Generally, there is no legal requirement in the United States for nutritional supplements (as opposed to drug products) to be tested and/or approved for use by any governmental agency prior to their sale to consumers. While the Food and Drug Administration (FDA) does have some regulatory authority and responsibility as to nutritional products, and while certain "new dietary ingredient" products must be reported to the FDA before such products are marketed, such supplements are only subject to regulation after such products are determined to be dangerous or to the extent that claims are made that such products cure, mitigate, or treat various diseases. However, companies are required to report serious adverse events associated with some products.

Due to the present lack of pre-sale regulation of these products, some such products may not be "pure," or in other words, of a certain formula or strength; and some, potentially, may not contain what is actually on the product label. Since nutritional products are not sold as prescriptions by healthcare providers, the legal doctrine applicable in some states and known as the "learned intermediary doctrine" does not limit the duty of producers and manufactures to warn consumers of adverse consequences associated with such products. Moreover, those who sell, provide, or recommend such products necessarily do so with only limited information, as compared to the information that is available for prescription drug products, which are subject to extensive testing and research before being approved by the FDA for sale to consumers.

Due to all of the foregoing, those recommending nutritional supplement products to consumers, and those actually involved in providing or selling such products to consumers, may well have increased ethical, professional, and legal duties and responsibilities to ensure that the products they recommend, sell, or provide are relatively safe for consumption and/or are beneficial to the user. This conclusion is due in part to the fact that such products are not "sanctioned" by any government agency and that there is often only limited information and research findings available from non-manufacturer sources as to the safety and efficacy of many of these products.

Since some nutritional supplements have been deemed by the FDA to be associated with certain adverse health effects, AFAA strongly discourages professionals from making any favorable recommendations to clients related to these specific products or from providing or selling same. Dietary Supplement Warnings and Safety Information can be obtained from the US FDA Internet site at http://www.cfsan.fda.gov/~dms/ds-warn.html. AFAA also discourages professionals from making favorable product recommendations or from selling or providing products to clients when the available scientific evidence and research findings from sources other than manufacturers are insufficient to provide clear guidance as to whether such products are beneficial.

AFAA recognizes that some health/fitness facilities and professionals do not, as a matter of policy, sell or provide supplements or advice to others concerning nutritional products. Many believe it to be inappropriate and even unethical to do so. Others do not do so for fear of incurring additional legal exposure in the situation in which an untoward event occurs which is related to such products. These concerns are valid and must be given some deference by professionals.

In the event that any of these products are sold, provided, or recommended by professionals to consumers to treat, cure, or beneficially impact a disease process or infirmity, or perhaps even for preventive purposes, such professionals could be exposed to criminal and/or civil claims related to the unauthorized practice of medicine or other similar licensed health-care provider practices such as those reserved for provision by dietitians. If an untoward event occurred which is associated with a practice violating any of the foregoing kinds of statutes, a fitness professional who recommends, provides, or sells nutritional substances in the course of providing unauthorized advice could be exposed to rather substantial claims.

To illustrate what can happen in regard to advice given to a fitness client about nutritional supplements readers should consider what was alleged in a lawsuit that was filed in the state of New York. The suit arose from the 1998 death of a 37-year-old facility patron who allegedly took five nutritional supplements at the claimed, written recommendation of a personal trainer employed by a health and fitness facility. The suit sought $320 million in damages against the trainer, the facility, the named retail seller of the supplements, and five nutritional supplement manufacturers. The suit was based upon negligence, willful, wanton, malicious, and reckless conduct, improper and dangerous product use instructions, failure to warn, and the sale of unreasonably dangerous products. The action was resolved in 2004 for an undisclosed, confidential settlement but reported at an amount exceeding $4 million paid by certain of the parties.

Based upon the foregoing concerns the following basic principles should be considered by professionals as to the sale, recommendation, or provision of nutritional supplement products to clients.

1   Health and fitness facilities and fitness professionals should not sell, recommend, or provide nutritional supplement products, including vitamins, minerals, herbs, and/or hormones ("nutritional supplements"), to their employees and/or members/guests/clients unless the sale, recommendation, or provision of such products is justified by existing scientific and medical research, which is derived independently from those who manufacture such products and which demonstrates some benefit or potential benefit to consumers who ingest such products.

2   Such facilities and personnel should not provide nutritional supplements unless there is adequate, independent, scientifically-based information other than manufacturer information available as to the use of such supplements to indicate that use is preferably beneficial or at least reason-

ably safe when taken in proper quantities and subject to health-care provider approval, review, and monitoring.

3   Nutritional supplements which have been determined by the FDA to be harmful or those which have been associated with certain adverse health effects should not be provided by fitness professionals to clients.

4   If the provision of nutritional supplements is deemed by health/fitness facilities or fitness professionals to be appropriate based upon the foregoing principles, consumers of such products should be provided with certain information. This information should be specific and individual warnings and/or disclaimers advising the consumer of the potential adverse consequences associated with certain supplements should be included. Provided information should also include a statement about the limitations of present knowledge as to some products, and the unknown risks or adverse potential reactions or consequences that might be associated with the use of some products, either when ingested alone or in conjunction with other similar products, drugs, other substances, some foods or beverages, or when some such products are used prior to surgical procedures. Those products that may not provide anticipated or advertised benefits should also be identified for consumers. Products that may be inadequately labeled or those whose quality or purity cannot be verified independently should not be recommended, provided, or sold to consumers.

5   In conjunction with the provision of any nutritional supplement, scientifically formulated and derived information should be provided in writing to the consumer/purchaser of such supplements that is based upon information obtained from scientifically/medically reliable sources apart from the manufacturers or wholesalers of such products. These authoritative sources might include the FDA or organizations such as the American Medical Association (AMA) or the American Dietetic Association. Fitness professionals must stay current as to developments in this area and provide reasonably current information to clients, including manufacturer information. Fitness professionals who decide to provide nutritional supplement products to clients while also providing information related to those products must be aware of and fully comply with applicable requirements related to such practices as provided by regulations issued under the Dietary Supplement Health and Education Act of 1994 (DSHEA) and as those regulations and statutes may be amended or changed from time to time. Under the latest revisions to the regulations promulgated pursuant to the DSHEA, the FDA has established new rules as to what kinds of information may be supplied (and how and in what context) to consumers associated with the sale of dietary supplement products. As a consequence, fitness professionals providing products and information must review the Act and the regulations promulgated there under as same may be amended or changed from time to time to determine what is permissible and what is not permissible in that regard. It may also be helpful for such professionals to review Federal Trade Commission (FTC) requirements dealing with claims in advertising (including direct marketing materials) and even state/local law/regulations that may impact the provision of such products and information. Consequently, based upon all of the foregoing, professionals must independently determine how, when, and in what manner and context relevant information may be provided to

consumers about nutritional supplement products.

6 The provision of nutritional supplements by health/fitness facilities/professionals should not under any circumstances be used to treat, cure, mitigate, or otherwise attempt to beneficially impact any condition. disease, or infirmity with which an individual is afflicted in violation of state health-care provider licensing and/or practice statutes, or be used in any way on the recommendation of a fitness professional, which would violate state practice of medicine acts or other similar statutes or laws. No exercise or fitness professional should ever recommend any supplement or even any activity under circumstances where the practice could be deemed to be the unauthorized practice of medicine or some other health-care discipline including those services reserved for provision by licensed nutritionists or dietitians.

7. Nutritional supplements must have appropriate and accurate labeling information that properly describes product purity, weight/size, quantity, and recommended dosages. Product information as required by law must be provided. Health claims associated with nutritional products must not be made unless specifically allowed by law.

8. The provision of nutritional supplements by health and fitness facilities/professionals should not be made for the purposes of enhancing or attempting to enhance athletic performance or the athletic condition of those clients participating in such activities.

9. Before a consumer begins using or ingesting a nutritional supplement that is provided by a fitness facility or professional, that individual's use of any nutritional supplement should be reviewed and approved by the consumer's health-care provider, especially when such supplements are provided to individuals who are taking other forms of prescription or over-the-counter medications or supplements. Moreover, an individual's use of such supplements should be monitored by his/her health-care provider. Due to the foregoing, fitness facilities and professionals must make such a recommendation to their members/guests/clients in writing before the provision of such a supplement product to seek such clearance, advice, guidance, and monitoring. Written documentation as to the client's receipt of such advice, and preferably the written acknowledgement of same by the recipient, should be secured if possible.

10. Health and fitness facilities and exercise professionals should document all of the foregoing in their written records. Such records should be maintained for a period of time coexistent with advice provided by their independent legal/professional advisors. The use of waivers, releases, or assumption-of-risk documents by fitness professionals to be executed by clients who are provided with nutritional supplements should be considered where warranted and as fitness personnel are advised by their individual professional/legal advisors.

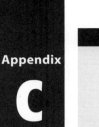

Glossary

abduction	Movement away from the midline of the body.
abduction	Movement away from the midline of the body.
acidosis	Too much acid in the blood and body fluids.
actin	A contractile protein of muscle fiber.
acute	Having a sudden onset, characterized by sharpness, severity and brief duration.
adaptive shortening	Shortening of muscle fibers and decreased range of motion due to inactivity.
adduction	Movement toward the midline of the body.
adipose tissue	Connective tissue in which fat is stored.
adolescent onset obesity	After puberty, when an individual acquires too much fat due to the sudden increase in the number of fat cells.
adrenaline (epinephrine)	A hormone secreted by the medulla of the adrenal glands, especially under conditions of stress that induces physiologic symptoms, such as accelerated heart rate, increased arterial blood pressure, and increase in blood sugar concentration.
AED	An automated external defibrillator.
aerobic	Means literally, with oxygen, or in the presence of oxygen.
aerobic capacity	The ability of the body to remove oxygen from the air and transfer it through the lungs and blood to the working muscles; related to cardiorespiratory endurance.
aerobic exercise	A method of conditioning the cardiorespiratory system by using a variety of activities that create an increased demand for oxygen over an extended period of time.
agility	The ability to change the body's position and direction with quickness and accuracy.
agonist	A muscle that is a prime mover, directly responsible for a particular action.
alkalosis	When the blood has a lower hydrogen ion concentration than normal and an excessive base (bicarbonate ions) in the extracellular fluids.
amenorrhea	Absence of menstruation.
amino acids	Building blocks of protein; organic compounds containing nitrogen, hydrogen, and carbon.
amphiarthrodial	A type of articulation joined by hyaline cartilage, classified as either permanent or stationary joints and slightly moveable.
anaerobic	Requiring no oxygen; usually short-spurt, high-energy activities.
anaerobic threshold	The point at which the body can no longer meet its demand for oxygen and anaerobic metabolism is accelerated.
anemia	A condition in which there is a reduced number of erythrocytes or decreased percentage of hemoglobin in the blood.
angina pectoris	Chest pains caused by insufficient supply of oxygen to the heart muscle.
anorexia nervosa	A psychological eating disorder, usually seen in young women who intentionally starve themselves.
anoxemia	A deficiency of oxygen in the blood.
anoxia	A deficiency of oxygen, most frequently occurring when blood supply to any part of the body is completely cut off.

antagonist	A muscle that acts in opposition to the action produced by a prime mover.
anterior	To the front.
aorta	The largest artery in the body that delivers oxygenated blood from the left ventricle to the entire body.
aortic stenosis	A narrowing of the valve opening between the lower left chamber of the heart and the aorta.
aponeurosis	A flat broad tendon that is a shiny, whitish-silvery color, sparingly supplied with blood vessels and nerves with a primary function to join muscle and the body part the muscle acts upon.
arrhythmia	An abnormal rhythm of the heart beat.
arteriole	Small arteries that regulate the flow of blood into the capillaries.
arteriosclerosis	Abnormal thickening or hardening of the arteries that causes the artery walls to lose their elasticity.
artery	Large vessel with smooth middle muscle layer that carries oxygenated blood away from the heart to the body tissues.
arthritis	Inflammation of the joints.
assistors	Muscles that help to perform the same task.
asthma	A common chronic disorder of the airways characterized by variable and recurring symptoms, airflow obstruction, broncospasm, and an underlying inflammation that is treatable and reversible.
atherosclerosis	A type of arteriosclerosis in which the inner layer of the artery wall becomes thick and irregular due to fat deposits, decreasing the inner diameter of the artery.
ATP (adenosine triphosphate)	Intracellular carrier of chemical energy produced by the body for muscular work.
atrophy	A reduction in size or wasting away of any organ cell, resulting from disease or disuse.
autonomic nervous system	Division of the nervous system that functions involuntarily and is responsible for innervating cardiac muscle, smooth muscle, and the glands.
axial skeleton	The bones of the head and the trunk: skull, vertebral column, thorax, and sternum.
balance	The ability to maintain equilibrium (or certain posture) while moving or stationary.
ballistic	Bounce or explosive movement, unsustained.
basal metabolic rate	The energy requirements necessary for maintenance of life processes, such as heart beat, breathing, and cell metabolic activities; referred to as BMR.
beta oxidation	The process by which fatty acids are broken down in mitochondria.
bilateral	Affects both sides of the body equally.
blood pooling	A condition caused by ceasing vigorous exercise too abruptly so that blood remains in the extremities and may not be delivered quickly enough to the heart and brain.
blood pressure	The pressure of the blood in the arteries.
body composition	Refers to the percentages of fat, bone, and muscle within the human body.
Body Mass Index (BMI)	One of several methods to assess body composition. The BMI is determined by the formula: weight in kilograms divided by height in meters squared.
bradycardia	Abnormally slow heart rate.
bronchus	One of two large passageways between the trachea and the lungs.
bulimia nervosa	A psychological eating disorder characterized by food gorging then induced vomiting after eating, as a means of weight control.

bursa	A fluid-filled sac or cavity, located in the tissue at points of pressure or friction, mainly around joints.
bursitis	Inflammation of the bursa sac; can be an overuse syndrome.
calisthenic exercises	Part of a workout that emphasizes specific muscular work, utilizing resistance.
calorie	The amount of heat necessary to raise the temperature of one gram of water 1° C.
cancellous bone	Inner, spongy portion of bone tissue.
capillary	Small, thin-walled blood vessels connecting arterial and venous blood systems that allow the exchange of materials between blood and tissues.
carbohydrate	Organic compounds containing carbon, hydrogen, and oxygen; when broken down, the main energy source for muscular work and one of the basic foodstuffs.
cardiac	Pertaining to the heart.
cardiac cycle	The contraction/relaxation pattern produced in the heart by the ventricles.
cardiac muscle	Involuntary muscle found only in the heart.
cardiac output	The volume of blood pumped by each ventricle in one minute.
carotid pulse	Pulse located on the carotid artery down from the corner of the eye, just under the jawbone; used for taking heart rate.
cartilage	White, semi-opaque fibrous connective tissue; cushions and prevents wear on articular surfaces.
catecholamine	A hormone that is a neurotransmitter, released under conditions of stress; includes epinephrine and norepinephrine.
cervical spine	Refers to the neck; the first seven vertebrae of the spine.
cholesterol	A chemical compound found in animal fats and oils; higher levels of cholesterol are often associated with high risk of atherosclerosis.
chondromalacia	Softening of chondral cartilage on patella (backside); first symptoms usually clicking or grating sound in knee.
chronic	Persisting for a long period of time.
chronic obstructive pulmonary disease (COPD)	A progressive disease that makes it hard to breathe.
circuit training	A combination of high-intensity aerobics and resistance training stations.
circumduction	Movement in which the extremity describes a 360° circle.
compact bone	Hard portion of bone that forms the diaphysis and epiphysis.
concentric contraction	Muscle shortens as positive work is done against gravity (e.g., lifting a weight).
condyle	A rounded projection at the end of a bone that articulates with another bone.
connective tissue	Primary tissue characterized by cells separated by intercellular fluid that supports and binds together other tissues and forms ligaments and tendons.
coordination	The ability of the body to utilize the senses and body parts in a harmonious relationship to perform a task smoothly and with accuracy.
coronary arteries	Two main arteries, arising from the aorta, arching down over the top of the heart and carrying blood to the heart muscle.
coronary heart disease	Occurs when fatty material and a substance called plaque build up on the walls of arteries causing them to narrow; slowing or restricting blood flow. This can cause chest pain, shortness of breath, heart attack, and other symptoms.
coronary thrombosis	An obstruction, generally a blood clot, within a coronary artery that hinders the flow of blood to a part of the heart.

couch potato	A side-lying position with head resting in palm of support arm causing a misalignment of the cervical spine.
CPR	Cardiopulmonary resuscitation. First-aid measure to aid an individual who is not breathing and without a pulse.
cross-training	Training in a variety of ways to improve overall performance.
cueing	Verbal technique using small words or phrases that describe upcoming exercises or body alignment positions.
dendrite	Nerve-cell process that transmits impulse to cell body.
detraining	The partial or complete loss of training-induced adaptations, in response to an insufficient training stimulus. Detraining characteristics may be different depending on the duration of training cessation or insufficient training.
diabetes	A metabolic disease in which the body does not produce or properly use insulin.
diaphysis	Shaft of a long bone, consisting of a hollow cylinder of compact bone that surrounds a medullary cavity.
diaphragm	Dome-like sheet of skeletal muscle that separates the thoracic and abdominal cavities; contraction during inspiration expands the thoracic (chest) cavity.
diarthrodial joint (synovial joint)	Freely moveable joint with movement limited only by ligaments, muscles, tendons, and adjoining bones.
diastolic pressure	Blood pressure within the arteries when the heart is in relaxation between contractions.
distal	End of any body part that is further from the midline of the body or from point of attachment.
diuretic	A drug that stimulates increased renal water excretion.
dorsal	Pertaining to the back.
dynamic flexibility	Having responsive muscles that are conditioned for their elastic properties in order to move a joint throughout full range of motion at varying speeds and forces.
DRI	Dietary Reference Intakes were established by the Food and Drug Administration to improve existing RDAs and provide new nutrient reference values.
dyslipidemia	An elevation of blood (plasma) cholesterol, triglycerides, or both, or a low high-density lipoprotein level contributing to atherosclerosis.
dysmenorrhea	Painful menstruation.
dyspenea	Shortness of breath.
eccentric contraction	Muscle lengthens while contracting, developing tension as when the muscles oppose the force of gravity.
ectomorph	Body type, characterized by frail and delicate bone structure, lean musculature, and usually very little fat.
edema	An abnormal accumulation of fluid in body parts or tissues; swelling.
electrocardiogram	A graphic record of the electrical activity and heart beat pattern; EKG, ECG.
electrolyte imbalance	Inappropriate concentration of ions in body fluids.
embolism	Sudden blocking of artery or vein by a clot brought to its place by the blood current.
empty calories	A term used to denote food-contributing calories that are void of nutrients, protein, vitamins, and minerals, such as alcohol, sugar, and fat.
endocrine glands	Ductless glands that empty their secretions directly into the blood stream; these secretions contain specific hormones that influence growth and reproduction.

endomorph	Body type characterized by a large block-shaped body, wider at hips and abdominals; a predominance of fat tissue, but not necessarily obese.
endorphin	A natural substance that can be produced by the body during extended exercise periods that may exhibit "morphine-like," pain-inhibiting qualities.
endurance	The ability for an individual to perform work over an extended period of time.
enzyme	A protein catalyst that stimulates and accelerates the velocity of chemical changes in the body.
epicardium	Thin, transparent outer layer of the heart wall.
epiphysis	Enlarged ends of bones where the growth centers for long bones are located (growth plate).
EPOC (excess post-oxygen consumption)	Excess post-exercise oxygen consumption, traditionally known as oxygen debt, refers to oxygen uptake remaining elevated above resting levels for several minutes during exercise recovery.
ergometer	An apparatus for measuring workloads by an individual (e.g., bicycle).
essential amino acids	The nine amino acids that the body cannot manufacture in sufficient amounts to meet physiologic need.
eversion	Movement of the foot so that the sole is turned outward (sometimes referred to as pronation).
extension	A motion of increasing the angle between two bones; straightening of a muscle previously bent in flexion.
fascia	Layer of fibrous tissue under the skin or covering and separating muscles.
fascicle	Bundles of nerve, muscle, or tendon fibers, separated by connective tissue.
fat	Stored as adipose tissue in the body, it serves as a concentrated source of energy for muscular work; a compound containing glycerol and fatty acids.
fatigue	A diminished capacity for work as a result of prolonged or excessive exertion.
fast twitch muscle fibers	Are able to generate quick, high-intensity contractions.
fatty acid	See triglyceride.
fibril	Fine thread-like structure that gives cells stability.
fibroblast	Connective tissue cell located near collagenous fibers that develop into fibers.
fibrous joint	See synarthrodial.
fixator	A muscle acting to immobilize a joint or bone; fixes the origin of prime movers so that occurring muscle action is exerted at the insertion.
flexion	Bending of a joint between two bones that decreases the angle between the two bones.
frequency	As related to exercise, how often work is performed.
frontal	A plane, vertical to the median line, that divides the body into anterior and posterior parts.
fructose	A monosaccharide, sometimes known as fruit sugar, that does not stimulate insulin production.
glottis	Opening between the vocal cords; entrance to the larynx.
glycogen	Form in which digested carbohydrates are stored in the muscles and liver and utilized as energy for aerobic activities.
glycogenolysis	Body's breakdown of glycogen to glucose.
glycolysis	The breakdown of glucose to simpler compounds, such as lactic acid; occurs in muscle.

glucose	A simple sugar; form in which carbohydrates are transported in the blood and in tissues; other sugars are converted into glucose by enzymes in the body before they can be used as an energy source.
golgi tendon organ (GTO)	A proprioceptor that protects the muscle from excessive shortening or lengthening.
HDL	High-density lipoproteins that return unused fat to the liver for disposal; are beneficial due to their "removal" effect on harmful lipoproteins.
heart attack	Damage (tissue death) of the heart muscle due to blockage of a coronary artery by either an embolus or thrombus.
heart failure	Congestion or accumulation of fluid in various parts of the body result from the inability of the heart to pump out all the blood that returns to it.
heart rate reserve (HRR)	A theoretical estimation of VO_{2max} utilizing resting heart rate and maximum heart rate.
heat exhaustion	The collapse of an individual, characterized by prolonged sweating and inadequate replacement of salt and fluid without failure of the body's heat regulating system.
heat stroke	Acute medical emergency characterized by rectal temperature at 105° F or higher and no sweating, caused by failure of the body's heat-regulating system.
hemoglobin	Oxygen-carrying protein of red blood cells.
herniated disc	A condition that occurs when the nucleus pulposus distends outside of the intervertebral disc; usually quite painful.
homeostasis	A state of equilibrium and internal balance of the body.
hormone	A chemical agent secreted by the endocrine glands; each affects a specific organ and elicits a specific response.
hyaline cartilage	Translucent bluish-white cartilage with a homogeneous matrix, present in joints and respiratory passage, and forms most of the fetal skeleton.
hyper	Beyond normal limits, excessive.
hyperextension	To increase the angle of a joint past the normal range of motion.
hyperplasia	Increase in the number of cells produced in an organ or body tissues.
hypertension	High blood pressure; unstable or persistent elevation of blood pressure above normal ranges. 140/90 and above is considered high blood pressure.
hypertrophy	Increase in size of tissue, organ, or cell, independent of general body growth.
hyperventilate	Excessive rate and depth of respiration, leading to abnormal loss of carbon dioxide from the blood; can cause dizziness.
hypo	Less than normal.
hypoglycemia	An abnormally low blood glucose concentration, characterized by a number of symptoms, such as dizziness, nausea, headache, heart palpitations, confusion, and forgetfulness.
inferior	Below or the lower half of the body.
insertion	The place or mode of attachment of a muscle; the moveable part of a muscle during action.
insulin	The hormone produced in the pancreas that regulates carbohydrate and fat metabolism and causes increased cellular uptake of glucose.
intensity	Degree of strength, energy, or difficulty; as related to a workout: the class level.
interval training	Combines high- and low-intensity timed intervals in a single workout.
intervertebral disc	Fibrocartilage cushion between the vertebrae.

inversion	Movement of the foot so that the sole is turned inward (sometimes referred to as supination).
ischemia	A local, usually temporary decrease in blood supply in some part of the body resulting from obstruction of arterial flow.
isokinetic	Contraction in which the tension developed by the muscle while shortening at constant speed is maximal over the full range of motion.
isometric contraction	A muscle contraction in which the tension increases, but muscle length remains the same.
isometric exercise	Force is applied to an immovable resistance (e.g., holding a flexed muscle in a stationary position or pushing against a brick wall).
isotonic contraction	A muscle contraction in which the tension remains constant as the muscle shortens or lengthens.
isotonic exercise	Movement of a resistance while maintaining constant tension; differs from isometric exercise in that there is movement of the joint during muscle contraction with constant tension (e.g., weight training with dumbbells and barbells).
ketone	A compound formed during the incomplete oxidation of fatty acids.
ketosis	An abnormal increase in ketone production and accumulation in the blood; occurs especially in protein-sparing diets or fasting.
kinesthetic awareness	Body sense; ability of individuals to "feel" where their bodies are in relation to space.
Krebs cycle	A series of chemical reactions occurring in the mitochondria, during which energy is produced from metabolism of carbohydrates, fats, and amino acids and the complete oxidation of acetyl coA is accomplished.
kyphosis	Abnormal rounding of the thoracic portion of the spine, usually accompanied by rounded shoulders.
lactic acid	The by-product of anaerobic metabolism of glucose or glycogen in muscle.
lactose	A disaccharide composed of glucose and galactose; milk sugar.
lateral flexion	Movement of head and/or trunk, bending to either side.
lateral movement	Any side-to-side movement away from the midline of the body.
LDL	Low-density lipoproteins; manufactured in the liver, they circulate throughout the body, making their fat available to all body cells; contain 45% cholesterol.
ligament	Bands or sheet-like fibrous tissues that connect bone to bone and reinforce joints from dislocation; they are nonelastic and have limited range of motion.
lipids	Fats; organic chemicals made up of carbon, oxygen, and hydrogen that are insoluble in water.
lordosis	Sway back; increased or excessive lumbar curve.
lumbar spine	The largest five vertebrae between the thorax and the pelvis; the area that needs the most protection during exercise.
maintenance	When dieting, caloric intake equals caloric expenditure.
marrow	A soft, highly vascular and specialized connective tissue found in the medullary cavity of most bones; capable of producing blood cells.
maximum heart rate (MHR or HR$_{max}$)	Theoretical maximum rate at which your heart can beat at your age; in a healthy individual, 220 minus your age is a formula used to calculate the maximum heart rate; do not exercise at this rate.

maximum oxygen	The maximum level of oxygen an individual can consume and utilize per minute during consumption (VO_{2max}) incremental exercise. Also referred to as maximal oxygen uptake or aerobic capacity.
medial	Toward the midline of the body.
meniscus	Crescent-shaped fibrocartilage within a joint (e.g., shock absorbers in the knee). A common knee injury caused by trauma or fast rotation movements.
mesomorph	Body type characterized by a solid muscular build.
metabolic equivalent (MET)	A unit of energy expenditure.
metabolic syndrome	A combination of medical disorders that increase the risk of developing cardiovascular disease and diabetes; also referred to as Syndrome X and Insulin Resistance Syndrome.
metabolism	The chemical reaction of a cell or living tissue that transfers usable materials into energy.
metatarsalgia	Pain in the forefoot in the region of the heads of the metatarsals.
mitochondria	Spherical or rod-shaped organelles, found outside the nucleus, that produce energy for cells through cellular respiration.
monosaccharide	Simple sugar (e.g., glucose, fructose, lactose) found in fruits, vegetables, milk, honey, and cane sugar; end-product of all digestible forms of carbohydrates.
Morton's syndrome	A condition in which the second toe is longer than the first, throwing more weight on the third and fourth toes, causing irritation of the nerves.
motor neuron	A nerve cell that directly or indirectly controls muscle contraction.
motor unit	One motor neuron and all the myofibers that it stimulates.
muscle spindle	A type of receptor, located among the fibers of a skeletal muscle that responds to muscle contraction (stretch).
muscular endurance	The ability to perform repetitive work over a prolonged period of time.
muscular strength	The ability to generate maximal force for one repetition.
myelin	Fatty, white substance forming medullary sheath around nerve.
myocardial infarction	The damage or death of an area of the heart muscle, resulting from a reduction of blood supply to the area; also called a "heart attack."
myocardium	The thick, muscular layer forming the heart wall.
myofascial release	A form of soft tissue therapy intended for pain relief and increasing range of motion.
myofibril	The longitudinally arranged contractile elements, composed of actin and myosin of a skeletal muscle.
myosin	Motor protein found in muscle fiber (myofibril) responsible for actin-based motility (the ability to move spontaneously and actively).
myotatic stretch reflex	The body's automatic protective mechanism against severe injury and abuse. If a muscle is stretched too quickly or with force, the reflex causes the muscle to contract; stretch threshold.
negative balance	In weight control, caloric intake is less than caloric expenditure.
negligence	A failure to conform your conduct to a generally accepted standard of care.
neuromuscular	Pertaining to the relation between nerves and muscles.
neuron	Nerve cell that transmits messages throughout the body.
obesity	A chronic disease that is associated with an abundance of body fat determined by a Body Mass Index (BMI) calculation of ≥ 30.

osteoporosis	A silent disease of the bones where they become thin and brittle (or porous) leading to fracture.
oxygen deficit	A period in which the level of oxygen consumption is below what is necessary to supply appropriate ATP production required of any exercise.
plyometrics	A form of training that uses fast eccentric contractions, followed by concentric contractions to increase muscular power.
posterior	To the back or behind, as opposed to the anterior.
power	The ability or rate at which one can exert strength to perform work quickly.
pressor response	The heart rate and blood pressure are elevated disproportionately to the oxygen cost of the activity.
progression	A gradual increase in frequency, intensity, time, and/or type of physical activity/exercise.
pronation	Medial movement of the forearm, with the palm in a downward position so the radius lies diagonally across the ulna.
prone	Lying face down.
proprioceptors	Sensor receptors in muscles, joints, and tendons that give information concerning movement and position of the body.
proximal	Nearer to any body part that is closer to the midline of the body or from point of attachment.
pulmonary ventilation	The rhythmic movement of air in and out of the lungs.
pulse pressure	The difference between the systolic and diastolic blood pressures.
radial pulse	Pulse found on the inside of the wrist on the thumb side near the wrist bone.
RDA	Recommended Dietary Allowances are the average daily dietary intake levels for nutrients that would adequately meet the nutritional needs and ward off disease in healthy persons.
reciprocal innervation	A stretching technique in which an individual contracts the opposite muscle he or she wants to stretch.
recovery heart rate	Heart rate taken at the end of class after a stretch cool-down to gauge when the heart rate has returned to pre-exercise pulse.
red blood cell	Erythrocyte; blood cells responsible for oxygen transport.
residual volume	The volume of air that remains in the lungs after the deepest possible expiration.
respiration	Interchange of oxygen and carbon dioxide between an organism and its environment.
resting heart rate	Pulse rate while still lying down in the morning before arising.
resting metabolic rate	The rate at which you burn energy or calories at rest.
rhythmic limbering	Low-intensity exercises, performed at a low to moderate pace that help prepare the body for more vigorous exercise by providing an increase in the flexibility of tendons and ligaments, raising muscle temperature, and stimulating muscle function.
RICE	Immediate injury treatment: rest, ice, compress, elevate.
risk factors	Factors known to be related to disease, but cannot be proven to be the actual cause.
ROM	Range of motion.
rotation	Movements around an axis.
sagittal	Plane that divides the body into right and left parts.
SAID principle	"Specific adaptations to imposed demand;" training must be relative to the activity for physiological change to take place.

sarcomere	The contractile unit of a myofibril.
saturated fat	A fatty acid carrying the maximum possible number of hydrogen atoms.
scanning	Teaching technique of observation; looking for incorrect body alignment and positioning in a group fitness class.
scoliosis	Abnormal lateral twisting or rotating of the spine.
shin splint	Delayed pain on the front or sides of lower legs caused by inflammation of the fascia connecting to the leg bones or muscle tears.
side stitch	Sharp pain in the side, thought to be caused by a spasm in the diaphragm, due to insufficient oxygen supply and improper breathing.
skeletal muscle	Is attached to bone via tendons and allows voluntary movement of the body.
smooth muscle	Involuntary muscles consisting of nonstriated, spindle-shaped muscle cells, found in the walls of hollow viscera.
specificity of training	To improve muscular endurance and strength, applied resistance and range of motion must be specific to the muscle or muscle groups being worked; also applies to endurance training.
speed	The ability to move the entire body quickly.
sphygmomanometer	Instrument used to measure arterial blood pressure.
spirometer	Instrument used for the collection, measurement, or storage of gas.
spot reducing	A popular, but false assumption, that an individual can "burn" fat only in desired areas.
sprain	Wrenching or twisting of a joint in which ligaments are stretched past their normal limits.
stabilization	Occurs by means of a static contraction of a muscle(s) that anchors or supports the movement, maintaining a stable position, so that movement of other primary muscle(s) can be performed.
static stretch	Static stretches are sustained in a supportive position that allows the muscle being stretched to relax and elongate.
steady state	After the first 3–4 minutes of exercise, oxygen uptake has reached an adequate level to meet the oxygen demand of the tissues; heart rate, cardiac output, and pulmonary ventilation have attained fairly constant levels.
strain	"Muscle pull;" a stretch, tear, or rip of the muscle or adjacent tissue, such as fascia or muscle tendon.
strength	Maximum force or tension that a muscle or muscle group can produce against resistance.
stress fracture	Fracture caused by stress, overuse, or pathologic weakness of the bone in the foot or leg.
strength plateau	A period of time that usually follows significant physical gains in which progressive increase in strength training effects ceases.
striated muscle	Skeletal voluntary muscle that attaches to and moves the skeleton.
stroke volume	The volume of blood ejected by each ventricle of the heart during a single systole.
stroke	A sudden, often severe impairment of body functions brought on by a disruption of blood flow to the brain.
subluxation	Dislocation or disarticulation of a joint.
submaximal work	Workload performed below maximum heart rate; aerobic exercise is submaximal.
superior	Above or the upper half of the body.

supination	The lateral movement of the forearm, with the palm in an upward position so the radius and ulna are parallel.
supine	Lying face up.
synarthrodial joint	All articulations in which bones are held together tightly by fibrous connective tissue in a nonmoveable fashion (e.g., sacroiliac).
synergist	Muscle that combines with another and aids in its action.
synovial joint	(See diarthrodial joint.)
systolic pressure	The highest level to which arterial blood pressure rises, following the systolic ejection of blood from the left ventricle.
tendon	Band of dense fibrous tissue forming the termination of a muscle and attaching muscle to bone with a minimum of elasticity.
tendonitis	Continuous, low-grade inflammation of a tendon, with pain on movement; can lead to partial or complete rupture of tendon.
thoracic spine	Twelve vertebrae from the neck to lumbar area.
tibial torsion	Twisting of the tibia, usually associated with supinated or pronated feet.
tonus	A slight, sustained muscle contraction.
torque	Amount of twist around an axis.
training effect	Physiologic adaptation that occurs as a result of aerobic exercise of sufficient intensity, frequency, and duration to produce beneficial changes in the body.
trans fatty acids	A compound formed during food processing when manufacturers change the chemical structure of unsaturated fats to make them semisolid at room temperature.
transient ischemic attack (TIA)	Sometimes called a mild stroke, TIAs manifest themselves with the same signs and symptoms of a stroke, but to a lesser degree and for a shorter time frame.
transverse	Plane that divides the body into upper and lower halves.
triglyceride	A compound composed of glycerol fatty acids; varies in degrees of saturation and the primary fats stored in the body.
unsaturated fats	Contain double bonds between carbon atoms; usually are vegetable rather than animal fat.
Valsalva maneuver	A dangerous condition that can occur if an individual holds his or her breath, causing the glottis to close and stomach muscles to contract, forming an unequal pressure in the chest cavity, reduced blood flow to the heart, and insufficient oxygen supply to the brain. Dizziness, temporary loss of consciousness may occur.
vasoconstriction	Narrowing of blood vessels as a result of smooth muscle contraction.
vasodilatation	Dilation of blood vessels due to the relaxation of smooth muscles.
vein	Vessel carrying blood toward the heart.
venous return	The "pumping action" of the muscles in the extremities and respiratory system along with venoconstriction to move oxygen-poor blood back to the heart.
ventral	Towards the stomach; anterior (front).
ventricle	Blood-dispensing chambers of the heart.
vertebrae	Bony or cartilaginous segments, separated by discs that form the spinal column.
vital capacity	The greatest volume of air that can be forcibly exhaled after the deepest inspiration.
vocal nodules	Growths that develop on the vocal cords due to overuse injury, resulting in severe, chronic hoarseness.

volume	A weight training concept defined as the total number of repetitions performed multiplied by the total amount of weight or resistance used during a single training session.
warm-up	A balanced combination of static stretches and rhythmic limbering exercises that prepare the body for more vigorous exercise.
wellness	A healthy state of well-being (the physical, mental, emotional, and spiritual states) free from disease.

Index